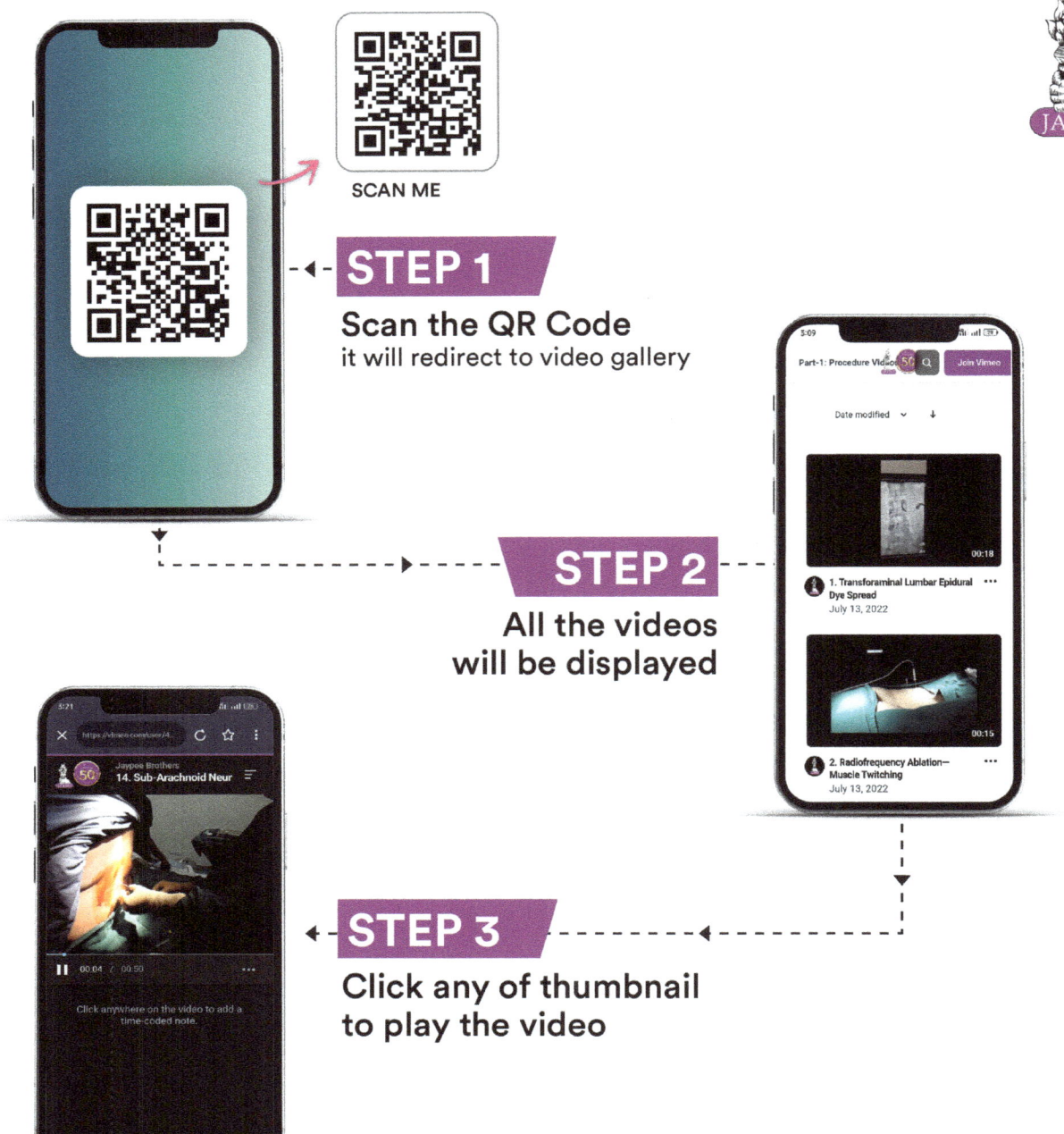

Jaypee Brothers allows you an exclusive, non-transferable right to access and use the digital assets for your own personal educational use during the period as determined by the Publisher. You shall not -

a) Create derivative works
b) Remove, obscure, or change Jaypee's or its licensor's copyright notices, policies, disclaimers, terms or other means of identification
c) Systematically download or print any part of the Publication or the Supplementary materials
d) Include, mount or distribute any of the Publication & Videos in other works
e) Use or distribute the Publication or Supplementary Videos for commercial use

Atlas of
Interventional Pain Management Procedures
A Stepwise Approach

VIDEO CONTENTS

PART 1: Routine Procedures

1. **Transforaminal Lumbar Epidural Dye Spread**
   Dwarkadas K Baheti
2. **Radiofrequency Ablation—Muscle Twitching**
   Dwarkadas K Baheti
3. **Trigeminal Nerve Block**
   Yashwant Laxman Nankar
4. **Stellate Ganglion Block**
   Preeti P Doshi
5. **Intra-Pleural Block**
   Dwarkadas K Baheti
6. **Celiac Plexus Block—CT Guided**
   Dwarkadas K Baheti
7. **Lumbar Median Branch Block**
   Annu Navani, Irina Melnik, Richard Derby, Jeong-Eun Lee
8. **Transforaminal Lumbar Epidural**
   Sanjay Bakshi, Gerard W Abrahamsen
9. **Interlaminar Lumbar Epidural Block**
   Sanjay Bakshi, Gerard W Abrahamsen
10. **Caudal Epidural Block**
    Sanjay Bakshi, Gerard W Abrahamsen
11. **Coccygeal Nerve Block**
    Yashwant Laxman Nankar
12. **Popliteal Block of Sciatic Nerve**
    Yashwant Laxman Nankar
13. **Piriformis Muscle Block**
    Yashwant Laxman Nankar
14. **Sub-Arachnoid Neurolysis**
    Kritika Doshi
15. **Trigger Point Injection**
    Vince Si, Mona Mirchandani, Kevin K Bernard, Emilia Ravski, Dellene E Troy, Christopher V Boudakian
16. **Transforaminal Endoscopic Discectomy**
    Kailash M Kothari

PART 2: Ultrasound Guided Blocks

1. **Ultrasound Guided Dry Needling**
   Lakshmi Vas
   A. Needle coming through spinalis. Iliocostalis (IC) quadratus lumborum (QL). Longissimus (L) Facet (F)
   B. Needle going through biceps femoris and semitendinosus
   C. Needle passing from gluteus maximus to piriformis
   D. Needle passing from the right ileocostalis (IC) to quadratus lumborum (QL). Spinalis (Sp) Longissimus (L) Facet (F)
   E. Needle Withdrawal
   F. back_7826
   G. back_7828
   H. USGDN tensor fascia lata (TFL) and rectus femoris (RF), sartorius (S)
2. **Brachial Plexus Block**
   Ritesh Roy, Gaurav Agarwal
3. **Supraclavicular Brachial Plexus Block**
   Ritesh Roy, Gaurav Agarwal
4. **Interscalene Brachial Plexus Block**
   Ritesh Roy, Gaurav Agarwal
5. **Lateral Femoral Cutaneous Nerve Block**
   Ritesh Roy, Gaurav Agarwal
6. **Parasacral Taha's Approach**
   Ritesh Roy, Gaurav Agarwal
7. **PENG Block**
   Ritesh Roy, Gaurav Agarwal
8. **Sacral Plexus Block (PSPS Approach)**
   Ritesh Roy
9. **TAP Block**
   Ritesh Roy, Gaurav Agarwal
10. **Subcostal TAP Block**
    Ritesh Roy, Gaurav Agarwal
11. **Lumbar Plexus Block**
    Ritesh Roy, Gaurav Agarwal

PART 1 PART 2

Scan the QR code to access the videos

Atlas of
Interventional Pain Management Procedures
A Stepwise Approach
(With Procedures Videos)

Editors

Dwarkadas K Baheti
MD
Head of Unit of Pain
Department of Anesthesia, Critical Care and Pain
Lilavati Hospital and Research Centre
Mumbai, Maharashtra, India
Consultant Pain Physician
Raheja, Shushrusha and Holy Family Hospitals
Mumbai, Maharashtra, India

Sanjeeva Gupta
MBBS MD Dip NB FRCA FIPP FFPMRCA
Consultant
Bradford Teaching Hospitals
NHS Foundation Trust
Bradford, UK

Sanjay Bakshi
MD MBA
Pain Physician
Interventional Pain Management
PRC Pain Relief Centers
Daytona Beach, Florida, USA
Former Treasurer
American Society of Interventional Pain Physicians
Past President, New York Society of Interventional Pain Physicians
Former Director of Pain Management, Lenox Hill Hospital, New York

RP Gehdoo
MD DA
Professor and Head
Department of Anesthesia
Dr DY Patil Medical College
Navi Mumbai, Maharashtra, India

Foreword

Subhash Jain

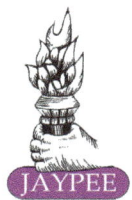

JAYPEE BROTHERS MEDICAL PUBLISHERS
The Health Sciences Publisher
New Delhi | London

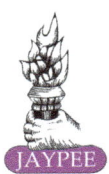 **Jaypee Brothers Medical Publishers (P) Ltd**

Headquarters

Jaypee Brothers Medical Publishers (P) Ltd
EMCA House, 23/23-B
Ansari Road, Daryaganj
New Delhi 110 002, India
Landline: +91-11-23272143, +91-11-23272703
+91-11-23282021, +91-11-23245672
Email: jaypee@jaypeebrothers.com

Corporate Office

Jaypee Brothers Medical Publishers (P) Ltd
4838/24, Ansari Road, Daryaganj
New Delhi 110 002, India
Phone: +91-11-43574357
Fax: +91-11-43574314
Email: jaypee@jaypeebrothers.com

Overseas Office

JP Medical Ltd
83 Victoria Street, London
SW1H 0HW (UK)
Phone: +44 20 3170 8910
Fax: +44 (0)20 3008 6180
Email: info@jpmedpub.com

Website: www.jaypeebrothers.com
Website: www.jaypeedigital.com

© 2023, Jaypee Brothers Medical Publishers

The views and opinions expressed in this book are solely those of the original contributor(s)/author(s) and do not necessarily represent those of editor(s) or publisher of the book.

All rights reserved. No part of this publication may be reproduced, stored or transmitted in any form or by any means, electronic, mechanical, photocopying, recording or otherwise, without the prior permission in writing of the publishers.

All brand names and product names used in this book are trade names, service marks, trademarks or registered trademarks of their respective owners. The publisher is not associated with any product or vendor mentioned in this book.

Medical knowledge and practice change constantly. This book is designed to provide accurate, authoritative information about the subject matter in question. However, readers are advised to check the most current information available on procedures included and check information from the manufacturer of each product to be administered, to verify the recommended dose, formula, method and duration of administration, adverse effects and contraindications. It is the responsibility of the practitioner to take all appropriate safety precautions. Neither the publisher nor the author(s)/editor(s) assume any liability for any injury and/or damage to persons or property arising from or related to use of material in this book.

This book is sold on the understanding that the publisher is not engaged in providing professional medical services. If such advice or services are required, the services of a competent medical professional should be sought.

Every effort has been made where necessary to contact holders of copyright to obtain permission to reproduce copyright material. If any have been inadvertently overlooked, the publisher will be pleased to make the necessary arrangements at the first opportunity. The **CD/DVD-ROM** (if any) provided in the sealed envelope with this book is complimentary and free of cost. **Not meant for sale**.

Inquiries for bulk sales may be solicited at: jaypee@jaypeebrothers.com

Atlas of Interventional Pain Management Procedures: A Stepwise Approach

First Edition: **2023**

ISBN: 978-93-5465-547-0

Dedicated to
*Chronic Pain Patients for being
Guide and Teacher to
Pain Physician*

Contributors

Allen Pinto MBChB FRCA FFPMRCA
Consultant in Anesthesia and Chronic Pain Management
Directorate of Anesthesia
Sheffield Teaching Hospitals NHS Foundation Trust
Sheffield, South Yorkshire, UK

Anil Sharma MD
Interventional Pain Management
President
Spine and Pain Centers of NJ and NY, Wall, New Jersey, USA

Archana Areti MD FRA
Assistant Professor
Department of Anesthesiology
Mahatma Gandhi Medical College and Research Institute
Puducherry, India

Babita Ghai
MD DNB FAMS and Commonwealth Fellowship in Pain Management QMUL, London
Professor and Consultant
In-charge, Pain Clinic
Postgraduate Institute of Medical Education and Research
Chandigarh, India

Dwarkadas K Baheti MD
Head of Unit of Pain
Department of Anesthesia
Critical Care and Pain
Lilavati Hospital and Research Centre
Mumbai, Maharashtra, India
Consultant Pain Physician
Raheja, Shushrusha and Holy Family Hospitals
Mumbai, Maharashtra, India

Ganesan Baranidharan
MBBS FRCA PG Dip Anes FFPMRCA
Consultant (Pain Medicine)
Leeds Teaching Hospitals NHS Trust
Leeds, UK

Gaurav Agarwal
DNB FIPM FPM FRA PGDHA CCEPC
Senior Consultant
Anesthesiology, Critical Care and Pain Management
Department of Anesthesiology and Pain Management
CARE Hospitals
Bhubaneswar, Odisha, India

Harun Gupta MBBS MD DNB MRCP FRCR
Consultant
Department of Musculoskeletal Radiology
Leeds Teaching Hospitals
Leeds, UK

Hemkumar Pushparaj
MBBS MD FFPMRCA
Pain Medicine and Neuromodulation
Clinical Fellow in Pain Medicine and Neuromodulation
Clinical Fellow
Department of Pain Medicine
The Walton Centre NHS Foundation Trust
Liverpool, L9 7LJ, Merseyside, UK

James Baren MBChB FRCR
Consultant
Musculoskeletal Radiology
Department of Musculoskeletal Radiology
Leeds Teaching Hospitals NHS Trust
Leeds, UK

Kailash M Kothari MD FIAPM
Interventional Spine and Pain Management
Director
Interventional Pain Management and Spinal Endoscopy
Pain Clinic of India Pvt Ltd
Mumbai, Maharashtra, India

Kenneth Lupton MBChB FRCR
Fellow
Musculoskeletal Radiology
Department of Musculoskeletal Radiology
Leeds Teaching Hospitals NHS Trust
Leeds, UK

Kritika Doshi MD DA ISSP-Pain Fellowship
Consultant Chronic Pain
Jupiter Hospital, Bethany Hospital
Thane, Maharashtra, India

Lakshmi Vas MD
Interventional Pain Specialist
Director
Ashirvad Institute of Pain Management and Research Center
Mumbai, Maharashtra, India

Manish Raj MD DA FIAPM
Director
Spine and Pain Management
Yatharth Hospital
Noida, Uttar Pradesh, India

Manohar Sharma MD FRCA MSc FFPMRCA
Consultant in Pain Medicine and Neuromodulation
Department of Pain Medicine
The Walton Centre NHS Foundation Trust
Liverpool, Merseyside, UK

Nick Plunkett
MBChB FRCA FFPMANZCA FFPMRCA
Consultant in Pain Medicine
Musculoskeletal Care Group
Sheffield Teaching Hospitals NHS Foundation Trust
Sheffield, South Yorkshire, UK

Preeti Doshi MD FRCA FIPP FIAPM
Director and Head
Department of Pain Medicine
Jaslok Hospital and Research Centre
Mumbai, Maharashtra, India

Quyen Van Truong MD
Attending Physician
Physical Medicine and Rehabilitation
Pain Medicine
PRC Associates, Lake Mary, FL, USA

Rathi Joseph DO
Physician
Physical Medicine and Rehabilitation, Sports Medicine and Pain Management
Department of Pain Management
PRC Alliance Pain Management
Daytona Beach, FL USA

Ritesh Roy MD FPM FRA
Associate Director and Head
Department of Anesthesiology and Pain Management
CARE Hospitals
Bhubaneswar, Odisha, India

RP Gehdoo MD DA
Professor and Head
Department of Anesthesia
Dr DY Patil Medical College
Navi Mumbai, Maharashtra, India

Samir Ranjit Jani
MD MPH Diplomate American Board of
Anesthesiology with certification in Pain Medicine
Attending Physician, Anesthesiology/
Pain Medicine
Garden State Medical Center
Whiting, NJ, USA

Sanjay Bakshi MD MBA
Pain Physician
Interventional Pain Management
PRC Pain Relief Centers
Daytona Beach, Florida, USA
Former Treasurer
American Society of Interventional
Pain Physicians
Past President, New York Society of
Interventional Pain Physicians
Former Director of Pain Management
Lenox Hill Hospital, New York

Sanjeeva Gupta
MBBS MD Dip NB FRCA FIPP FFPMRCA
Consultant
Bradford Teaching Hospitals NHS
Foundation Trust
Bradford, UK

Satish Kamath MD DMRE DMRT (Mumbai)
Consultant Radiologist
Lilavati Hospital and Research Centre
Mumbai, Maharashtra, India

Sherdil Nath MBBS DRCOG FRCA
Consultant
The Pain Clinic
University Hospital (Retired)
Östra Esplananden 6, 903
30 Umeå, Sweden

Shiraz Ahmed Munshi
MBBS D Ortho DNB Anesthesia
Director
Department of Spine and Pain
Management
Cheers Hospital
Ahmedabad, Gujarat, India

Timothy Ray Deer MD FIPP DAPBM
President and CEO
The Spine and Nerve Center
of the Virginias
The Center for Pain Relief
Charleston, West Virginia, USA

Yashwant Laxman Nankar
MD (Anesthesia) Chronic Pain Fellowship
Program Director and
Assistant Professor
Pain Clinic
Department of Anesthesia
Dr DY Patil Medical College and Hospital
Pune, Maharashtra, India

Yehia Kamel
MBBCh MSc FRCA FFPMRCA FIPP CIPS EDRA
Staff Anesthesiologist and
Pain Physician
Department of Anesthesia and Pain
Management Unit
Queen Elizabeth II Health Sciences Centre
Halifax, Nova Scotia, Canada

Foreword

When I was a medical student in Jaipur in the 1960s, pain management was not known to us as a distinct discipline of medicine. To be sure, we were consumed with the alleviation of suffering of our patients—but the notion that pain management was a specialty and foreign to us and virtually unheard of.

There were no textbooks of pain, no pain management faculty, and no pain management rotations. There were scant medications to alleviate pain—and the notion of interventional procedures was more the stuff of science fiction than of real-world practice. Some would say it was, at the time, an undiscovered discipline. More than 50 years later, that I can write the foreword of a book such as this one, is special and meaningful.

This book is not just an opus worthy of great attention and acclaim for its contributions to our field—but it also heralds the breath-taking degree of sophistication of the pain management profession in India and abroad.

In retrospect, the science and practice of pain management, was built brick-by-brick by a number of innovators who were consumed with the idea that pain was not an unchangeable companion of a wide range of diseases—but instead a disease with its own pathophysiology and associated treatments.

The insights of these innovators form the foundation of this text and patients will benefit significantly from the contents contained herein. It is especially meaningful that the Lead Editor of this textbook is Dr Dwarkadas K Baheti. In my years leading the pain service at New York's Memorial Sloan-Kettering Cancer Centre, I regularly hosted a number of observers, fellows, and students from around the world, who promised to take what they learned and apply it in service of others.

Among the many who made this promise, Dr Baheti stands out for having fulfilled it. Ever-curious, Dr Baheti, a natural leader, had a thirst for knowledge that was unquenchable—and second only to his desire to share what he learned with others.

This book—assembled by Dr Baheti and his collection of thoughtful and brilliant Co-Editors—is the culmination of Dr Baheti's commitment to his field—and for that, we are all in his debt.

Subhash Jain MD
Former Chief
Pain Service Memorial
Sloan Kettering Cancer Center
Former Chairman
Department of Pain Management
Hackensack University Medical Center
Professor, Weil Cornell Medical Center
New York, NY 10065, USA

Preface

The team of Editors including Dwarkadas K Baheti, Sanjay Bakshi, Sanjeeva Gupta and RP Gehdoo have been working tirelessly to bring out newer books in the field of pain management for the past twelve years. As the time goes on, this team has responded to pressing medical needs and brought out many books in the field of pain management.

The same team presents their dream project titled, *Atlas of Interventional Pain Management Procedures: A Stepwise Approach,* which will complement the previous publications written by the Editors. Such an Atlas from this part of the world was a much-needed one. Pain management as a specialty is advancing by leaps and bounds. Nowadays many young physicians are opting for pain management as a profession. Thus, the timing for such a book is apt.

Atlas of Interventional Pain Management Procedures: A Stepwise Approach has 57 chapters spread over 11 sections from basics to advanced pain management. In addition, it has 16 videos of routine procedures and 11 videos of ultrasound-guided procedures. Most of the authors have an international reputation in the field of pain medicine. All of them have done an excellent job. We, the editors, express our heartfelt gratitude to all of them.

We also express our heartfelt gratitude to our readers for the stupendous response to our previous books which gave us the much-needed encouragement and responsibility to bring out the Atlas.

We have taken the utmost care to bring out this book of international standards at an affordable price. We hope that our efforts to come out with this book will benefit pain physicians as well as chronic pain patients.

Last but not least M/s Jaypee Brothers Medical Publishers (P) Ltd, New Delhi, India, have been publishing these books of international standard at an affordable cost. We express our heartfelt thanks to the publishers and the editorial team.

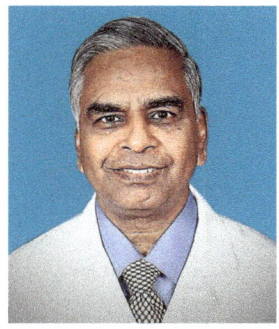
Dwarkadas K Baheti

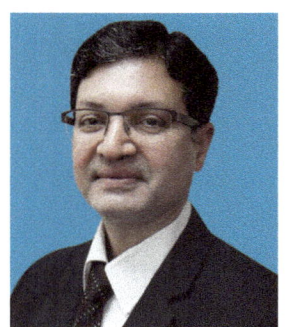
Sanjeeva Gupta

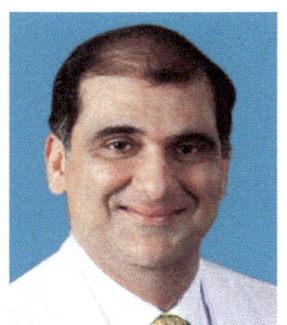
Sanjay Bakshi

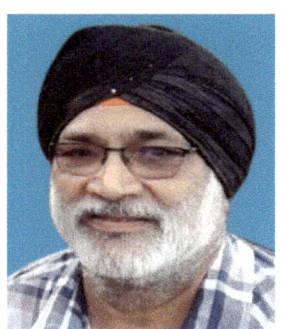
RP Gehdoo

Contents

SECTION 1 — BASICS: INTERVENTIONAL PAIN MANAGEMENT

1. Fluoroscopy for Minimally Invasive Spinal and Trigeminal Procedures 3
   Sanjeeva Gupta, Ganesan Baranidharan, Manohar Sharma, Harun Gupta

2. Understanding of Radiological Anatomy 27
   Kenneth Lupton, James Baren, Harun Gupta

3. Understanding Common Image-guided Procedures 36
   Kenneth Lupton, Jamen Baren, Harun Gupta

4. Understanding the Pathology of Common Conditions through Magnetic Resonance Imaging for the Pain Physician 40
   Harun Gupta, James Baren, Kenneth Lupton

5. Radiation Protection 44
   Satish Kamath, Dwarkadas K Baheti

6. Informed Consent for Interventional Pain Management Procedures 50
   Dwarkadas K Baheti

7. Protocol for Interventional Pain Management Procedures 52
   Dwarkadas K Baheti

8. Role of Investigations for Interventional Pain Treatment Procedures 54
   Dwarkadas K Baheti

9. Medications Used for Interventional Pain Procedures 59
   Kritika Doshi, RP Gehdoo

SECTION 2 — HEAD AND NECK

10. Trigeminal Nerve Block 67
    Hemkumar Pushparaj, Manohar Sharma

11. Percutaneous Cervical Cordotomy 72
    Manohar Sharma, Hemkumar Pushparaj

SECTION 3 — CERVICAL SPINE

12. Interlaminar Cervical Epidural Block 79
    Rathi Joseph

13. Cervical Medial Branch Block 82
    Sanjeeva Gupta, Babita Ghai

14. Cervical Medial Branch Radiofrequency Ablation 88
    Quyen Van Truong

15. Cervical Radiofrequency Denervation in Lateral Patient Position 91
    Sherdil Nath, Sanjeeva Gupta

SECTION 4 — CHEST AND THORAX

16. Intercostal Nerve Block 103
    Dwarkadas K Baheti

17. Intrapleural Block 105
    Dwarkadas K Baheti

SECTION 5 — LUMBOSACRAL SPINE

18. Interlaminar Lumbar Epidural Block 109
    Sanjay Bakshi

19. Transforaminal Lumbar Epidural Block 111
    Dwarkadas K Baheti, Sanjeeva Gupta

20. Lumbar Transforaminal Epidural Steroid Injections: Technical Challenges 121
    Sanjeeva Gupta, Dwarkadas K Baheti, Sanjay Bakshi

21. Lumbar Medial Branch Block and Radiofrequency Ablation 132
    Anil Sharma, Sanjeeva Gupta

22. Caudal Epidural Block 146
    Sanjay Bakshi

23. S1 Nerve Root Block and Technical Challenges 148
    Sanjeeva Gupta, Manohar Sharma, Sanjay Bakshi

24. Sacroiliac Joint Block 153
    Sanjeeva Gupta, Babita Ghai

25. Sacroiliac Joint Radiofrequency Denervation 156
    Samir Ranjit Jani, Sanjeeva Gupta, Ganesan Baranidharan

26. Sacroiliac Joint Fusion: A Minimally Invasive Posterior Approach 170
    Samir Ranjit Jani

27. Piriformis Tendon and Muscle Injection............175
    Yashwant Laxman Nankar, Dwarkadas K Baheti

28. Pudendal Nerve Block and Pulsed
    Radiofrequency Procedure 177
    Sanjeeva Gupta, Babita Ghai

29. Coccygeal Nerve Block...........................179
    Yashwant Laxman Nankar, Dwarkadas K Baheti

SECTION 6 — NEUROMODULATION

30. Sacral Nerve Stimulation 185
    Hemkumar Pushparaj, Manohar Sharma

SECTION 7 — PERIPHERAL BLOCKS

31. Radiofrequency Neurotomy of Suprascapular
    Nerve for Refractory Shoulder Joint Pain 193
    Nick Plunkett, Allen Pinto

32. Tennis or Golfer's Elbow..........................197
    Dwarkadas K Baheti

33. Hip Joint Injection.................................200
    Yehia Kamel

34. Greater Trochanteric Bursa Injection 203
    Yehia Kamel

35. Popliteal Nerve Block 206
    Yashwant Laxman Nankar, Dwarkadas K Baheti

36. Calcaneal Spur Injection 210
    Dwarkadas K Baheti

SECTION 8 — SYMPATHETIC BLOCK

37. Stellate Ganglion Block............................215
    Preeti Doshi

38. Splanchnic Plexus Block: Fluoroscopy Guided...220
    Dwarkadas K Baheti

39. CT-guided Splanchinc Plexus Block 223
    Dwarkadas K Baheti

40. CT-guided Celiac Plexus Block 225
    Dwarkadas K Baheti

41. Celiac Plexus Block: Fluoroscopy Guided 229
    Dwarkadas K Baheti

42. Lumbar Sympathetic Plexus Block.................232
    Dwarkadas K Baheti

43. Superior Hypogastric Plexus Block 235
    Dwarkadas K Baheti, Yashwant Laxman Nankar

44. Ganglion of Impar Block............................238
    Dwarkadas K Baheti

SECTION 9 — ULTRASOUND GUIDED BLOCK

45. Suprascapular Nerve Block........................243
    Ritesh Roy, Gaurav Agarwal

46. Brachial Plexus Block
    (Supraclavicular Approach) 249
    Ritesh Roy, Gaurav Agarwal

47. Thoracic Paravertebral Block......................253
    Archana Areti, Ritesh Roy, Gaurav Agarwal

48. Ultrasound-guided Transversus Abdominis
    Plane Block 258
    Gaurav Agarwal, Ritesh Roy

49. Lumbar Plexus Block 262
    Ritesh Roy, Gaurav Agarwal

50. Lateral Femoral Cutaneous Nerve Block...........268
    Ritesh Roy, Gaurav Agarwal

51. Sacral Plexus Block................................270
    Ritesh Roy, Gaurav Agarwal

52. Pericapsular Nerve Group Block
    (For Hip Joint).....................................276
    Ritesh Roy, Gaurav Agarwal

SECTION 10 — ULTRASOUND-GUIDED DRY NEEDLING

53. Ultrasound-guided Dry Needling..................283
    Lakshmi Vas

SECTION 11 — ADVANCED PAIN MANAGEMENT

54. Spinal Cord Stimulation............................291
    Timothy Ray Deer

55. Intrathecal Drug Delivery System 294
    Samir Ranjit Jani, Dwarkadas K Baheti

56. Transforaminal Endoscopic Discectomy............298
    Kailash M Kothari, Manish Raj, Shiraz Ahmed Munshi

57. Kyphoplasty 317
    Samir Ranjit Jani

    Index..321

SECTION 1
Basics: Interventional Pain Management

- **Fluoroscopy for Minimally Invasive Spinal and Trigeminal Procedures**
  Sanjeeva Gupta, Ganesan Baranidharan, Manohar Sharma, Harun Gupta

- **Understanding of Radiological Anatomy**
  Kenneth Lupton, James Baren, Harun Gupta

- **Understanding Common Image-guided Procedures**
  Kenneth Lupton, Jamen Baren, Harun Gupta

- **Understanding the Pathology of Common Conditions through Magnetic Resonance Imaging for the Pain Physician**
  Harun Gupta, James Baren, Kenneth Lupton

- **Radiation Protection**
  Satish Kamath, Dwarkadas K Baheti

- **Informed Consent for Interventional Pain Management Procedures**
  Dwarkadas K Baheti

- **Protocol for Interventional Pain Management Procedures**
  Dwarkadas K Baheti

- **Role of Investigations for Interventional Pain Treatment Procedures**
  Dwarkadas K Baheti

- **Medications Used for Interventional Pain Procedures**
  Kritika Doshi, RP Gehdoo

CHAPTER 1

Fluoroscopy for Minimally Invasive Spinal and Trigeminal Procedures

Sanjeeva Gupta, Ganesan Baranidharan, Manohar Sharma, Harun Gupta

INTRODUCTION: BASIC PRINCIPLES

- Understanding neuroanatomy of the different structures that can cause spinal pain is essential before attempting interventions.
- We can only see bony structures on fluoroscopy (X-ray) and have to construct a 3D image in our mind and consider the different structures in relation to the bone.
- Bony anatomy and the surrounding structures may not be the same in every patient, especially if they have significant spondylosis, osteophytes, spondylolisthesis, scoliosis, etc.
- Bones are our FRIEND and our EYES. Try to contact the bone before navigating the needle deeper as this will increase safety.
- If you are a beginner, always start with simple lumbar spine interventions and then consider cervical and thoracic followed by trigeminal interventions.
- If you are having difficulty in identifying the target point (TP), look at the TPs one level above and below as this can help identify the TP. In some patients, changing the position can help identify the TP, e.g., lateral to prone position for cervical interventions in patients with short neck.
- Use a standardized terminology to identify the structures for the procedure being done.
- Neural axis safe iodinated contrast should be used where necessary (e.g. epidural, transforaminal injections, etc.).
- *Get the level correct*:
  - *Lumbar level*:
    - Count levels from T12 downward. Be aware of transitional vertebra at the L5/S1 level.
    - When performing transforaminal epidural injection, compare the sagittal MRI image with the lateral fluoroscopic view to confirm that the procedure is being performed at the correct level.
  - *Cervical level*:
    - Count levels from C2 (largest spinous process) downward and/or
    - C7 upward [C7 transverse process (TP) slanting down and T1 TP slanting up]

PATIENT POSITIONS FOR PROCEDURES

- *Prone position*:
  - All lumbar, sacral, and thoracic procedures
  - Cervical epidural, lower cervical medial branch block (MBB)/RFD
- *Supine position*:
  - Cervical MBB and radiofrequency denervation (RFD)
  - Cervical nerve root block
  - Cervical disc procedures
- *Lateral position*:
  - Cervical MBB and RFD
- *Sitting position on a trolley or operating table (not on a chair)*:
  - Cervical MBB and RFD. May be helpful in patients with very short neck. Very rarely used (try prone position instead). Be aware that a vasovagal episode can occur and have a plan to manage.
  - Cervical epidural

FLUOROSCOPY

- Radiation safety standards should be followed.
- Agree the terminology to be used when operating fluoroscopic C-arm with the radiographer to decrease unnecessary X-ray exposure.
- *Agree that the top end of the fluoroscope is the reference point*:
  - Antero-posterior (AP) view
  - Moving the top end toward the head—cephalic tilt
  - Moving the top end toward the foot—caudal tilt
  - Rotating the top end to the right—right oblique
  - Rotating the top end to the left—left oblique
  - Lateral view
  - Moving the fluoroscope C-arm in either direction in the lateral view to square the vertebral endplates/disc—wig-wag

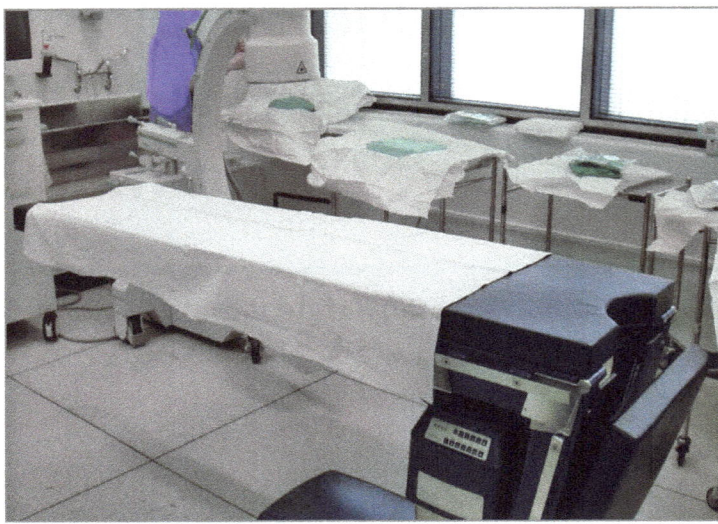

Fig. 1: Appropriate procedure table is essential to facilitate spinal interventional procedures. Radiolucent carbon fiber table may avoid any metal artifacts, especially when oblique rotation and tilt of the C-arm is required, e.g., for L5/S1 disc access.

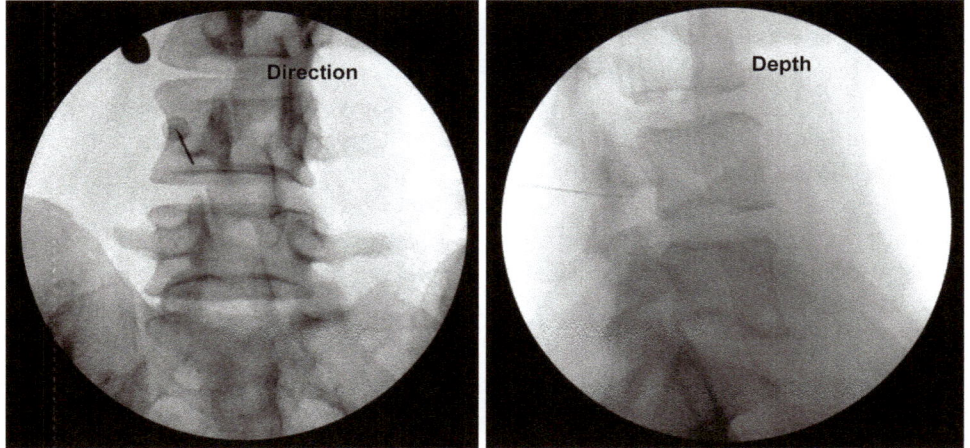

Fig. 2: Fluoroscopy—basic principles. Target point should be in the center of the screen. Look at one level above and below. *3D principle: In prone position*: Antero-posterior (AP) and oblique views guide the *Direction* of the needle; lateral view guides the *Depth* of the needle. If the depth is not satisfactory, return back to antero-posterior/oblique view to advance the needle in the correct *Direction* and check the *Depth* in the lateral view.[1]
Source: Reproduced with permission from M/s Jaypee Brothers Medical Publishers. Stimulation-guided pan mapping. In: Baheti DK, Bakshi S, Gupta S, Gehdoo RP (Eds). Interventional Pain Management: A Practical Approach, 2nd edition; 2016. p. 82 [Figures 1 and 2]

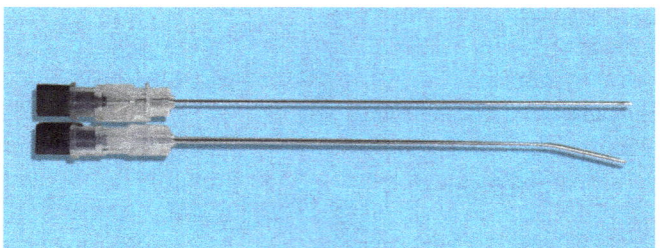

Fig. 3: *Block needle*: Using a curved tipped needle or bending/curving the distal few millimeters of the needle manually (away from the hub OR in the direction of the bevel) can assist in navigating the needle to the target point.

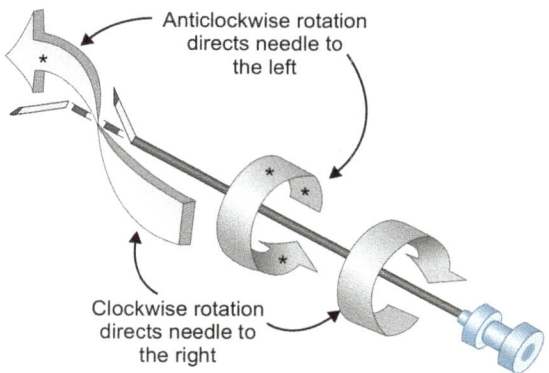

Fig. 4: *Block needle*: Diagrammatic representation of how a curved tip spinal/block needle can assist in navigating the tip to the target point.[2]
Source: Reproduced with permission from Oxford University Press. Drugs, equipment and basic principles of spinal interventions. In: Simpson K, Baranidharan G, Gupta S (Eds). Spinal Interventions in Pain Management. 2012. p. 27 [Figure 3.1].

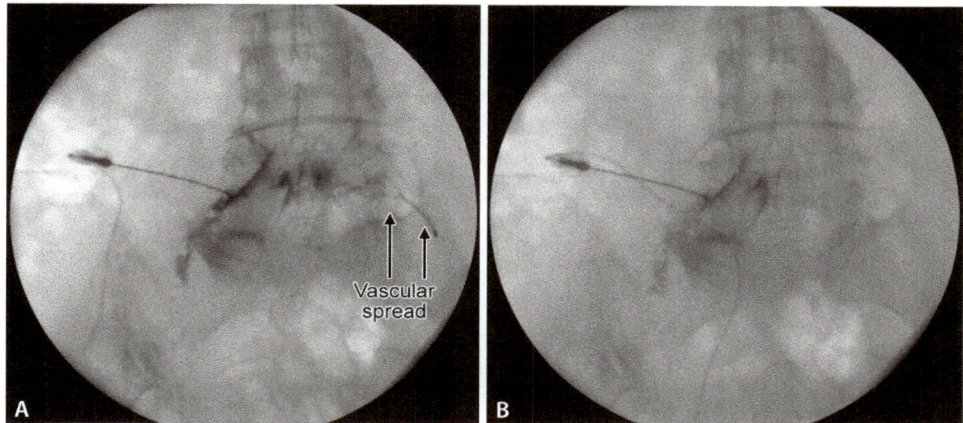

Figs. 5A and B: If fluoroscopy is used for transforaminal epidural injection, the contrast should be injected in antero-posterior view (not lateral view) under continuous imaging to rule out vascular spread. (A) Contrast under continuous fluoroscopy (vascular spread seen); (B) Static image after contrast injection (vascular spread missed).

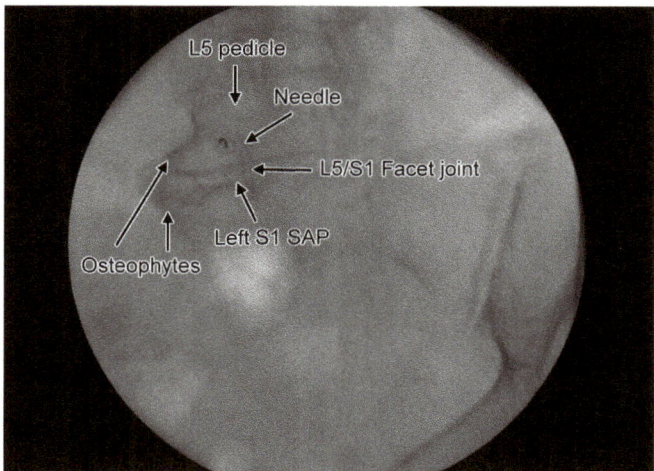

Fig. 6: *Fluoroscopy*: Knowing the depth of the different spinal structure in relation to the skin entry point of the needle is essential. The image shows vertebral body/disc osteophytes at the left L5/S1 level which produce a shadow in the area of the target for a left L5/S1 transforaminal epidural procedure. However, as we are aware that the vertebral body is anterior to the target point (deeper from skin entry site), we can safely place a curved tip needle over the left L5 pedicle and then navigate below the pedicle and into the intervertebral foramen. (SAP: superior articular process)

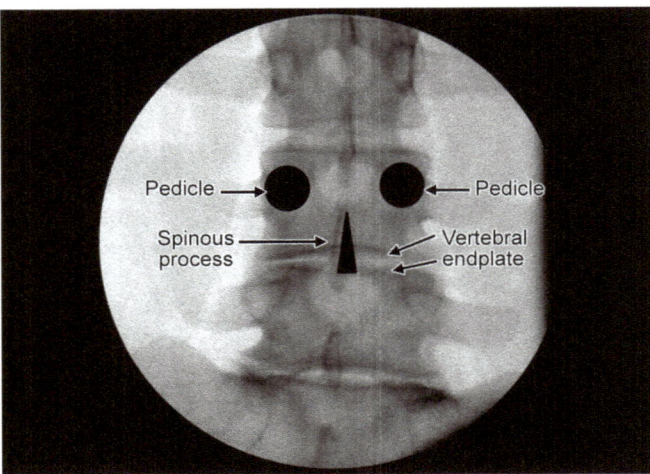

Fig. 7: *Fluoroscopy—lumbar level*: First, obtain a true antero-posterior view in which the spinous process is seen between the two pedicles. Then cephalic or caudal tilt to "square off" the vertebral endplate (the image will appear like the face of an owl). Normally for lower lumbar/upper sacral levels—cephalic tilt; upper lumbar/lower thoracic—caudal tilt; upper thoracic and cervical—depends on patient position. Try both caudal and cephalic tilt and then decide.

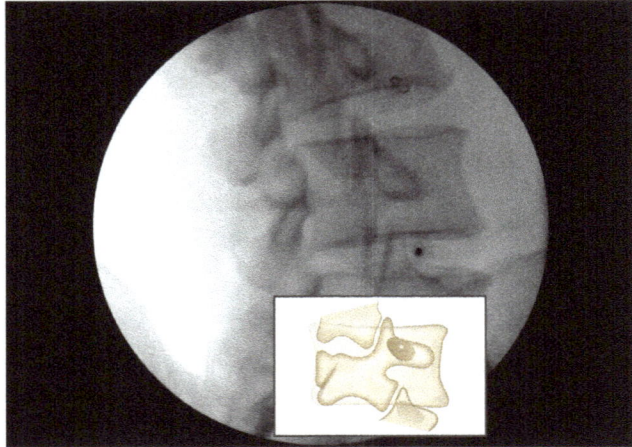

Fig. 8: *Fluoroscopy—lumbar level*: Once the true antero-posterior view is obtained, then rotate the C-arm in the right or the left oblique direction to obtain a "scotty view" as shown in the image. As a general rule, the structures closest to the C-arm move in the direction of the C-arm and the structures away from the C-arm move in the opposite direction.
Source: Reproduced with permission from Oxford University Press. Applied anatomy and fluoroscopy for spinal interventions. In Simpson K, Baranidharan G, Gupta S (Eds). Spinal Interventions in Pain Management. 2012; p. 6. [Figure 1.4]

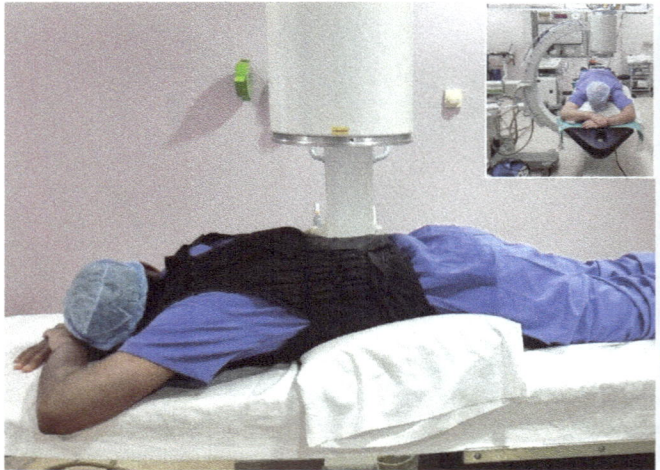 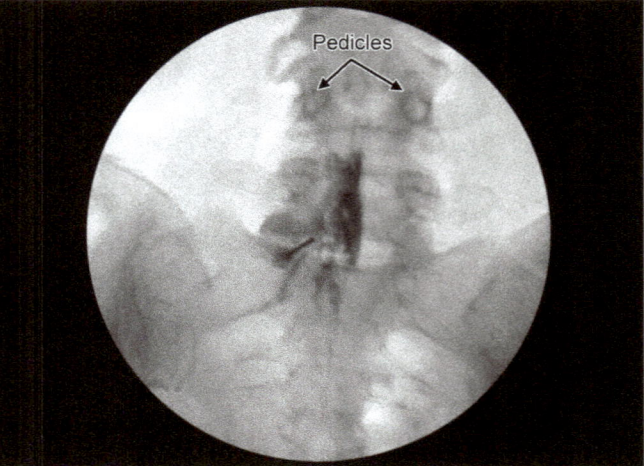

Fig. 9: *Fluoroscopy*: C-arm—antero-posterior (AP) view: Pillow under the lower abdomen/pelvis to decrease lumbar lordosis. Identify the structure of the lumbar spine. The inset shows the C-arm view from head end. In AP view, the spinous process is in the middle of the two pedicles.

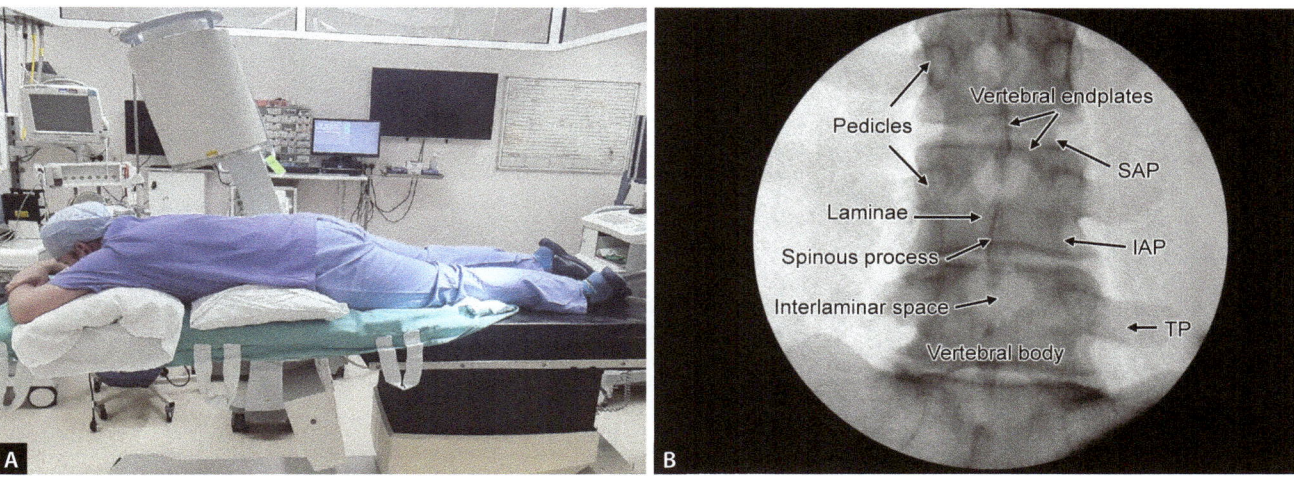

Figs. 10A and B: *Fluoroscopy*: C-arm—cephalic tilt: C-arm view from the side. The L4/5 and the L5/S1 vertebral end plates are squared showing the disc space at lower lumbar levels; (B) Identify the structures of the spine relevant to the procedure once the AP view is obtained and the vertebral end plates are "squared off" by cephalic or caudal tilt. (IAP: inferior articular process; SAP: superior articular process; TP: transverse process)

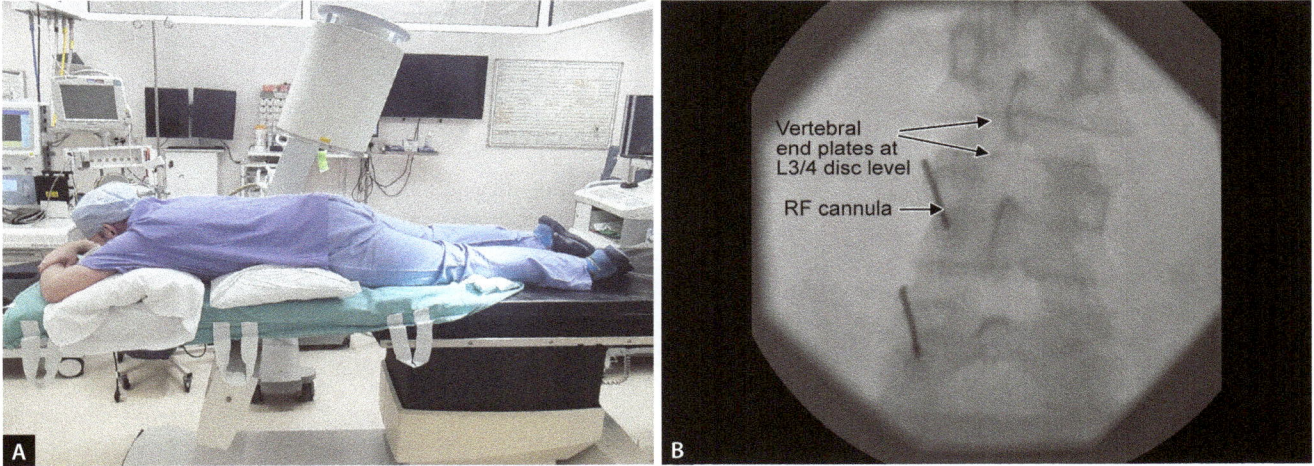

Figs. 11A and B: *Fluoroscopy*: (A) C-arm—caudal tilt: C-arm view from the side; (B) At the upper lumbar and lower thoracic level the C-arm may need to be tilted 5° to 7° caudad to square the vertebral endplates (ignore the RF cannula in this image).

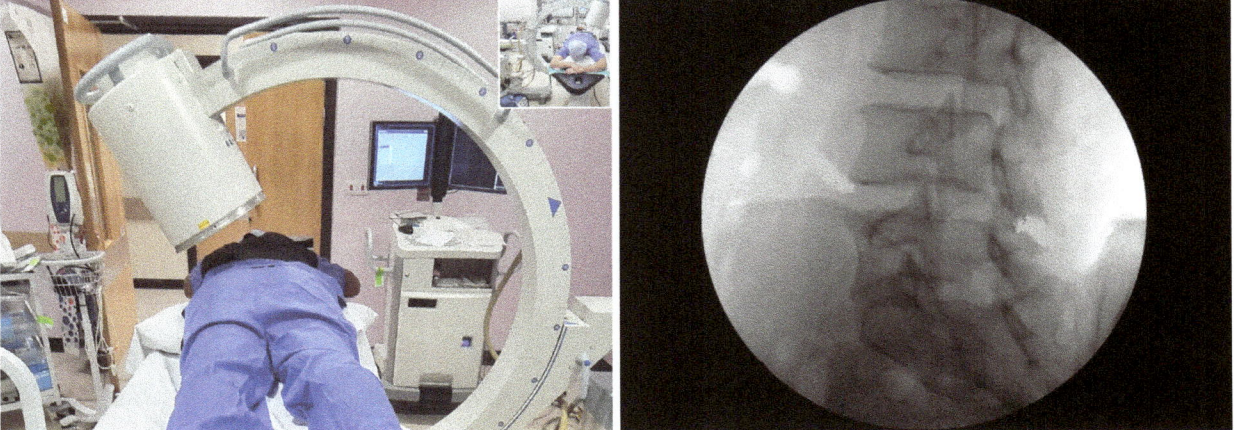

Fig. 12: *Fluoroscopy*: C-arm in left oblique view: After obtaining the antero-posterior view, the C-arm is tilted cephalic to square the vertebral endplates and then rotated left oblique to obtain a "scotty view." The inset shows the C-arm view from head end.

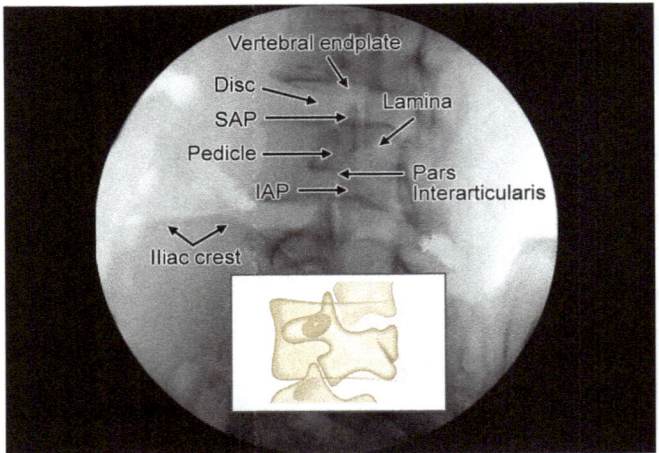

Fig. 13: *Fluoroscopy*: Left oblique view of the lumbar spine creates the "scotty view." Identify the structures of the spine before starting the procedure. The area of the junction between the superior articular process (SAP) and the inferior articular process (IAP) is known as pars interarticularis (PI) and a fracture at PI can lead to spondylolisthesis which is more common at the L5/S1 level.

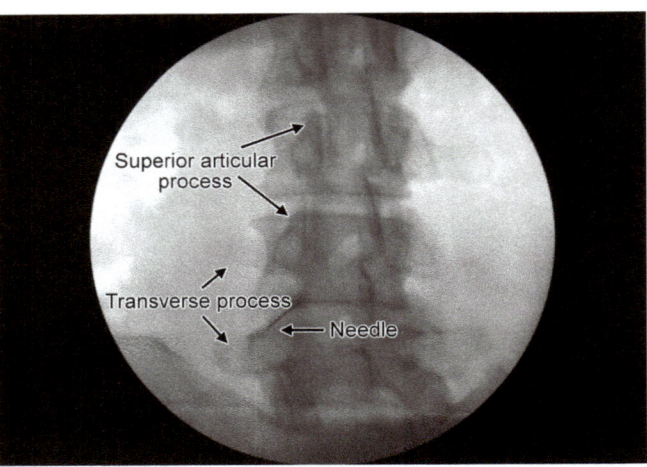

Fig. 14: *Fluoroscopy*: Identify the junction of the L4 superior articular process (SAP) and the transverse process (TP). Place the needle just below the junction of the left L5 SAP and the TP for medial branch block.

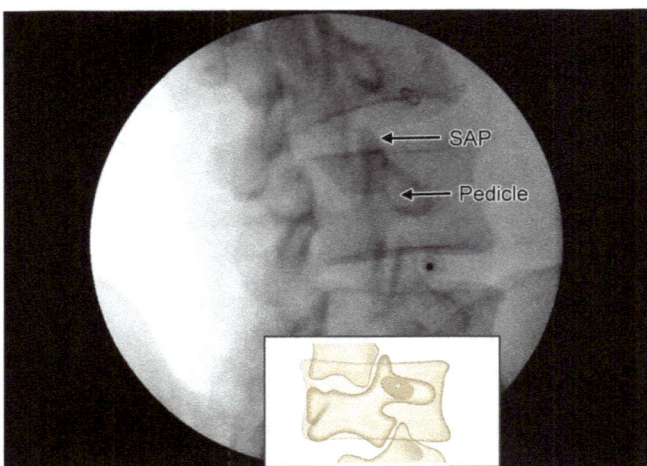

Fig. 15: Identifying two key structures on lumbar fluoroscopy can assist in performing most procedures. Superior articular process (SAP) for: Facet joint injection, medial branch block, medial branch radiofrequency, discogram, disc interventions and infraneural/retrodiscal transforaminal epidural injection. Pedicle for: Selective nerve root block and vertebroplasty. End-on view (gun barrel technique) of spinal needle just infront of the L5 SAP and in the middle of the disc space for L4/5 disc access.
Source: Reproduced with permission from Oxford University Press. Applied anatomy and fluoroscopy for spinal interventions. In Simpson K, Baranidharan G, Gupta S (Eds). Spinal Interventions in Pain Management. 2012. p. 6 [Figure 1.4].

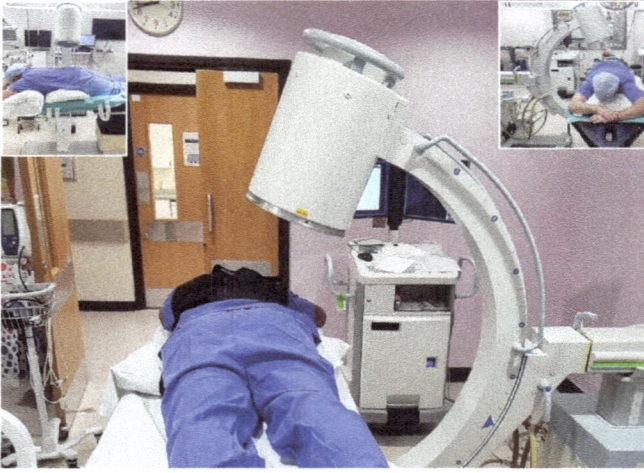
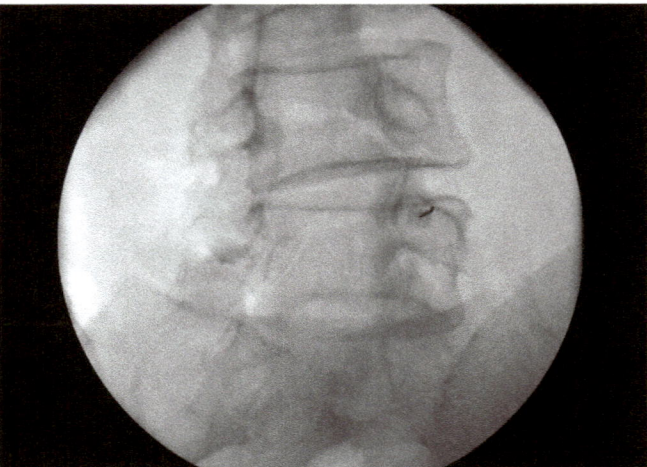

Fig. 16: *Fluoroscopy*: C-arm in right oblique view. After obtaining the antero-posterior view, the C-arm is tilted cephalic to square the vertebral endplates of lower lumbar vertebra and then rotated to the right to obtain a "scotty view." The inset shows the C-arm view from head end and the side.

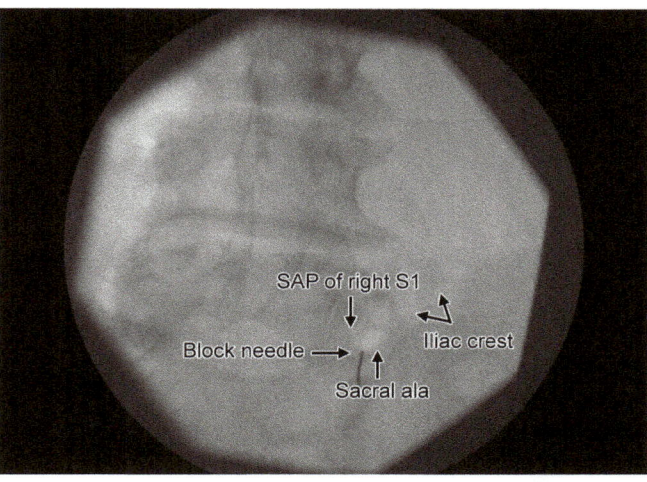

Fig. 17: *Fluoroscopy*: Tip of the needle at the junction of the right superior articular process (SAP) of the S1 vertebra and the ala of the sacrum for L5 dorsal rami (DR) block. If the fluoroscopy C-arm is rotated further oblique, the iliac crest will overshadow the L5 DR target.

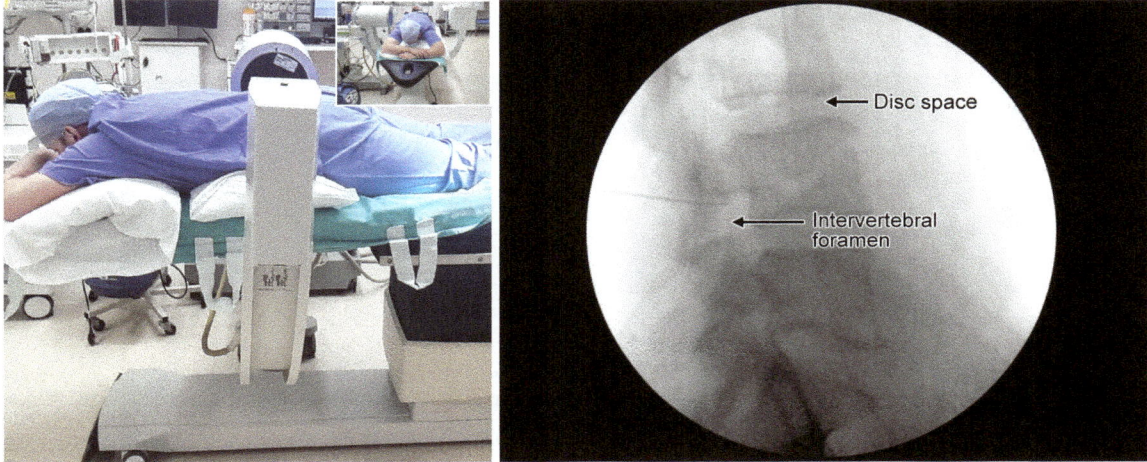

Fig. 18: *Fluoroscopy*: In the lateral view, the vertebral end plates are squared off with the disc space and intervertebral foramen visible. The inset shows the C-arm view from the head end.
Source: Gupta S. Stimulation guided pan mapping. In: Baheti DK, Bakshi S, Gupta S, Gehdoo RP (Eds). Interventional Pain Management: A Practical Approach, 2nd edition. New Delhi: Jaypee Brothers Medical Publishers; 2016. pp. 81-3.

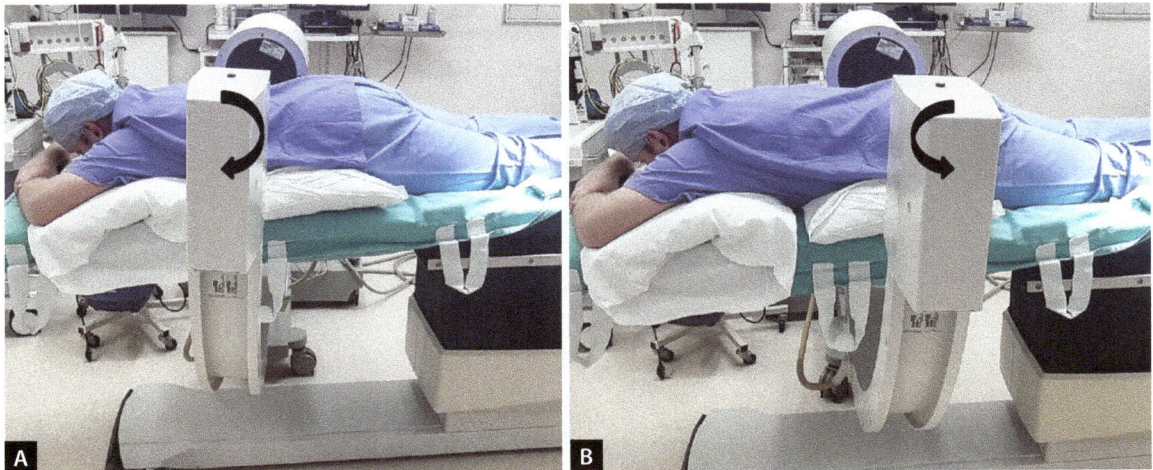

Figs. 19A and B: Fluoroscopy: In some patients, it can be difficult to identify/outline the disc space and/or the intervertebral foramen in the lateral view. Moving the C-arm in either direction in the lateral view to "square off"" the vertebral end plates is commonly known as "wig-wag." These movements help to identify the disc space and intervertebral foramen at thoracic spine levels and also in some cases at the lumbar and cervical spine levels. The black curved arrows in the image indicate the direction of the C-arm movements.

FLUOROSCOPY FOR PROCEDURES AT THE LUMBOSACRAL AREA

Figures 20 to 43 will show fluoroscopic images of some procedures at the lumbosacral level with the anatomy/bony landmarks identified.

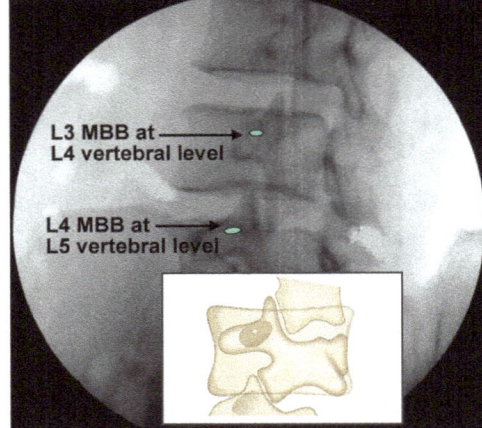

Fig. 20: *Fluoroscopy:* Targets for left L3 medial branch block (MBB) at the "eye" of the "scotty dog" at L4 level and L4 MBB at L5 level to block the nerve supply to the left L4/5 facet joint.

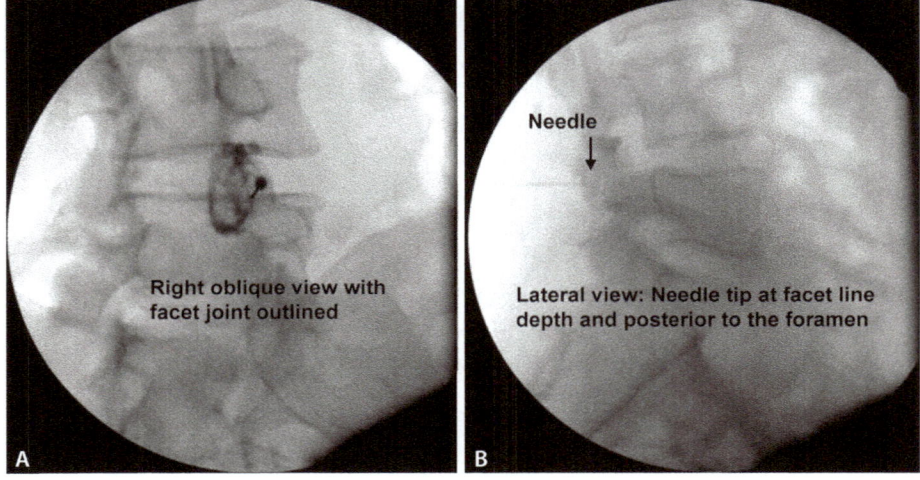

Figs. 21A and B: Facet joint injection (not commonly performed): Sometimes, the needle can pass through the facet joint and contact the nerve root posteriorly. Lateral view is rarely needed.

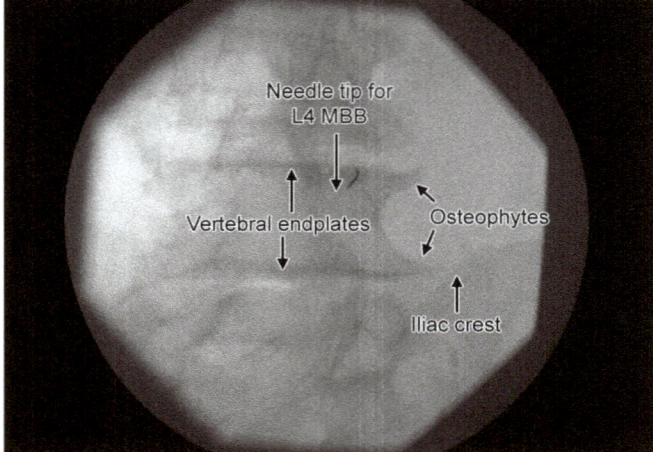

Fig. 22: Right oblique view—challenges encountered: Identify the junction of the superior articular process and the transverse process at L4 level. Needle in position for L3 medial branch block (MBB) at L4 level. The target for the left L5 dorsal rami block is obscured by the iliac crest—decreasing the right obliquity of the C-arm will expose the target area for the left L5 DR block. The junction of the SAP and the vertebral endplate can sometimes be mistaken to be the junction of SAP and transverse process.

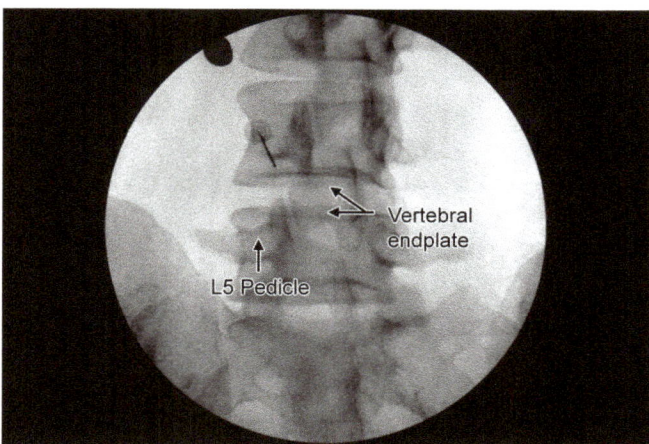

Fig. 23: Left oblique view for left L4/5 transforaminal epidural injection (subpedicular technique). First, obtain an antero-posterior view followed by cephalic tilt to square the *vertebral endplate closest to the target point* and then left oblique view to obtain the image shown below (3D principle: Direction, Depth, Direction).
Source: Gupta S. Stimulation guided pan mapping. In: Baheti DK, Bakshi S, Gupta S, Gehdoo RP (Eds). Interventional Pain Management: A Practical Approach, 2nd edition. New Delhi: Jaypee Brothers Medical Publishers; 2016. pp. 81-3.

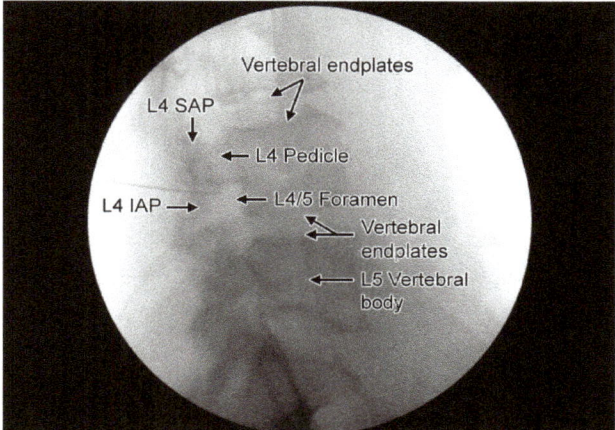

Fig. 24: Lateral view for L4/5 transforaminal epidural injection (subpedicular technique). If there is difficulty in identifying the intervertebral foramen, then moving the fluoroscopy C-arm in a sideward direction in lateral view (wig-wag: see Figure 19) to square the vertebral endplates will improve the view of the intervertebral foramen. (IAP: inferior articular process; SAP: superior articular process).
Source: Gupta S. Stimulation guided pan mapping. In: Baheti DK, Bakshi S, Gupta S, Gehdoo RP (Eds). Interventional Pain Management: A Practical Approach, 2nd edition. New Delhi: Jaypee Brothers Medical Publishers; 2016. pp. 81-3.

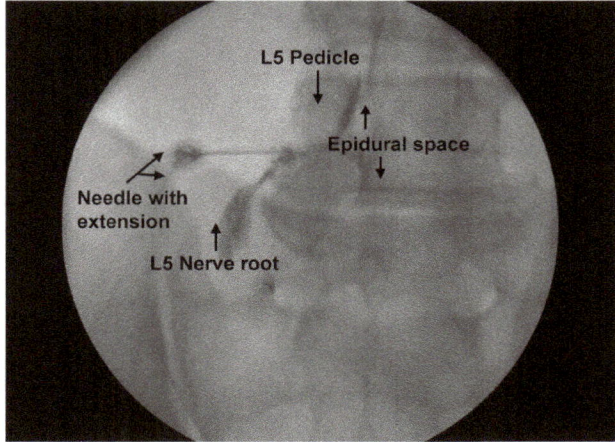

Fig. 25: Antero-posterior (AP) view—needle with low-volume extension tubing attached in position for left L5/S1 transforaminal epidural injection. Contrast injected under continuous fluoroscopy in AP view. Contrast spread can be seen along the left L5 nerve root, inferior and medial to the pedicle and into the epidural space.

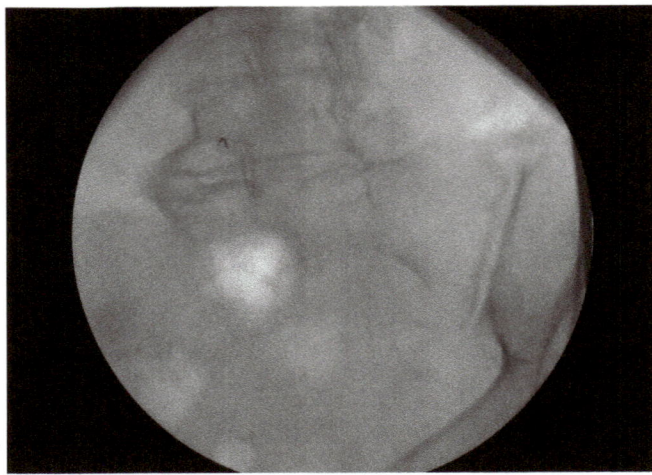

Fig. 26: Procedures at L5/S1 level can be technically difficult. Identify the structures of the lumbar spine relevant to left L5/S1 transforaminal epidural injection. Identify the right sacroiliac joint.

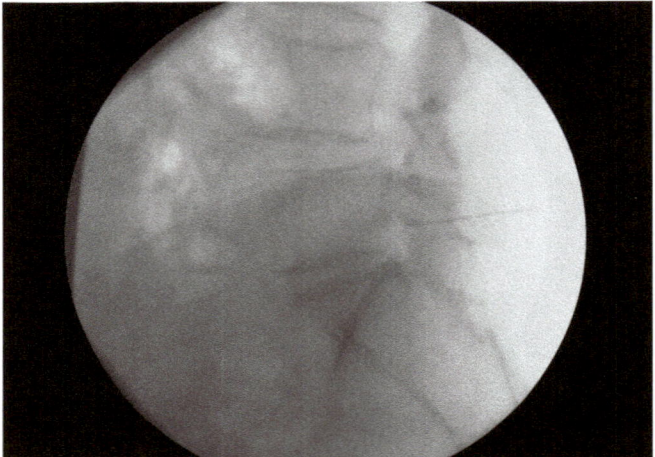

Fig. 27: Lateral view with needle tip in the L5/S1 intervertebral foramen. Identify the L4 and L5 pedicles, L4 and L5 vertebral endplates, L4 and L5 vertebral bodies, and L4/5 and L5/S1 intervertebral foramina.

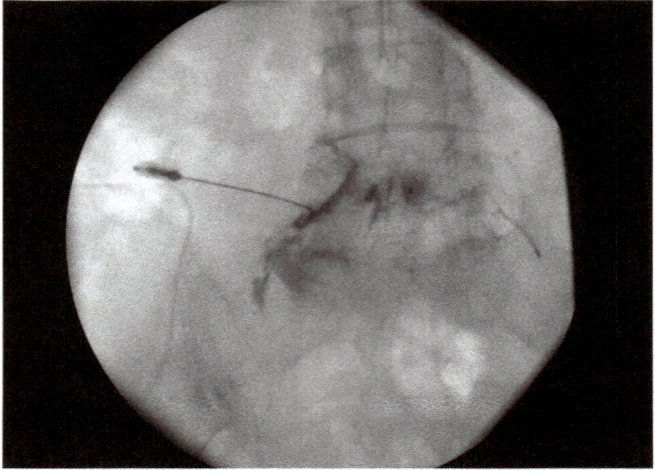

Fig. 28: Contrast injected in AP view under continuous fluoroscopy: What can you see? Would you inject steroid?

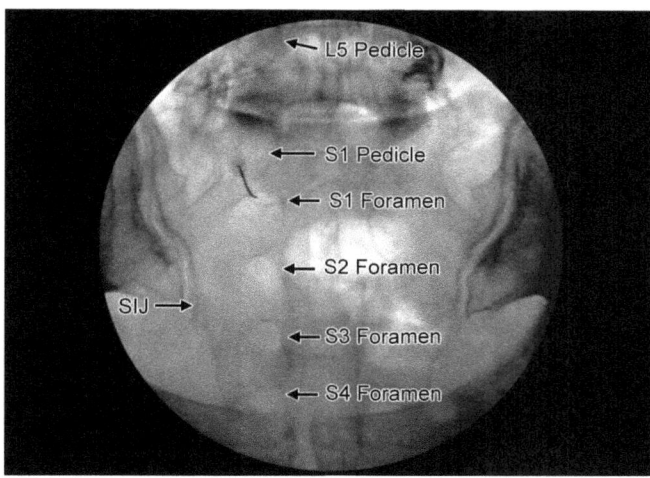

Fig. 29: *Antero-posterior view of the sacrum:* Left S1 foramen. The S2, S3, S4 foramina can also be seen. There are anterior and posterior foramina and they must be overlapped and are often difficult to visualize. Cephalic tilt in an attempt to identify the L5/S1 disc space can facilitate visualizing the S1 foramen. Normally, the S3 foramen is at the level of the lower end of the sacroiliac joint (SIJ).

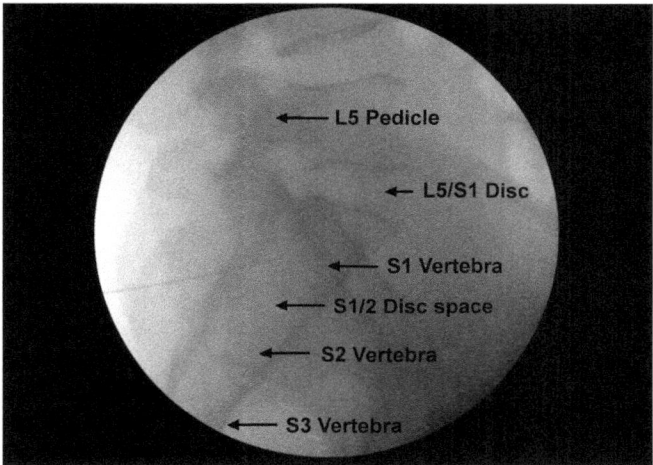

Fig. 30: Lateral view showing the needle in the epidural space at S1 level. If the disc space/landmarks are not clearly visible, then moving the C-arm in either direction in the lateral position "wig-wag" can square the vertebral endplates defining the bony anatomy better.

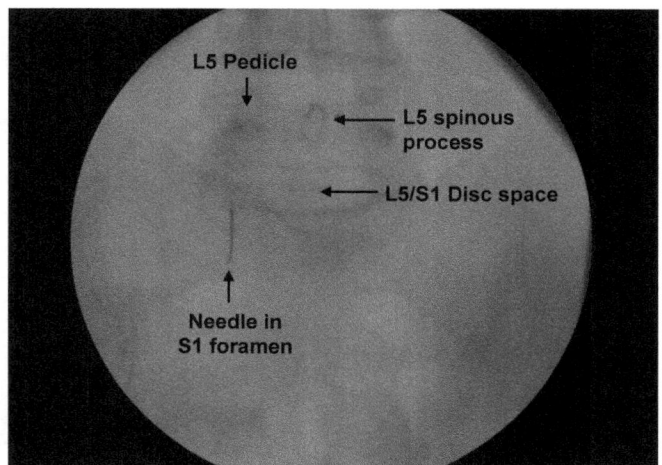

Fig. 31: AP view. Needle is directed toward the S1 foramen.

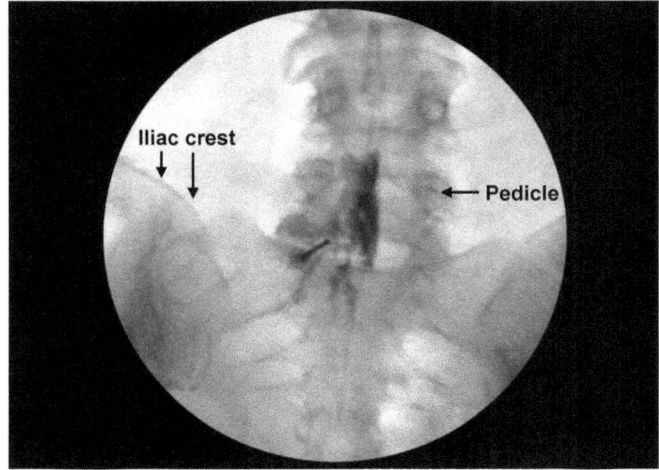

Fig. 32: Targeted left-sided L5/S1 interlaminar epidural.

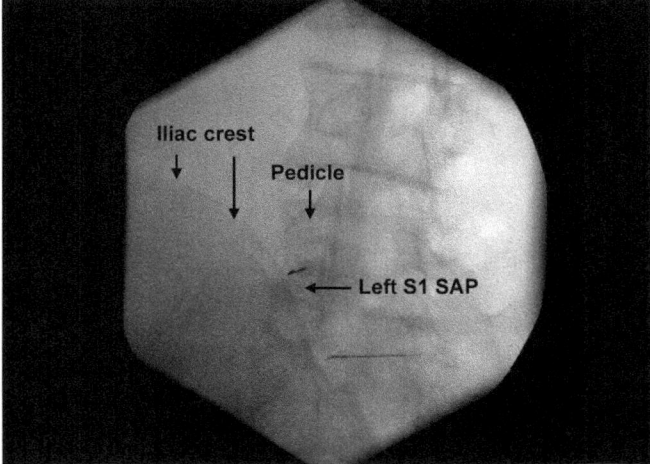

Fig. 33: Left oblique view showing the needles in place at the left S1 foramen and at L5/S1 foramen (retrodiscal/infraneural technique) levels. The curved tip needle is just lateral to the lower part of the left S1 superior articular process (SAP). The left iliac crest is overlying the target for L5 dorsal rami.

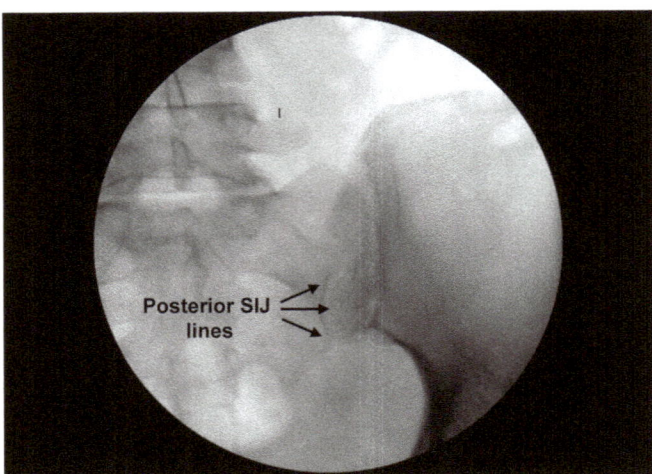

Fig. 34: Antero-posterior view of the right sacroiliac joint (SIJ). Normally, the medial joint lines are the posterior joint lines (arrows) that can be accessed.[3]
Source: Gupta S, Richardson J. Sacroiliac joint block. In: Baheti DK, Bakshi S, Gupta S, Gehdoo RP (Eds). Interventional Pain Management: A Practical Approach, 1st edition. New Delhi: Jaypee Brothers Medical Publishers; 2009. pp. 198-203.

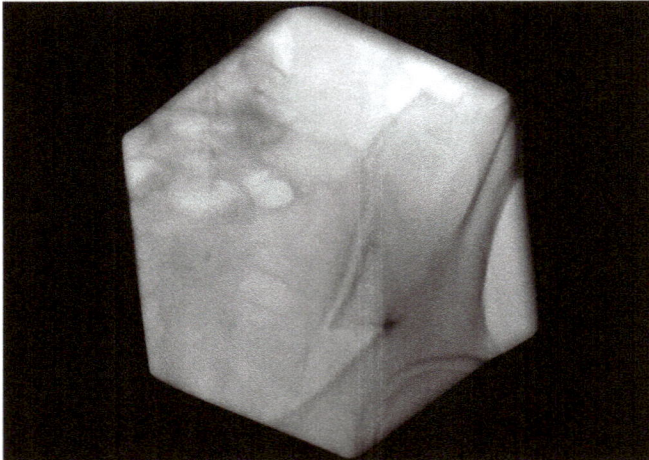

Fig. 35: The anterior and posterior joint lines of the right sacroiliac joint have been superimposed by contralateral oblique rotation of the C-arm.[3]
Source: Gupta S, Richardson J. Sacroiliac joint block. In: Baheti DK, Bakshi S, Gupta S, Gehdoo RP (Eds). Interventional Pain Management: A Practical Approach, 1st edition. New Delhi: Jaypee Brothers Medical Publishers; 2009. pp. 198-203.

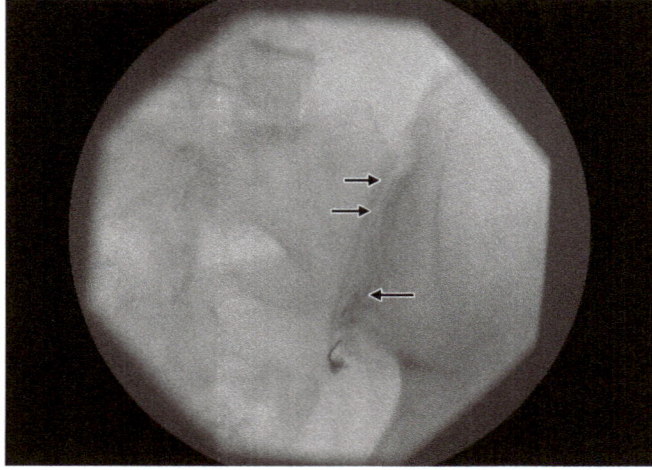

Fig. 36: If the needle is in the sacroiliac joint, then contrast spread can be seen like a thin line along the joint line (arrows).

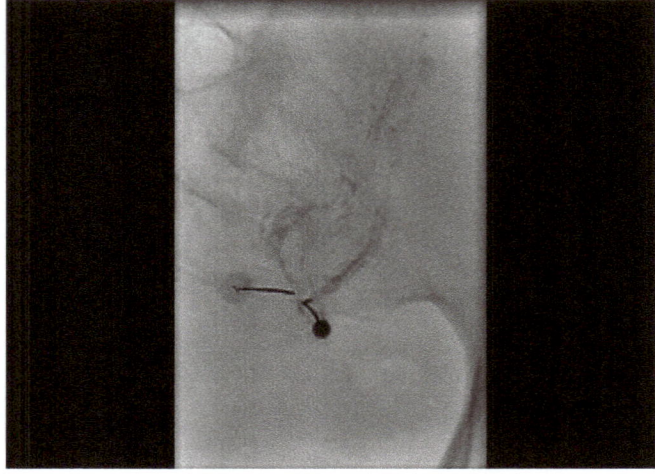

Fig. 37: Double-needle technique for sacroiliac joint injection [Refer to Chapter 24 (Sacroiliac Joint Block) for more details].

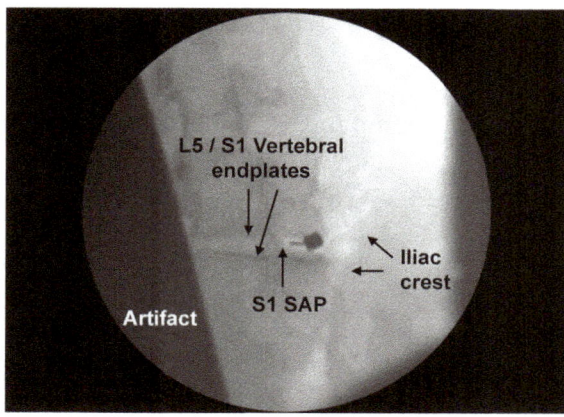

Fig. 38: L5/S1 intervertebral disc access can be challenging as the iliac crest, which is posterior to the disc, can overshadow the target area/skin entry area due to the cephalic tilt and the oblique rotation that is necessary to access the L5/S1 disc space. The artifact is due to suboptimal operating table. (SAP: superior articular process)

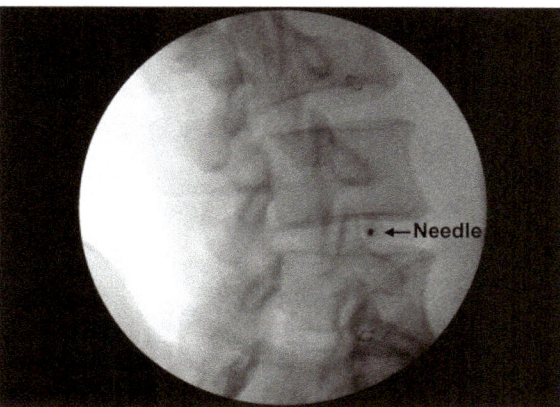

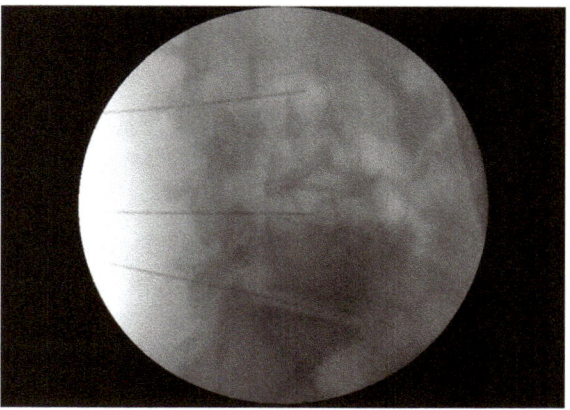

Fig. 39: L4/5 disc access—first obtain a true antero-posterior (AP) view with the spinous process in the middle of the two pedicles. Then cephalic tilt to square off the vertebral plate closest to the target area followed by right oblique rotation to obtain the required image. The disc is accessed using the "gun-barrel technique." The skin entry point is in the middle of the disc space just lateral to the superior articular process. This image determines the *Direction* of the needle.
Source: Reproduced with permission from Oxford University Press. Applied anatomy and fluoroscopy for spinal interventions. In: Simpson K, Baranidharan G, Gupta S (Eds). Spinal Interventions in Pain Management; 2012. p. 6 [Figure 1.4].

Fig. 40: Disc access—the lateral view helps to assess the *Depth* of the needle and if the tip is in the center of the disc (not close to the vertebral endplates). The image shows needles in place for three-level lower lumbar discogram. If the disc space is not clearly visible, moving the C-arm in either direction (wig-wag) in lateral view can improve disc visibility.
Source: Reproduced with permission from Oxford University Press. Applied anatomy and fluoroscopy for spinal interventions. In: Simpson K, Baranidharan G, Gupta S (Eds). Spinal Interventions in Pain Management; 2012. p. 6 [Figure 1.4].

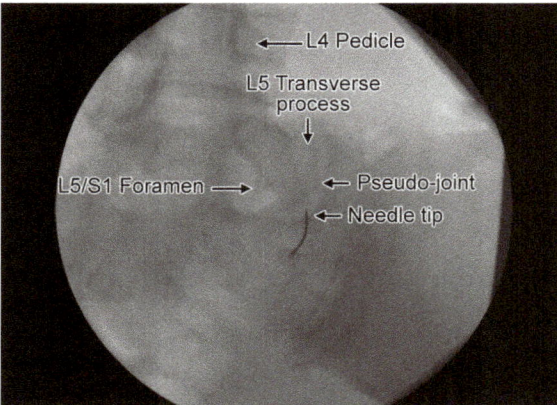

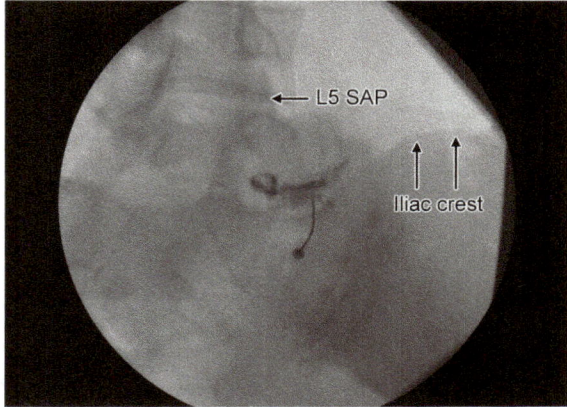

Fig. 41: *Right oblique view:* The tip of the needle is in the pseudojoint between the abnormal right L5 transverse process and ala of the sacrum over which the patient had pain on palpation. There appears to be an L5/S1 foramen formed due to the changes. To rule out transitional vertebra, count from T12 downward if a plain X-ray of lumbar spine is not available.

Fig. 42: *Right oblique view:* Contrast injection into the pseudo-joint provoked concordant pain.

FLUOROSCOPY FOR PROCEDURES IN THE CERVICAL SPINE AREA

General Considerations

- Procedures at the cervical level are considered more riskier than at the lumbar levels.
- Before performing procedures at the cervical level, it may be advisable to attend/observe some cervical spine procedures being performed by some colleagues experienced in performing such procedures.
- It is advisable to use a shorter spinal needle, e.g., 5 cm long.
- Cervical procedures can be done in lateral, supine, prone, or rarely sitting position.
- In patients with short neck prone position is better but if sitting position is chosen, this has to be done with the patient sitting on an operating table or a trolley (not on a chair) and one should be prepared to manage a vasovagal episode if this occurs.
- Upper cervical procedures can be done in lateral or supine position and prone position may be considered for lower cervical procedures.
- The head, neck, and chest should be positioned appropriately.
- Fluoroscopic image of C-spine should be obtained to identify the target points before scrubbing for the procedure. If target points are not visible please consider changing the position of the patient e.g. lateral position to prone position.
- Generally, upper cervical procedures are done one side at a time, especially 3rd occipital nerve block.
- Consider the risk of pneumothorax when performing procedures at lower cervical levels.

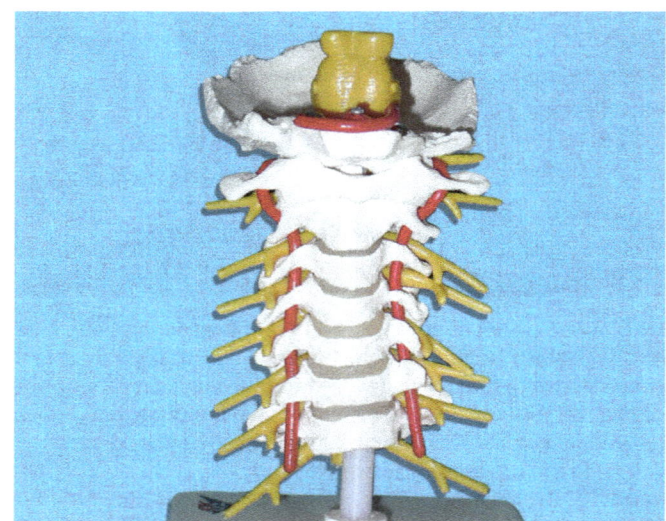

Fig. 43: *C-spine model:* Cervical procedures are riskier as many important structures are close to each other in a narrow space.

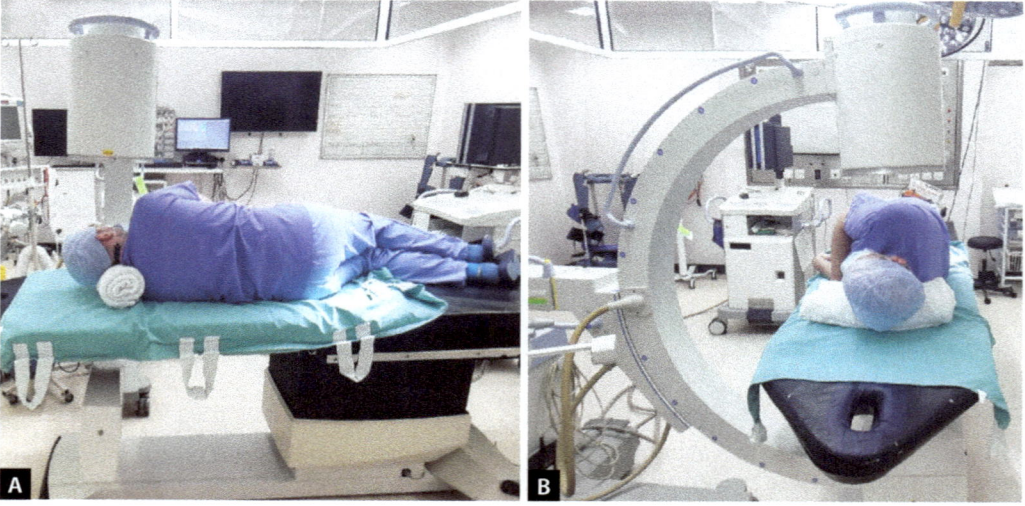

Figs. 44A and B: *Cervical spine:* Lateral position viewed from the (A) back and (B) head-end. The neck is supported on a roll of sheets/blankets. Both the shoulders are pulled as low as possible so that the target areas in the lower cervical spine are visible. Both knees are bent toward the abdomen/chest and both hands hold the knees, to increase the visibility of the cervical spine.

CHAPTER 1 | Fluoroscopy for Minimally Invasive Spinal and Trigeminal Procedures

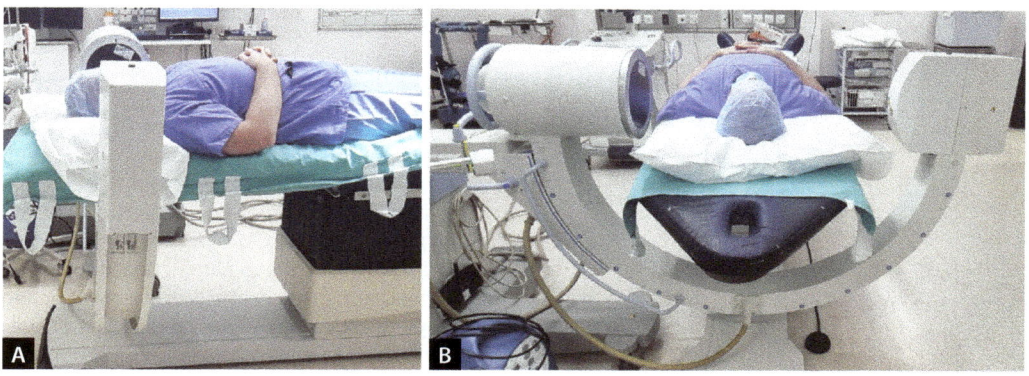

Figs. 45A and B: *Cervical spine*: Supine position—lateral view from the (A) side and (B) head-end of the operating table. The head/neck area is placed on a pillow or folded sheets.

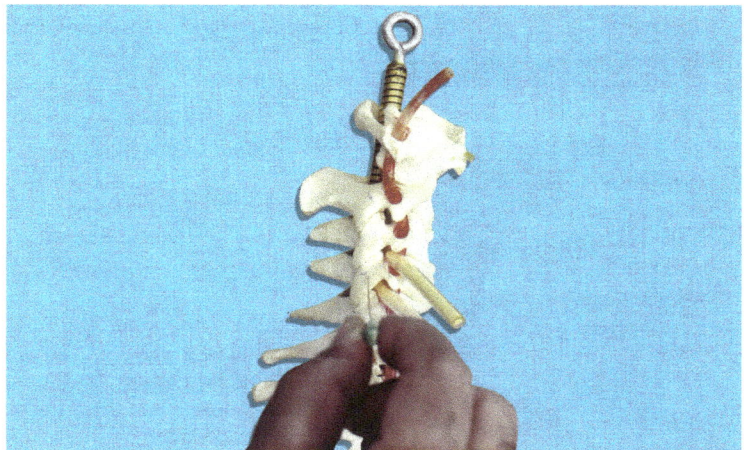

Fig. 46: Lateral view of the cervical spine model with the needle tip showing the target point for C4 medial branch block.
Courtesy: Dr Sherdil Nath, FRCA, Consultant in Pain Medicine, Umeå, Sweden.

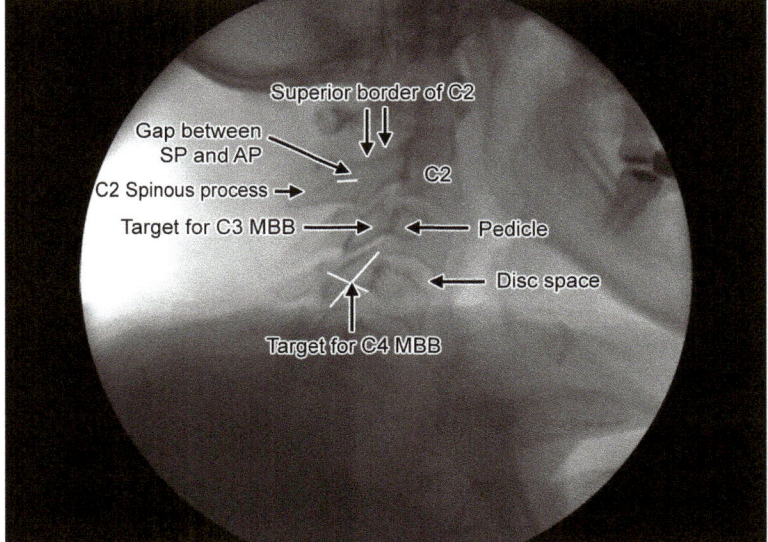

Fig. 47: *Lateral view*: After appropriate oblique rotation of the C-arm to the right or left under continuous fluoroscopy and then tilting the C-arm in cephalic or caudal direction, the right and the left articular pillars are superimposed. The facet joint lines appear crisp with the vertebral bodes and disc spaces outlined. The upper largest spinous process is the C2 level, and this helps in identifying the levels. This image is good to identify the target point for C3 medial branch block (MBB). The C-arm will need to be adjusted again if other level MBB are planned. Target is in the center of the rhomboid formed by the articular pillar as shown at C4 level. The pedicle is normally at the posterosuperior area of the vertebral body. There should be a gap between the spinous process (SP) and the articular pillar (AP) as shown by the horizontal white line at C2 level.[4]
Source: Gupta S, Varma S. Cervical medial branch block. In: Baheti DK, Bakshi S, Gupta S, Gehdoo RP (Eds). Interventional Pain Management: A Practical Approach, 2nd edition. New Delhi: Jaypee Brothers Medical Publishers; 2016. pp. 220-9.

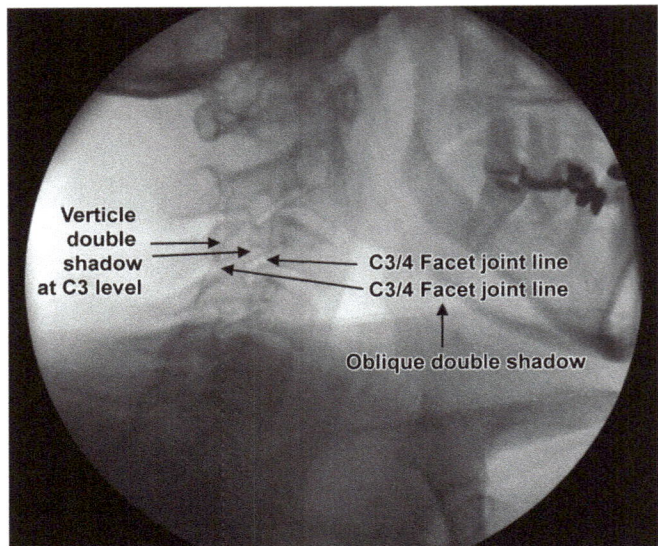

Fig. 48: Lateral view of cervical spine. The right and the left articular pillars (APs) and the facet joint lines are not super-imposed and double shadows (parallax) can be seen. To get the correct image (true lateral view) observe the movement of the vertical lateral margins of the APs with right or left oblique C-arm rotation under continuous fluoroscopy to super-impose them thus eliminating the vertical double shadows. Then tilt the C-arm in the cephalic or caudal direction under continuous fluoroscopy to superimpose the oblique/horizontal margins of the APs (facet joint lines) to eliminate the oblique/horizontal double shadow (parallax). This gives a true lateral view with the right and the left articular pillars superimposed which will decrease the risks of performing cervical medial branch procedures.
Source: Gupta S, Varma S. Cervical medial branch block. In: Baheti DK, Bakshi S, Gupta S, Gehdoo RP (Eds). Interventional Pain Management: A Practical Approach, 2nd edition. New Delhi: Jaypee Brothers Medical Publishers; 2016. pp. 220-9.[4]

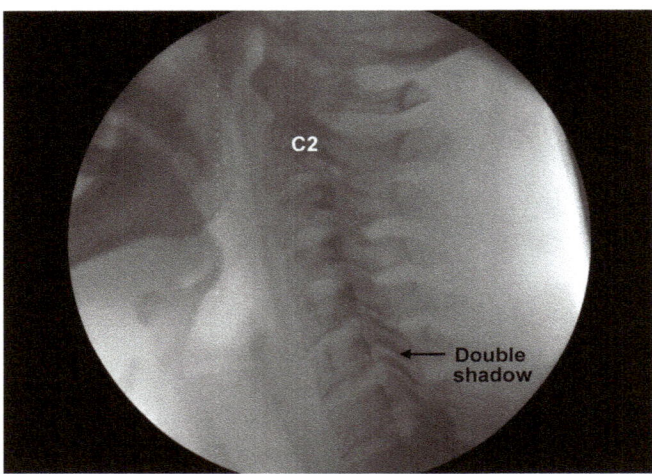

Fig. 49: *Double shadow (parallax)*: In this image, there is oblique double shadow (parallax) at the C6/7 level. Tilting the C-arm in the cephalic or caudal direction under continuous fluoroscopy will eliminate the double shadow (parallax). Once the oblique double shadow (parallax) is eliminated, the C-arm may have to be rotated in the right or left oblique direction to eliminate the vertical double shadow (parallax) that may have appeared.[5]
Source: Gupta S, Varma S. Cervical medial branch block. In: Baheti DK, Bakshi S, Gupta S, Gehdoo RP (Eds). Interventional Pain Management: A Practical Approach, 2nd edition. New Delhi: Jaypee Brothers Medical Publishers; 2016. pp. 220-9

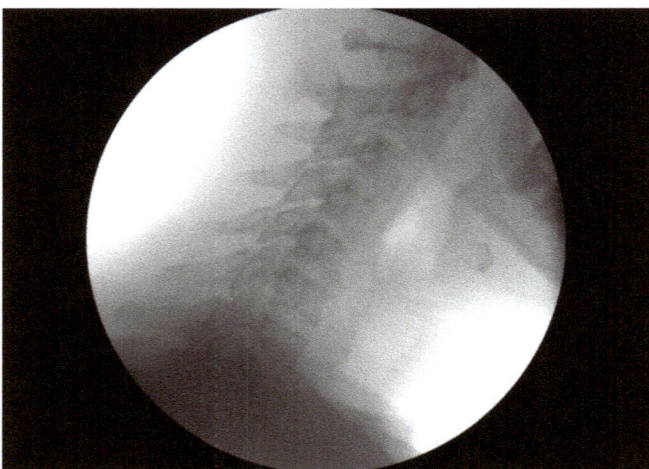

Fig. 50: *Cervical spine lateral view:* Identify the double shadow (parallax).
Source: Reproduced with permission from Oxford University Press. Applied anatomy and fluoroscopy for spinal interventions. In: Simpson K, Baranidharan G, Gupta S (Eds). Spinal Interventions in Pain Management. 2012. p. 9 [Figure 1.8].

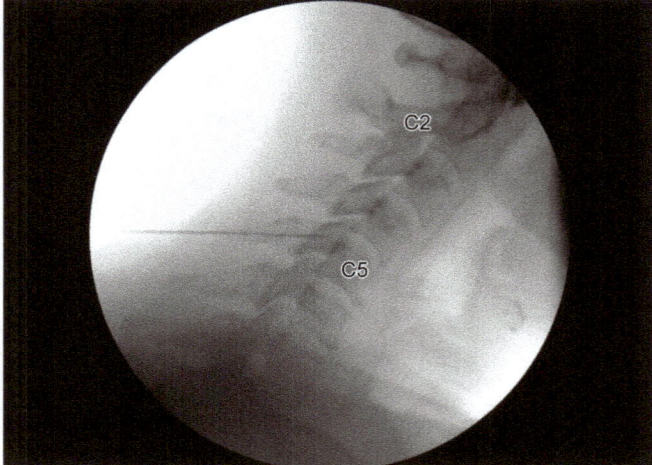

Fig. 51: *Fluoroscopy:* Cervical lateral view with double shadow (parallax) eliminated after oblique rotation. Count the vertebral levels from C2 (largest spinous process) downward. The tip of the needle is at the centroid of the C5 articular pillar.
Source: Reproduced with permission from Oxford University Press. Applied anatomy and fluoroscopy for spinal interventions. In: Simpson K, Baranidharan G, Gupta S (Eds). Spinal Interventions in Pain Management. 2012. p. 9 [Figure 1.8].

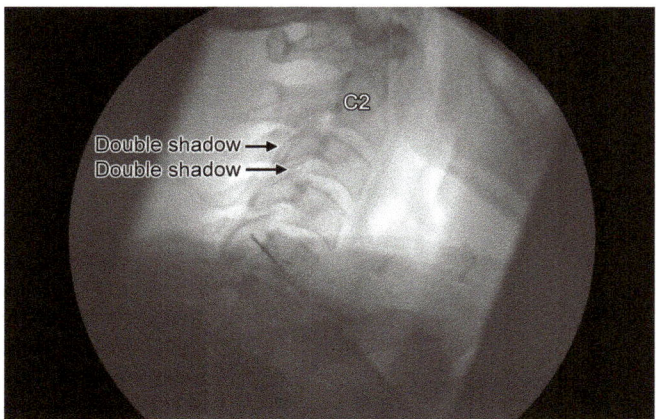
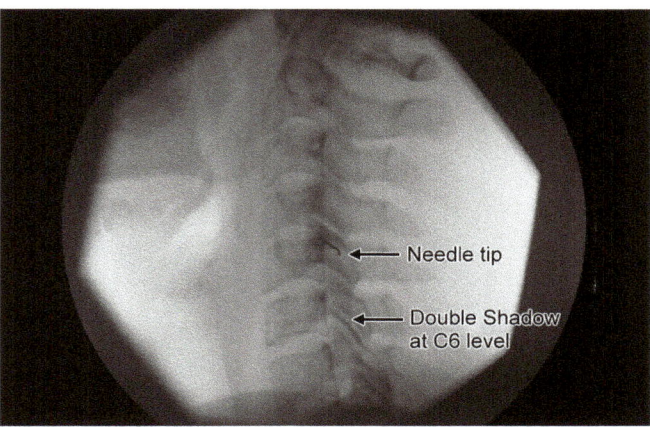

Fig. 52: *Lateral view*: Needle tip is at the target point for a C5 medial branch block (MBB). Note that there is double shadow (parallax) at the C3 and C4 levels. The horizontal double shadow (parallax) along the C3/4 facet joint line can be eliminated by cephalic or caudal tilt and the vertical double shadow (parallax) at C3 level can be eliminated by right or left oblique rotation before performing C4 and C3 MBB, respectively.[4]
Source: Gupta S, Varma S. Cervical medial branch block. In: Baheti DK, Bakshi S, Gupta S, Gehdoo RP (Eds). Interventional Pain Management: A Practical Approach, 2nd edition. New Delhi: Jaypee Brothers Medical Publishers; 2016. pp. 220-9.

Fig. 53: In some patients, the entire cervical spine can be seen. Appropriate patient position and collimation can enhance the image. Needle tip in place for C5 medial branch block (MBB). The C-arm will need to be tilted to eliminate the oblique/horizontal double shadow (parallax) for C6 MBB.[4]
Source: Gupta S, Varma S. Cervical medial branch block. In: Baheti DK, Bakshi S, Gupta S, Gehdoo RP (Eds). Interventional Pain Management: A Practical Approach, 2nd edition. New Delhi: Jaypee Brothers Medical Publishers; 2016. pp. 220-9.

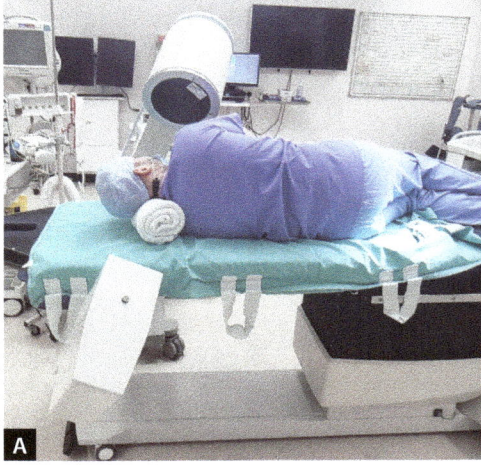
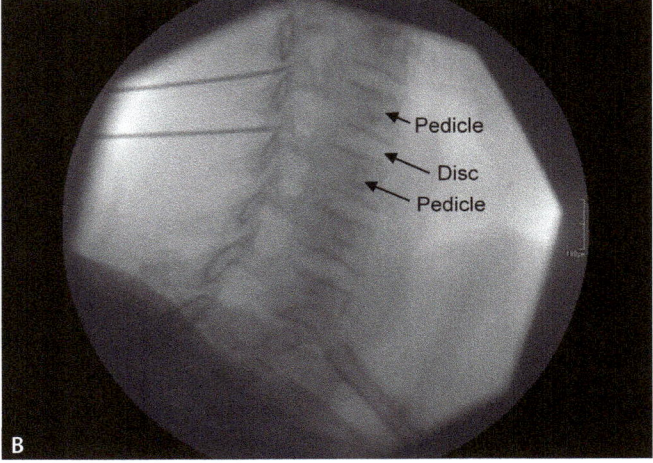

Fig. 54: (A) Anterior inferior oblique view. Patient in lateral position with the C-arm rotated anteriorly with a caudal tilt; (B) Anterior inferior oblique view. The optimal view is when the opposite pedicles appear in the middle of the vertebral bodies (short arrows) and the intervertebral disc appear well defined.

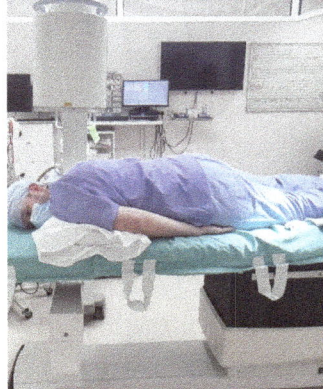
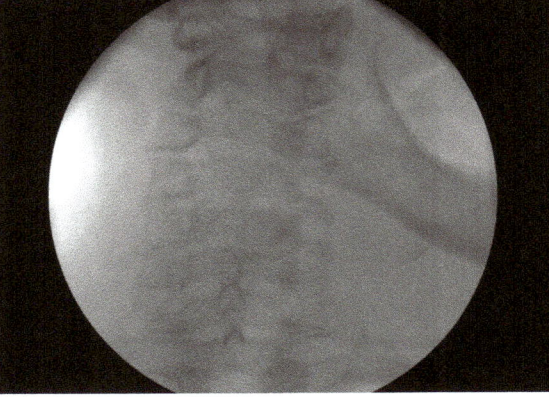

Fig. 55: *Cervical spine*: Prone position: Antero-posterior (AP) view. The upper chest is supported on pillows or sheets. Both the shoulders are pulled as low as possible with the upper limbs to the side of the body. The head is supported on a ring or a wedge. For cervical medial branch block, the neck is turned to the opposite side of the target areas, thus moving the jaw away from the target areas. For interlaminar epidural, the neck is kept straight and chin tucked under to eliminate the skin folds in the lower neck area.

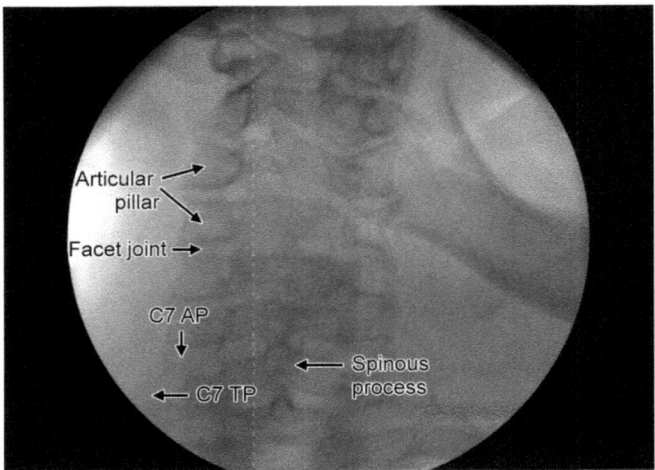

Fig. 56: *Cervical spine:* Prone position: Antero-posterior (AP) view with tilt. (AP: articular pillar; TP: transverse process)

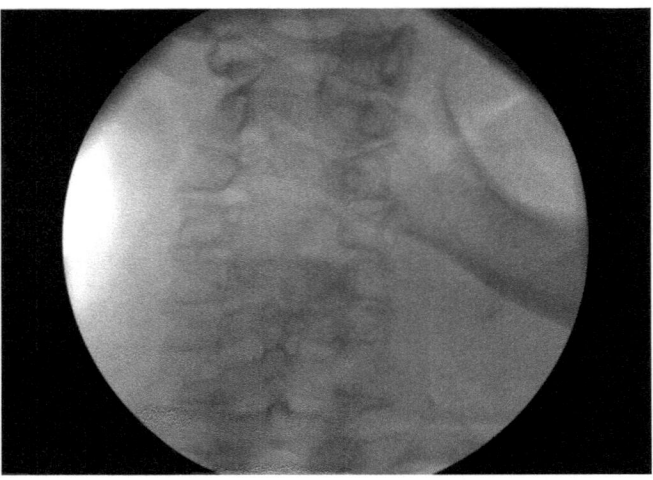

Fig. 57: *Cervical spine:* An antero-posterior (AP) view. Identify the left C7 transverse process. Is this an optimal image for left C7 medial branch block? (Suboptimal image as the C7 not in the center of the screen).

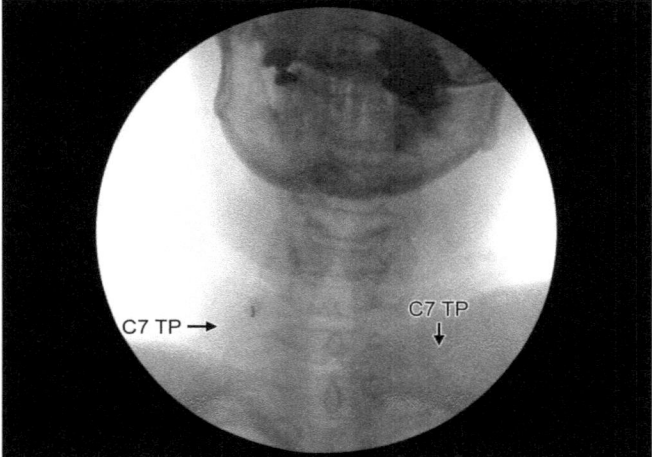

Fig. 58: Antero-posterior (AP) view showing the needle tip at the junction of C7 superior articular process (SAP) and the transverse process (TP).
Source: Reproduced with permission from Oxford University Press. Applied anatomy and fluoroscopy for spinal interventions. In: Simpson K, Baranidharan G, Gupta S (Eds). Spinal Interventions in Pain Management. 2012. p. 9 [Figure 1.8].

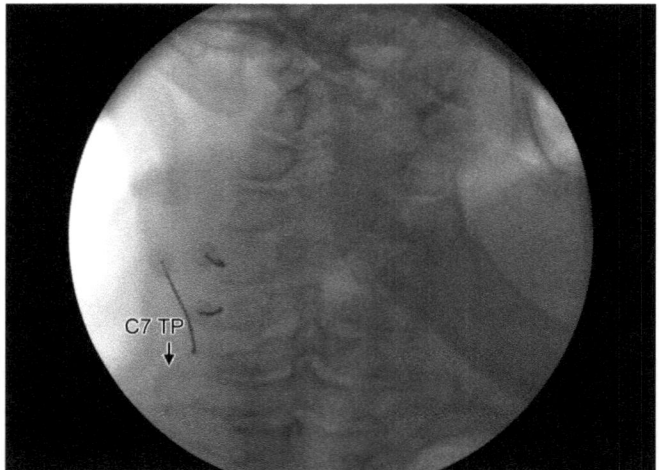

Fig. 59: Antero-posterior fluoroscopic image of cervical spine with needle tip in position for left C5, C6, and the first target point for the C7 medial branch block. The junction of the C7 transverse process and superior articular process appears like a "ski boot."
Source: Gupta S, Varma S. Cervical medial branch block. In: Baheti DK, Bakshi S, Gupta S, Gehdoo RP (Eds). Interventional Pain Management: A Practical Approach, 2nd edition. New Delhi: Jaypee Brothers Medical Publishers; 2016. pp. 220-9.

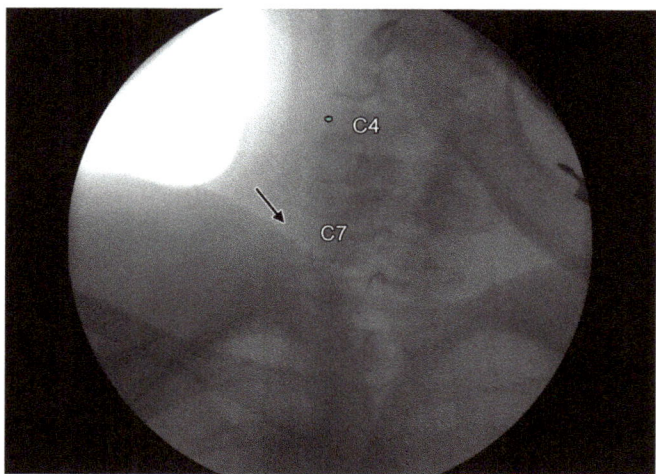

Fig. 60: Antero-posterior view of the cervical spine. The target point for the MBB is the most medial aspect on the waist of the respective articular pillar. This image is appropriate for left C4 medial branch block (MBB). The arrow points to the junction of the superior articular process and the transverse process of C7 which appears like a front of a "ski boot."
Source: Gupta S, Varma S. Cervical medial branch block. In: Baheti DK, Bakshi S, Gupta S, Gehdoo RP (Eds). Interventional Pain Management: A Practical Approach, 2nd edition. New Delhi: Jaypee Brothers Medical Publishers; 2016. pp. 220-9.

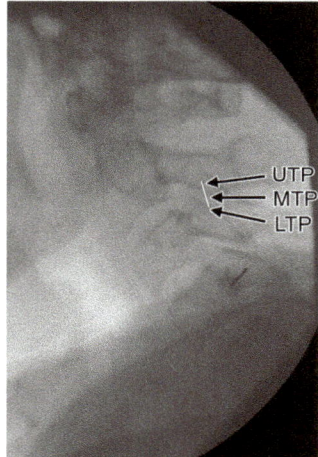

Fig. 61: Imaginary line bisecting the C2–3 facet joint line. The upper target point (UTP), middle target point (MTP), and lower target point (LTP) along the bisecting line for the third occipital nerve block are shown by the arrows. The middle target point is at the C2/3 facet joint level along the bisecting line.[4]
Source: Gupta S, Varma S. Cervical medial branch block. In: Baheti DK, Bakshi S, Gupta S, Gehdoo RP (Eds). Interventional Pain Management: A Practical Approach, 2nd edition. New Delhi: Jaypee Brothers Medical Publishers; 2016. pp. 220-9.

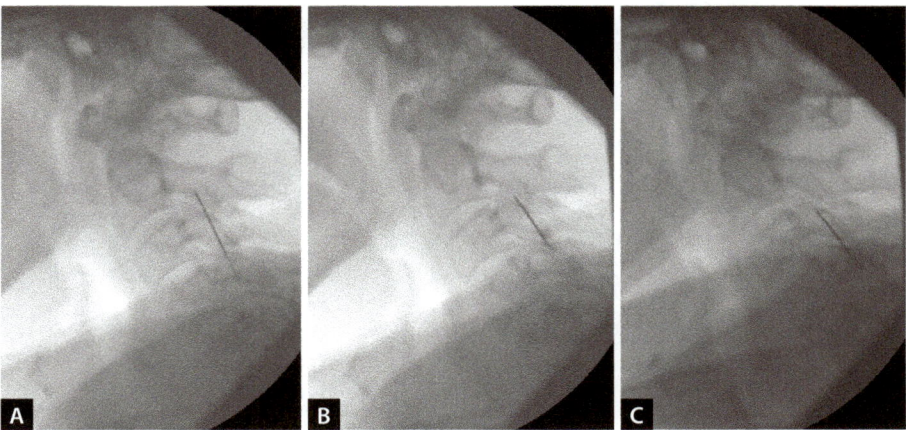

Figs. 62A to C: *Cervical spine:* Lateral view: Needle tip in position for (A) upper, (B) middle, and (C) lower targets for the third occipital nerve block.[4]
Source: Gupta S, Varma S. Cervical medial branch block. In: Baheti DK, Bakshi S, Gupta S, Gehdoo RP (Eds). Interventional Pain Management: A Practical Approach, 2nd edition. New Delhi: Jaypee Brothers Medical Publishers; 2016. pp. 220-9.

FLUOROSCOPY FOR PROCEDURES AT THE THORACIC SPINE AREA

General Considerations

- Procedures at the thoracic level are considered more riskier than at the lumbar level.
- Before performing procedures at the thoracic level, it may be advisable to attend/observe some thoracic spine procedures being performed by some colleagues experienced in performing such procedures.
- Consider the risk of pneumothorax when performing procedures at the thoracic levels.
- It may be challenging to identify bony landmarks in some patients due to the presence of ribs and air shadow of the lungs.

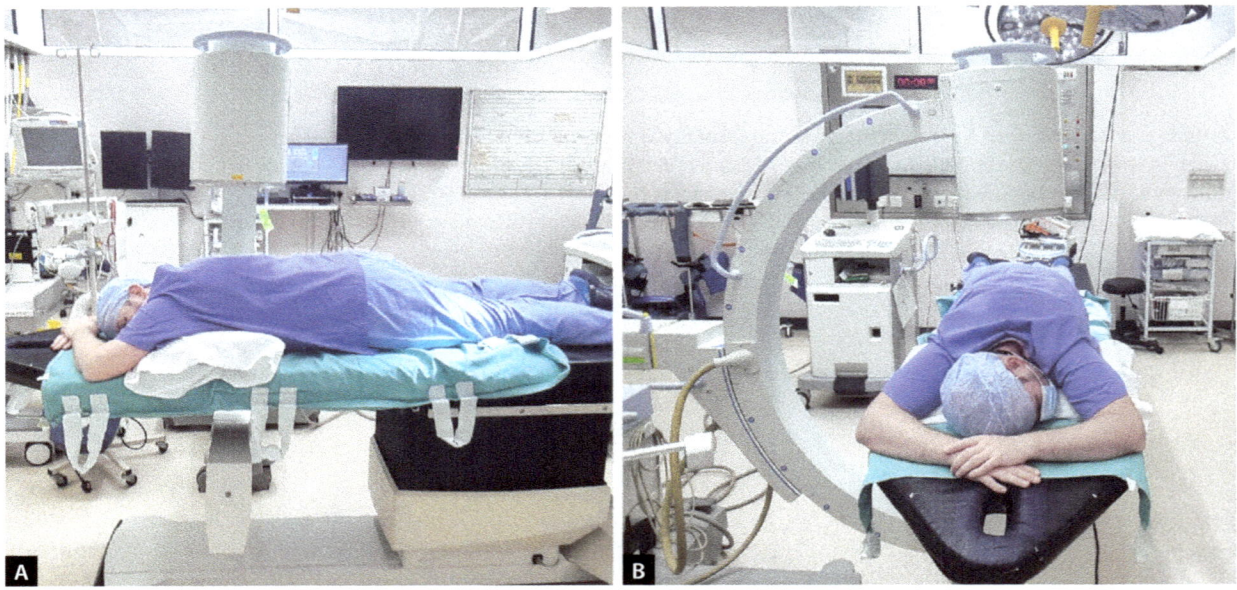

Figs. 63A and B: *Thoracic fluoroscopy*: Antero-posterior view: C-arm viewed from the (A) side and (B) head end. Upper limbs are placed in front of the head to facilitate lateral view if necessary.

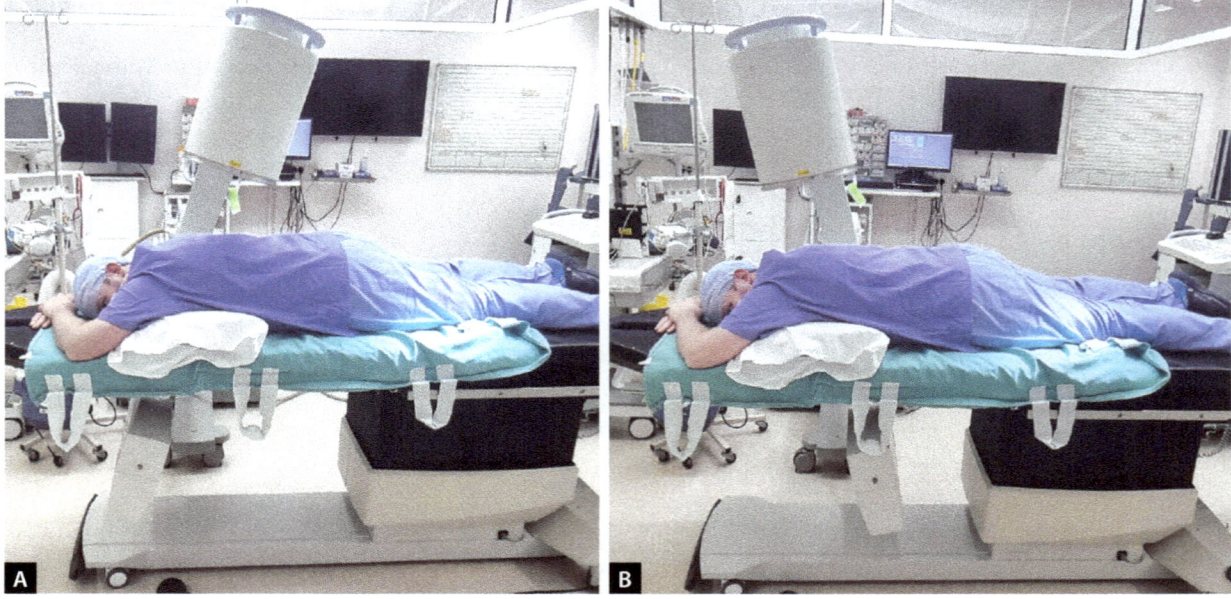

Fig. 64: *Thoracic fluoroscopy*: C-arm (A) caudal tilt; (B) cephalic tilt.

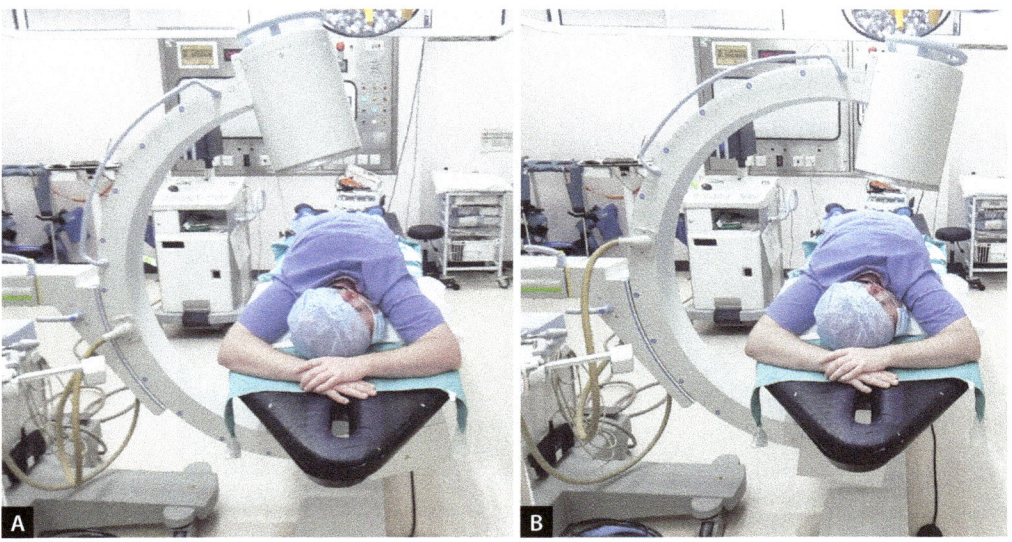

Figs. 65A and B: *Thoracic fluoroscopy:* C-arm (A) right oblique rotation; (B) left oblique rotation.

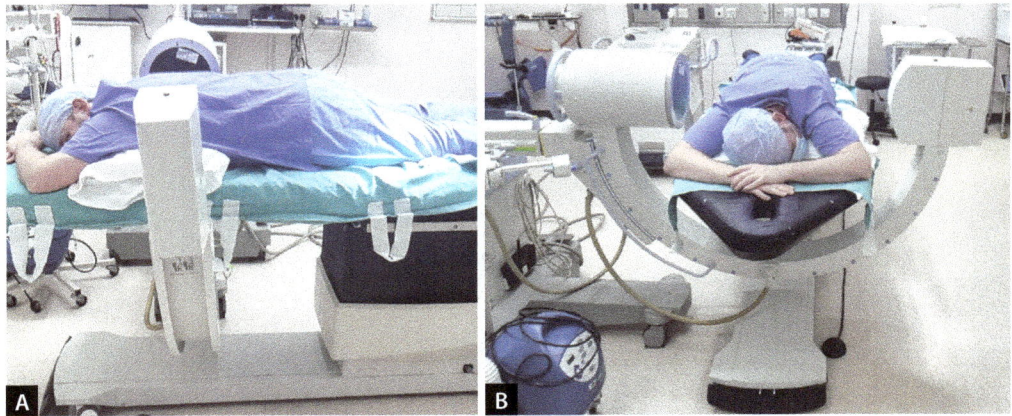

Figs. 66A and B: *Thoracic fluoroscopy:* C-arm lateral view from the (A) side and the (B) head end. The C-arm may need to be moved in either direction (wig-wag) in lateral view to square the vertebral end plates to make to disc and the intervertebral foramen visible as the ribs and other structures around the spine can overlap making it difficult to define the bony anatomy/landmarks.

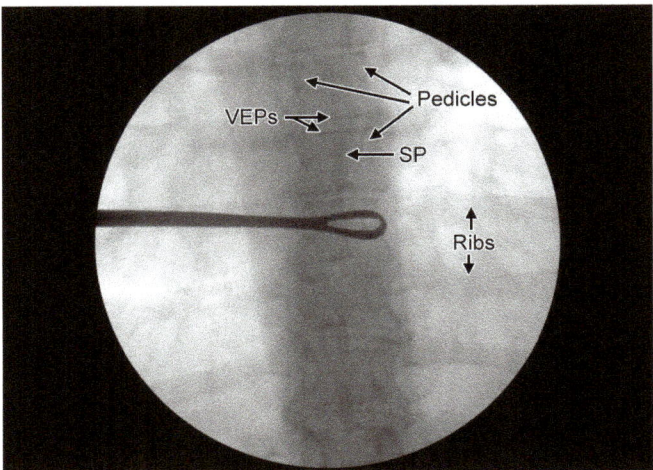

Fig. 67: *Thoracic fluoroscopy:* Antero-posterior (AP) view. The spinous process (SP) is in the middle of the two pedicles with the vertebral end plates (VEPs) "squared off" by tilting the C-arm.

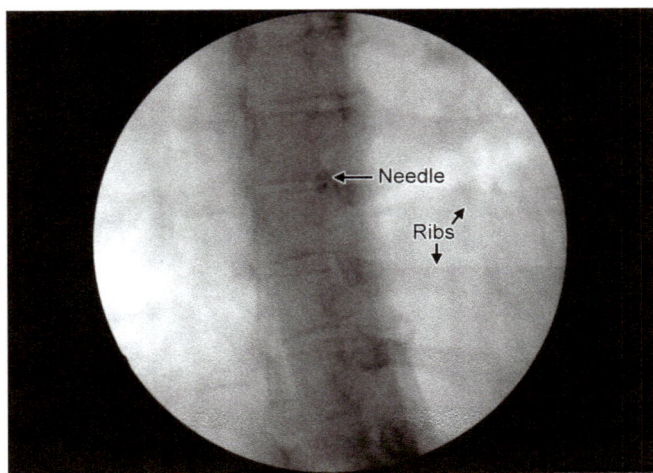

Fig. 68: *Thoracic fluoroscopy*: Right oblique view. Identify the pedicle at the appropriate level for a transforaminal epidural injection. The arrow points to the "end on" view of the needle when performing a transforaminal epidural injection *(Direction of the Needle)*.

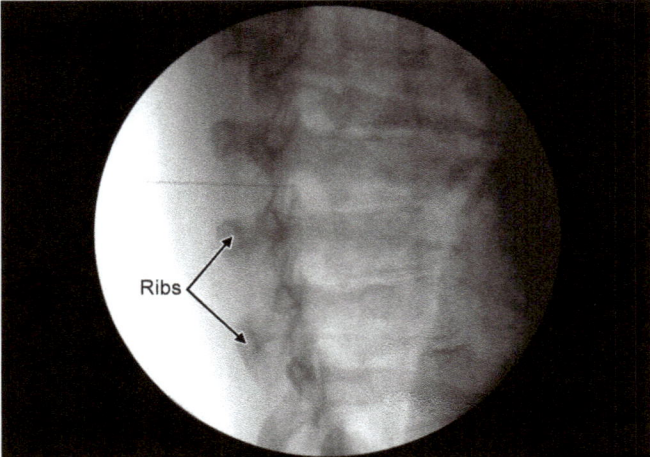

Fig. 69: *Thoracic fluoroscopy*: Lateral view. The tip of the needle is in the intervertebral foramen. Although the foramen is visible, the disc space is not clear (the disc space is seen better in the Figure 70).

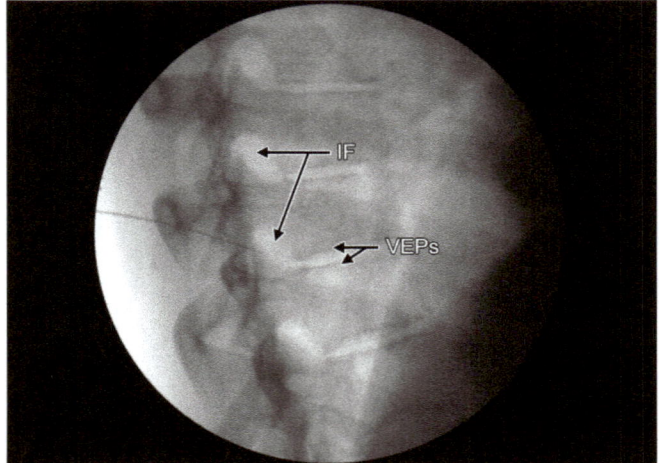

Fig. 70: At the thoracic spine level, it can be difficult to identify the intervertebral foramen in the lateral view due to the ribs and air (lung) shadow. Moving the C-arm side-ward direction in the lateral C-arm position (wig-wag) to square the vertebral end plates (VEPs) to make to disc space crisp improves the view of the intervertebral foramen (IF).

FLUOROSCOPY FOR TRIGEMINAL GANGLION INTERVENTIONS

General Considerations

- Trigeminal ganglion interventions can be riskier than procedures at spinal levels.
- Before performing trigeminal ganglion intervention, it may be advisable to attend/observe some trigeminal ganglion procedures being performed by some colleagues experienced in performing such procedures.
- Consider the risk of injuring extra- or intracranial blood vessels.
- It can be challenging to identify bony landmarks.

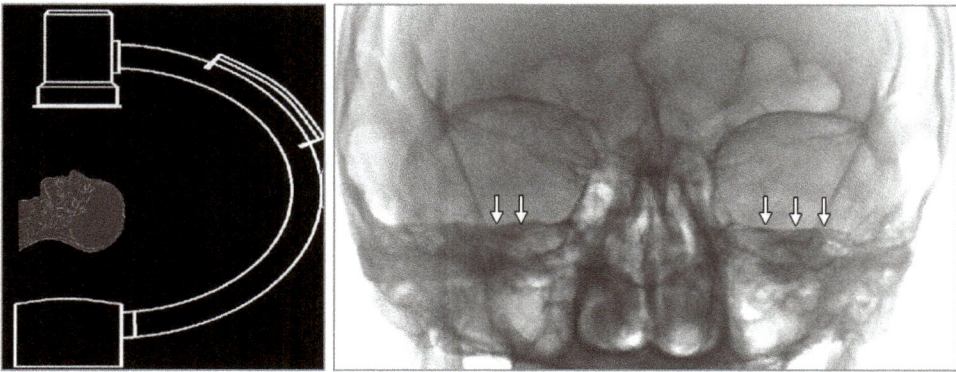

Fig. 71: *Foramen ovale imaging for trigeminal interventions:* Positioning the fluoroscope is of prime importance. Straight posteroanterior (PA) projection is obtained with the petrous ridge seen through the orbit (white arrow).

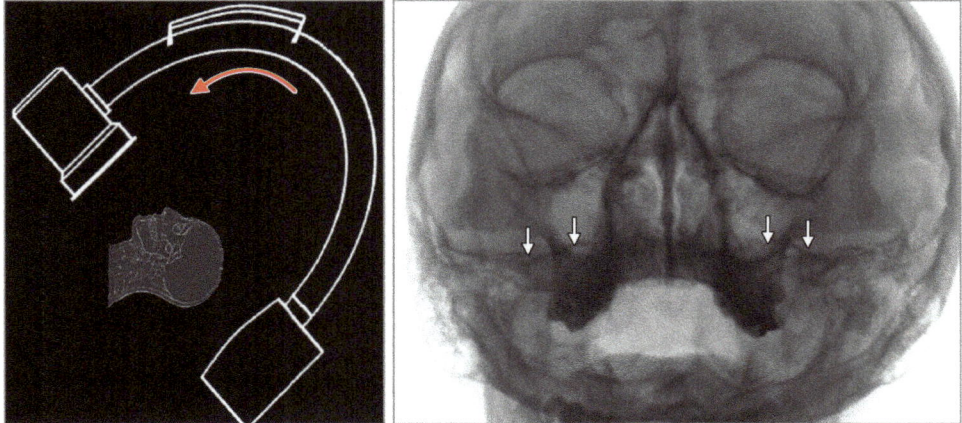

Fig. 72: *Foramen ovale imaging for trigeminal interventions:* The fluoroscope is then tilted caudad to see the superior border of petrous ridge projected at the inferior border of the maxillary sinus (white arrows).

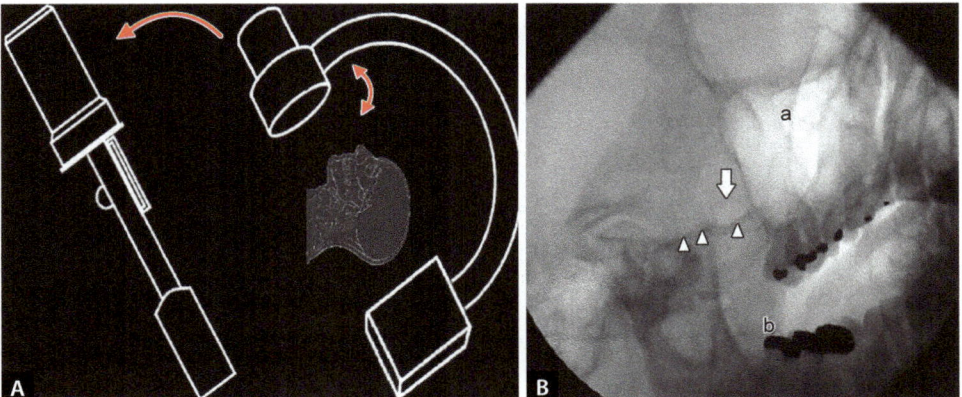

Figs. 73A and B: *Foramen ovale imaging for trigeminal interventions:* Ipsilateral oblique rotation is then performed by 10–25° to visualize the petrous ridge below maxillary sinus (A) and above the jawline (B) [white pointer—petrous ridge, white arrow—foramen ovale (FO)]. Only minimal movement in sagittal plane is required to visualize the FO. This modified submental view is best to visualize FO.

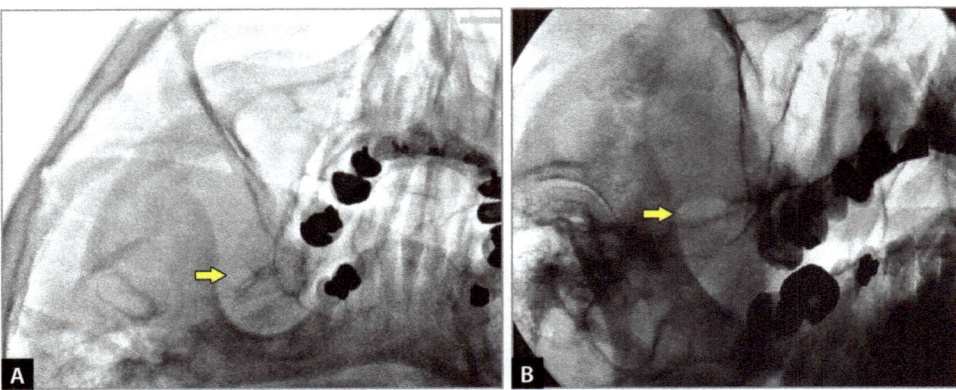

Figs. 74A and B: Foramen ovale imaging for trigeminal interventions. (A) Increased caudal tilt changes the orientation of FO to a circle whereas (B) cephalad tilt makes the foramen flat like a slit. A flatter/elliptical orientation is preferred rather than circular as a coaxially oriented needle would be directed to the floor of middle cranial fossa.

REFERENCES

1. Gupta S. Stimulation guided pan mapping. In: Baheti DK, Bakshi S, Gupta S, Gehdoo RP (Eds). Interventional Pain Management: A Practical Approach, 2nd edition. New Delhi: Jaypee Brothers Medical Publishers; 2016. pp. 81-3.
2. Gupta S, Dhandapani K. Drugs, equipment and basic principles of spinal interventions. In: Spinal Interventions in Pain Management. Simpson K, Baranidharan G, Gupta S. Oxford University Press; 2012. pp. 1-10.
3. Gupta S, Richardson J. Sacroiliac joint block. In: Baheti DK, Bakshi S, Gupta S, Gehdoo RP (Eds). Interventional Pain Management: A Practical Approach, 1st edition. New Delhi: Jaypee Brothers Medical Publishers; 2009. pp. 198-203.
4. Gupta S, Varma S. Cervical medial branch block. In: Baheti DK, Bakshi S, Gupta S, Gehdoo RP (Eds). Interventional Pain Management: A Practical Approach, 2nd edition. New Delhi: Jaypee Brothers Medical Publishers; 2016. pp. 220-9.

CHAPTER 2

Understanding of Radiological Anatomy

Kenneth Lupton, James Baren, Harun Gupta

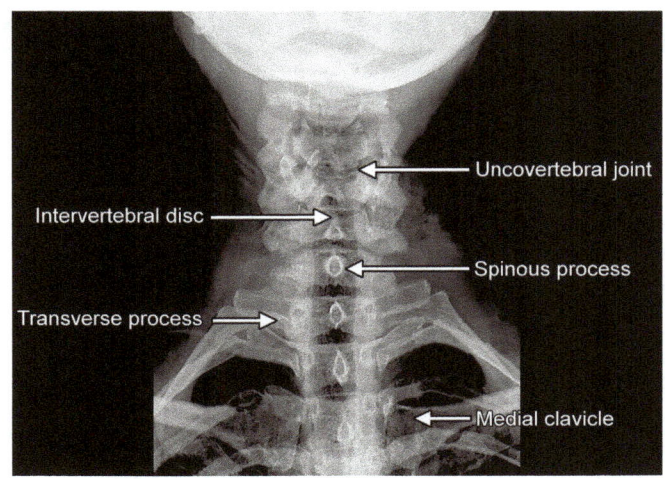

Fig. 1: Cervical spine radiograph anteroposterior (AP) projection.

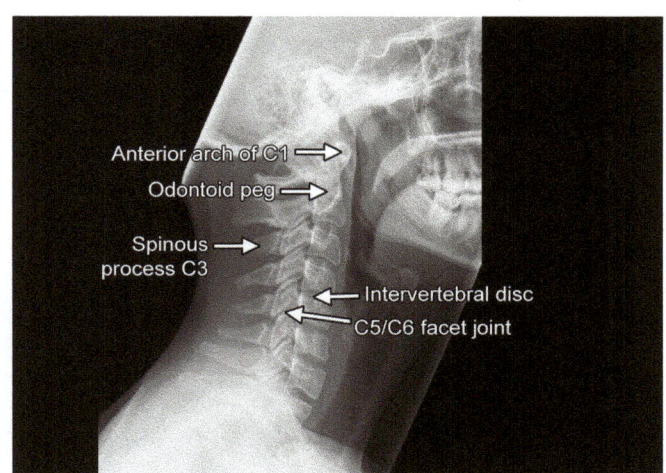

Fig. 2: Cervical spine radiograph lateral projection.

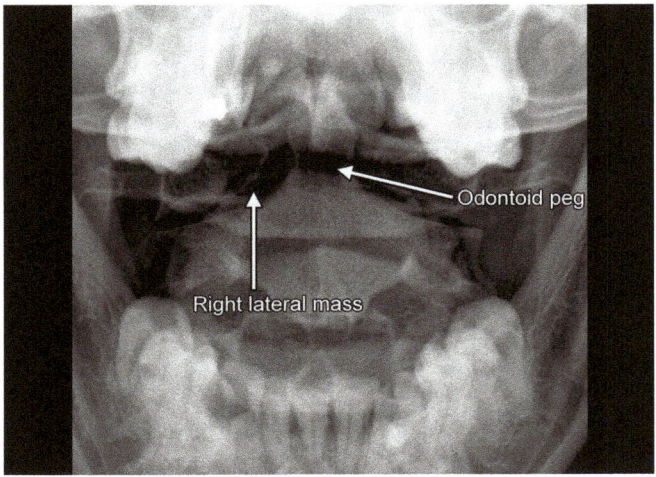

Fig. 3: Cervical spine radiograph peg projection.

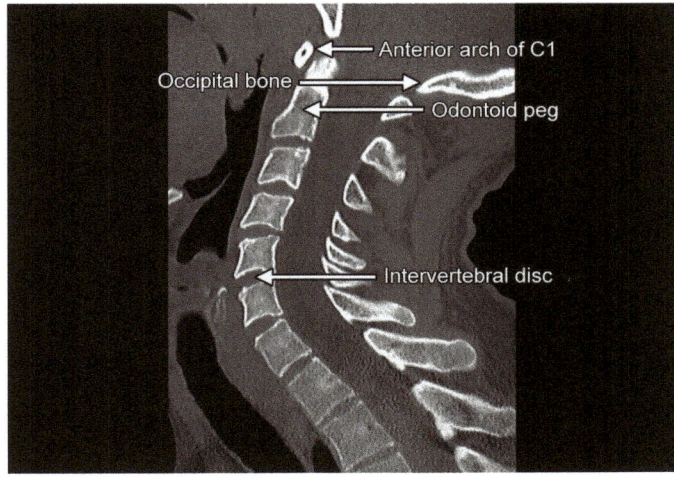

Fig. 4: Cervical spine CT sagittal reformat.

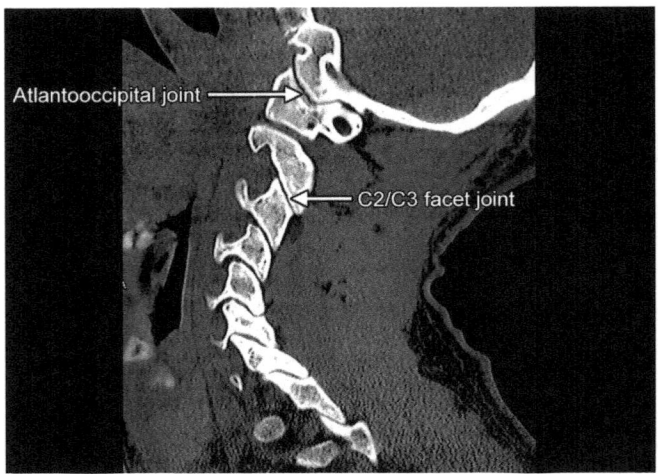

Fig. 5: Cervical spine CT sagittal reformat off midline revealing the facet and atlantooccipital joints.

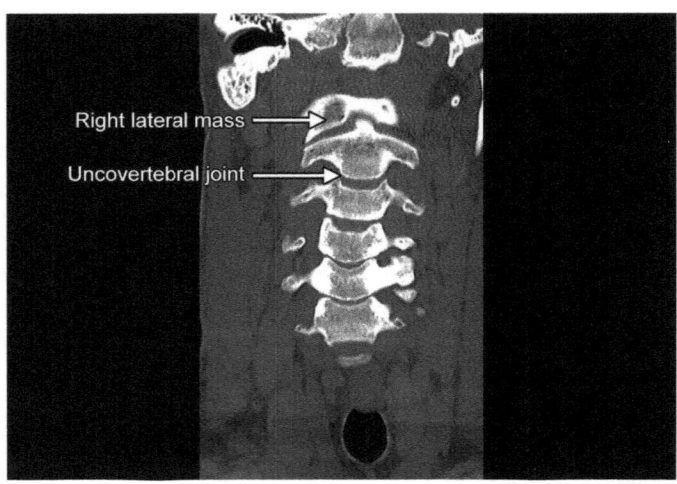

Fig. 6: Cervical spine CT coronal reformat.

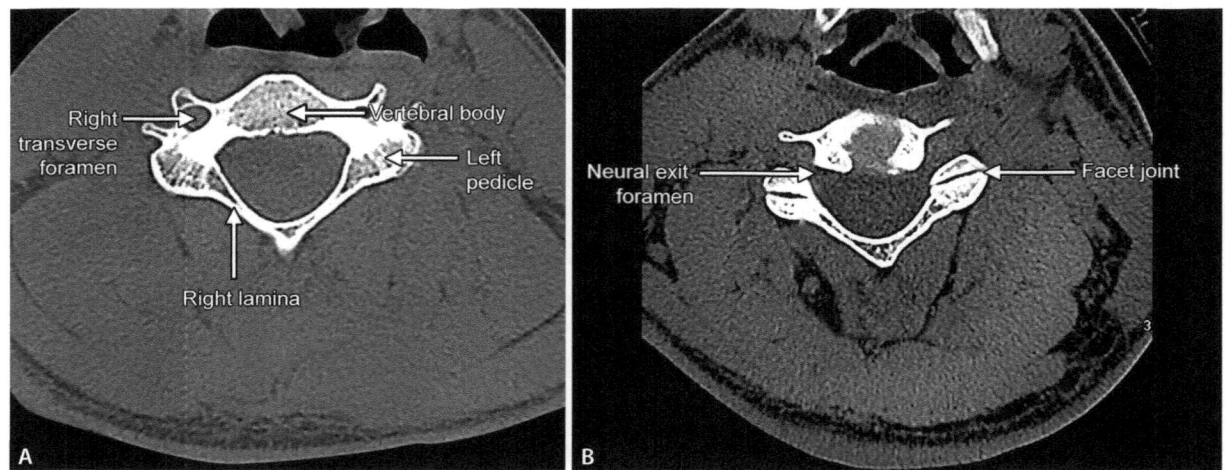

Figs. 7A and B: (A) Cervical spine CT axial reformat showing gross vertebral anatomy; (B) Cervical spine CT axial reformat showing the facet joints and neural exit foramina.

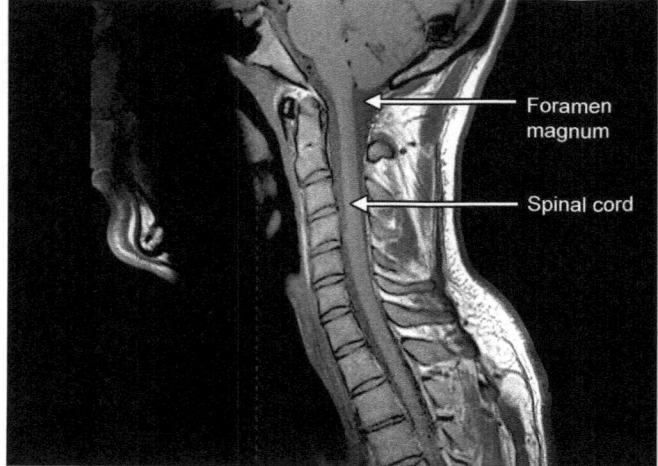

Fig. 8: MRI cervical spine sagittal T1-sequence.

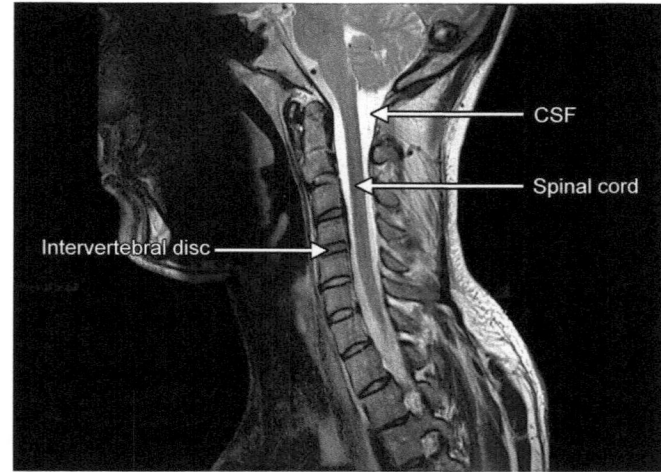

Fig. 9: MRI cervical spine sagittal T2 sequence.

CHAPTER 2 | Understanding of Radiological Anatomy

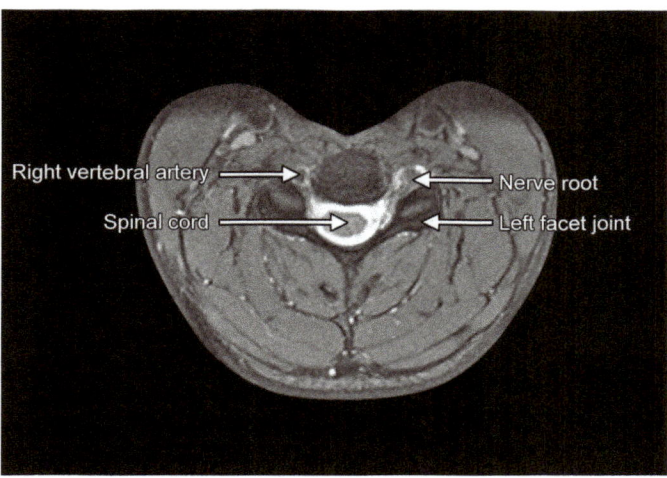

Fig. 10: MRI cervical spine axial T2 sequence at the level of the neural exit foramina. (CSF: cerebrospinal fluid)

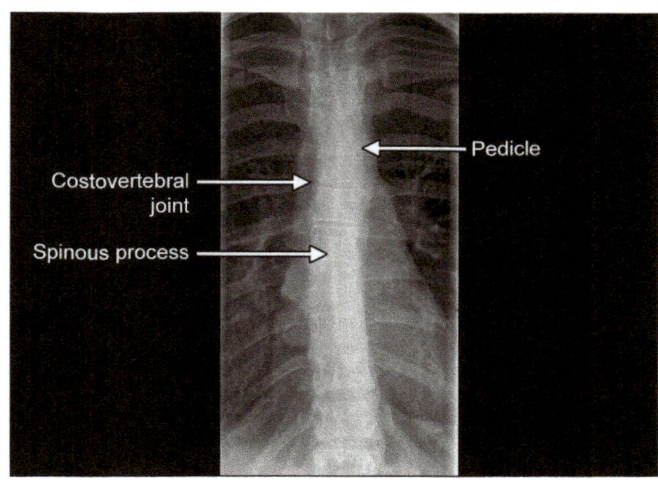

Fig. 11: Thoracic spine radiograph anteroposterior (AP) projection.

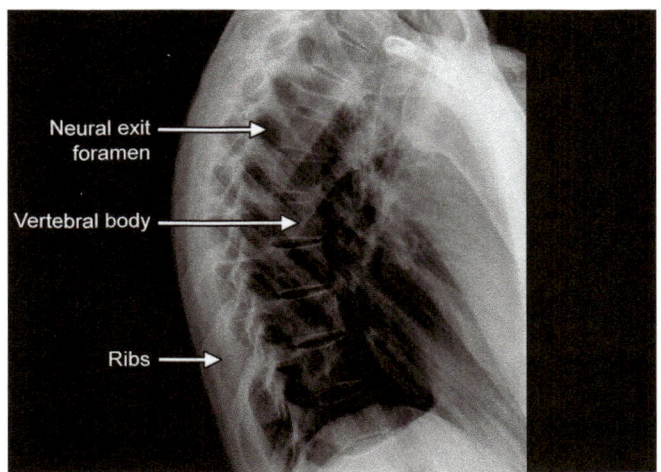

Fig. 12: Thoracic spine radiograph lateral projection.

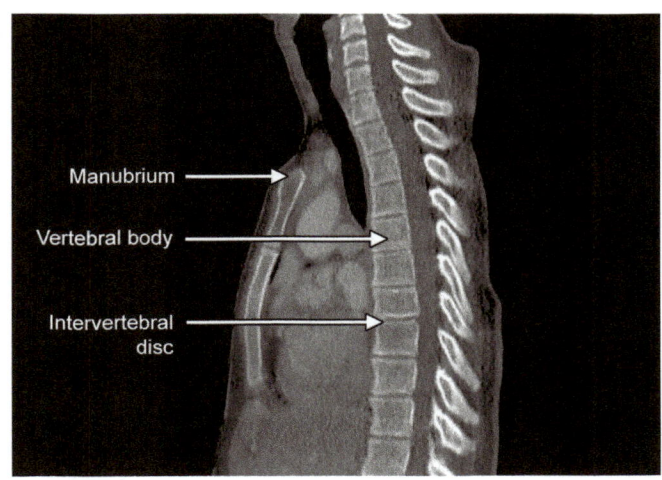

Fig. 13: Thoracic spine CT sagittal reformat.

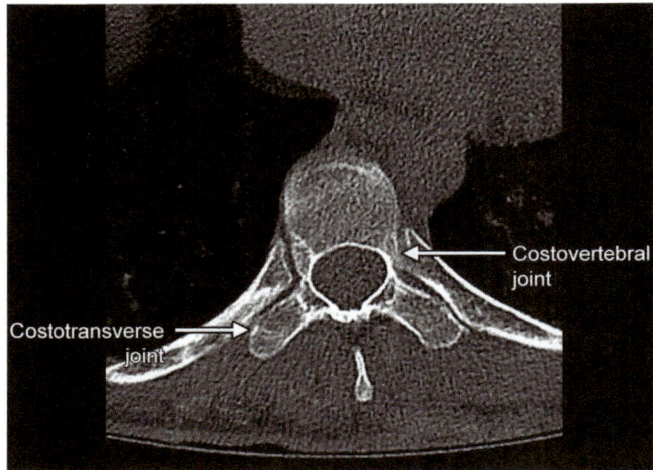

Fig. 14: Thoracic spine CT axial reformat showing the costovertebral and costotransverse joints.

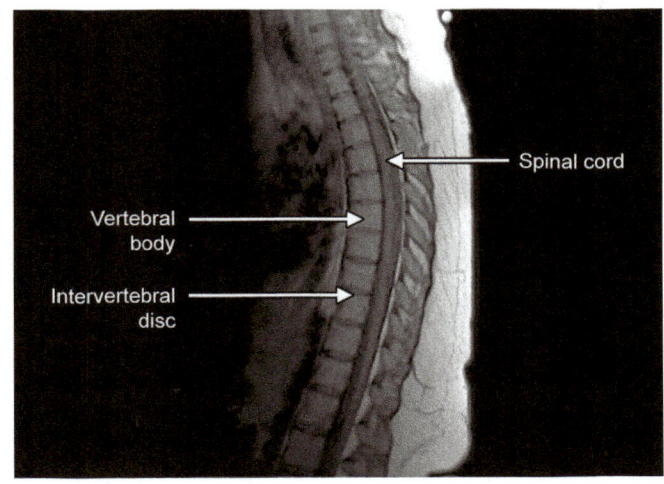

Fig. 15: Thoracic spine MRI sagittal T1 sequence.

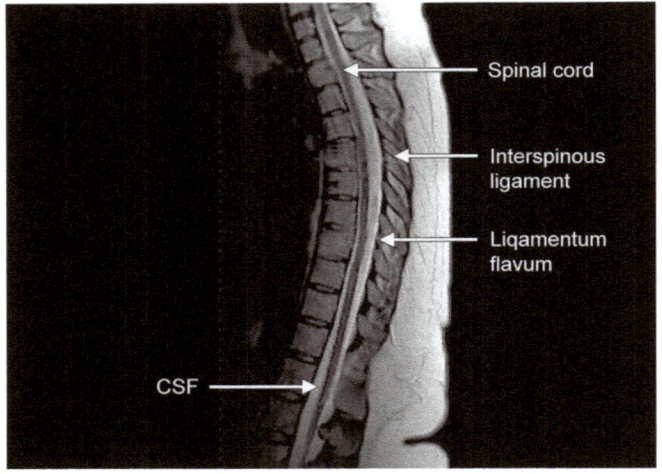

Fig. 16: Thoracic spine MRI sagittal T2 sequence. (CSF: cerebrospinal fluid)

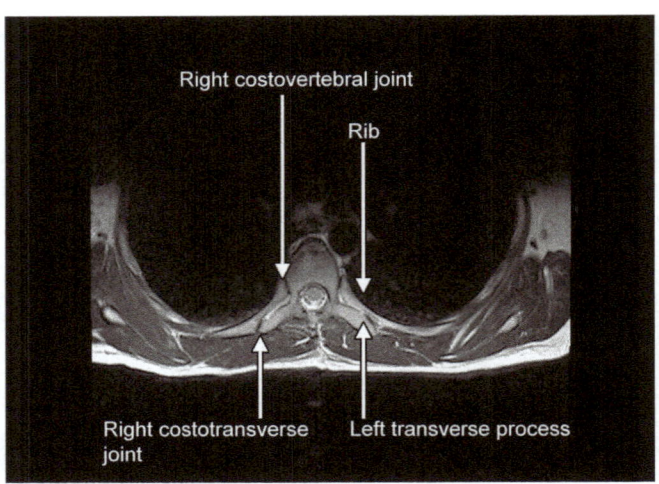

Fig. 17: Thoracic spine MRI axial T2 sequence.

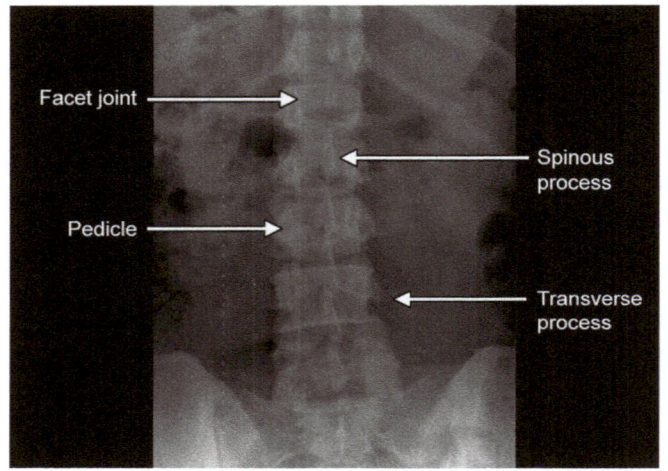

Fig. 18: Lumbar spine radiograph anteroposterior (AP) projection.

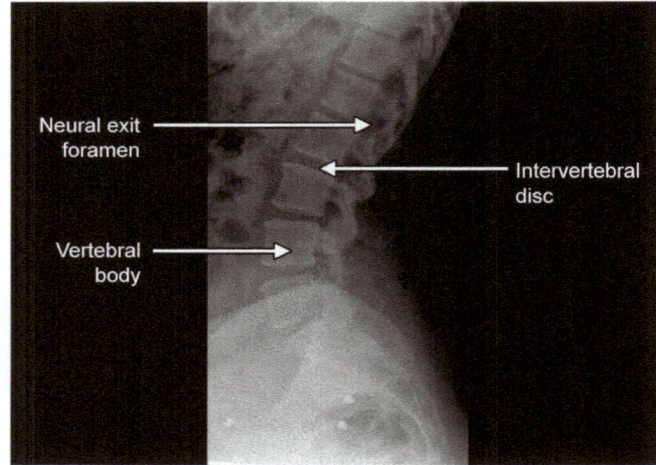

Fig. 19: Lumbar spine radiograph lateral projection.

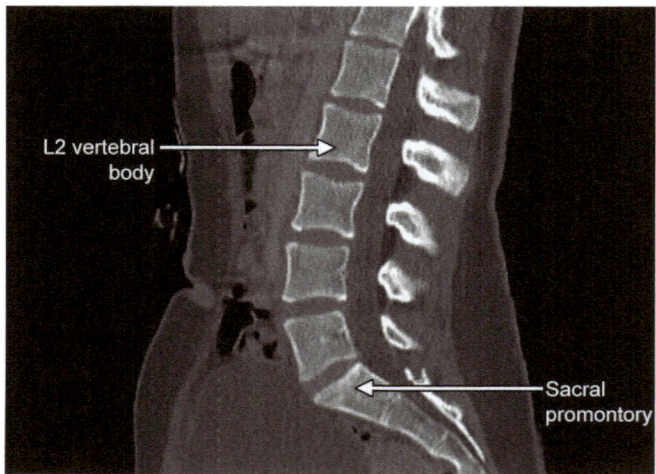

Fig. 20: Lumbar spine CT sagittal reformat.

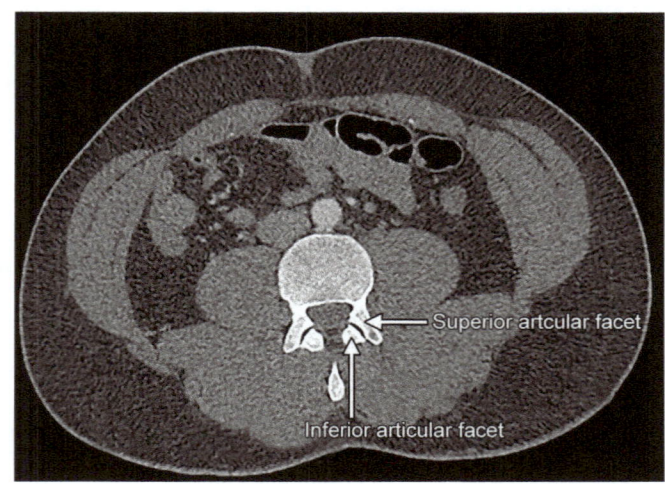

Fig. 21: Lumbar spine CT axial reformat.

CHAPTER 2 | Understanding of Radiological Anatomy

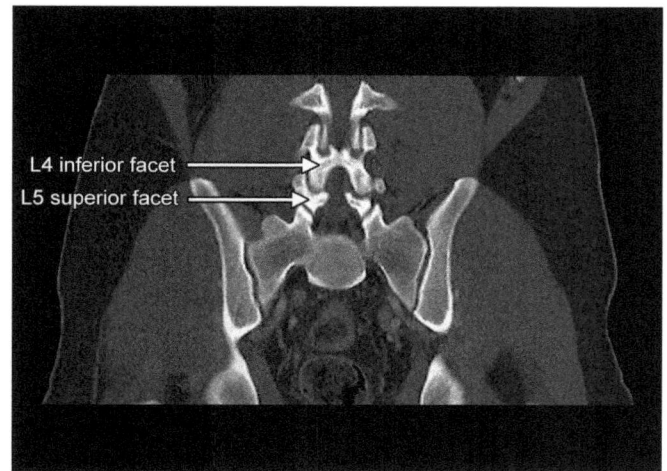

Fig. 22: Lumbar spine coronal reformat.

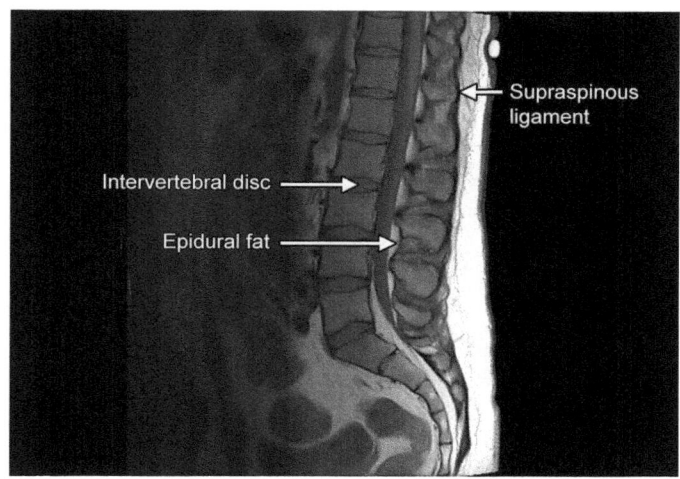

Fig. 23: Lumbar spine sagittal T1 sequence.

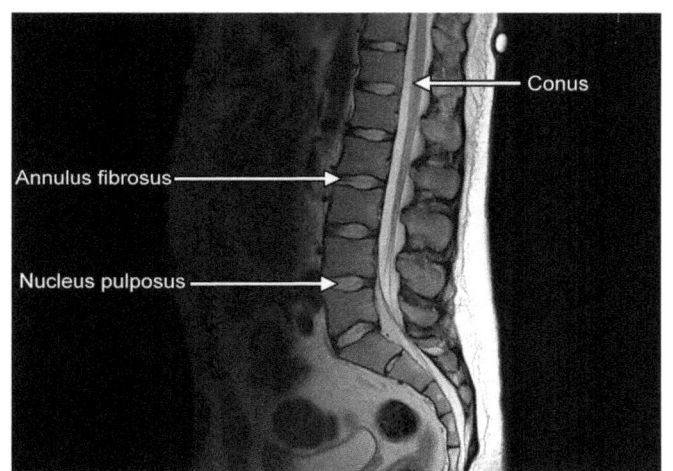

Fig. 24: Lumbar spine sagittal T2 sequence.

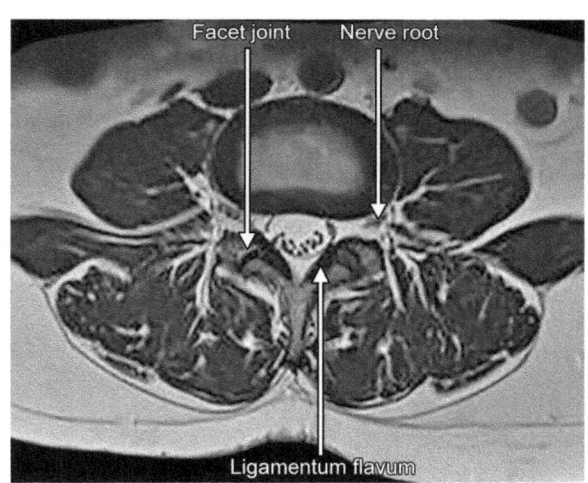

Fig. 25: Lumbar spine axial T2 sequence.

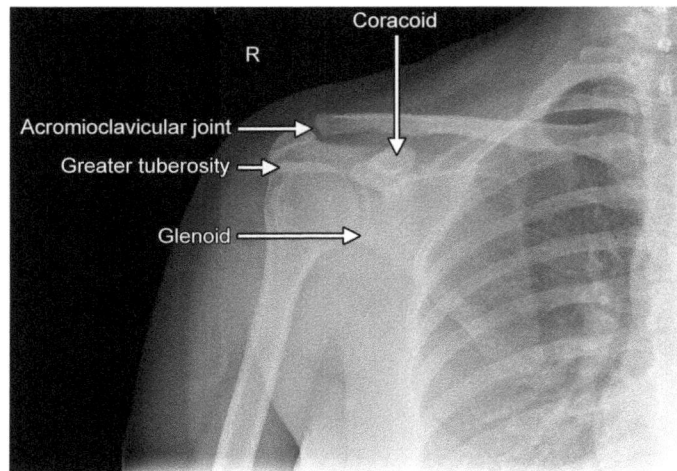

Fig. 26: Shoulder radiograph anteroposterior (AP) projection.

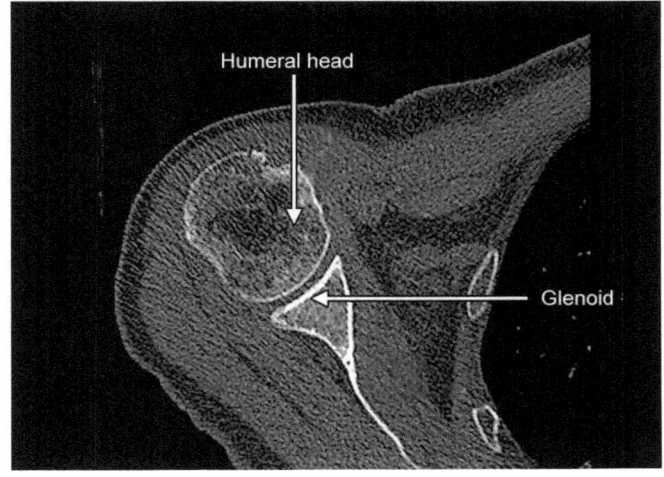

Fig. 27: Shoulder CT axial reformat.

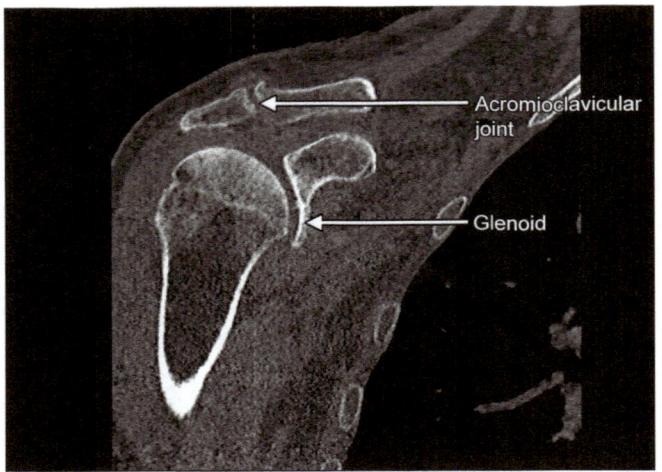

Fig. 28: Shoulder CT coronal reformat.

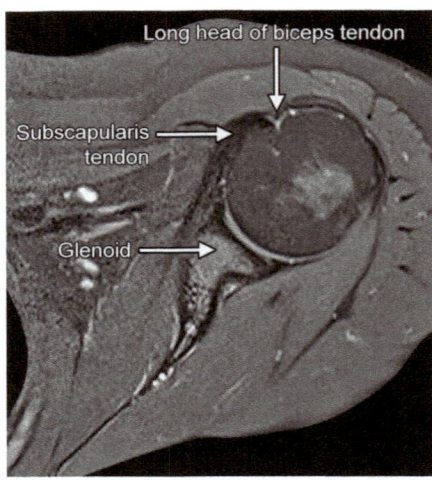

Fig. 29: Shoulder MRI axial proton-density fat-saturated sequence.

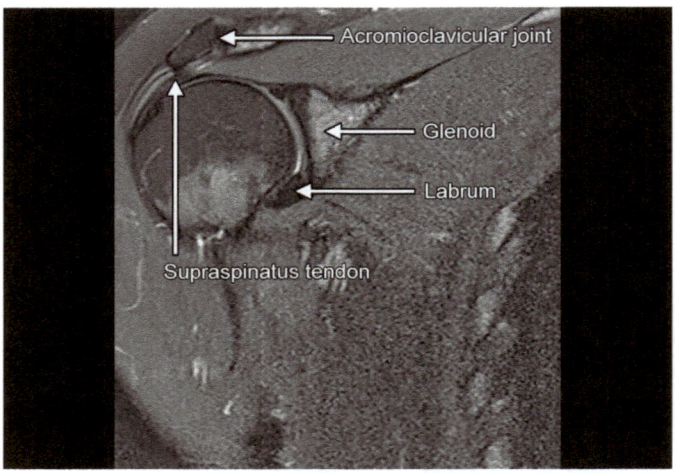

Fig. 30: Shoulder MRI coronal proton-density fat-saturated sequence.

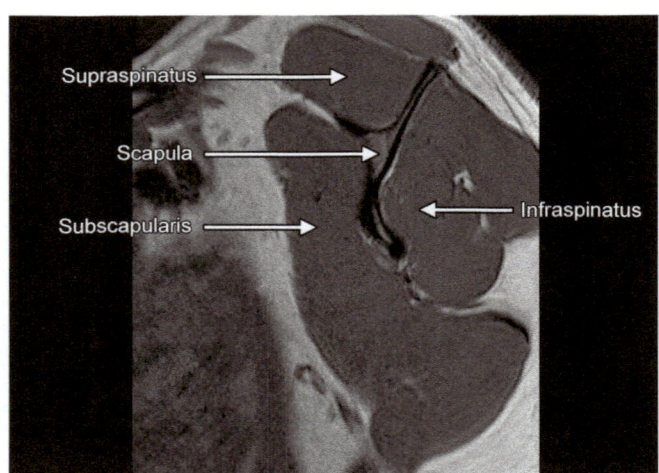

Fig. 31: Shoulder MRI sagittal T1 sequence.

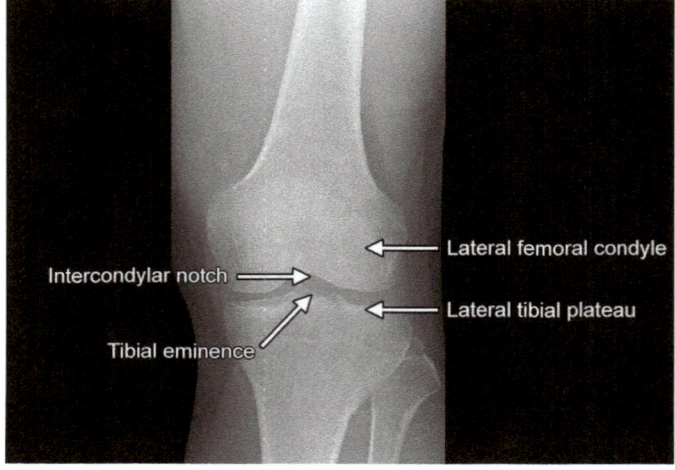

Fig. 32: Knee radiograph anteroposterior (AP) projection.

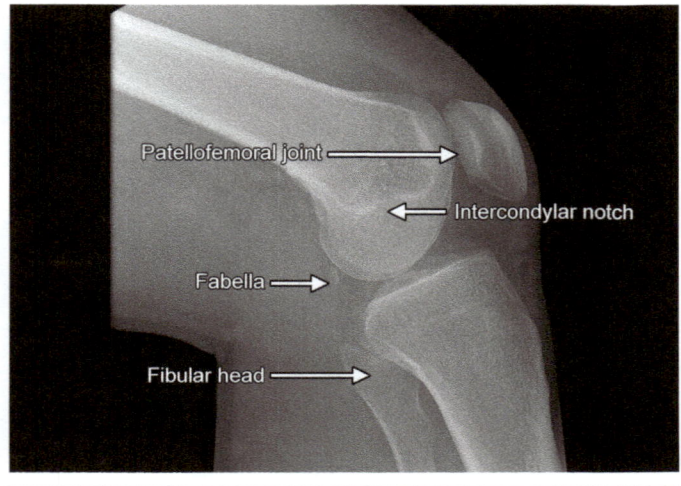

Fig. 33: Knee radiograph lateral projection.

CHAPTER 2 | Understanding of Radiological Anatomy

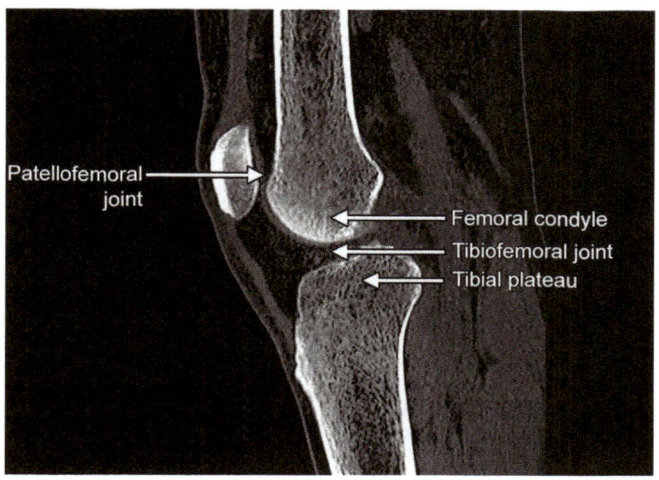

Fig. 34: Knee CT sagittal reconstruction.

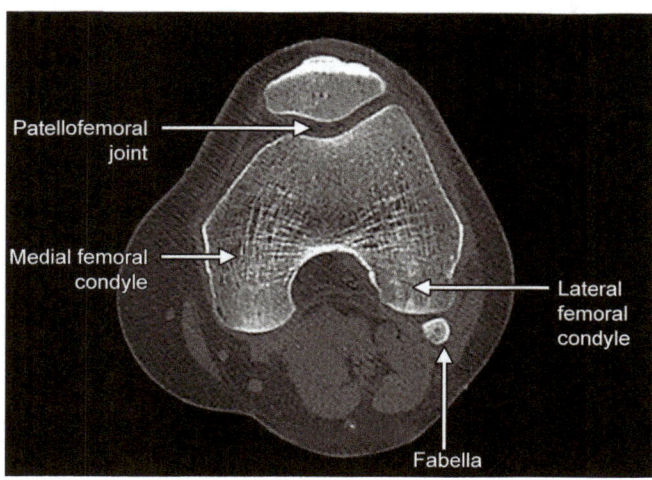

Fig. 35: Knee CT axial reconstruction.

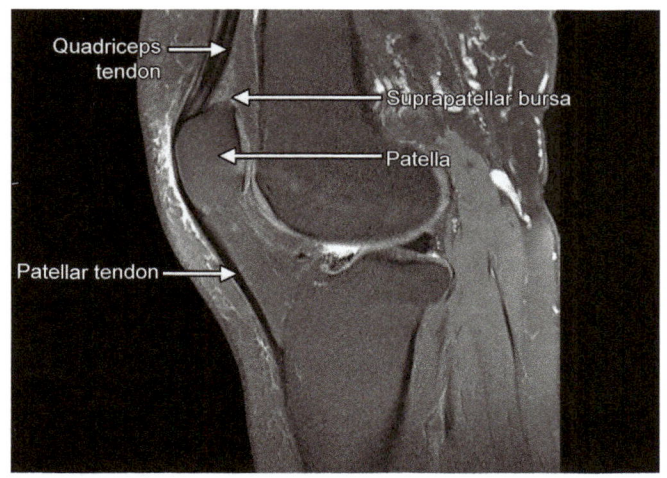

Fig. 36: Knee MRI sagittal proton-density fat-saturated sequence.

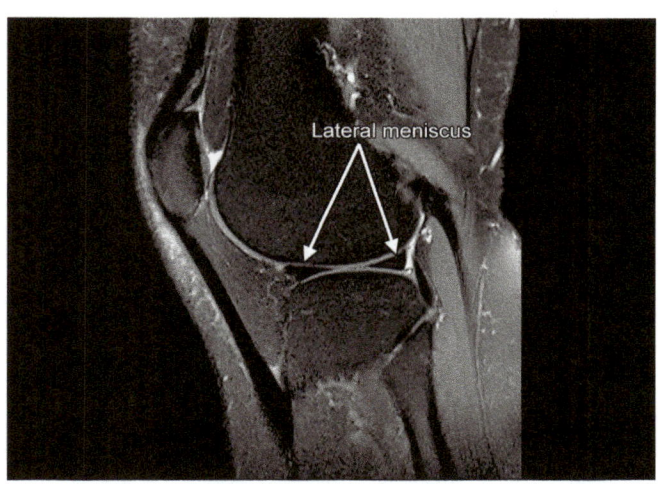

Fig. 37: Knee MRI sagittal proton-density fat-saturated sequence (lateral meniscus view with "bow-tie" appearance).

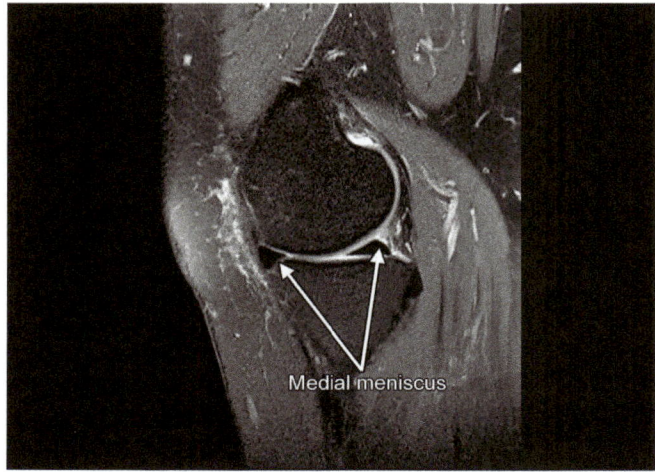

Fig. 38: Knee MRI sagittal proton-density fat-saturated sequence (medial meniscus view with "bow-tie" appearance).

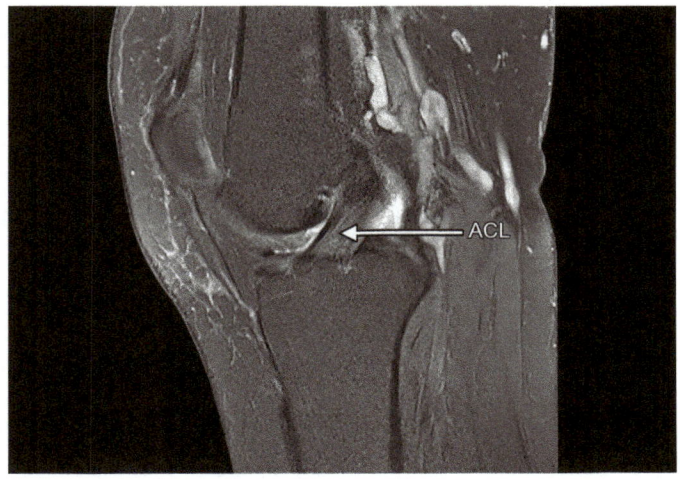

Fig. 39: Knee MRI sagittal proton-density fat-saturated sequence (ACL view). (ACL: anterior cruciate ligament)

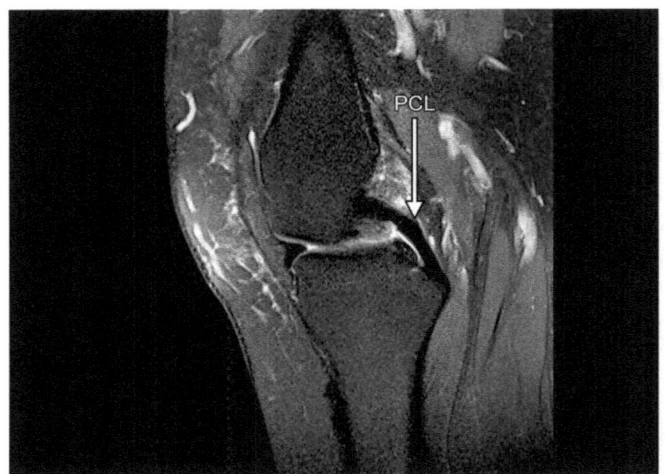

Fig. 40: Knee MRI sagittal proton-density fat-saturated sequence (PCL view). (PCL: anterior cruciate ligament)

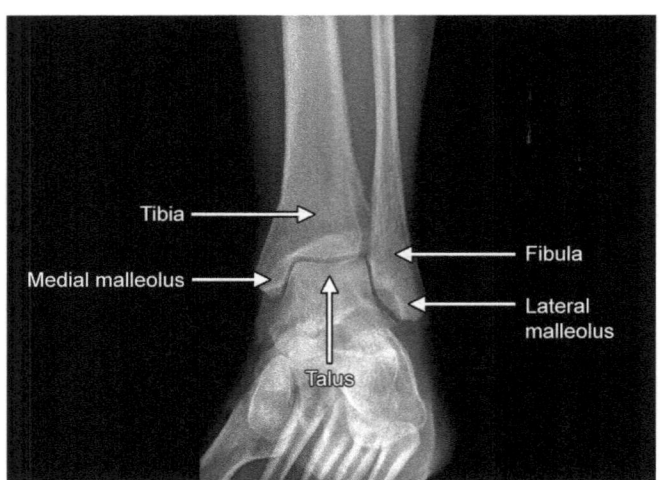

Fig. 41: Ankle radiograph anteroposterior (AP) projection.

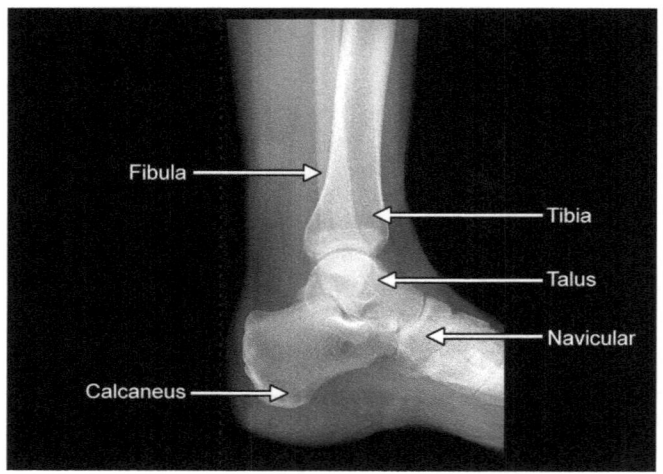

Fig. 42: Ankle radiograph lateral projection.

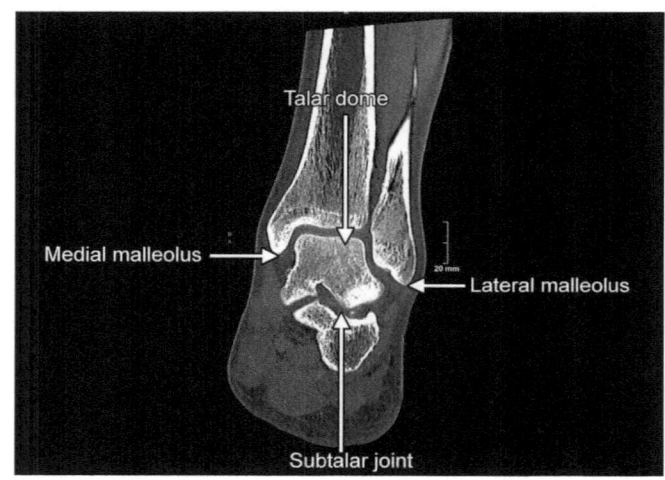

Fig. 43: Ankle CT coronal reconstruction.

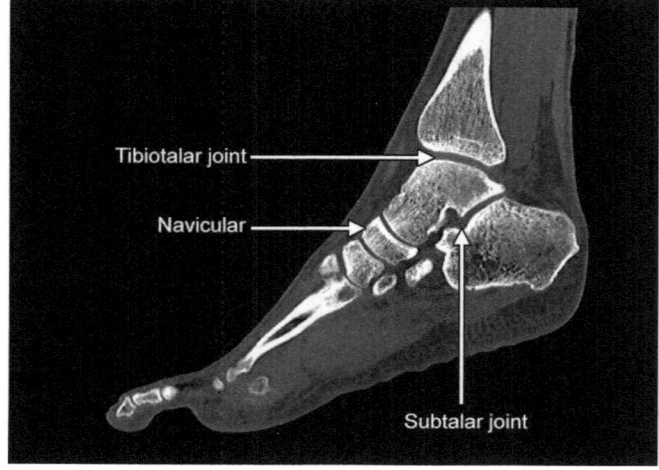

Fig. 44: Ankle CT sagittal reconstruction.

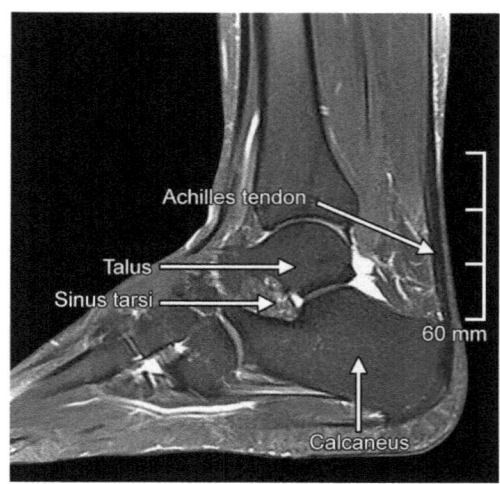

Fig. 45: Ankle MRI sagittal proton-density fat-saturated sequence.

CHAPTER 2 | Understanding of Radiological Anatomy | 35

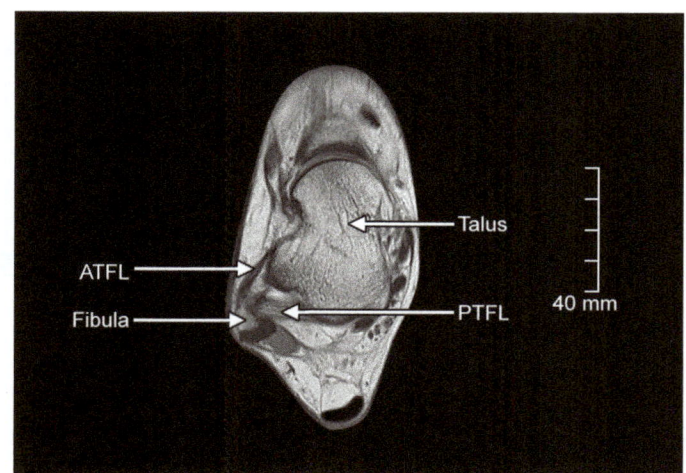

Fig. 46: Ankle MRI axial proton-density fat-saturated sequence showing the anterior and posterior talofibular ligaments.

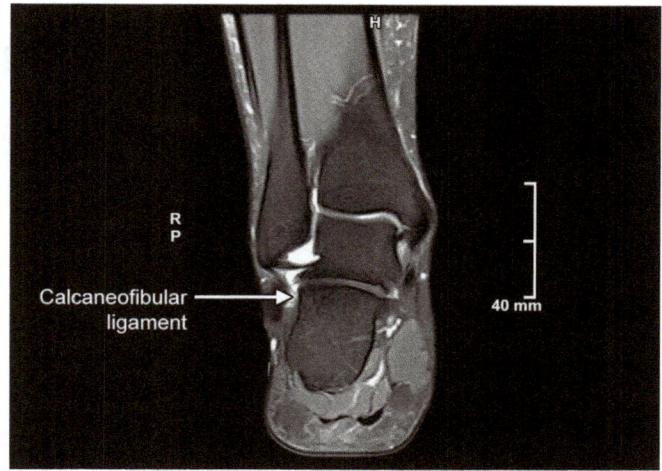

Fig. 47: Ankle MRI coronal proton-density fat-saturated sequence showing the calcaneofibular ligament.

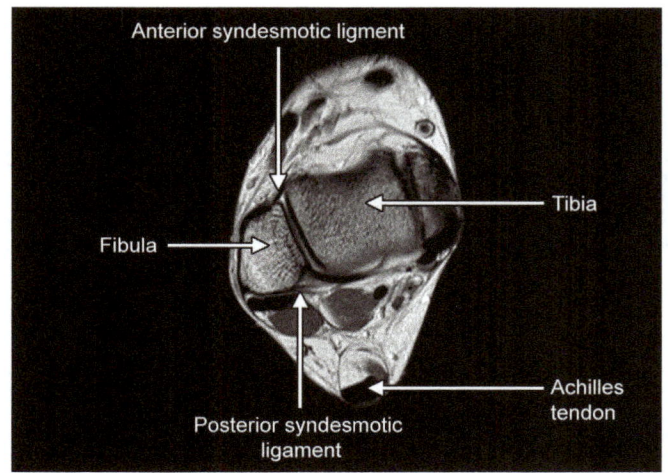

Fig. 48: Ankle MRI axial proton-density fat-saturated sequence showing the anterior and posterior syndesmotic ligaments.

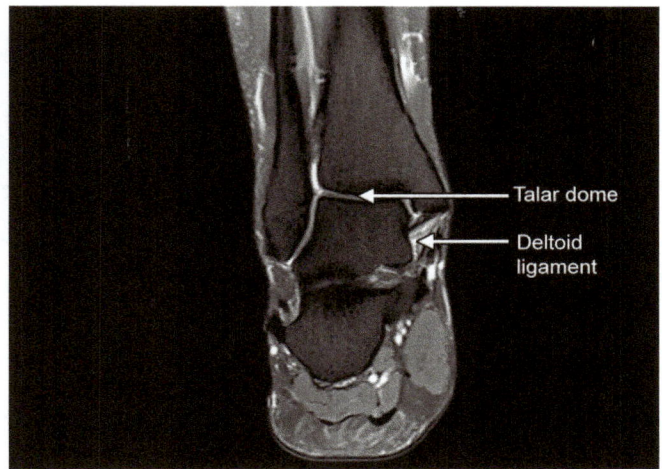

Fig. 49: Ankle MRI coronal proton-density fat-saturated sequence showing the deltoid ligament.

CHAPTER 3
Understanding Common Image-guided Procedures

Kenneth Lupton, Jamen Baren, Harun Gupta

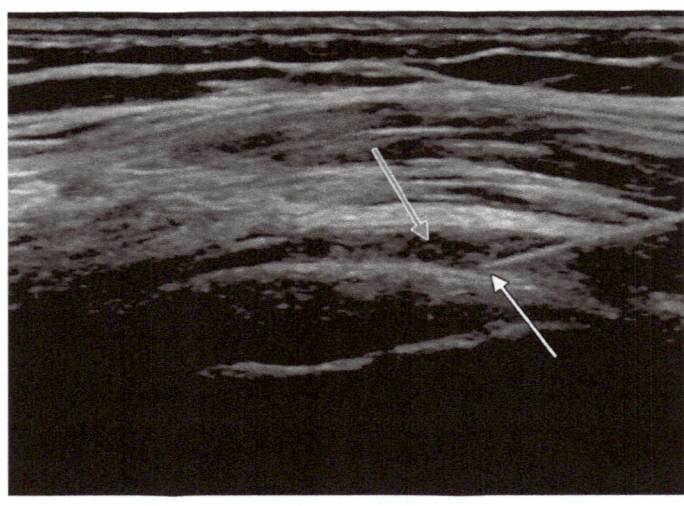

Fig. 1: Ultrasound-guided injection with tip of needle (white arrow) lying within the subacromial subdeltoid bursa (gray arrow).

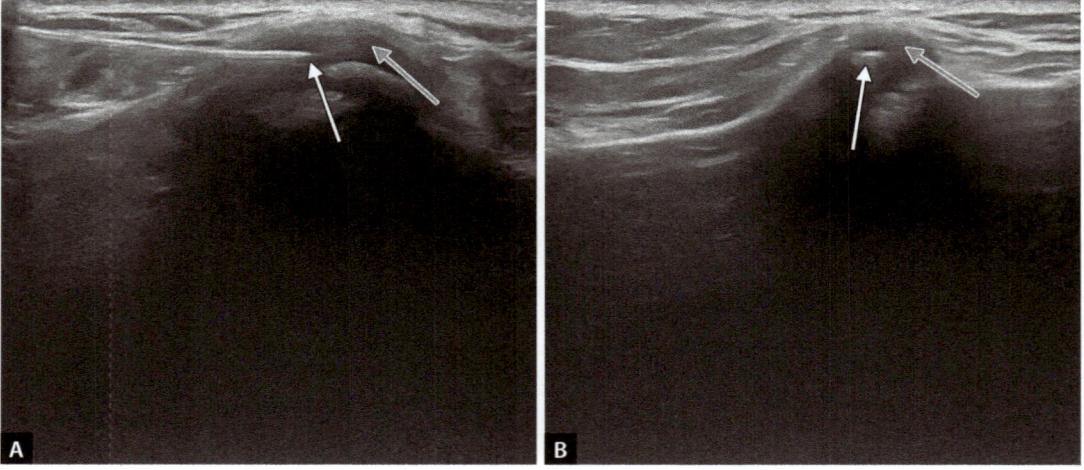

Figs. 2A and B: Ultrasound-guided acromioclavicular joint injection in both the (A) in-plane and (B) out-of-plane approaches. The needle tip (white arrow) is seen to lie within the joint space where there is a degree of capsular thickening (gray arrow).

CHAPTER 3 | Understanding Common Image-guided Procedures

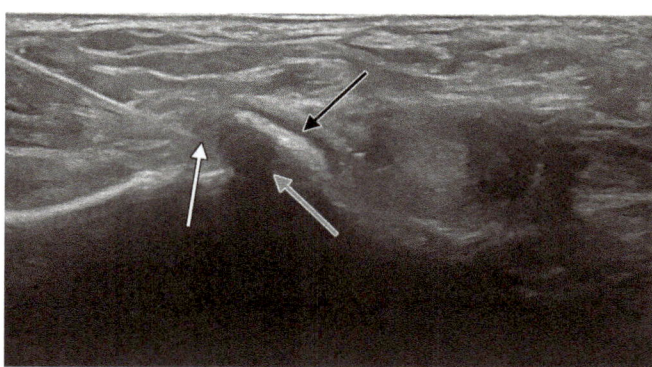

Fig. 3: Ultrasound-guided calcaneocuboid joint injection. The needle tip (white arrow) can be seen approaching the joint space (gray arrow) with a prominent osteophyte (black arrow) at the joint margins.

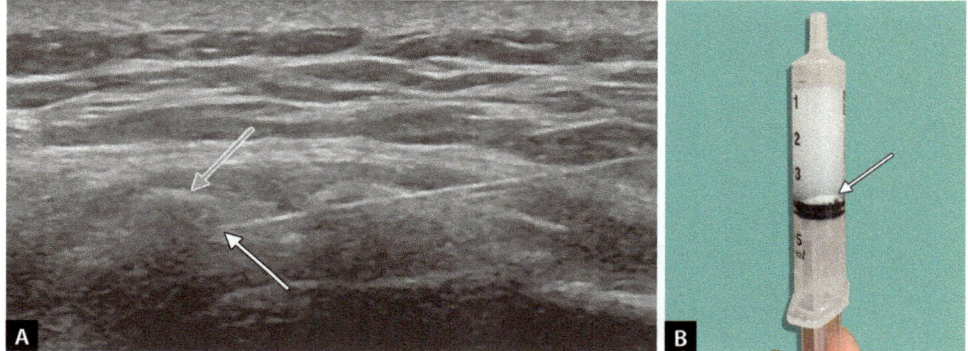

Figs. 4A and B: (A) Ultrasound-guided barbotage of calcific tendinopathy affecting the gluteus medius tendon. The needle tip (white arrow) can be seen within the region of the tendon calcification (gray arrow); (B) Successful aspiration of calcium which is layering (white arrow) within the barbotage injectate.

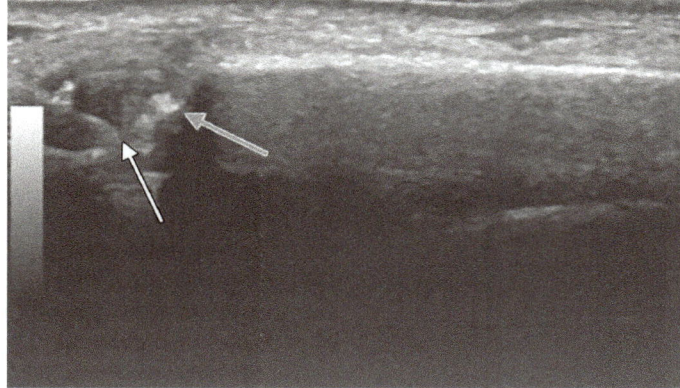

Fig. 5: Ultrasound-guided carpometacarpal (CMC) joint injection. The needle tip (white arrow) can be seen approaching the base of the first metacarpal (gray arrow) using an in-plane longitudinal approach where there is prominent bony irregularity in keeping with degenerative change.

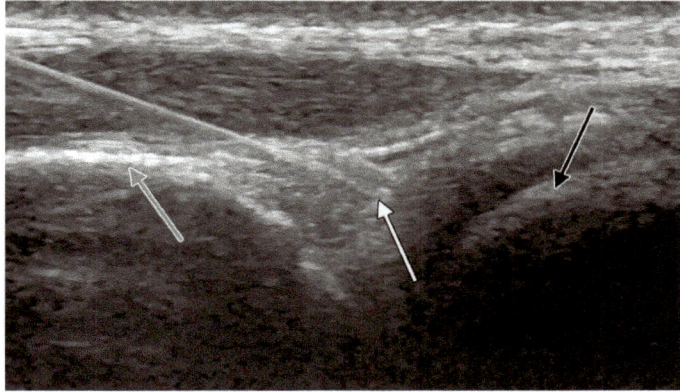

Fig. 6: Ultrasound-guided tibiotalar joint injection using a longitudinal in-plane approach. The needle tip (white arrow) can be seen within the joint space between the tibia (gray arrow) and the talus (black arrow).

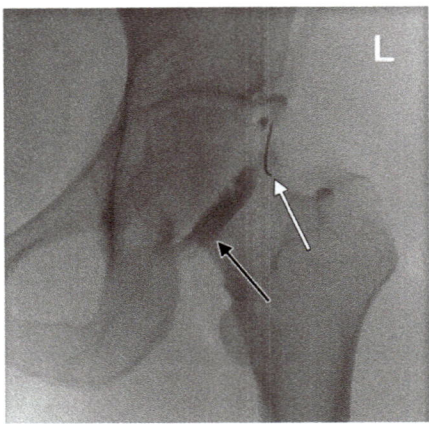

Fig. 7: Fluoroscopic-guided hip joint injection. The needle tip is positioned at the femoral head–neck junction (white arrow) and subsequent injection of contrast (black arrow) reveals the desired extension away from the needle in an elliptical configuration corresponding with the hip joint capsule.

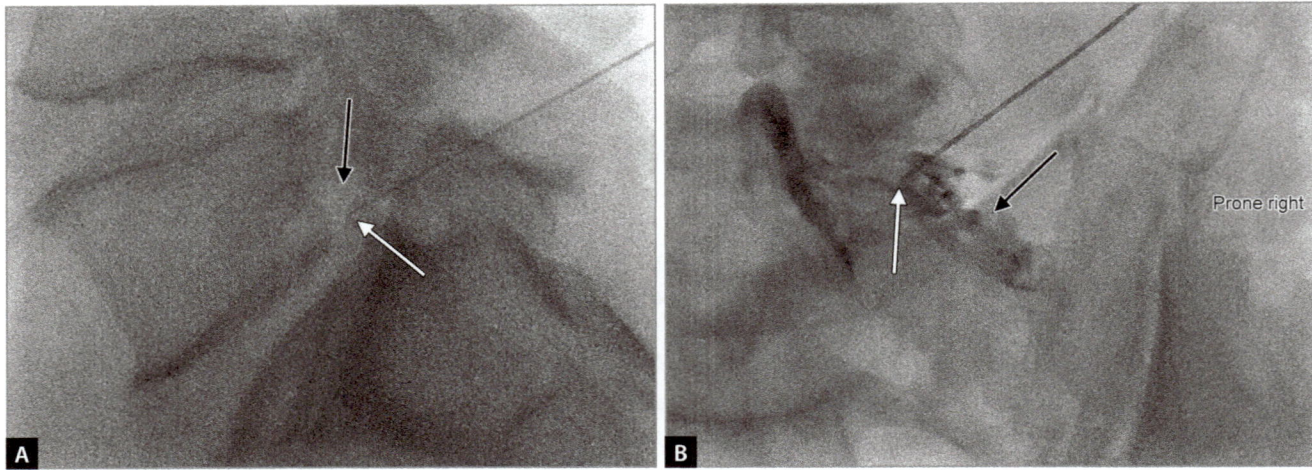

Figs. 8A and B: Fluoroscopic-guided right L5 nerve root injection with (A) lateral and (B) anteroposterior (AP) views. In (A), the needle tip (white arrow) is seen positioned within the neural exit foramen (black arrow). In (B), the needle tip (white arrow) is again shown in the neural exit foramen with contrast extending along the L5 nerve root (black arrow) and medially toward the vertebral canal confirming satisfactory positioning.

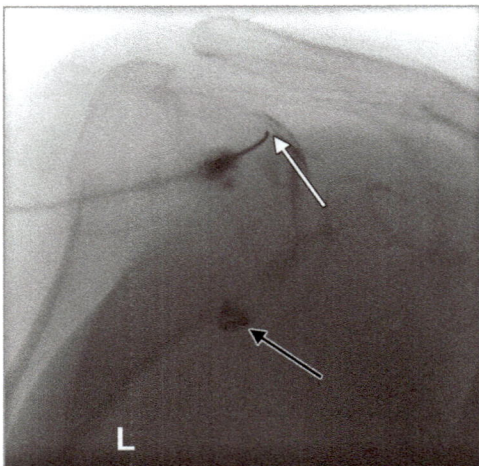

Fig. 9: Fluoroscopic-guided shoulder hydrodistension using the posterior approach. The needle tip (white arrow) is inserted down to the superomedial aspect of the humeral head. Contrast can be seen to have extended away from the needle tip to lie in a satisfactory position in the axillary recess (black arrow).

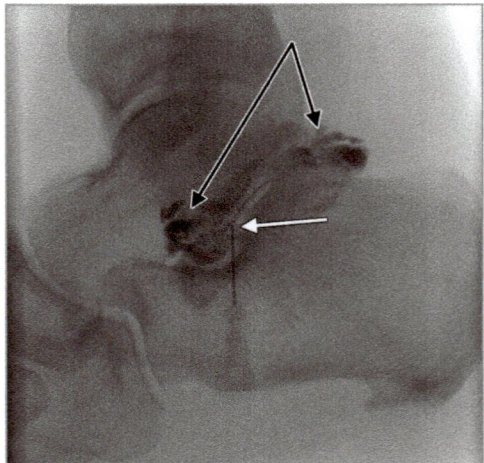

Fig. 10: Fluoroscopic-guided subtalar joint injection. The needle tip (white arrow) is positioned within the mid-subtalar joint with contrast (black arrows) extending satisfactorily into the anterior and posterior subtalar joints indicating satisfactory position.

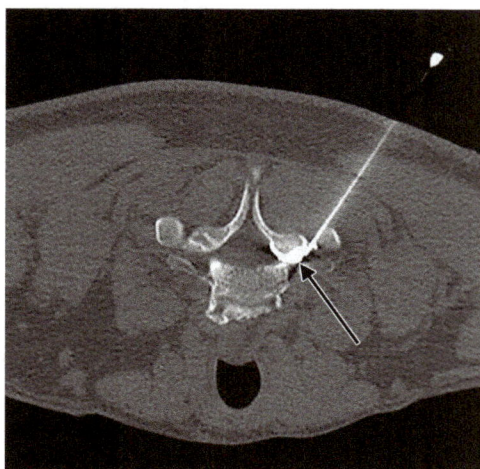

Fig. 11: CT-guided right C8 nerve root injection. The needle tip is positioned close to the nerve root within the epidural fat of the exit foramen. Subsequent injection of contrast reveals satisfactory extension along the nerve root into the vertebral canal (black arrow).

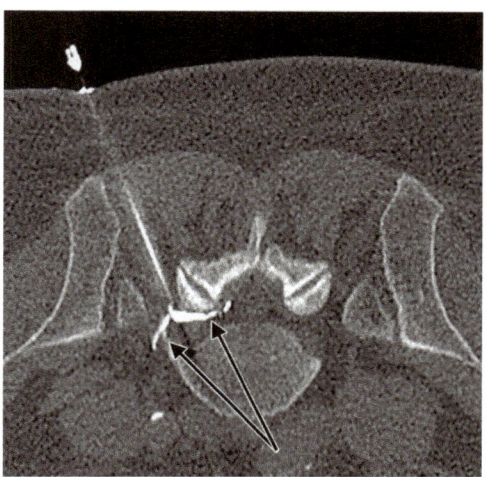

Fig. 12: CT-guided left L5 nerve root injection. The needle tip is again positioned within the epidural fat of the exit foramen close to the exiting nerve root. Contrast injection confirms extension along the nerve root proximally and distally indicating satisfactory position (black arrows).

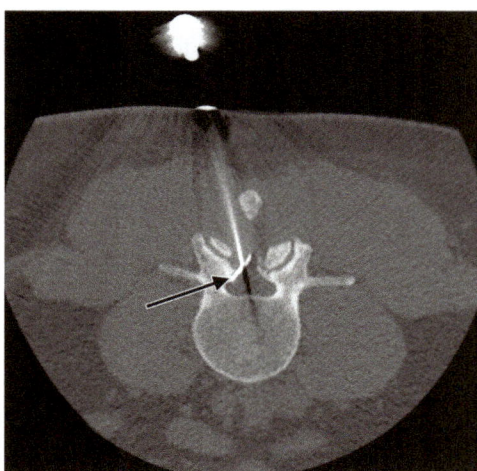

Fig. 13: CT-guided epidural injection using a translaminar approach. Contrast (black arrow) can be seen extending along the epidural space.

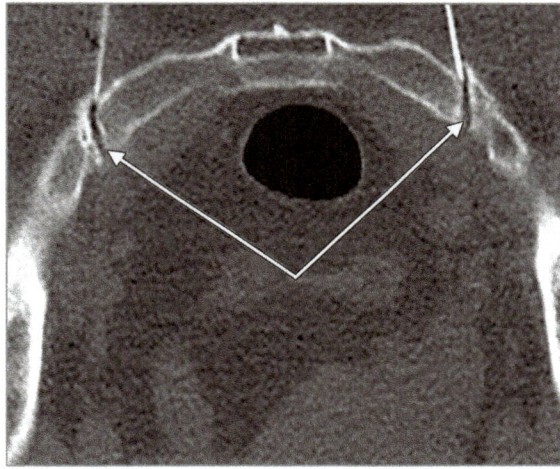

Fig. 14: CT-guided bilateral sacroiliac joint injections. The needles are inserted down to the inferior aspect of the sacroiliac joints at the synovial portion (white arrows).

CHAPTER 4

Understanding the Pathology of Common Conditions through Magnetic Resonance Imaging for the Pain Physician

Harun Gupta, James Baren, Kenneth Lupton

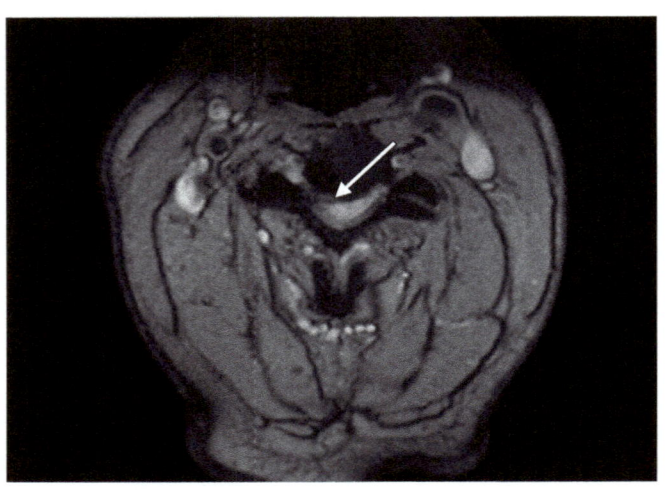

Fig. 1: Axial proton-density weighted MRI cervical spine sequence. A posterior disc-osteophyte bar (white arrow) causes central and right foraminal stenosis.

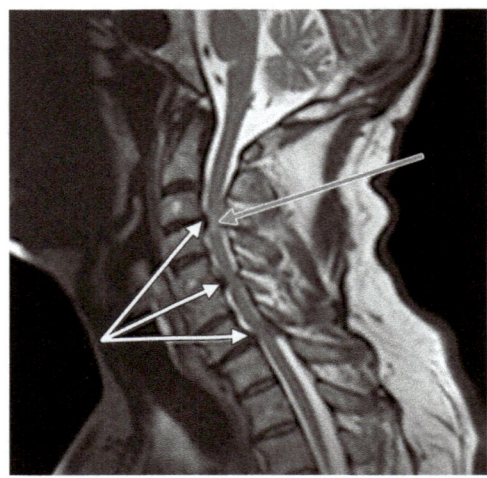

Fig. 2: Sagittal T2-weighted MRI cervical spine sequence. Multilevel disc-osteophyte bars (white arrows) cause central canal stenosis and efface the underlying thecal sac. Increased signal within the cord at the level of C3–C4 is consistent with myelopathic change (gray arrow).

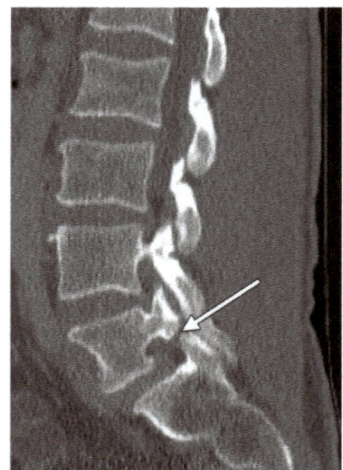

Fig. 3: CT lumbar spine sagittal reformat showing L5 pars defect (white arrow) with grade 1 spondylolisthesis of L5 on S1.

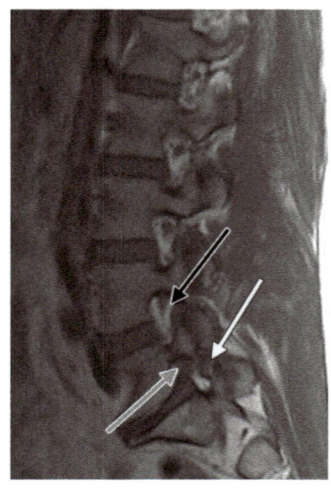

Fig. 4: Sagittal T1-weighted MRI lumbar spine sequence. An L5 pars defect (white arrow) with grade 1 spondylolisthesis of L5 on S1 is evident. There is also effacement of the epidural fat surrounding the L5 root in the exit foramen indicating foraminal stenosis (grey arrow). A normal neural exit foramen (black arrow) is noted at L4.

CHAPTER 4 | Understanding the Pathology of Common Conditions through Magnetic Resonance Imaging for the Pain Physician

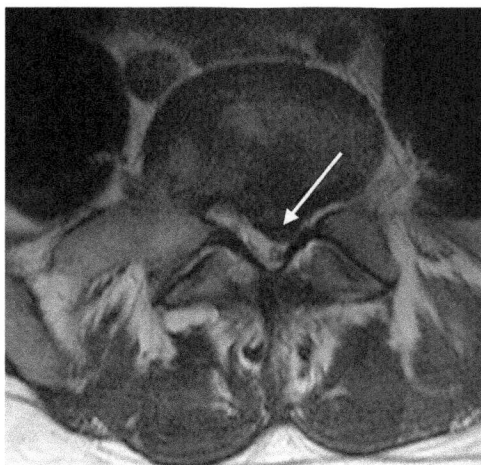

Fig. 5: Axial T2-weighted MRI lumbar spine sequence. Left central/subarticular disc protrusion (white arrow) causing left lateral recess stenosis and compromising the transiting left nerve root.

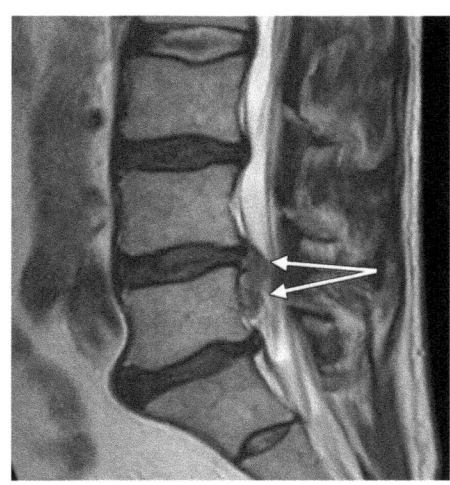

Fig. 6: Sagittal T2-weighted MRI lumbar spine sequence. L4–L5 disc extrusion (white arrows) with extension posteroinferior to lie at the level of the posterior L5 vertebral body.

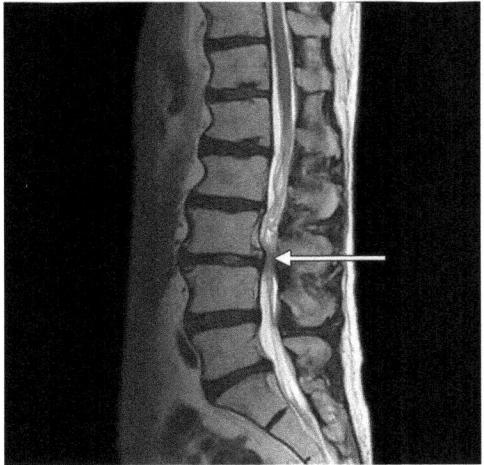

Fig. 7: Sagittal T2-weighted MRI lumbar spine sequence. Severe central canal stenosis (white arrow) at L3–L4 with grade 1 anterolisthesis of L3 on L4.

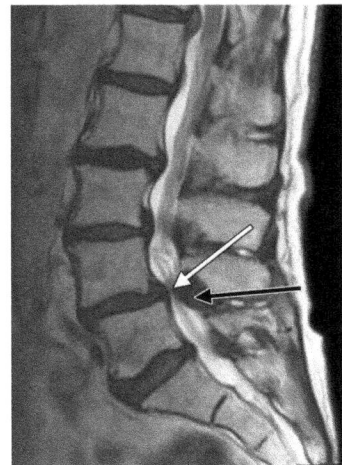

Fig. 8: Sagittal T2-weighted MRI lumbar spine sequence. Severe central canal stenosis (white arrow) at L4–L5 secondary to disc bulge, facet and ligamentous hypertrophy (black arrow) with grade 1 degenerative spondylolisthesis.

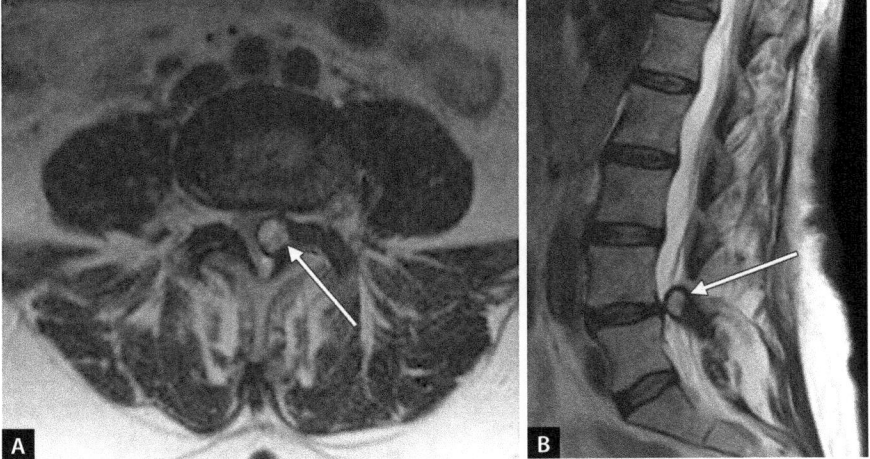

Figs. 9A and B: (A) Axial T2-weighted and (B) sagittal T2-weighted sequences of the lumbar spine. A facet joint cyst (white arrows) causes severe central stenosis with thecal effacement and neural compromise.

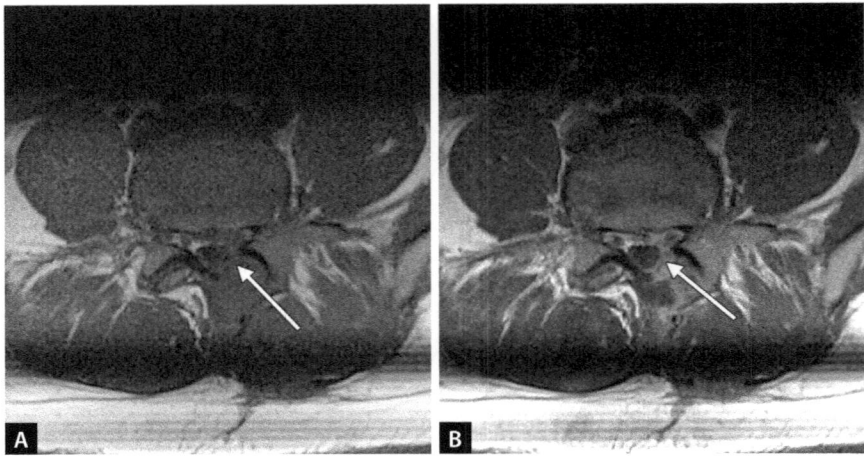

Figs. 10A and B: (A) Pre-contrast and (B) post-contrast T1-weighted axial lumbar spine sequences in a patient who had undergone microdiscectomy and left laminectomy. On the pre-contrast scan, there is low signal (white arrow) within the left epidural region. This enhances on the post-contrast scan (white arrow in B) and is consistent with post-operative scar tissue.

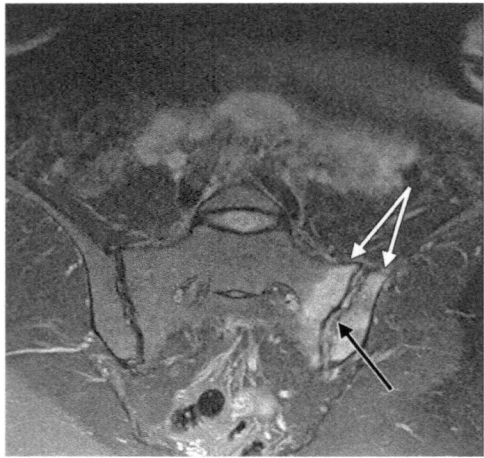

Fig. 11: Coronal oblique T2 fat-saturated sequence of the sacroiliac joints. There is marked edema (white arrows) of the left sacroiliac joint on both the iliac and sacral surfaces of the joint with bony irregularity (black arrow) reflecting erosions. The appearances are typical of sacroiliitis.

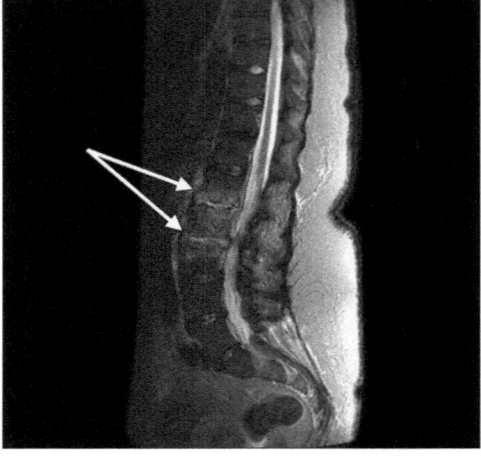

Fig. 12: Sagittal short T1 inversion recovery (STIR) MRI lumbar spine sequence. High signal is seen centered around the discs of L1–L2 and L2–L3 reflecting fluid within the discs and adjacent endplate edema (white arrows). The appearances are typical for infective spondylodiscitis.

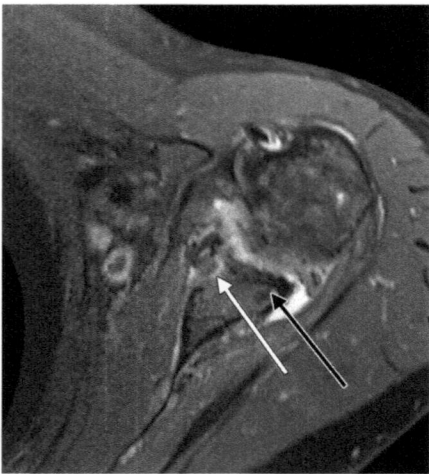

Fig. 13: Axial proton-density fat-saturated MRI shoulder sequence. A bony Bankart lesion is shown with a cleft of high signal undercutting the anteroinferior glenoid (white arrow). The posterior glenoid (black arrow) is marked for reference.

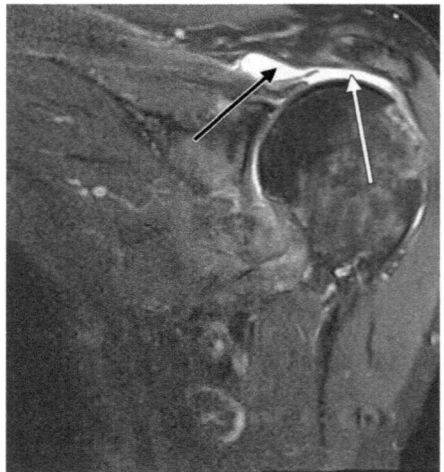

Fig. 14: Coronal proton-density fat-saturated MRI shoulder sequence. A full-thickness supraspinatous tear is demonstrated with no tendon fibers visible at the expected position superior to the humeral head (white arrow). There is also florid subacromial subdeltoid bursitis (black arrow).

CHAPTER 4 | Understanding the Pathology of Common Conditions through Magnetic Resonance Imaging for the Pain Physician

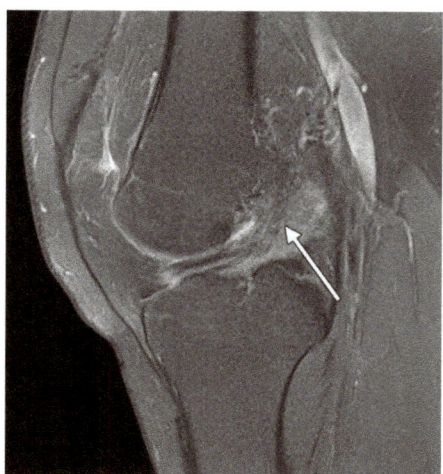

Fig. 15: Sagittal proton-density fat-saturated MRI knee sequence. There is a full thickness anterior cruciate ligament (ACL) tear with poor ligament fiber definition within the ligament (white arrow).

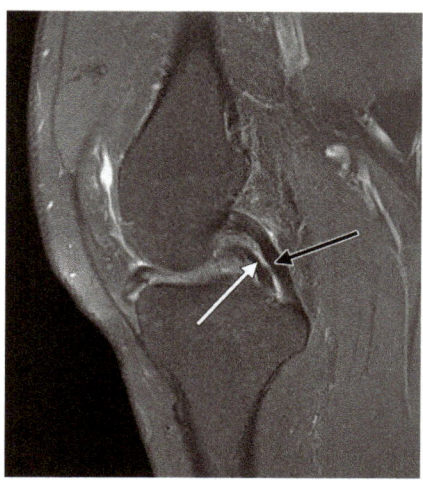

Fig. 16: Sagittal proton-density fat-saturated MRI knee sequence. There is a bucket-handle tear of the medial meniscus (white arrow) with the so-called double posterior cruciate ligament (PCL) sign present. This represents the flipped meniscal fragment (the handle) lying anterior to the normal PCL (black arrow) giving the impression of two ligaments.

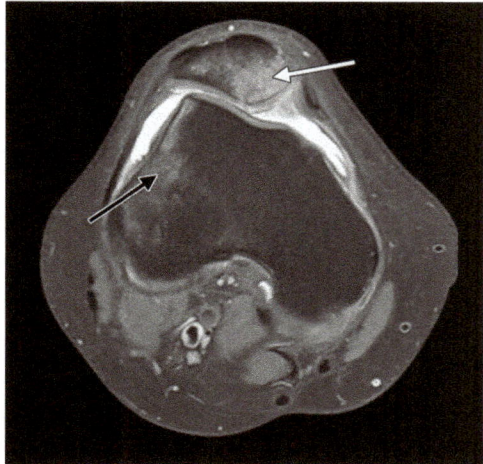

Fig. 17: Axial proton-density fat-saturated MRI knee sequence. Marked subchondral edema is seen at the medial aspect of the patella (white arrow) and the lateral aspect of the lateral femoral condyle (black arrow). This pattern is typical of lateral patellar dislocation.

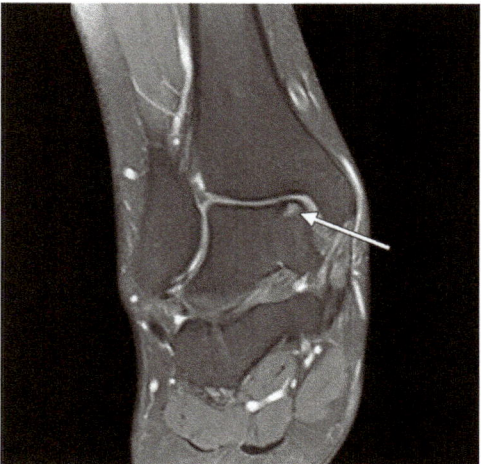

Fig. 18: Coronal proton-density fat-saturated MRI ankle sequence. A focus of high signal (white arrow) is present at the medial aspect of the talar dome in keeping with an osteochondral injury. This is considered stable given the lack of a rim of high signal demarcating the deep aspect of the injury from the adjacent bone.

CHAPTER 5

Radiation Protection

Satish Kamath, Dwarkadas K Baheti

Myth: The dose of radiation used in the performance of interventional pain procedures is inconsequential, and few measures are required to maintain radiation safety.

Fact: Radiation exposure at any dose carries some risk for both the patient and the healthcare team. Mitigation strategies for radiation exposure are governed by the principles of ALARA (as low as reasonably achievable). Adoption of simple and inexpensive tactics may reduce radiation exposure by >90%.

Radiation protection, sometimes known as radiological protection, is the science of protecting people and the environment from the harmful effects of ionizing radiation, which include both particle radiation and high-energy electromagnetic radiation.

X-rays were discovered by Wilhelm Roentgen in 1895. Subsequently Gamma rays, proton beam, electron beam and radioisotope are used in diagnosis, treatment and palliative care of patients.

The knowledge of effects of different types of radiation on human tissues and protection from ill effects of radiation is quite essential. Radiation protection has progressed hugely in recent times. Hence understanding the biological effects of radiation is essential **(Flowchart 1 and Fig. 1)**.

Flowchart 1: Biological effects of radiation.

```
                    Biological effects of radiation
                              │
              ┌───────────────┴───────────────┐
              ▼                               ▼
        X-rays and gamma rays          Ionizing radiations
                                    (α-, β- proton and electron)
              │                               │
              └───────────────┬───────────────┘
                              ▼
                Ionization and excitation in tissues
                              │
                              ▼
                Chemical change (free radical formation)
                              │
                              ▼
                Biological change (DNA damage)
                              │
          ┌───────────────────┼───────────────────┐
          ▼                   ▼                   ▼
      Mutation          Malignant           Inhibition of
                       transformation       cell division
          │                                       │
          ▼                                       ▼
   Genetic defects                            Cell death
```

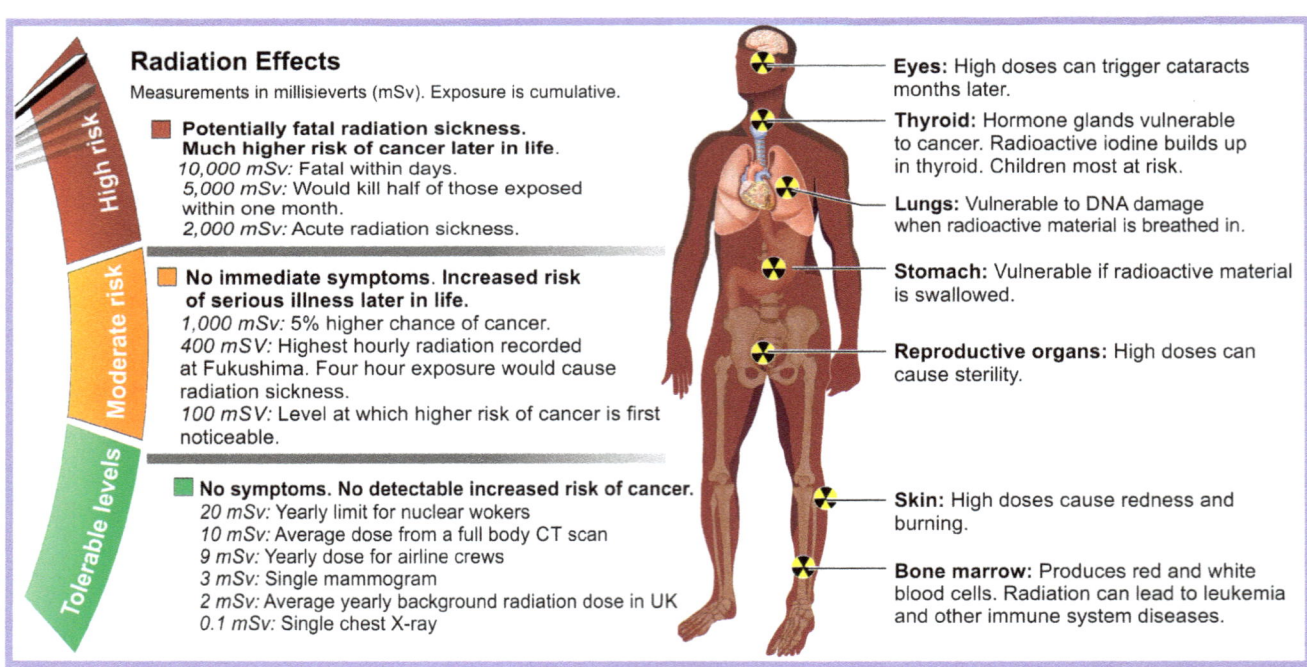

Fig. 1: Radiation effects of organs.
Courtesy: Kiran Medical Systems

Flowchart 2: Radiation exposure can lead to.

```
                        Radiation exposure
                       /                  \
        Stochastic change, e.g.,        Non-stochastic change
        Cancers, Genetic defects                |
        1. Leukemia—Latent period—5–20 years   Results in organ atrophy and fibrosis
           Other tumors—10–30 years             |
        2. Genetic defects may manifest after   1. Eye lens opacities
           several generation                   2. Fall in blood count
                                                3. Fall in sperm count

        Effects on blood                    Effects in pregnancy
       /       |         \                 /         |            \
Platelet   WBC          RBC            Fetal    Intrauterine    Congenital
depletion  depletion    depletion      defect   growth          malformation
               |            |                   retardation
           Causing      Causing
           infection    anemia
```

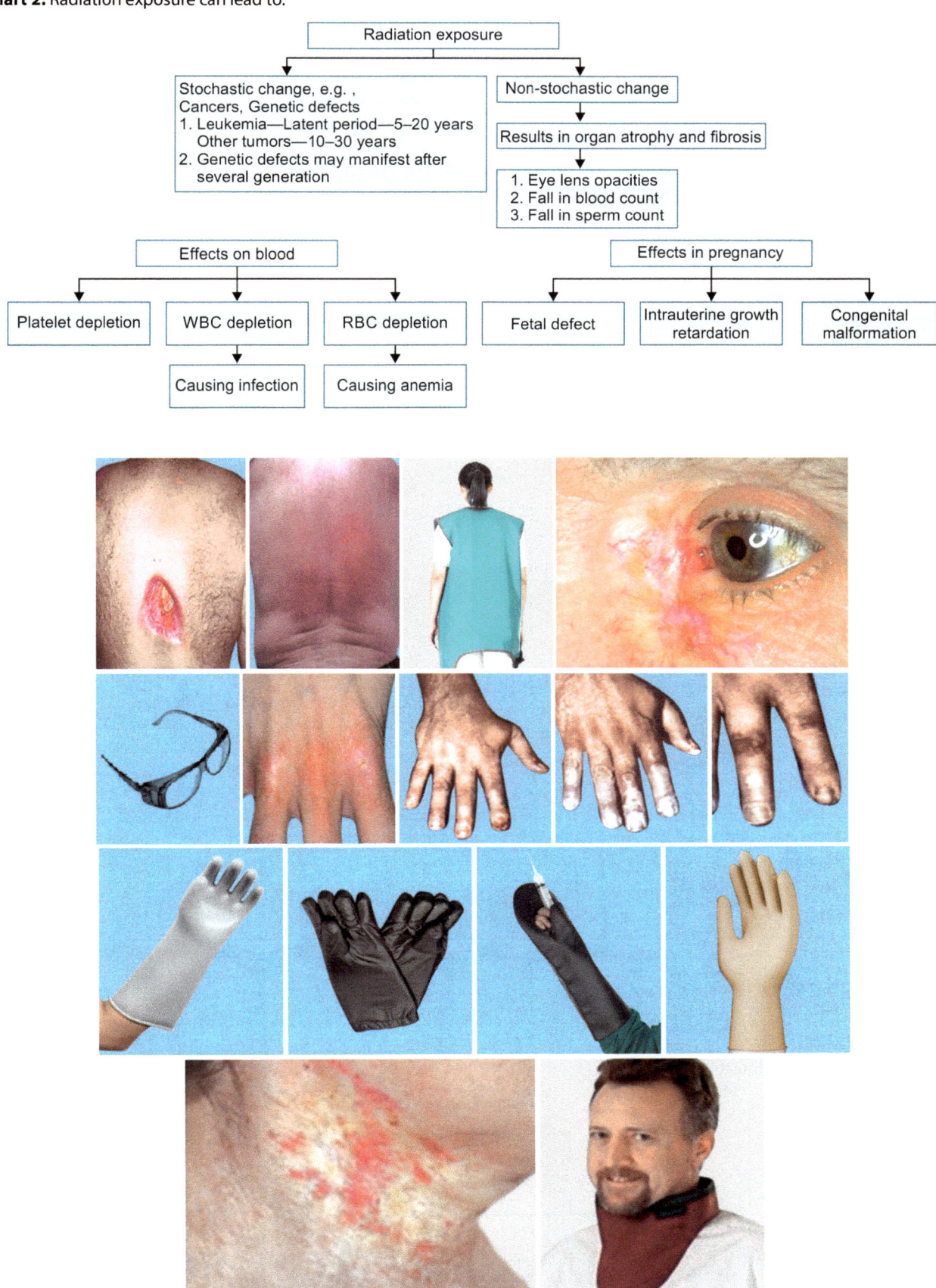

Fig. 2: Effects of radiation.

AERB (ATOMIC ENERGY REGULATORY BOARD) (FLOWCHART 3)

- Lays down guidelines for medical equipment room layout for installation.
- Lays down responsibilities of radiation personnel and Radiation Safety Officer (RSO)
- Regulatory control over new models of X-ray equipment.
- Commissioning and decommissioning of X-ray installation.

Radiation Protection

General Information

Rad: Unit of absorbed dose
Gray: SI unit of absorbed dose
1 Gray = 100 rads
Rem: Measure of biological effect of radiation
1 Sievert = 100 rem

Principles of Radiation Protection

- Justification of practice
- Optimization of protection (**Flowchart 4**)
  - Magnitude of individual doses
  - Number of people exposed should be kept as low as possible
- Dose limitation

Radiation Detection and Measurement

- Radiation detection devices
- Radiation measuring devices

Personnel Monitoring Devices

- Pocket dosimeter
- SIPM badge
- TLD—Thermoluminescent dosimeter
- OSL—Optically stimulated luminescent
- Electronic dosimeter

AERB Dosimeter

Occupational Workers (Effective dose):

- 20 mSv/year average over 5 years
- 30 mSv in a year
- Public 1 mSv/year

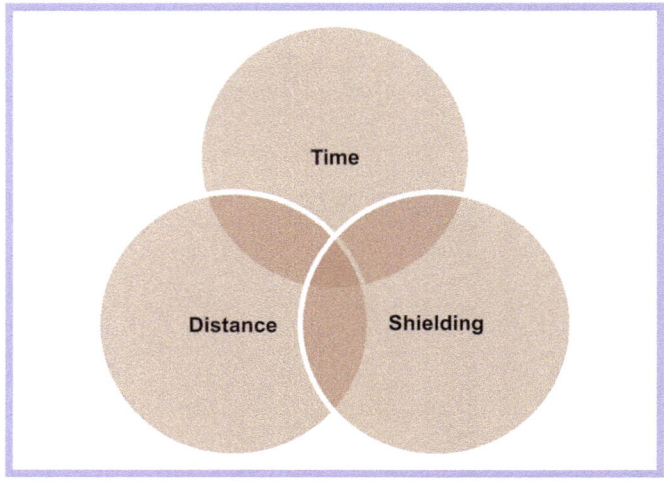

Fig. 3: Cardinal rules of radiation protection.
Courtesy: Kiran Medical Systems

Flowchart 3: Regulatory bodies.

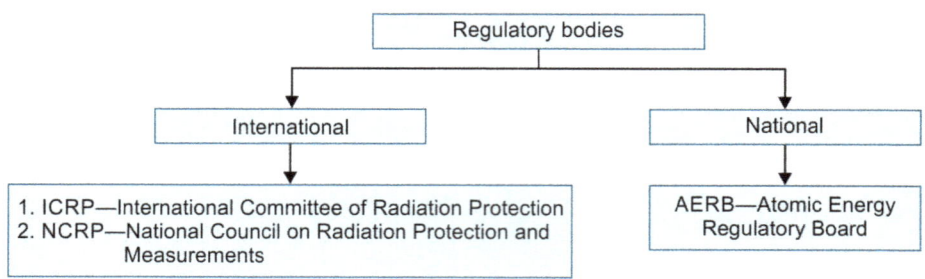

Flowchart 4: Optimization of protection.

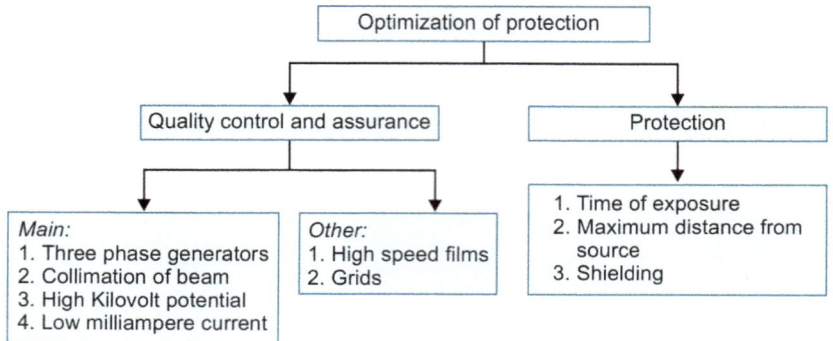

- Cardinal rules of radiation protection are **time, distance, and shielding.**
- Lead apron is to protect from secondary radiation.
- Lead equivalence, lead compounding, lead migration.
- X-ray should not be focused on a single point for longer time.
- Lead apron should be checked every quarter.

Fig. 4: *Rule 1*—Protection of radiation.
Courtesy: Kiran Medical Systems.

- Distance is the most effective means of radiation protection.
- Maintain safe distance from the source of radiation.
- Try and position yourselves in a place wherein the X-ray reaches you after scattering twice.

Fig. 5: *Rule 2*—Protection of radiation.
Courtesy: Kiran Medical Systems.

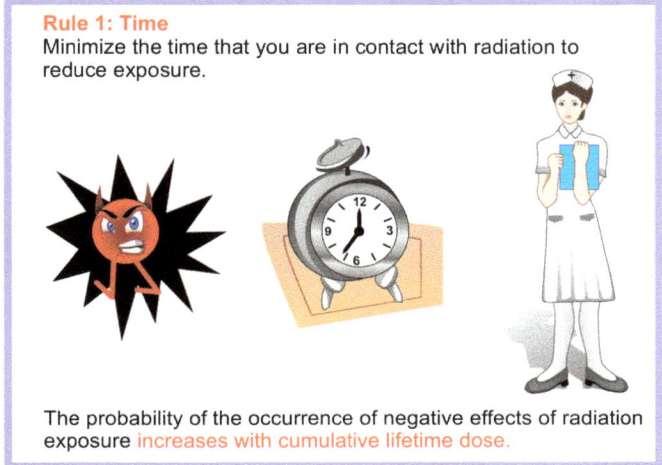

Fig. 6: *Rule 1*—To minimize radiation exposure.
Courtesy: Kiran Medical Systems

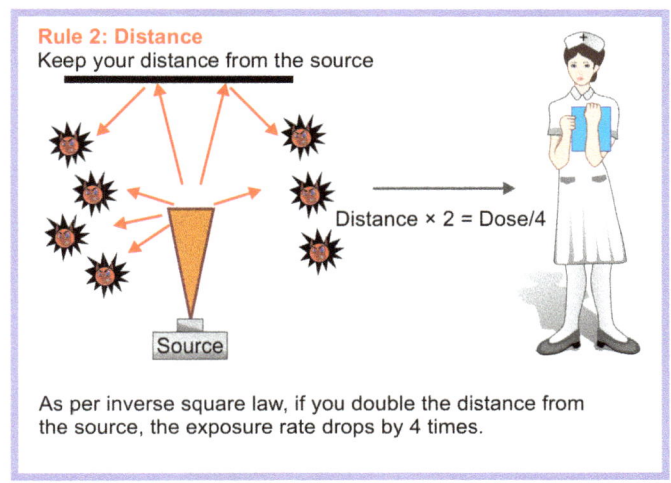

Fig. 7: *Rule 2*—Safe distance from the source.
Courtesy: Kiran Medical Systems

Rule 3: Shielding
- Shielding is only from scattered radiation and not for primary radiation.
- A properly worn lead apron can protect up to 80% active blood-forming organs.

A well-chosen apron should cover from the manubrium of the sternum down to include the symphysis pubis and mid thigh.

Fig. 8: *Rule 3*—Shielding.
Courtesy: Kiran Medical Systems

Shielding requirements according to NCRP recommendations are:
- Lead aprons—0.35 mm lead equivalency
- Lead gloves—0.25 mm lead equivalency
- Protective curtain—0.25 mm lead equivalency
- Thyroid shield—0.25 mm lead equivalency
- Aprons for pregnancy—total 1.0 mm Pb equivalency at fetal level
- Bucky slot cover 0.5 mm lead equivalency
- Eyewear—0.75 mm lead equivalency

Radiation Protections Equipment or Gears (Figs. 9 to 12)

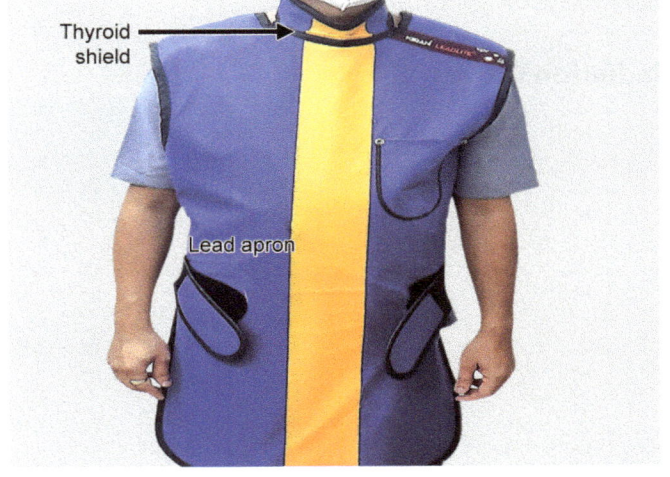

Fig. 9: Lead apron.

Thyroid Shield

Thyroid Shield

The thyroid gland is especially sensitive to radiation. Our range of thyroid shields provide complete protection to your neck and sternum so that you never have to feel unsafe.

Lead equivalence: 0.35 mm Pb or 0.50 mm Pb

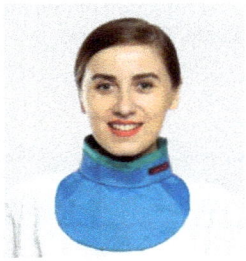

Class
- All time popular design
- Wide coverage area
- One size fits all

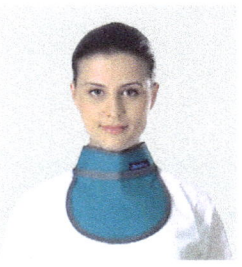

Elegant
Easily attaches to our double-sided apron and vest adjustable fastener

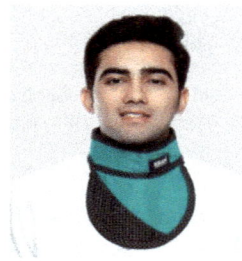

Slimline
- Provides perfect fit and protection
- Easily attaches to all aprons

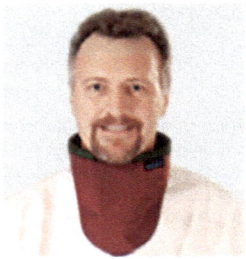

Harmony
Collar design which perfectly thyroid gland wide coverage

Fig. 10: Thyroid shield.
Courtesy: Kiran Medical Systems

Radiation Gloves

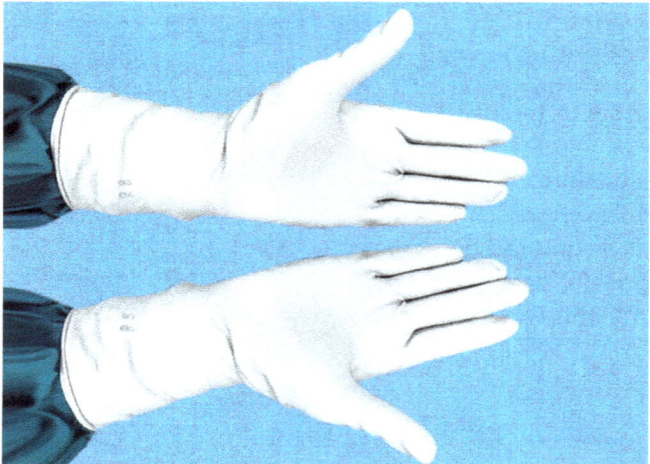

Fig. 11: Radiation gloves.

Eye Protection

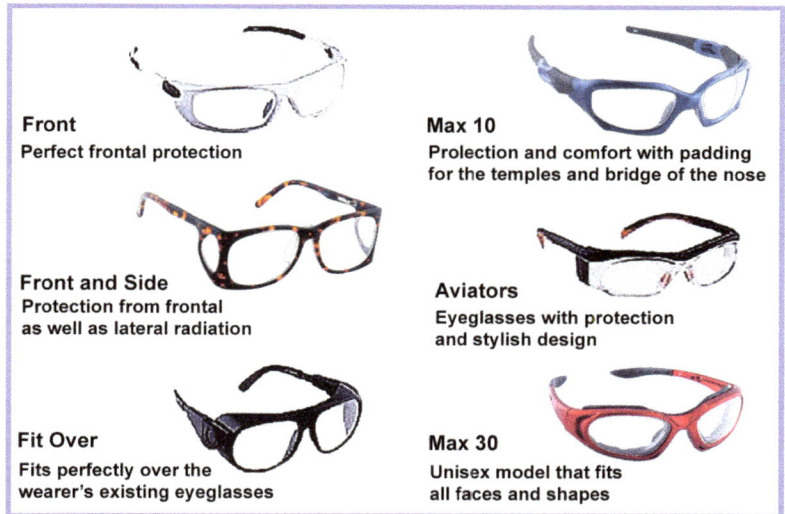

Fig. 12: Eye protection.
Courtesy: Kiran Medical Systems

Storage Systems

Poor storage reduced the shelf life of protective apparel and also takes up excessive space. Perfectly crafted range of storage systems can help safely store multiple pairs of apparel and accessories in a compact unit that is space efficient and easy to install and comes in stainless steel grade.

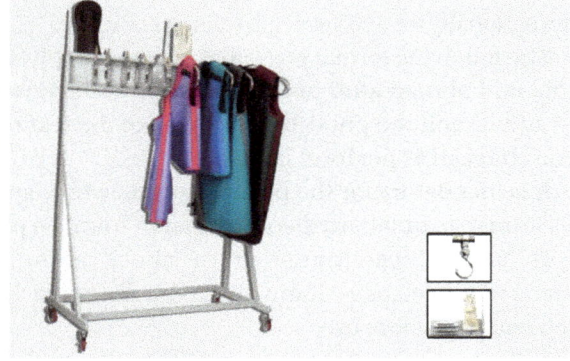

Mobile Storage System with Hangers
- Convenient mobile storage system with brakes
- Stainless steel hangers for hygienic storage
- Compact unit for storing apparel, gloves, and shields
- Detachable hooks for more storage options

Available Models
- *5 Hangers and glove holder:* Stores up to 5 pairs of apparel
- *10 Hangers and glove holder:* Stores up to 10 pairs of apparel
- Glove holder and hooks are available for fixing on the mobile system.

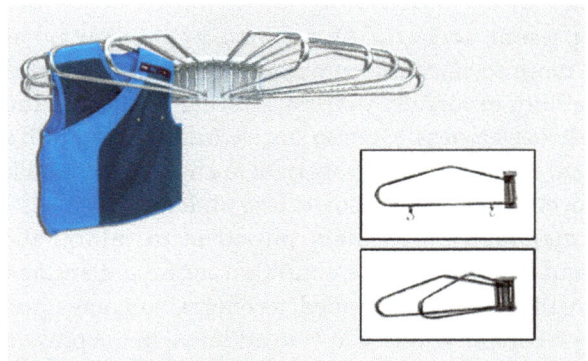

Mounted Wall Racks
- Swivel hangers for ease of hanging and removing
- Stainless steel hangers for hygienic storage
- Space-saving racks store apparel close to a wall
  Wall bracket can be right- or left-sided for optimum use of space.

Available Models
- Wall racks with one, two, three and five hangers.
- Hook are available for fixing on all wall racks.

Fig. 13: Storage system.
Courtesy: Kiran Medical Systems

- Radiation is of two types–Ionizing and non-Ionizing
- In Ionizing-Our interest is in X-rays
- We should use ALARA/ALARP principle to protect ourselves from radiation
- Radiation protection is from scattered radiation
- The probability of the occurrence of negative effects of radiation exposure increases with cumulative lifetime dose

Fig. 14: Summary.
Courtesy: Kiran Medical Systems

CHAPTER 6

Informed Consent for Interventional Pain Management Procedures

Dwarkadas K Baheti

It is a standard protocol to follow a multidisciplinary/modal approach for total pain management which includes pain relief, physiotherapy, and psychotherapy.

The pain management includes use of a battery of group of pain and other medications; however, the interventional pain treatment procedure or as pain block remains an important modality for relief of pain.

All precautions must be taken to make pain relief simpler, free of stress, devoid of any complications, and cost-effective. However, as pain management procedure is an invasive one, so unexpected, untoward side effects or complications can occur.

The present scenario of practice of medicine has changed more so since the corona pandemic. It has added accountability to already present Internet explosion and medicolegal awareness. More so since we are dealing with a live person, the patient has every right to know all the details of the procedure and treatment he is to undergo.

It is mandatory for a pain physician to inform the patient and his relatives the condition of the patient and procedure that is to be performed, its effects, outcomes, and unforeseen complications, if any. In addition, in the present corona pandemic, one needs to update about the risk of hospitalization and cost involved due to administrative guidelines.

In this pandemic, COVID-19 test and high-resolution computed tomography (HRCT) of chest are added cost and changed the protocol of the theater.

The sample draft of the informed consent form, which is different from the earlier one, used by the author for interventional pain procedures is given in the following text. He has used the following format in more than 5,000 pain-relief procedures at the Pain Management Clinic of Bombay Hospital and Medical Research Center and other centers nationally and internationally for >20 years into clinical practice.

The following format is used by many pain physicians in India and abroad after obtaining the written consent from the author and the publisher. The part of the text may have been changed as per local laws.

It is mandatory for the pain physician, who wants to use this format, to obtain written permission from the publisher.

It is also recommended to check about certain objectionable clauses, if any, with the notary or lawyer in their country before use.

INFORMED CONSENT FOR PAIN MANAGEMENT PROCEDURE

Sample Draft

Patient Name: _____

Age: _____ Sex: Male/Female Date: _____

Address: _____
_____

I hereby authorize Dr _____ to perform a Pain Management Procedure known as
_____
This procedure has been explained to me by Dr _____ and I completely Understand the nature and consequences of the said procedure in present Corona 19 pandemic.

The following points have been made particularly clear.
1. Complications that may follow a procedure with/without relief of pain are same as those that may follow any other type of surgical procedure, such as infection, hematoma formation and corona infection etc. These complications are enhanced in those cases where the patient is old and infirm, those with diabetes and hypertension as also with those who have earlier cardiac ailments and decompensation.
2. The drugs that are being used for this procedure are used in pain relief procedure. A patient may be allergic/idiosyncratic to this drug and may react to these drugs in an unpredictable fashion and rarely with unpredictable results.
3. Rarely in some procedures may be followed with paralysis of one or more limbs. The risk of this has been explained to me.
4. In some procedures, specially prepared long needles needed to be used. It is not always possible to use disposable needles in such cases. Though they are fully autoclaved the possibility of AIDS and B virus hepatitis cannot be excluded.
5. Specially prepared needles are known sometimes, though rarely to break and if this happens a foreign body still is within the body and will require surgery to remove it. If surgery need be done, then I allow Dr _____ to get such operation performed a surgeon of his choice. At times blood transfusions may be needed during or after surgery. Though the blood is fully tested it may give rise to mismatch, B virus, malaria as well as AIDS.
6. I understand that the Dr _____ relies on the qualified staff provided by the hospital or nominated by him for postoperative care of the patient. He personally may not be able to visit the patient everyday.

I am aware that during the procedure unforeseen condition may need other or different procedures that those set forth above. I therefore authorize and request that Dr _____ to perform such procedures as are, in this professional judgment, necessary; these includes but are not limited to, procedures said above. The Authority granted there, shall extend to remedying conditions that were unknown before the start of the operation.

I understand the risks of Local and General anesthesia. I consent to the administration of anaesthesia under the supervision of Dr _____ or such anaesthesiologist that he shall select, and to the use of such anaesthesia as he may think advisable.

The approximate recuperation time and the interval before I can return to work have been discussed with me. There is no guarantee when I shall be able to resume normal activities.

I consent to be photographed or filmed before, during and after treatment, and that these pictures will be property of Dr _____ and may be published inn scientific Journals and/or shown for scientific purpose.

I am known/not known allergic to any drug.

I agree to keep Dr _____ informed of any change of address so that he can let me know of any late findings, and I agree to cooperate with Dr _____ in the postoperative care until discharged.

I have read the above consent form/I have been explained the contents of this form in a language I understand _____
_____ and I understand the contents.

I have had sufficient opportunity to discuss my condition with Dr _____ and all my questions have been answered to my satisfaction. I have adequate knowledge on which to base an informed consent to the proposed treatment.

_____ _____
Witness **Patient**

I _____ (Relation _____) of the patient _____ have understood and been explained the contents of the above form. The patient cannot be explained as he/she is minor/is tense and cannot be explained as he/she is mentally disturbed, and I would rather sign the form.

_____ _____
Witness **Relative**

_____

Declaration

Part of the text and some images are taken with permission from M/s Jaypee Brothers Medical Publishers, New Delhi, from the chapter "Informed Consent" published in the book *Interventional Pain Management: Practical Approach* 2009 and 2018 edited by DK Baheti, Sanjay Bakshi, Sanjeeva Gupta, and RP Gehdoo.

CHAPTER 7
Protocol for Interventional Pain Management Procedures

Dwarkadas K Baheti

An interventional pain procedure stays the mainstay for the treatment protocol in relief of chronic pain and total pain management.

In the era of Internet explosion, the pain physician is accountable for his deeds while performing of the pain-relief procedure. In addition, the insurance agency needs to be satisfied of its queries before the reimbursement of the claim.

Hence, it is mandatory for a pain physician to follow a strict protocol while performing any interventional procedure. It will not only provide the safety and minimum or no morbidity but also ensure the credibility of the procedure and that of the physician.

In the present scenario of COVID-19 pandemic, many patients are anxious and concerned of COVID protocol and hospitalization for the procedures leave aside visiting hospital for consultation.

The suggested protocol is as follows:
- Assurance and safety about following of strict adherence to COVID-19 safety for patients and relatives
- Complete evaluation and documentation of pain problem, history, symptoms, signs, and investigations such as X-ray, computed tomography (CT) scan, magnetic resonance imaging (MRI), electromyography, nerve conduction study, real-time reverse transcription-polymerase chain reaction (RTPCR) and high-resolution computed tomography (HRCT) chest.
- Explain the patient and family members about the procedure details, side effects, and complications, if any.
- Obtaining of informed consent. This should be explained in the language in which the patient and his relatives understand and sign the informed consent willingly.
- Hospitalization for few hours to few days as the need be.
- Investigations such as bleeding time, clotting time, international normalized ratio (INR) ratio (if the patient is on anticoagulants), human immunodeficiency virus (HIV), Australia antigen, and RTPCR, and HRCT chest
- Interventional pain procedure should be done in either an operating room or a procedure room equipped with monitoring and resuscitation facilities.
- Preprocedure visit of Anesthesiologist and Physician for fitness
- Anesthesiologists' standby for monitoring of the patient-pulse, non-invasive blood pressure (NIBP), and oxygen saturation (SaO_2), and, if needed, sedation
- Aseptic precaution such as wearing of gown, gloves, and preparation of the area
- Radiation protection with lead apron, thyroid shield, and radiation gloves (if possible) to the pain physician and his assistant
- Radiation protection for all staff present in the procedure or the operating room.
- Radiation counter/measure monitor for pain physician and C-arm operating personnel
- Documentation in the form of printout and CD–one copy for record and one for patient
- Postprocedure monitoring of vital signs
- Follow-up advice must include:
  - Dosage and schedule of medications
  - Explain about the side effects of the drug
  - Date and time of the next visit
  - Driving instruction to the patient, if driving by himself

Additional Tips while Performing the Procedure
- Keep talking to the patient to allay the fear and anxiety.
- Follow rule of three Ds, i.e., direction, depth, and destination while doing fluoroscopy. Aim for tunnel vision (**Fig. 1**).

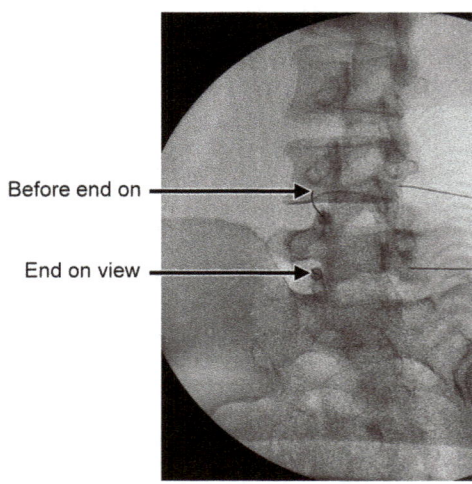

Fig. 1: Tunnel vision.

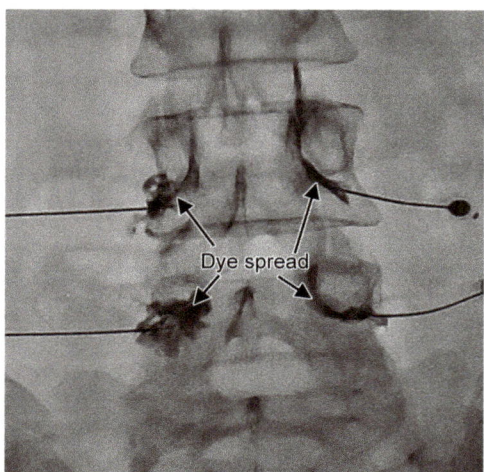

Fig. 2: Spread of dye—anteroposterior (AP) view. Transforaminal lumbar epidural showing dye in epidural space of multiple level lumbar nerve roots and outlining of pedicle.

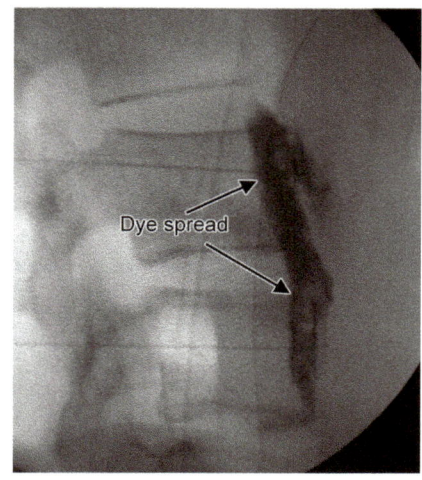

Fig. 3: Lumbar sympathetic block dye spread—lateral view.

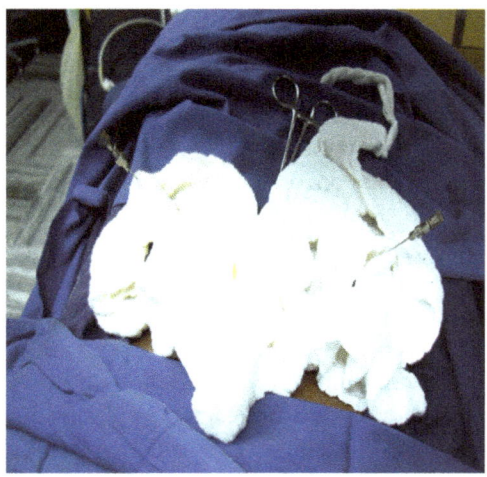

Fig. 4: Sponge around needles during celiac plexus block.

- At a regular interval, push the needle about 1 cm and confirm the direction, depth, and destination.
- Repeated negative aspiration after confirming the position of the needle, injection of dye and local anesthetic agent, steroid, and neurolytic agent
- Confirm the spread of dye **(Figs. 2 and 3)**.
- Before injecting a neurolytic agent, put a gauze piece or abdominal sponge around the needle. This will prevent spilling of the neurolytic agent on the skin and will prevent skin burns **(Fig. 4)**.
- Inject a local anesthetic agent into the track of needle while withdrawing the needle. This will reduce the postprocedure pain at the site of insertion of needles.

Declaration

Part of the text and some images are taken with permission from M/s Jaypee Brothers Medical Publishers, New Delhi, from the chapter, Protocol for Pain Management Procedures published in the book *Interventional Pain Management: Practical Approach* 2009 and 2018 edited by DK Baheti, Sanjay Bakshi, Sanjeeva Gupta, and RP Gehdoo.

CHAPTER 8

Role of Investigations for Interventional Pain Treatment Procedures

Dwarkadas K Baheti

INTRODUCTION

The history, thorough clinical examination well supported by investigations, and choice of proper interventional pain treatment procedure (IPTP) are key to pain relief. The battery of investigations provides a clue and supports the clinical judgment in a multimodal approach to total pain management in patients with chronic pain.

The following of a strict protocol provides maximum relief in pain and minimizes physiological and hemodynamic disturbances in body systems.

The IPTP is as good as any surgical procedure. So, it demands utmost care and precautions to make it safe. It can be repeated safely.

The author has highlighted the role of investigations earlier. However, it needs to be revised in the present COVID-19 pandemic and, on top of it, the complex nature of chronic pain, use of multimodal approach, possible drug interactions, and investigations before IPTP.

CLASSIFICATION OF INVESTIGATIONS

Investigations are classified as:
- Biochemical investigations
- COVID-19-related investigations
- Diagnostic investigations

Biochemical Investigations

These are mainly laboratory investigations such as:
- *Bleeding time, clotting time, and international normalized ratio:* The status of coagulation is vital as IPTP is a blind procedure, especially in patients on thrombolytic agents such as aspirin and clopidrogrel. There will be a high risk of bleeding and formation of hematoma during the passage of needle through various planes, the possibility of injury to vessel or organ cannot be ruled out.
- *Human immunodeficiency virus (HIV) and Australia antigen:* It would help to prevent the spread of HIV, Australia antigen, and other communicable diseases.
- *Complete blood count:* It will give us information about any underlying infection and anemia.
- *Serum creatinine:* It would help to know kidney function in view of use of nonsteroidal anti-inflammatory drugs (NSAIDs).

COVID-19-related Investigations

RT-PCR

RT-PCR is a brief description of the real-time reverse transcriptase-polymerase chain reaction (RT-PCR) test. It provides basic information on how this molecular biology test is used in laboratories to detect genetic material of a pathogen such as severe acute respiratory syndrome coronavirus 2 (SARS-CoV-2), the cause of COVID-19 disease.

The RT-PCR diagnostic tests can provide information on whether or not a patient has been infected with SARS-CoV-2 by detecting and measuring the virus' genetic material.

Cycle threshold (Ct) values are useful because they provide information about the patient's pathogen genetic material load (SARS-CoV-2). A low Ct value indicates high viral genomic load, whereas a high Ct value indicates low viral genomic load. Health professionals can use Ct values in conjunction with clinical symptoms and history to gauge a patient's stage of disease. Furthermore, serial C values generated from repeated testing can also help clinicians monitor the disease progression and predict stages of recovery and infection resolution. Contact tracers also utilize Ct values to prioritize their attention to patients with the highest viral genomic load, which indicates a high risk for transmissibility **(Table 1)**.

TABLE 1: Interpretation of CT values

Ct value	Indication	Interpretation
<25	High levels of SARS-CoV-2 genomic load	Patients with higher SARS-CoV-2 genomic loads are more likely to develop severe outcomes and require intubation and severe outcomes. Patient needs to be monitored.
25–30	Moderate levels of SARS-CoV-2 genomic load	
>30	Low levels of SARS-CoV-2 genomic load	Low SARS-CoV-2 genomic load can be found early in infection when viral replication has just begun.

Contd...

Contd...

Ct value	Indication	Interpretation
		Additionally, it can indicate the later phases of infection after the virus has been cleared and has left behind remnants of its genomic content. Interpretation requires clinical context.

(SARS-CoV-2: severe acute respiratory syndrome coronavirus 2)

Diagnostic Investigations

The diagnostic investigations are imaging studies, electromyography, nerve conduction studies, diskography, and thermography.

Imaging Studies

The commonly done imaging studies are plain radiography, computed tomography (CT), magnetic resonance imaging (MRI), dual-energy X-ray absorptiometry (DEXA) scan, myelography, nuclear medicine scanning (bone scan), arthrography, diskography, and thermography.

The choice of imaging modality depends upon the site of pain, type of the tissue involved and likely diagnosis; for example, a CT scan is for bony structures in trauma and related diseases and MRI for soft-tissue structures which needed more penetration.

Plain radiography lumbar spine **(Figs. 1 and 2)**: This is a commonly available, reliable, rapid, portable, and least expensive modality. It gives the information about musculoskeletal disorders including trauma, abnormality of joints, bony structure, and osteophytes.

Computed tomography: It provides information of the musculoskeletal system in comparison to plain radiography, especially for bone and joint spaces. It is an efficient, imaging-guided technique which can increase the precision of the pain procedures, to improve results and reduce the complications.

CT guidance allows exact needle positioning, avoids injury to nerve and other structures around, reduces complications, and improvises the result in celiac plexus block, cervical spine injections, and cranial nerve blocks.

High-resolution computer tomography **(Fig. 3)**: In the current COVID-19 pandemic, it is mandatory to have normal HRCT before IPTP. It is more precise than chest 2-rat in the diagnosis and monitoring of diseases of the lung tissue and the airways.

Magnetic resonance imaging **(Figs. 4 and 5)**: MRI is the modality of choice for deeper structures, degree, position, and extension of spinal cord compression due to disk protrusion and musculoskeletal and intracranial structures. The use of gadolinium contrast helps to identify early inflammatory and infectious process such as postprocedural diskitis and suspected intrathecal catheter tip granuloma. The gadolinium is iodine-free, so it scores over other agents in iodine-allergy patients.

MRI is contraindicated in ferromagnetic implants such as cardiac pacemakers, intracranial clips, or claustrophobic patients. It is mandatory to verify with the manufacturer for MRI compatibility, in patients with pacemaker or for implantation of intrathecal implants.

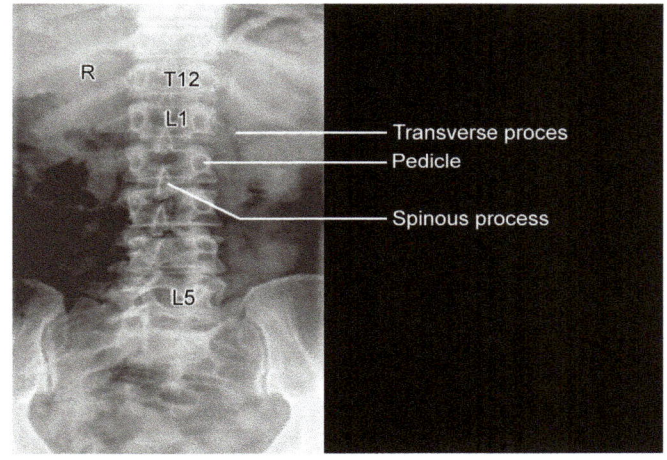

Fig. 1: Anteroposterior (AP) view of dorsolumbar spine.

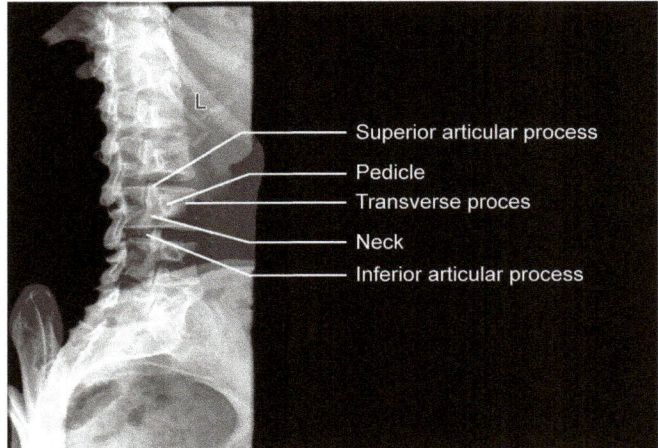

Fig. 2: Lateral view of lumbar spine.

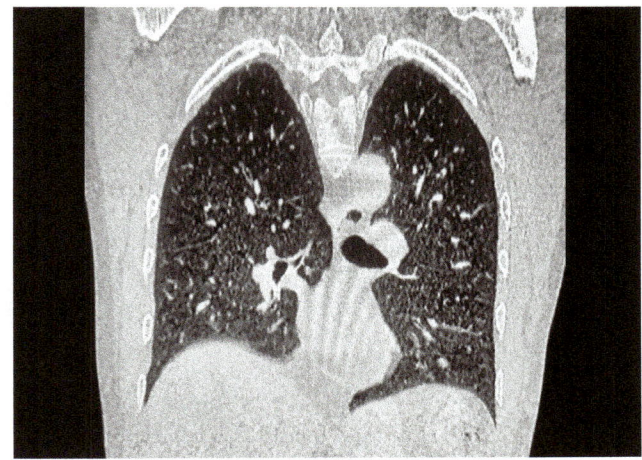

Fig. 3: Normal HRCT. (HRCT: high-resolution computed tomography)

DEXA scan: DEXA scan informs about the condition and strength of bones, which is a common cause of generalized body and musculoskeletal pain. It also provides the diagnosis of osteoporosis or osteopenia. The radiographs have low sensitivity to the changes of osteoporosis and irrespective of cause, the appearances are the same.

Osteopenia is a nonspecific and descriptive term, used for rarefaction of the skeleton as seen on radiographs. Osteoporosis is the result of prolonged, slow bone loss, and the pattern of loss is different for trabecular and cortical bone. In postmenopausal women, the annual remodeling rate is 25% for trabecular bone and 3% for cortical bone. Hence, osteoporosis is more obvious in the axial skeletons and ends of long bones where the trabecular bone is abundant. The structurally insufficient osteoporotic bone is predisposed to fractures. The cancellous bone fractures the most, with the spine being the most frequently affected site. The lifetime risk of osteoporotic fractures is estimated to be 40%, which is very close to the risk of cardiovascular disease.

Myelography: Myelography is to visualize spinal canal and thecal sac. With the advent of MRI, myelography is done in selective patients. It is indicated in the absence of an MRI facility, where MRI does not correlate with the clinical findings, and in a claustrophobic patient.

Nuclear medicine scanning: Nuclear medicine scanning (bone scan) **(Figs. 6 and 7)**: This is bone scintigraphy with technetium-99 (Tc-99) phosphate. It indicates bone turnover in bone metastases and other disorders involving bone metabolism.

Diskogram: Normal diskogram is seen in **Figure 8**. Diskography is done to confirm the back pain of diskogenic origin. Which can be the cause of pain due to disk herniation or degeneration.

It can be done in conjunction with CT and MRI. Diskography is invasive and has a risk of infection and neural injury, so it should be used as a confirmatory and not initially a diagnostic tool.

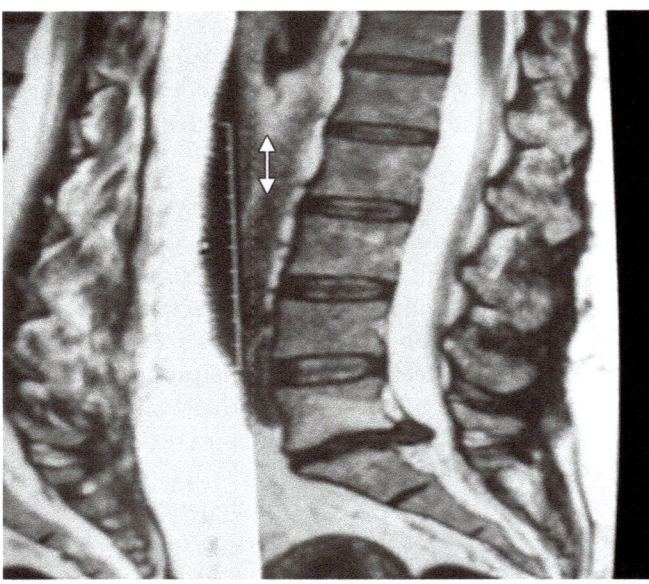

Fig. 4: Magnetic resonance imaging.

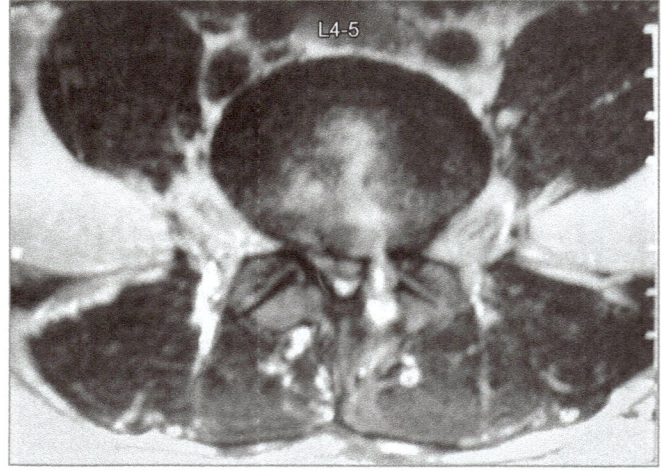

Fig. 5: Magnetic resonance imaging root disk protrusion at L5–S1 showing root compression at L4–5 nerve.

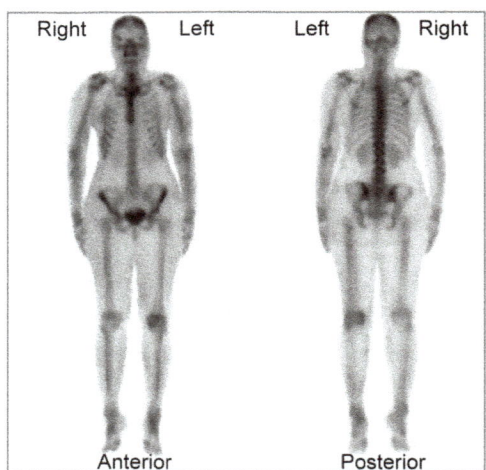

Fig. 6: Normal bone scan.

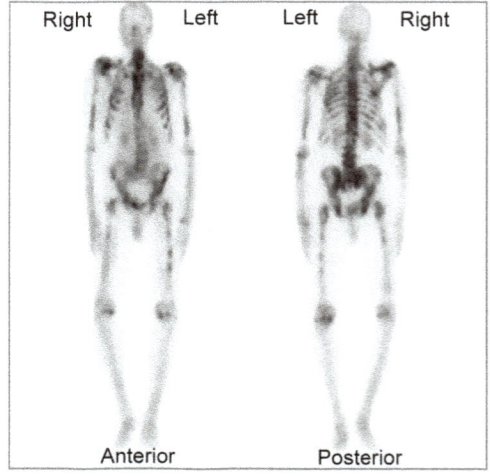

Fig. 7: Bone scan with secondaries.

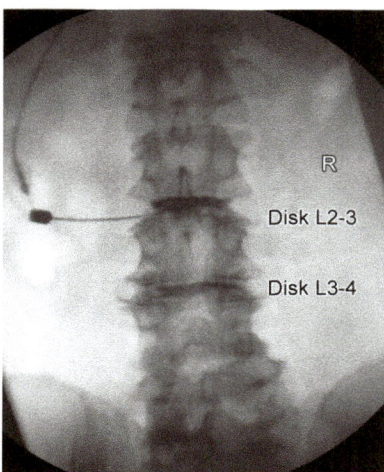

Fig. 8: Normal diskogram.

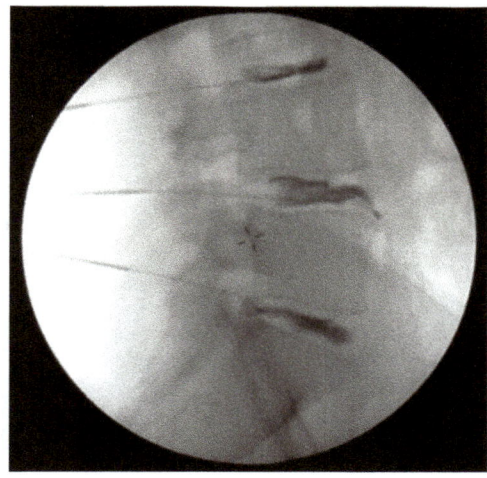

Fig. 9: Provocative diskogram.

Provocative diskogram: This is done for disk prolapse as seen in **Figure 9**. Dye leaking out confirms the disk prolapses as the possible cause of diskogenic pain.

ELECTROMYOGRAPHY AND NERVE CONDUCTION STUDIES: ELECTRO-DIAGNOSTIC STUDIES (FIGS. 10 AND 11)

Electromyography (EMG) and nerve conduction studies (NCS) are done in a patient with neurological or muscular symptoms such as shooting or burning pain, numbness, or weakness and are useful in the diagnosis of dorsal root ganglion lesion and its treatment.

In case of neuropathy, electrodiagnostic studies (EDX) will show the type—whether axonal or demyelinating, severity, and muscle involvement that may be present because of denervation of the muscle. Severe neuropathies may cause weakness. The carpel tunnel syndrome may be bilateral, with only one hand clinically involved. So, it is necessary to examine lower extremity as well as to rule out generalized neuropathy. For suspected neuropathies in tibialis anterior, EMG needle examination is recommended as it may show enervation.

To confirm radiculopathies, both EMG and NCS are necessary. As NCS may be normal, the needle EMG is diagnostic.

The temperature of extremity will significantly alter the NCS. In myasthenia gravis, antibody assays are helpful to confirm the diagnosis.

Contraindications: The contraindications for EMG studies are as follows:
- Uncooperative and unwilling patient
- Coagulopathies
- Lymph edema or anasarca
- Patient in which muscle biopsy is to be performed

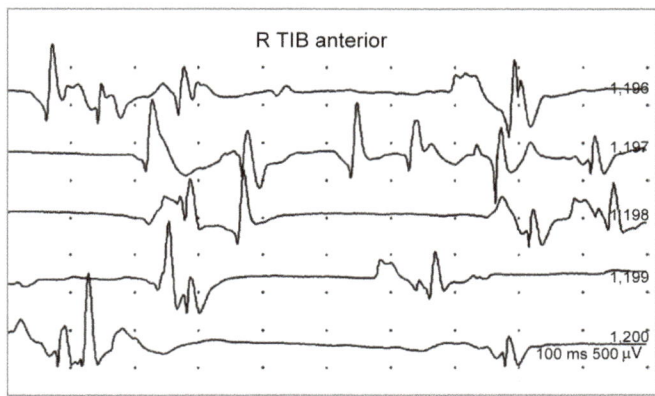

Fig. 10: Normal electromyography tracings.

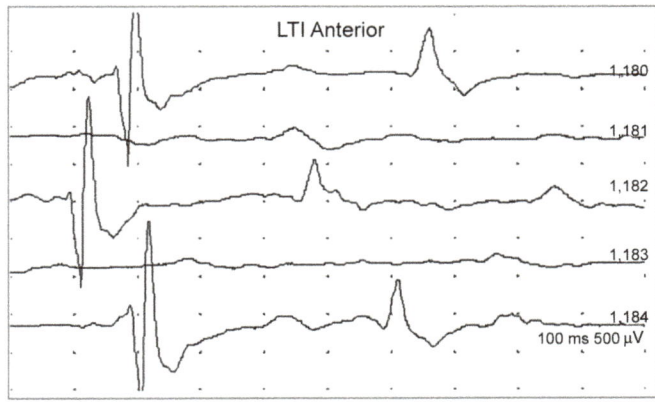

Fig. 11: Large wide triphasic units on needle electromyography of left tibialis anterior muscle in left L5 radiculopathy. (LTI: lateral trochlear inclination)

Thermography (Figs. 12 and 13)

This is a safe and noninvasive disease-screening technique that can detect abnormalities/dysfunction for the health of the whole body. The congestion, inflammation, and other conditions can be detected before any symptoms are given off by your body such as periodontal disease or infection

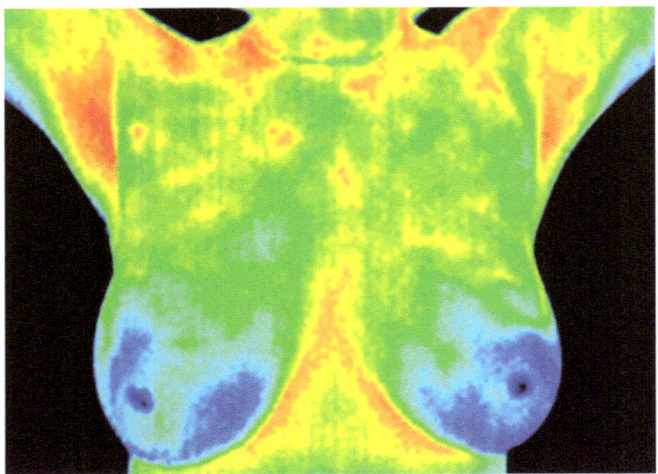

Fig. 12: Normal thermogram.

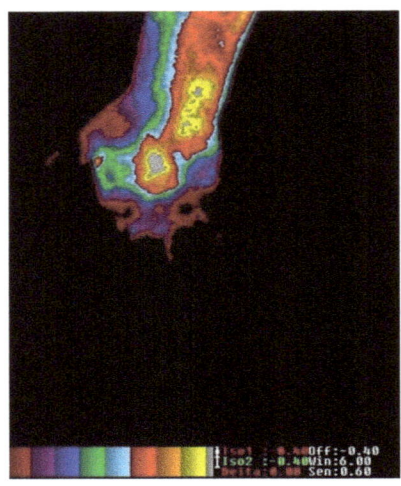

Fig. 13: Thermogram in complex regional pain syndrome.

that may go unnoticed by X-ray. It will guide a sympathetic component in sympathetically maintained pain (SMP). The qualitative data obtained reflect a quantitative temperature difference of up to 0.1°C.

The following criteria for examination room will provide precise information:
- Ambient temperature of room at 20°
- Carpeted floor
- Examination table in the center of room

The patient should wear light clothing and have not recently exercised, smoked, or taken vasoconstrictor medicines.

The clinical application of thermography is a functional test of physiology to detect autonomic nervous system and blood flow responses to evaluate the dynamic physiological changes that reflect the underlying pathology. The changes in the pattern of temperature will help in differential diagnosis of pain due to peripheral nerve injury, spinal root pathology, and complex regional pain syndrome (CRPS). For example, increase in sympathetic activity causes vasoconstriction and resultant decrease in skin temperature whereas decreased sympathetic flow causes increase in regional blood flow which results in rise in skin temperature.

Normal thermogram **(Fig. 12)** displays temperature differentials in the entire area scanned. These images reflect alterations in blood flow superficially or up to 27 mm deep.

Colder temperatures are reflected as blue to black hues and warmer temperatures as pink to red. The difference in temperature provides important diagnostic information. The mean temperature differential in peripheral nerve injury is 1.5°C.

In sympathetic dysfunctions such as reflex sympathetic dystrophy (RSD), SMP, and complex regional pain syndrome (CRPS) **(Fig. 13)**, temperature differentials ranging from 1 to 10°C depending on severity are not uncommon. Rheumatologic processes generally appear as "hot areas" with increased temperature patterns. The pathology is generally an inflammatory process, i.e., synovitis of joints and tendon sheaths, epicondylitis, capsular and muscle injuries.

Both hot and cold responses may coexist, if the pain associated with an inflammatory focus excites an increase in sympathetic activity. Also, vascular conditions are readily demonstrated by digital infrared thermal imaging (DITI) including Reynaud's disease, vasculitis, limb ischemia, deep vein thrombosis (DVT), etc.

CONCLUSION

Pain management is becoming a recognized specialty so it has added more accountability for a pain physician. The awareness amongst patients, medical fraternity, and electronic media—every step in pain relief—is vital. The complex nature of chronic pain widened the horizon of pain practice, and the accountability has become a top priority for all.

So, thorough clinical examination supported by investigations does help to know the hematological and biochemical status of patients. The detailed study and understanding of the above-mentioned investigations help in accurate diagnosis and in identifying the type of IPTP to be performed. This, in turn, will decide the safe outcome of IPTP for total pain relief.

Declaration

Part of the text and some images are taken with permission from M/s Jaypee Brothers Medical Publishers, New Delhi, from the chapter "Role of Investigations" published in the book, *Interventional Pain Management: Practical Approach* 2009 and 2018 edited by DK Baheti, Sanjay Bakshi, Sanjeeva Gupta, and RP Gehdoo.

CHAPTER 9

Medications Used for Interventional Pain Procedures

Kritika Doshi, RP Gehdoo

INTRODUCTION

Interventional pain treatment procedures are potent tools for the management of chronic pain. In acute pain, analgesic pharmacotherapy alone is adequate whereas chronic pain due to its complex pathophysiology explained by the biopsychosocial model needs multimodal polypharmacy for effective relief.

Interventional pain treatment procedures are image-guided using fluoroscopy, CT scan, ultrasound, or nerve stimulator techniques.

The common drugs used for these procedures include:
- Radiopaque contrast (dye)
- Steroid group of drugs
- Chemical neurolytic agents
- Local anesthetics

Radiopaque Contrast

Radiopaque contrast is an agent injected in the body to increase image differentiation of anatomical structures at the destination. In addition, also to confirm that contrast media or dye is not injected into the muscle or artery, intrathecally, or in any organ. It acts by increasing the differentiation between the areas containing contrast media and the areas not containing contrast media.

High Osmolar Contrast Media

These are composed of salts which dissociate in water into anions (Radiopaque) and cations (osmotically active). They have osmolality up to eight times that of serum and can be toxic if they enter the vascular compartment. They are used for the nonintravascular route—oral/rectal. They are not for use in subarachnoid space. For example, gastrografin, urografin, and isteropac.

Where is it Needed?
It is useful to exclude intravascular or intrathecal injection and to delineate anatomy as in sacroiliac joints, epidural spaces, sympathetic blocks, discography, etc.

TYPES OF CONTRAST AGENTS (FLOWCHART 1)

Negative Contrast

Negative contrast agents are so named as they yield a lower contrast than body tissues while positive contrast yields a higher attenuation compared to body tissues.

Iodinated Contrast Media

Iodinated contrast media are contrast agents that contain iodine atoms **(Flowchart 2)**. Under fluoroscopy, the image contrast depends upon Compton scattering and photoelectric absorption. As iodine has a high atomic number-53, compared to most tissues in the body, the administration of

Flowchart 1: Types of contrast agents.

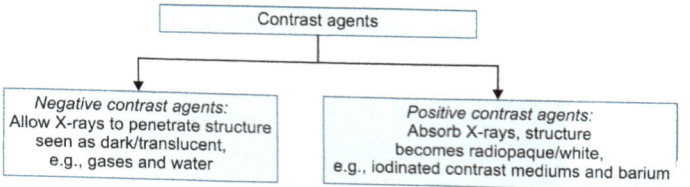

Flowchart 2: Iodinated contrast media.

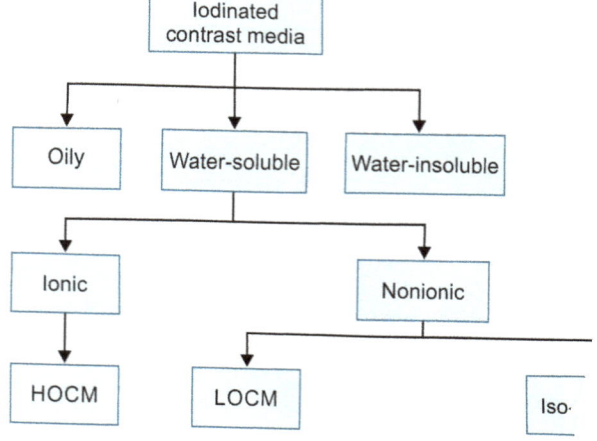

(HOCM: high osmolar contrast media; LOCM: low osmolality cor

iodinated material produces image contrast due to differential photoelectric absorption.

First generation: Iodinated-tri-iodinated benzoate anion **(Fig. 1)**.
- Limited by high osmolar concentration
- Up to 8 × physiologic level
- Higher osmolality → toxicity (hemodynamic and discomfort)

For interventional procedures, nonionic low osmolality contrast media (LOCM) are used. LOCM are nondissociating with only 2 × serum osmolality, have less side effects, and are less nephrotoxic, e.g., Ultravist, Omnipaque **(Fig. 2)**.

Nonionic LOCM are available in varying concentrations ranging from 240 to 400 mg/mL iodine.

The LOCM are usually named as "Name + number" where the name is the iodinated particle and the number is the concentration of the iodinated particle. For example, Omnipaque 180 = 180 mg/mL of iodine **(Figs. 3A and B)**. The recommended daily limit is 3 g/day.

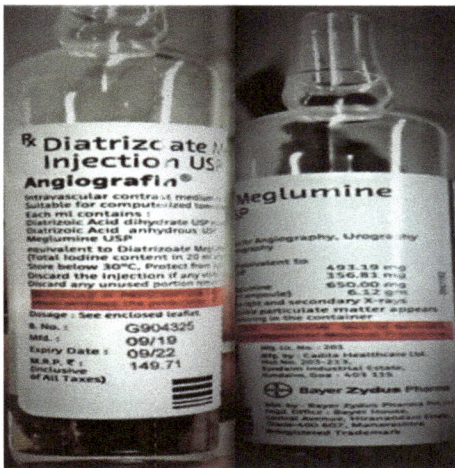

Fig. 1: Ionic contrast media.

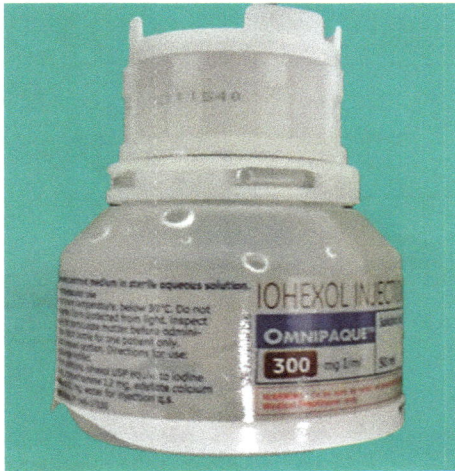

Fig. 2: Iohexol (Omnipaque -300).

Adverse reactions: About 90% of the adverse reactions occur within 15 minutes (recommended observation 30–60 minutes postprocedure). It is essential to have resuscitation equipment and drugs available before the start of the procedure.

The incidence of adverse reactions is higher with ionic agents. Most common adverse reactions include headache, nausea, and vomiting. Allergic reactions include vasomotor, cutaneous responses; bronchospasm; cardiovascular collapse; and vasovagal and anaphylactoid reactions.

Chemotoxic reactions may present as nephrotoxicity, arrythmias and rarely as thyrotoxicosis.

The hyperosmolality may cause erythrocyte damage, endothelial damage, thrombosis, vasodilation, hypervolemia, and cardiac depression.

Renal toxicity is seen with ionic agents and in patients with poorly controlled diabetes mellitus, dehydration/pre-renal azotemia, and chronic renal disease.

The following patients are at high risk for adverse reactions and need to be carefully evaluated:
- Proven/suspected hypersensitivity to iodine
- Previous severe reaction to contrast media
- Asthma/significant allergy history
- Heart disease
- Infants/children/elderly
- Liver failure
- Renal impairment (moderate-to-severe)—non-insulin dependent diabetes mellitus (NIDDM) on metformin
- Myelomatosis
- Poor hydration
- Sickle cell anemia
- Thyrotoxicosis
- Pregnancy
- Pheochromocytoma

Steroids or Glucocorticoids

In chronic pain, glucocorticoids are used to influence inflammatory and immune processes but they can also affect carbohydrate, protein, and fat metabolism.

They are normally produced by adrenal cortex (hydrocortisone, cortisol), are immunosuppressive, and possess

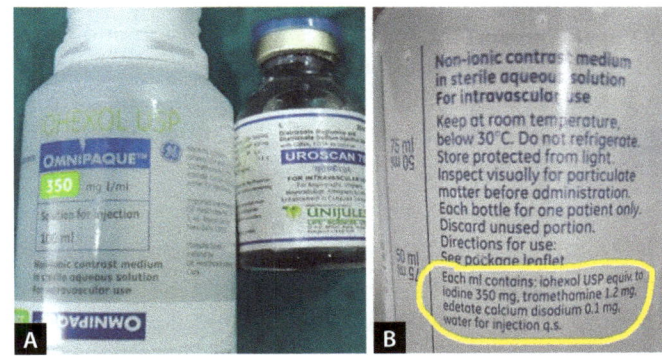

Figs. 3A and B: (A) Omnipaque-350 or uroscan; (B) Label indicating iodine content.

anti-inflammatory action against radiation, mechanical, chemical, infective, and immunologic stimuli.

The mechanisms of action are as follows:
- Inhibiting leukocyte function
- Has a weak local anesthetic action (by local membrane depolarization)
- Influences the activity of dorsal horn cells
- Reduces ectopic discharge from neuromas

Steroids can be divided as particulate or nonparticulate and short acting or long acting **(Fig. 4)**.

There are different types of steroids available as described in **Table 1**.

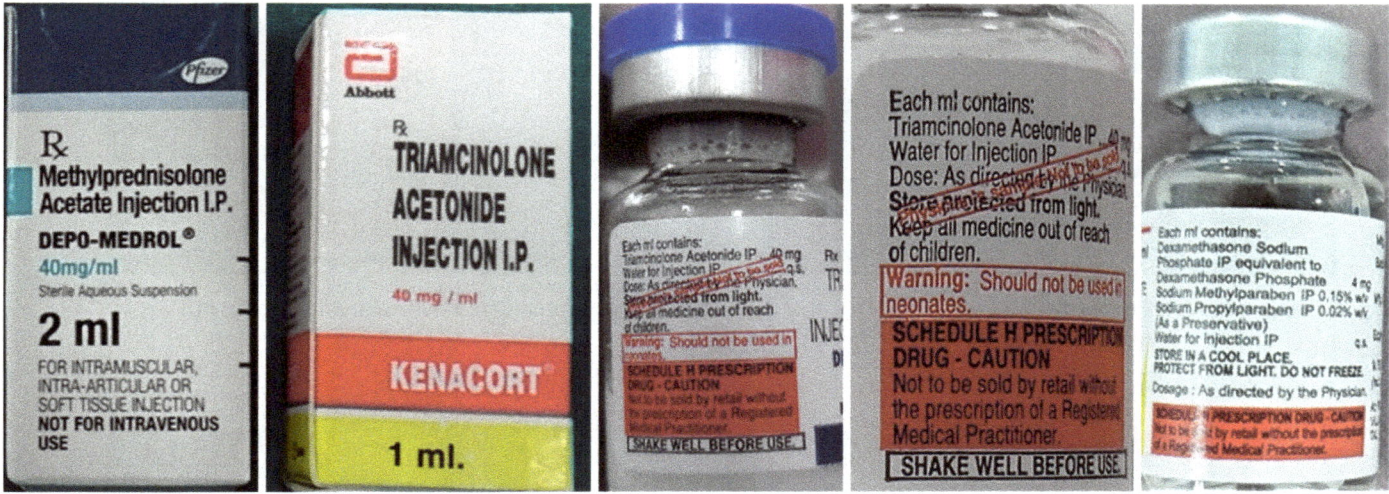

Fig. 4: Types of steroids—particulate (Methylprednisolone, Triamcinolone) and nonparticulate (Dexamethasone).

TABLE 1: Types of steroid agents—dosage and duration of action.				
Agent	Half-life (hr)/duration of action	Anti-inflammatory potency	Salt-retaining potency	Dose
Hydrocortisone	8–12 Short	1	1	
Triamcinolone (Particulate)	12–36 Long	5	0	40–80 mg
Methylprednisolone (Particulate)	12–36 Long	5	0.5	40–80 mg
Dexamethasone (Nonparticulate)	36–72 Long	25	0	4–8 mg

Local Anesthetics

Local anesthetics are commonly used for regional anesthesia techniques. Single-use ampoules as well as multidose vials are available. The multidose vials contain preservatives to prolong the shelf life. For interventional pain procedures, it is advisable to always use preservative-free local anesthetic as toxicity is related to additives. Though "multiuse vials" are a cost-saving method (preservative is added to prolong shelf life), bacterial contamination is common (despite the preservative). They usually contain methylparaben as a preservative, which is neurotoxic. Severe neurotoxicity has been reported when methylparaben has been given epidurally or spinally.

Usual Agents: Preservative Free

- Lignocaine **(Fig. 5)**—short duration of action 2–4 hours
- Bupivacaine intermediate duration of action 2–6 hours
- Ropivacaine **(Fig. 6)**—long duration of action 3–24 hours

Others

- *Adjuvants:* Fentanyl, ketamine, clonidine **(Fig. 7)**, midazolam
- *Hyaluronidase:* Used for epidural adhesiolysis; freeze-dried powder which is reconstituted just before use **(Fig. 8)**.
- *Opiates:* Morphine

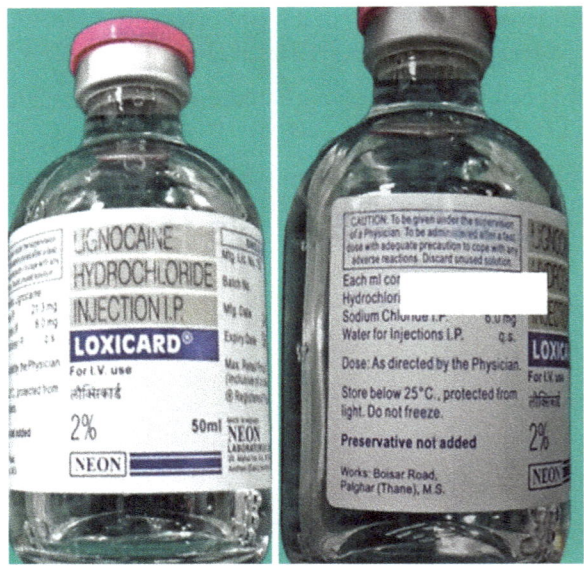

Fig. 5: Preservative-free lignocaine.

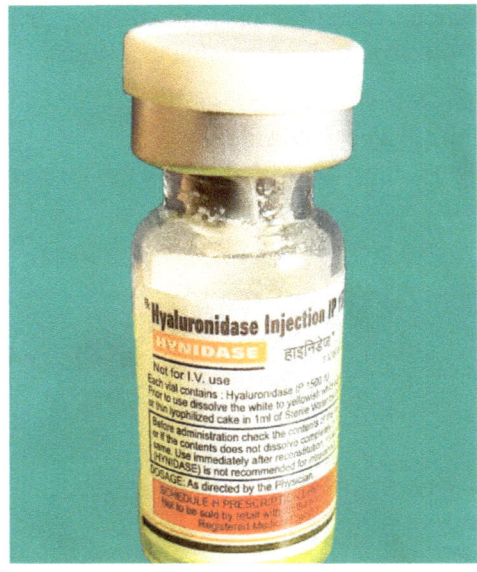

Fig. 8: Hyaluronidase 1,500 international units (IU) vial.

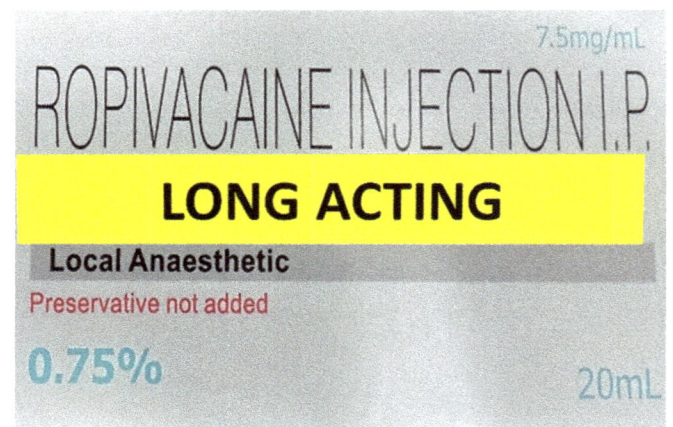

Fig. 6: Ropivacaine 0.75%.

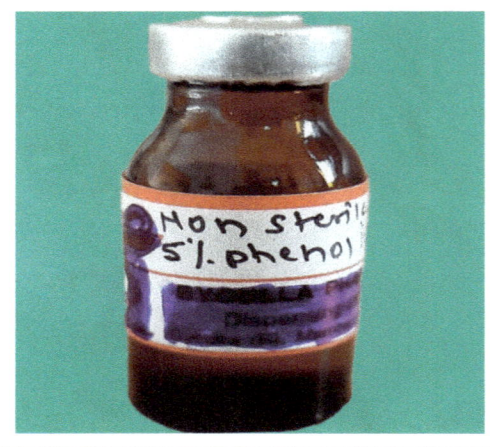

Fig. 9: Phenol in glycerine.

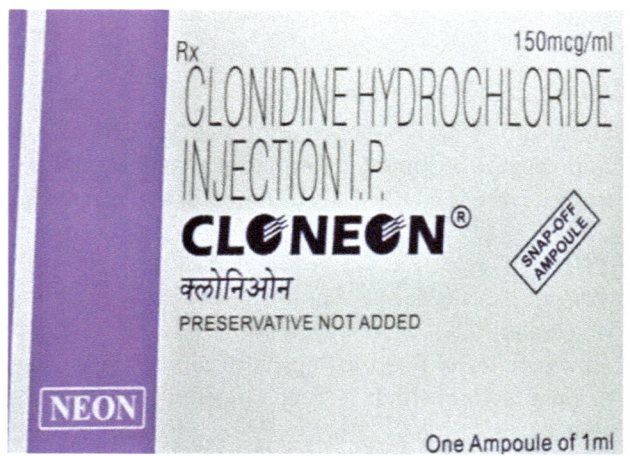

Fig. 7: Clonidine 150 µg.

Neurolytic Agents

Chemical neurolyses are indicated for prolonged interruption of pain pathway. They are cheap, easily available, and, in a country like India, a very useful option. Some of the agents used are phenol, ethyl alcohol, hypertonic saline, and glycerol (which has a special application in trigeminal neuralgia cases).

- *Ethyl alcohol:* It is colorless and hypobaric compared to cerebrospinal fluid (CSF). Use of absolute or 99% alcohol leads to complete denervation. A 33% alcohol concentration gives analgesia without any motor paralysis. It is a local irritant and can produce burning or dysesthesias. Hence, the injection of alcohol is preceded by injecting local anesthetic solution.

CHAPTER 9

Medications Used for Interventional Pain Procedures

Kritika Doshi, RP Gehdoo

INTRODUCTION

Interventional pain treatment procedures are potent tools for the management of chronic pain. In acute pain, analgesic pharmacotherapy alone is adequate whereas chronic pain due to its complex pathophysiology explained by the biopsychosocial model needs multimodal polypharmacy for effective relief.

Interventional pain treatment procedures are image-guided using fluoroscopy, CT scan, ultrasound, or nerve stimulator techniques.

The common drugs used for these procedures include:
- Radiopaque contrast (dye)
- Steroid group of drugs
- Chemical neurolytic agents
- Local anesthetics

Radiopaque Contrast

Radiopaque contrast is an agent injected in the body to increase image differentiation of anatomical structures at the destination. In addition, also to confirm that contrast media or dye is not injected into the muscle or artery, intrathecally, or in any organ. It acts by increasing the differentiation between the areas containing contrast media and the areas not containing contrast media.

High Osmolar Contrast Media

These are composed of salts which dissociate in water into anions (Radiopaque) and cations (osmotically active). They have osmolality up to eight times that of serum and can be toxic if they enter the vascular compartment. They are used for the nonintravascular route—oral/rectal. They are not for use in subarachnoid space. For example, gastrografin, urografin, and isteropac.

Where is it Needed?
It is useful to exclude intravascular or intrathecal injection and to delineate anatomy as in sacroiliac joints, epidural spaces, sympathetic blocks, discography, etc.

TYPES OF CONTRAST AGENTS (FLOWCHART 1)

Negative Contrast

Negative contrast agents are so named as they yield a lower contrast than body tissues while positive contrast yields a higher attenuation compared to body tissues.

Iodinated Contrast Media

Iodinated contrast media are contrast agents that contain iodine atoms **(Flowchart 2)**. Under fluoroscopy, the image contrast depends upon Compton scattering and photoelectric absorption. As iodine has a high atomic number-53, compared to most tissues in the body, the administration of

Flowchart 1: Types of contrast agents.

```
                    Contrast agents
                    /             \
Negative contrast agents:        Positive contrast agents:
Allow X-rays to penetrate        Absorb X-rays, structure
structure seen as                becomes radiopaque/white,
dark/translucent,                e.g., iodinated contrast
e.g., gases and water            mediums and barium
```

Flowchart 2: Iodinated contrast media.

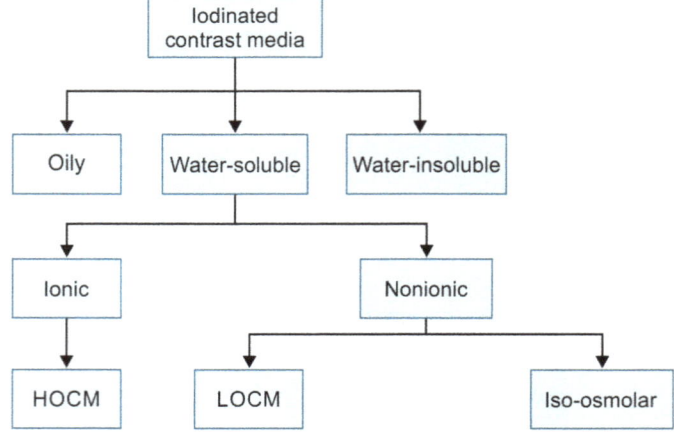

(HOCM: high osmolar contrast media; LOCM: low osmolality contrast media)

The alcohol acts by precipitating the cell membrane proteins, extracts lipid compounds, and results in demyelination and Wallerian degeneration. After subarachnoid injection of the rootlets, there may be mild meningeal inflammation and demyelination of post columns and dorsal roots.

- *Phenol or carbolic acid:* This is a combination of carbolic acid, phenic acid, phenylic acid, phenyl hydroxide, hydroxybenzene, and oxybenzene. It is not available commercially and has to be freshly prepared. It is soluble in alcohol, glycerol, and dye, and this is used to visualize the drug spread under fluoroscopy. It is usually mixed with glycerine forming a hyperbaric and viscous liquid which turns red on exposure to air. The concentration used is 6–10%. Solution >1% produces local anesthesia without risk of toxicity or neurolysis. Concentrations up to <5% cause protein denaturation; a 5–6% solution results in Wallerian degeneration. Concentrations >6% cause axon abnormalities, nerve root damage, spinal cord infarcts, arachnoiditis, and meningitis and are toxic. The block is less intense and has a shorter duration compared to alcohol **(Fig. 9)**.

SECTION 2

Head and Neck

- **Trigeminal Nerve Block**
  Hemkumar Pushparaj, Manohar Sharma

- **Percutaneous Cervical Cordotomy**
  Manohar Sharma, Hemkumar Pushparaj

CHAPTER 10

Trigeminal Nerve Block

Hemkumar Pushparaj, Manohar Sharma

INTRODUCTION

Glycerol gangliolysis, radiofrequency (RF) rhizotomy, and percutaneous balloon compression (PBC) of the gasserian ganglion (GG) are the minimally invasive interventions performed in trigeminal neuralgia (TN) which are pharmacologically refractory. PBC and RF are the most commonly used techniques.

Percutaneous balloon compression is preferred in the author's practice due to better outcomes and selective damage to the large myelinated fibers, thus preserving corneal reflex.

This chapter focusses primarily on fluoroscopy-guided PBC for TN.

TABLE 1: Characteristics of the trigeminal nerve.

Characteristics	Trigeminal neuralgia
Location	Mostly unilateral. Usually V2 and V3 areas
Quality	Intense, sharp, and shooting
Episodes	Few seconds to 2 minutes with refractory period between episodes
Provoked by	Brushing teeth, speaking, eating, chewing, and cold wind over face
Pain-free intervals	Weeks to months
Examination	No neurological deficit
Associated symptoms	Facial flushing

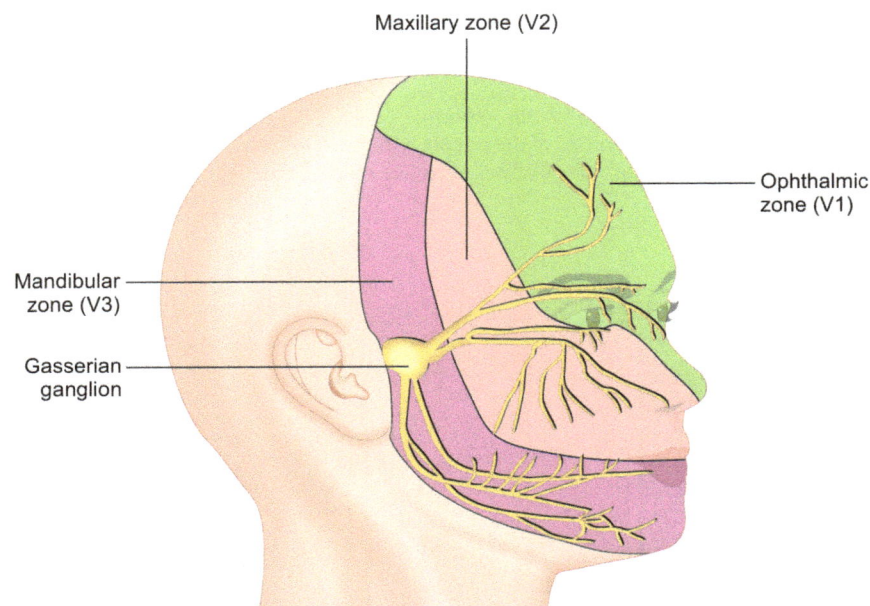

Fig. 1: Sensory innervation of trigeminal nerve.
Source: BruceBlaus, CC BY-SA 4.0 <https://creativecommons.org/licenses/by-sa/4.0>, via Wikimedia Commons) and patient characteristics of trigeminal neuralgia (TN).

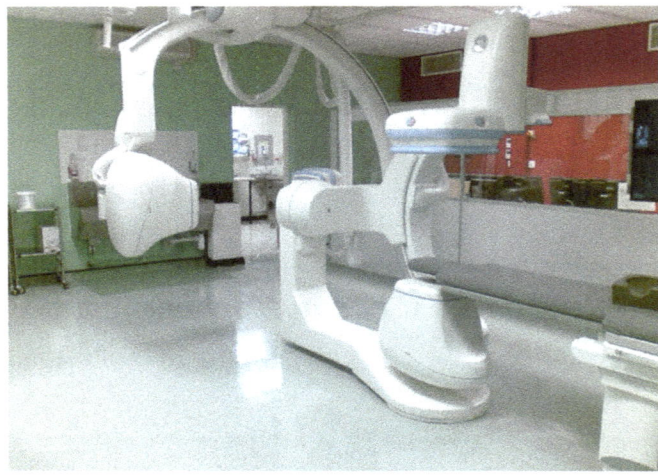

Fig. 2: Bipolar fluoroscope. Biplanar fluoroscopy is preferred by authors for ease of technique and real-time guidance into two planes—lateral and modified submental oblique views. The technique can be performed using a uniplanar fluoroscope as well, but exact angles of orientation should be noted to repeatedly change viewing planes.

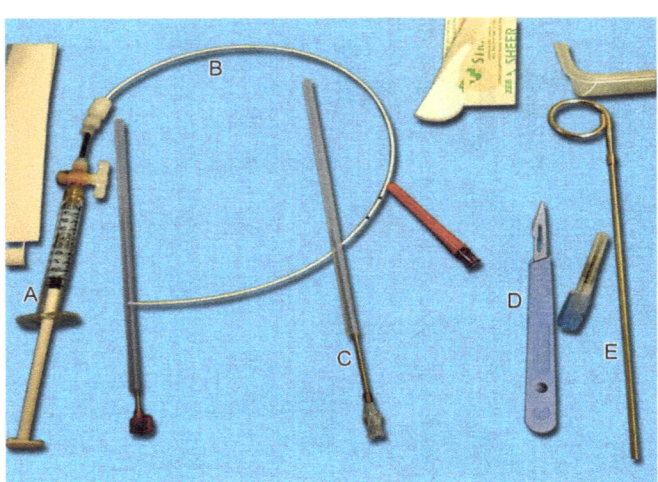

Fig. 3: Equipment for trigeminal percutaneous balloon compression. A—1 mL tuberculin syringe loaded with water-soluble contrast (Omnipaque 300), B—4 Fr (40 cm) Fogarty catheter, C—14 G (10 cm) needle to access foramen ovale (FO), D—Scalpel for skin incision at needle entry site, E—Radiopaque pointer.

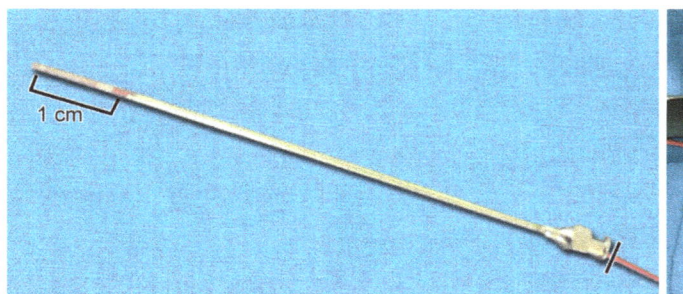
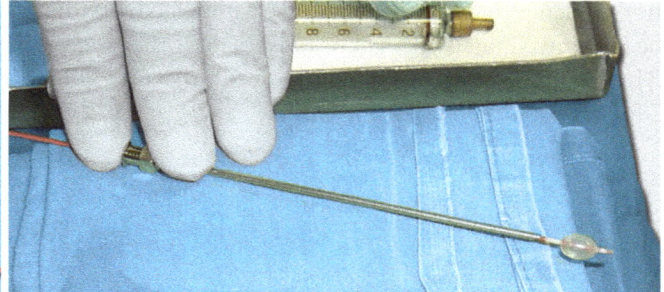

Fig. 4: *Step 1:* Check and mark the Fogarty catheter prior to intervention.
Note: The tip of the catheter is passed 1 cm ahead of the tip of the needle and the length at the proximal end of needle is marked for reference later. Catheter balloon is inflated to de-air and confirm integrity. The procedure might be ineffective if the Gasserian ganglion (GG) is compressed with air in the balloon.

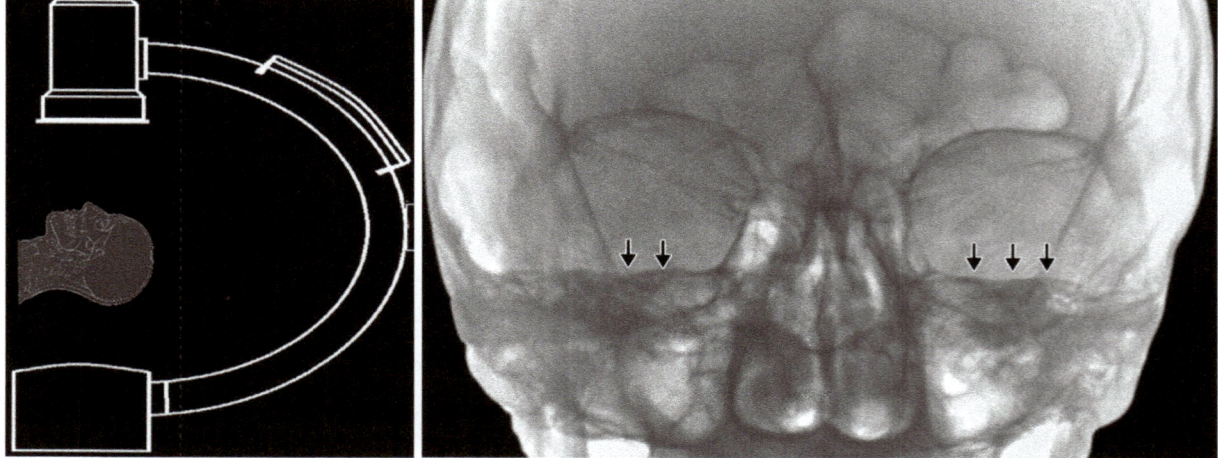

Fig. 5: *Step 2.1:* Positioning the fluoroscope is of prime importance. Straight posteroanterior (PA) projection is obtained with the petrous ridge seen through the orbit.
Source: ©Nevit Dilmen, CC BY-SA 3.0 (<https://creativecommons.org/licenses/by-sa/3.0>, via Wikimedia Commons).

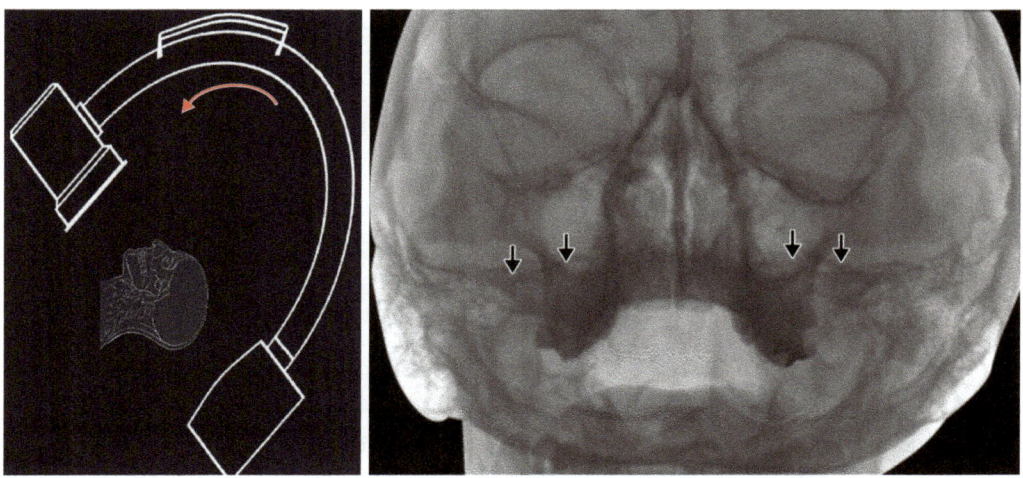

Fig. 6: *Step 2.2:* The fluoroscope is then tilted caudad (to about 40°) to see the superior border of petrous ridge projected at inferior border of the maxillary sinus.

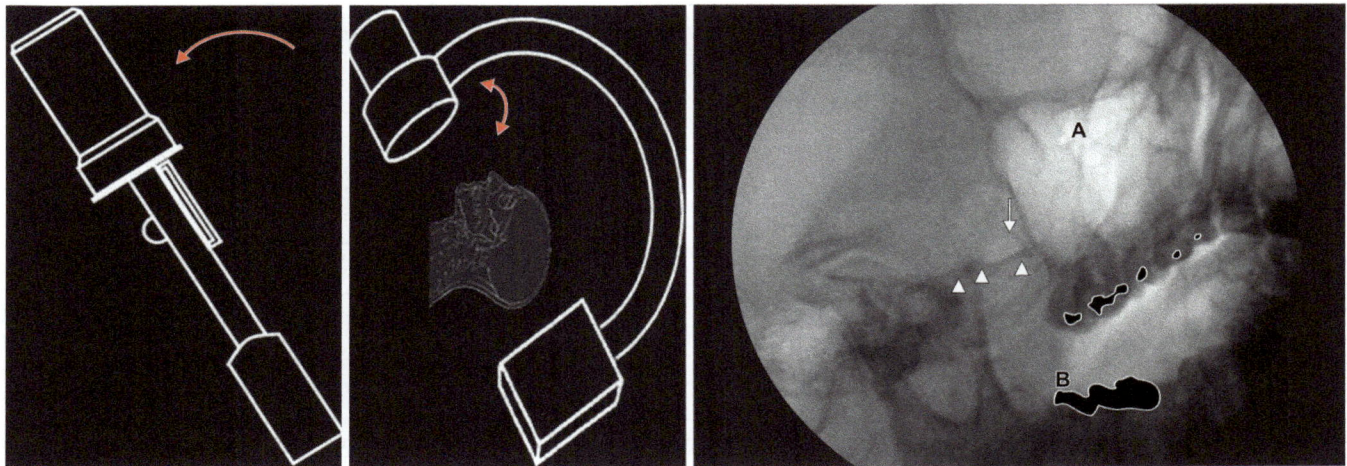

Fig. 7: *Step 2.3:* Ipsilateral oblique tilt is then performed by 10–25° to visualize the petrous ridge below maxillary sinus (A) and above the jawline (B) White pointer—petrous ridge, white arrow—foramen ovale (FO). Only minimal movement in sagittal plane is required to visualize the FO. This modified submental view is best to visualize FO.

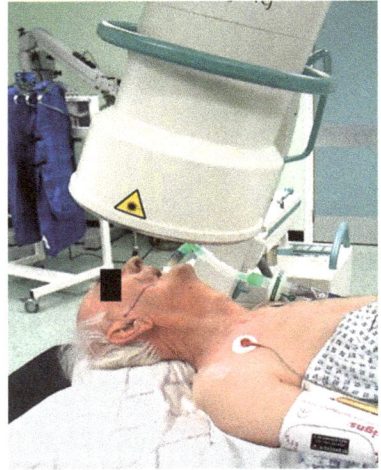

Fig. 8: *Step 3:* The procedure is performed under general anesthesia in our center to minimize patient discomfort. Brief intense pain is common during balloon compression. Patient positioned supine with head in neutral position. Note the position of the fluoroscope in modified submental view.

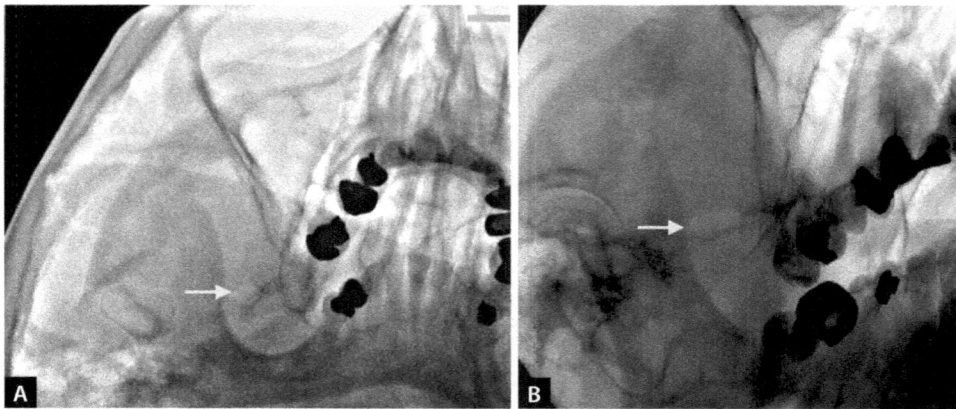

Figs. 9A and B: Increased caudal tilt changes the orientation of foramen ovale to a circle (A) whereas cephalad tilt makes the foramen flat-like a slit (B). A flatter/elliptical orientation is preferred rather than circular as a coaxially oriented needle would be directed to the floor of middle cranial fossa in increased caudal orientation.

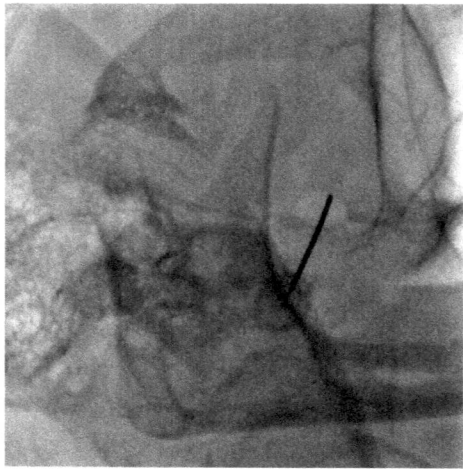

Fig. 10: *Step 4:* After anesthetizing the skin with local anesthetic, the needle is inserted in a perfectly coaxial technique. Note that the needle should be aimed to the middle or medial aspect of the foramen ovale. Lateral insertion will lead to direct access to the temporal lobe in middle cranial fossa.

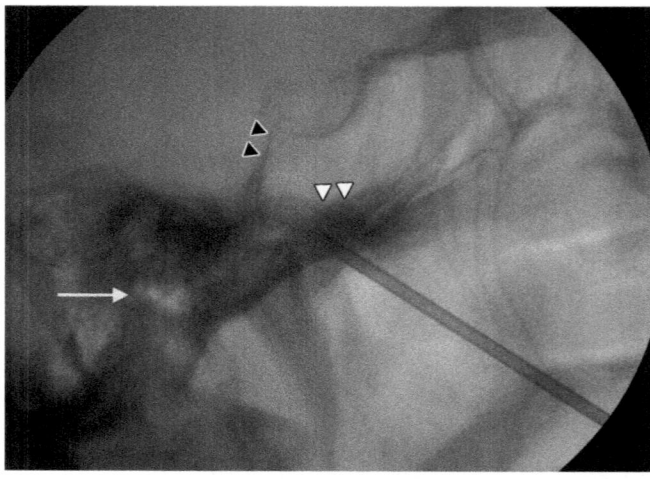

Fig. 11: *Step 5:* Once the needle is engaged, a lateral image should be taken showing the needle at the entry of foramen ovale (FO). Note that the needle is placed at the entry of FO. Further insertion might be needed but never beyond intersection of petrous ridge (white pointer) and clivus (black pointer). A true lateral view is attained when both external auditory meatus (arrow) are superimposed on each other without parallax.

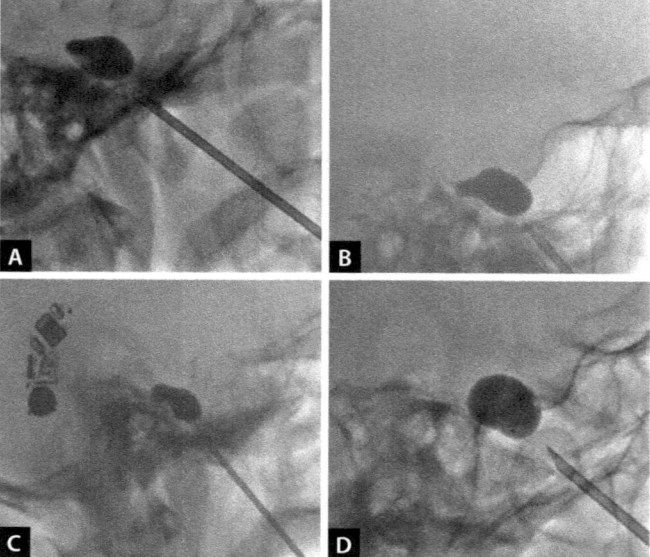

Figs. 12A to D: *Step 6:* Fogarty catheter is inserted up to the predetermined mark on the catheter. Slow expansion with the contrast should show a pear-shaped balloon (A and B) on lateral fluoroscopy imaging. An hourglass shape (C) of balloon denotes posterior placement into posterior cranial fossa whereas a circular/cylindrical shape (D) denotes extracisternal location of the balloon.

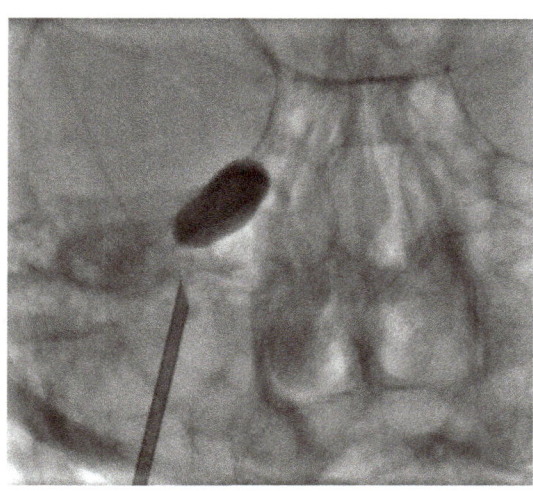

Fig. 13: *Step 7:* Posteroanterior image should show medial projection of the expanded balloon. After the procedure, needle and Fogarty catheter are withdrawn as a whole.

CLINICAL PEARLS

- General anesthesia is preferred to minimize patient discomfort.
- Balloon is inflated and deflated multiple times during the procedure. In the author's practice, usually three inflations are performed depending on the hemodynamic changes.
- Balloon is always inflated with contrast agent to visualize the shape of balloon.
- The duration of each inflation differs between different physicians. The authors inflate the balloon for 60 seconds and deflate in between inflations for 30 seconds.
- Ideally, a pear-shaped balloon is aimed for to confirm correct placement. In case of an "hourglass shape", the balloon is to be inflated at full capacity and withdrawn until a classical pear-shape is attained **(Fig. 12)**. Some traction might be needed to prevent it from herniating into the cerebellopontine angle.

FURTHER READING

1. Brown JA, McDaniel MD, Weaver MT. Percutaneous trigeminal nerve compression for treatment of trigeminal neuralgia: results in 50 patients. Neurosurgery. 1993;32(4):570-3.
2. De Córdoba JL, García Bach M, Isach N, Piles S. Percutaneous balloon compression for trigeminal neuralgia: imaging and technical aspects. Reg Anesth Pain Med. 2015;40(5):616-22.
3. Lichtor T, Mullan JF. A 10-year follow-up review of percutaneous microcompression of the trigeminal ganglion. J Neurosurg. 1990;72(1):49-54.
4. Mullan S, Lichtor T. Percutaneous microcompression of the trigeminal ganglion for trigeminal neuralgia. J Neurosurg. 1983;59:1007-12.
5. Tatli M, Satici O, Kanpolat Y, Sindou M. Various surgical modalities for trigeminal neuralgia: literature study of respective long-term outcomes. Acta Neurochirurgica. 2008; 150(3):243-55.

CHAPTER 11

Percutaneous Cervical Cordotomy

Manohar Sharma, Hemkumar Pushparaj

INTRODUCTION

There is a growing interest in percutaneous cervical cordotomy (PCC) as an effective pain-relief procedure because of an expected increase in mesothelioma cases and its role in otherwise difficult-to-control cancer pain in a small number of cases. Various publications have recommended access to cordotomy services for selected indications in difficult-to-manage cancer pain syndromes. Cordotomy is very effective for unilateral, medically refractory cancer pain below the 4th cervical dermatome. Essentially, cervical cordotomy means radiofrequency ablation of spinothalamic tracts on the side contralateral to the pain. There are several techniques described in literature, but this chapter will focus on the fluoroscopic method as this is practiced routinely by the authors.

PRACTICAL IMPLICATIONS OF SOMATOTOPY KNOWLEDGE FOR PREFORMING CORDOTOMY

- Cervical segments are ventral and medial in the anterior spinal quadrant.
- Sacral segments are posterior and lateral in the anterior spinal quadrant.
- Test with cold and with pinprick because of the possibility of dissociation of spinothalamic tract.
- With sacral segments, there is less distance to the tractus corticospinalis to lesion from surface of spinal cord.
- Spinal cord is mobile and this means that once the probe enters the cord, it may retract over the probe meaning you may end up slightly deeper in the spinal cord.

RADIOFREQUENCY LESIONING TIPS

- 75°C, 20–25 seconds each lesion
- Incremental lesion
- Check motor power (use to raise arm and leg)
- Check loss of spinothalamic sensation (temperature, pinprick)
- Check pain levels (incident pain)
- Increase up to 90°C if needed but titrate according to pain relief and sensory testing.
- Mirror pain with overzealous lesioning.
- Adjust probe position if unsure and repeat.

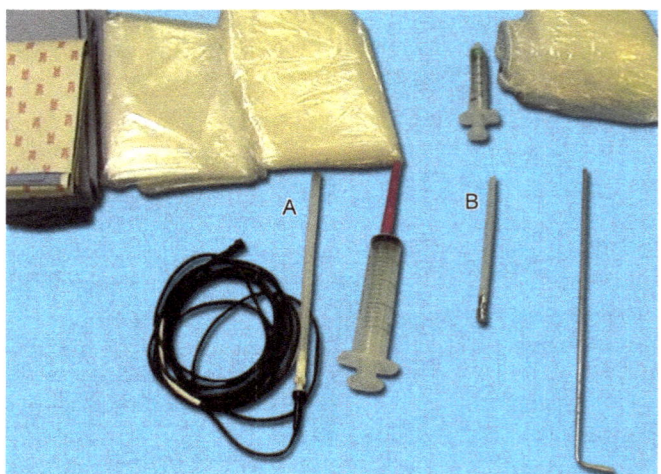

Fig. 1: Preparation for cervical cordotomy (A—cordotomy probe with 2 mm active tip; B—spinal needle).

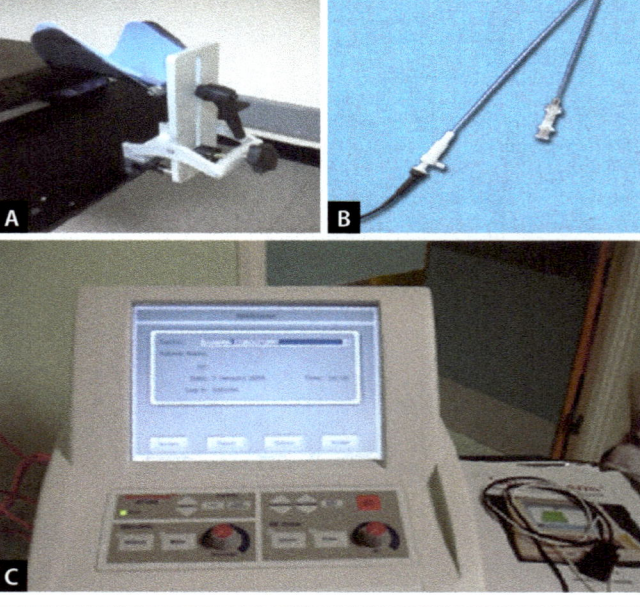

Figs. 2A to C: Images of equipment needed for cervical cordotomy. (A) Head rest; (B) Cordotomy probe; (C) Radiofrequency machine with cordotomy lesion settings.

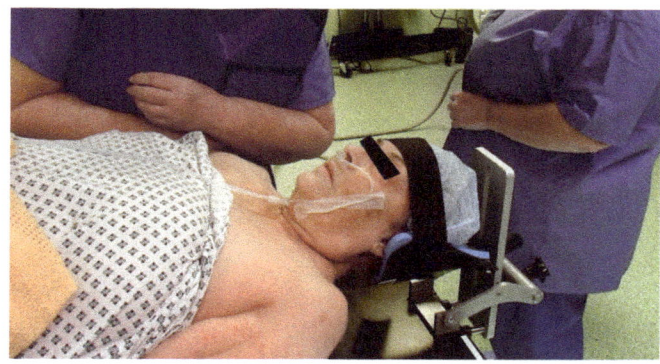

Fig. 3: Patient position on cordotomy head rest. Note position of nasal cannula to avoid image artifact in C1–2 areas.

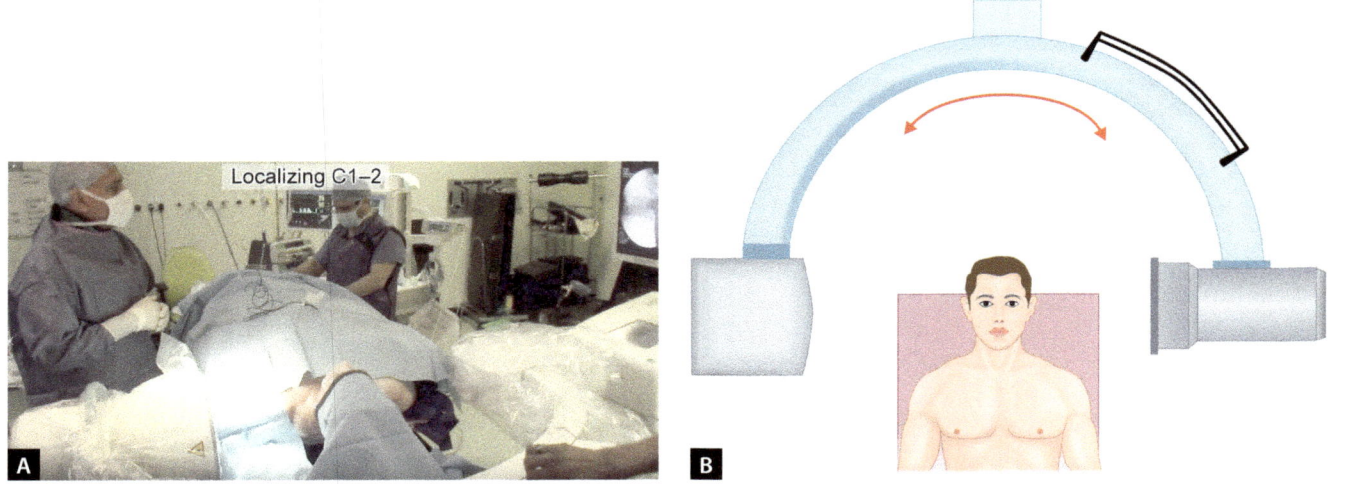

Figs. 4A and B: C-arm positioning for imaging through C1–2 foramen. C-arm can be adjusted in the coronal plane to obtain a true lateral image.

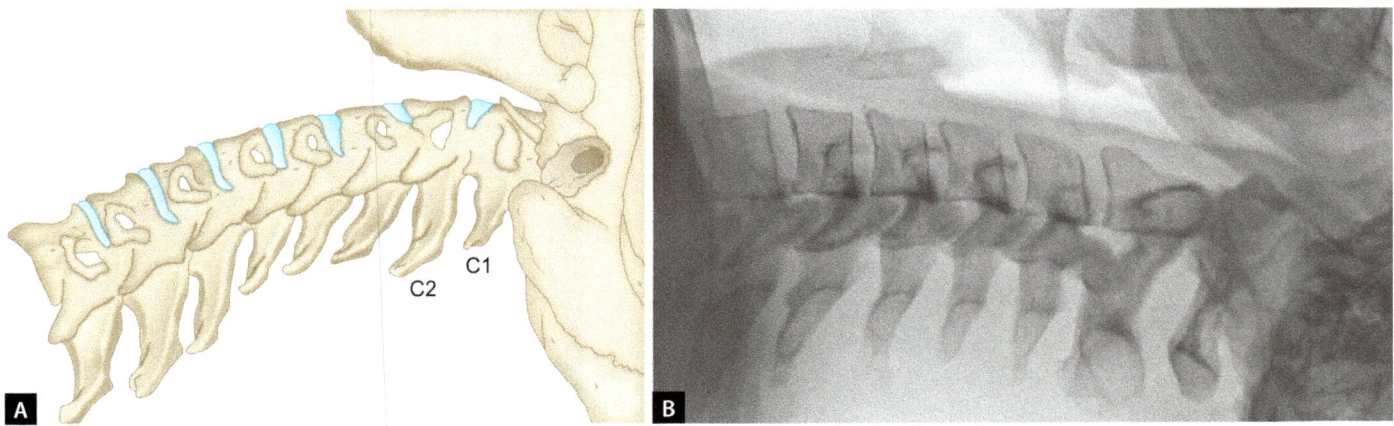

Figs. 5A and B: Lateral image of cervical spine showing C1, 2 cervical spine. Note a fairly good lateral image—transverse process over superior-posterior part of the vertebral body, minimal to no parallax of articular process.
Source: Patrick J Lynch, Medical Illustrator, CC BY 2.5 <https://creativecommons.org/licenses/by/2.5>, Hellerhoff, CC BY-SA 3.0 <https://creativecommons.org/licenses/by-sa/3.0>.

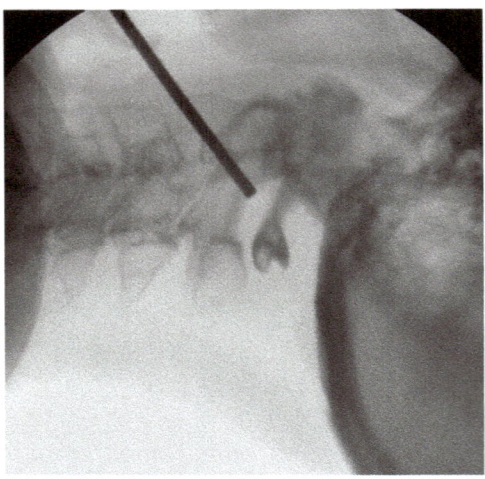

Fig. 6: Localizing the needle entry point on the skin.

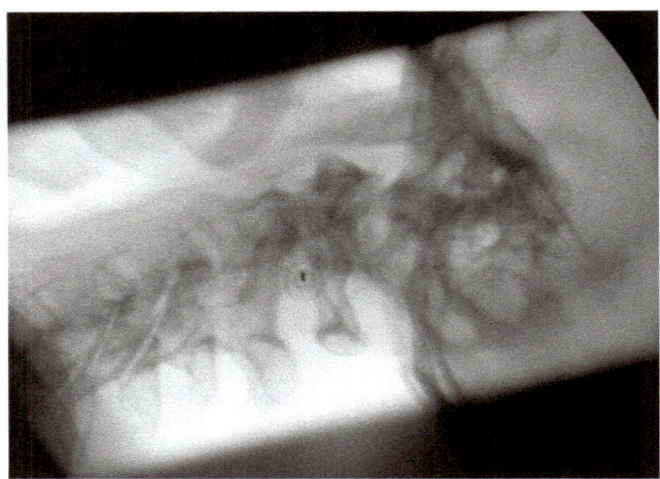

Fig. 7: Note the needle in good location but C1/2 end plates not squared (It can be squared by adjusting C-arm craniocaudal tilt).

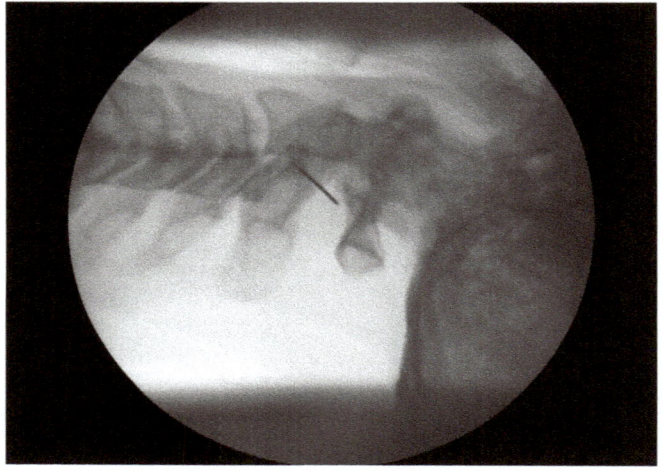

Fig. 8: Needle in the C1–2 foramen.

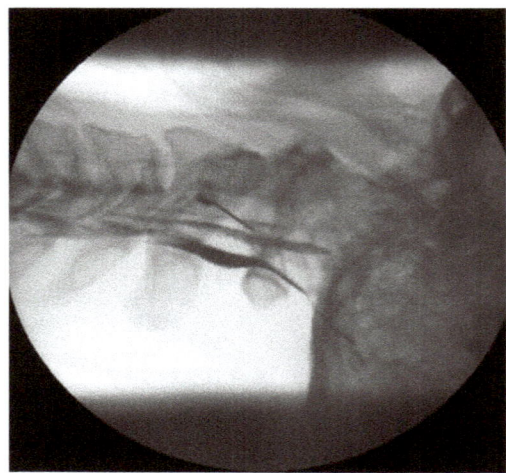

Fig. 9: Good myelogram picture.

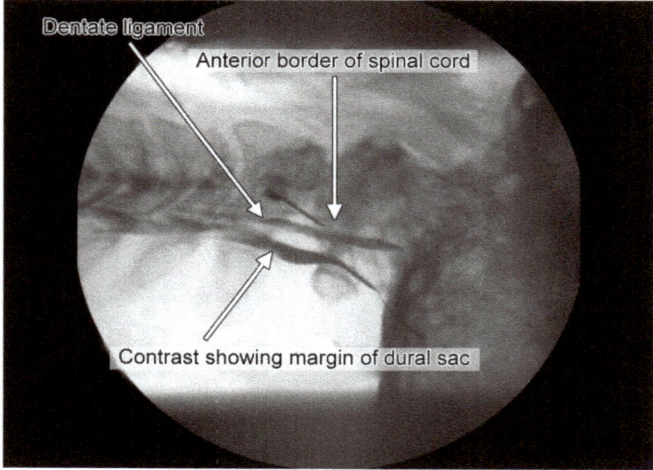

Fig. 10: Description of landmarks and myelogram.

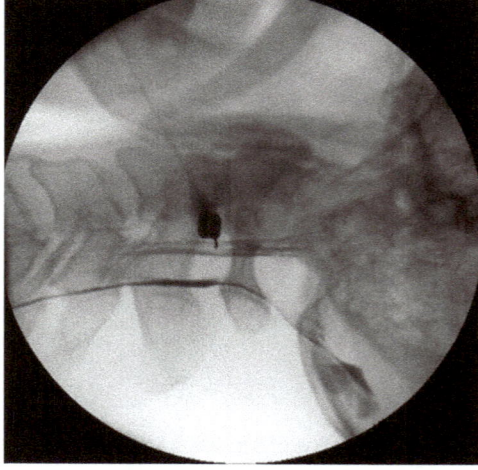

Fig. 11: Cordotomy probe in the correct location in the anterolateral quadrant of the spinal cord.

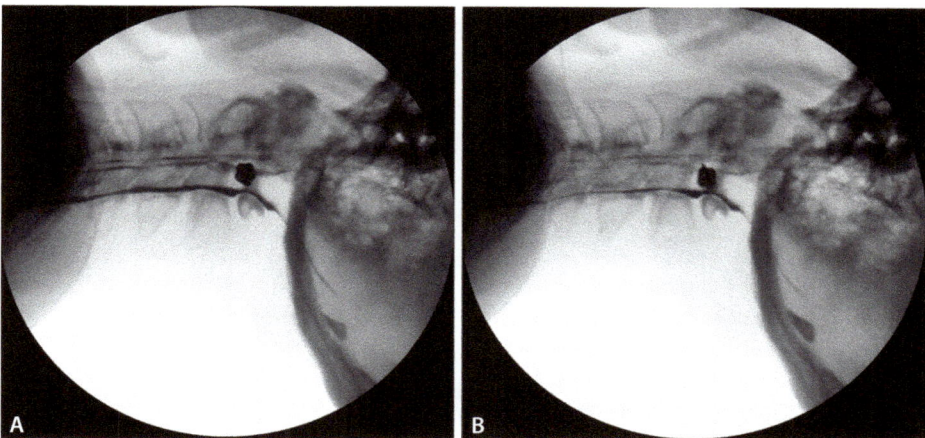

Figs. 12A and B: Further adjustment of the probe to localize spinothalamic tract before incremental radiofrequency lesion and sensory and motor testing (Further probe adjustment depends on the sensory motor stimulation parameters).

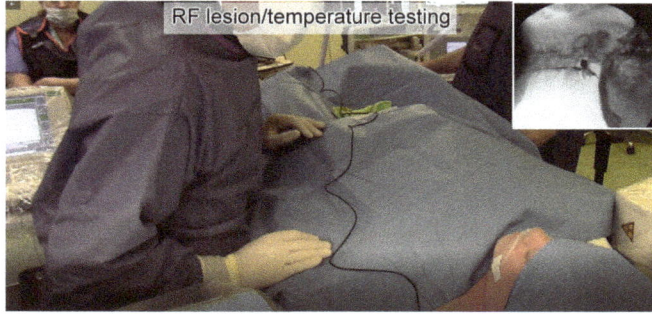

Fig. 13: Cordotomy probe is in the correct location and then radiofrequency (RF) lesioning (Note lifting of arm and leg to monitor signs of weakness while lesioning).

Additional Tips

- Do not rush; gentle sedation; talk to patient and your team.
- Separate anesthetist for sedation and monitoring.
- Do not inject contrast or probe if there is no cerebrospinal fluid (CSF) flow.
- If there is no flow of CSF, first withdraw needle.
- Once in the subarachnoid space, only small movements of the needle with probe should be performed.
- Do not lesion if unsure of stimulation pattern.

FURTHER READING

1. Bain E, Hugel H, Sharma M. Percutaneous cervical cordotomy for the management of pain from cancer: a prospective review of 45 cases. J Palliat Med. 2013;16(8):901-7.
2. Doyle A, Sharma ML, Gupta M, Goebel A, Marley K. Percutaneous cervical cordotomy for cancer-related pain: prospective multimodal outcomes evaluation BMJ Support Palliat Care. 2020. doi: 10.1136/bmjspcare-2019-002084. [Online] ahead of print.
3. Poolman M, Makin M, Briggs J, Scofield K, Campkin N, Williams M, et al. Percutaneous cervical cordotomy for cancer-related pain: national data. BMJ Support Palliat Care. 2020;10(4): 429-34.
4. Sharma M, Vishwanathan A. Cervical cordotomy technique (fluoroscopic and CT guided). In: Sharma M, Simpson KH, Bennett MI, Gupta S (Eds). Practical Management of Complex Cancer Pain, 2nd edition. New York: Oxford University Press; 2021.

SECTION 3

Cervical Spine

- **Interlaminar Cervical Epidural Block**
  Rathi Joseph

- **Cervical Medial Branch Block**
  Sanjeeva Gupta, Babita Ghai

- **Cervical Medial Branch Radiofrequency Ablation**
  Quyen Van Truong

- **Cervical Radiofrequency Denervation in Lateral Patient Position**
  Sherdil Nath, Sanjeeva Gupta

CHAPTER 12

Interlaminar Cervical Epidural Block

Rathi Joseph

BASIC INFORMATION

Indications
- Cervical nerve root compression
- Disk bulges with radicular pain
- Cervical radiculopathy

Contraindications
- Unwilling patient
- Bleed disorders or anticoagulant use
- Upper motor neuron signs

Risks
- Intrathecal injection
- Spinal cord injury
- Hematoma

Types of Injection
- One level, midline or just off midline
- Transforaminal approach more risk of stroke due to vertebral artery uptake, use digital subtraction to improve visualization

Medications Used
- *Steroids:* Non-particulated steroids 12 mg dexamethasone
- *Contrast:* Iodinated contrast up to 3 mL
- *Local anesthetic:* For superficial use only

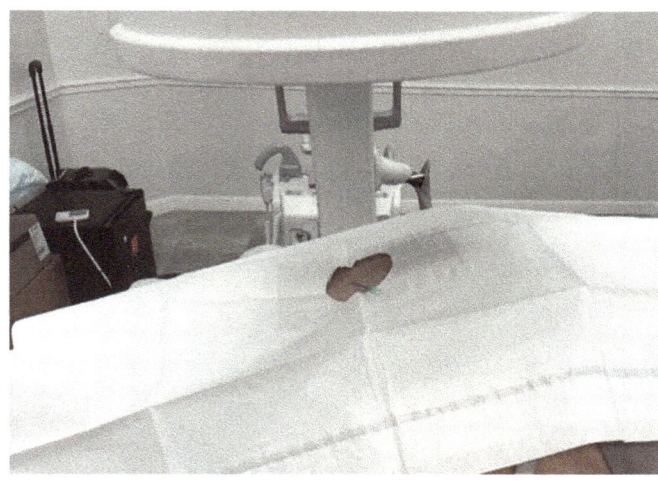

Fig. 2: Skin marking and local anesthetic introduction.

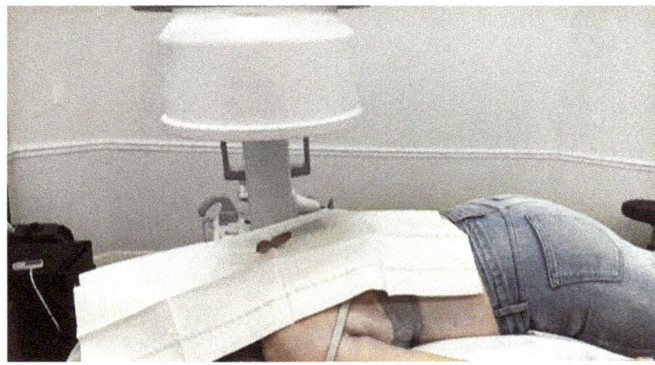

Fig. 1: Patient prone with pillow under the pelvis for comfort; chin tucked to patient tolerance.

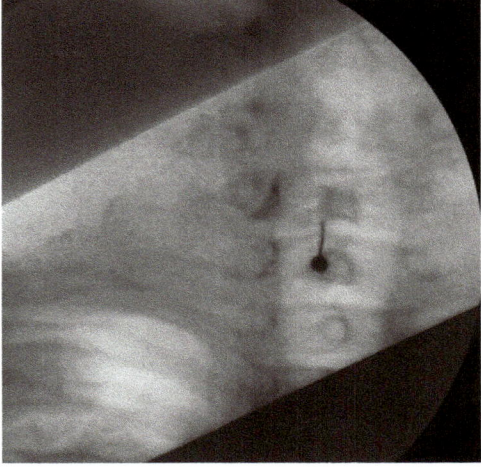

Fig. 3: Needle tip at lamina—anteroposterior (AP) view.

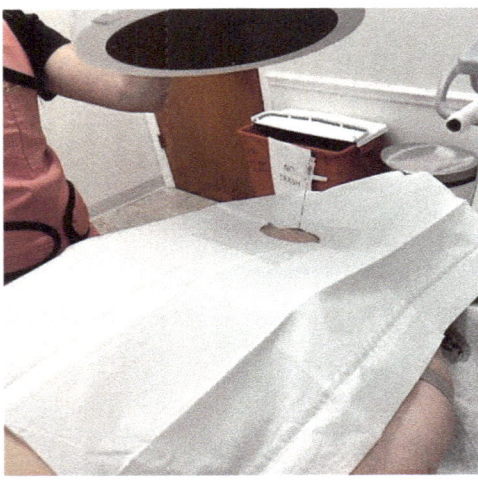

Fig. 4: Tuohy needle introduction until stable in the musculature.

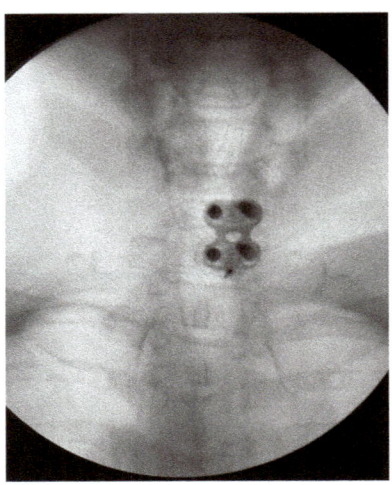

Fig. 5: End on view—needle in anteroposterior view at the C7--T1 interspace biased to the right.

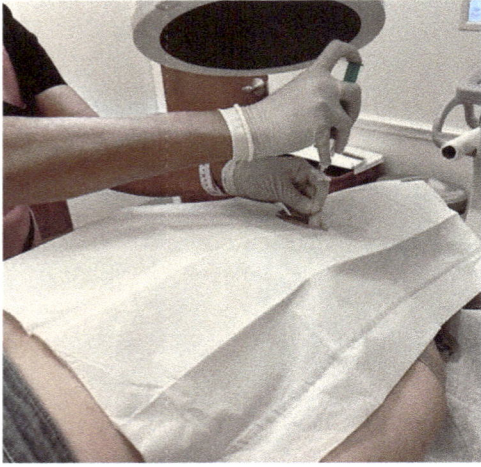

Fig. 6: Loss of resistance toggling the C-arm between AP and 45° contralateral oblique.

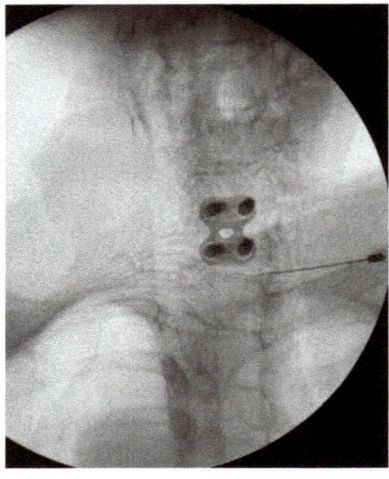

Fig. 7: Left contralateral oblique view for depth assessment.

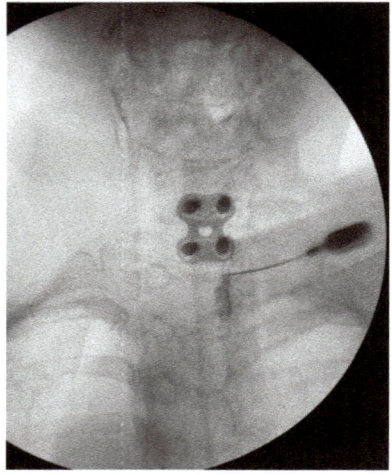

Fig. 8: Contrast flow after loss of resistance at the spinolaminar line with epidural fat stippling.

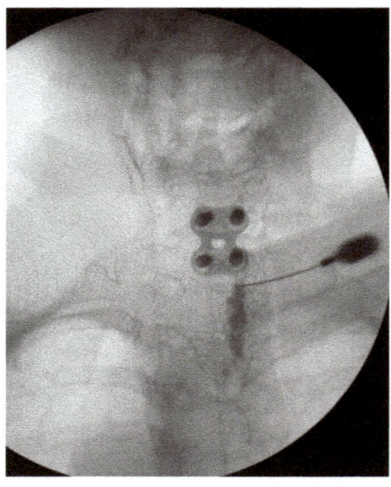

Fig. 9: Epidural contrast spread in contralateral oblique view.

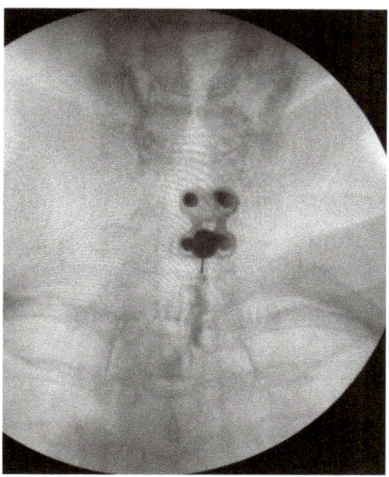

Fig. 10: Epidural contrast spread biased to the right in AP view.

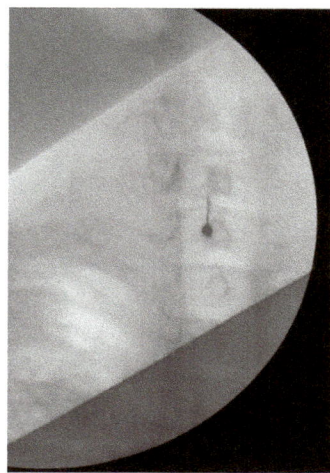

Fig. 11: AP view of the Tuohy needle at the C7-T1 biased to the left.

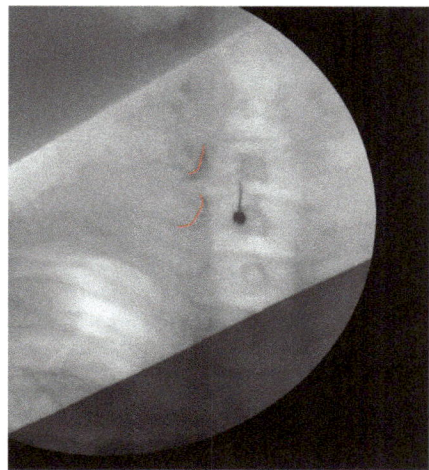

Fig. 12: AP view of the Tuohy needle at the C7-T1, medial pedicle borders outlined in red.

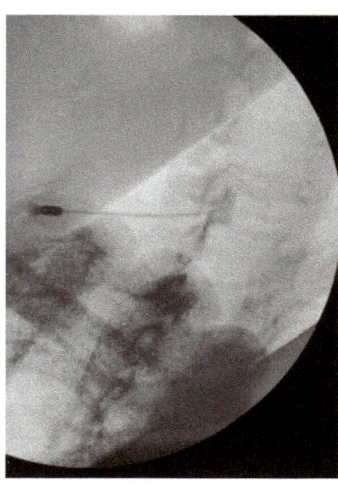

Fig. 13: Contralateral oblique right.

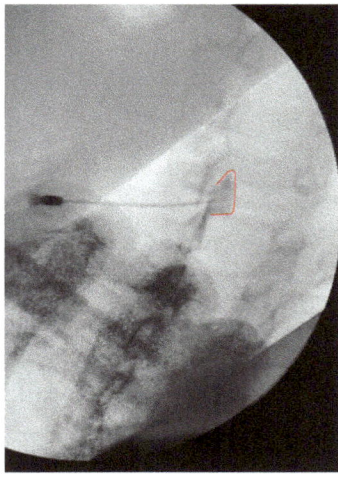

Fig. 14: Contralateral oblique right with lateral spread outlined in red.

CHAPTER 13

Cervical Medial Branch Block

Sanjeeva Gupta, Babita Ghai

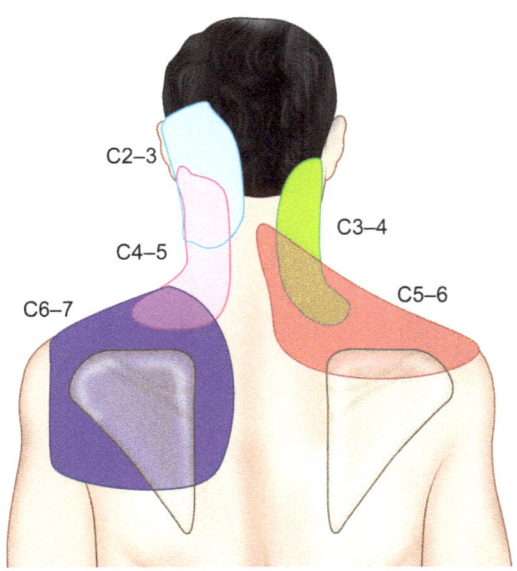

Fig. 1: Cervical somatic referral pattern.
C5–6 facet joint most commonly involved followed by C6–7.
One can localize to within +/– one joint on the basis of referral map.

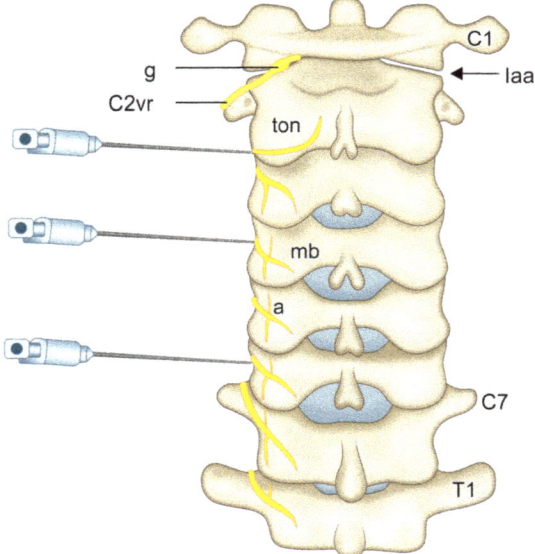

Fig. 2: Diagram showing the antero-posterior (AP) view of the cervical spine with medial branches (mb) and articular branches (a). For medial branch block the needle can be perpindicular to the medial branch (MB) but for radiofrequency denervaton the needle should be parallel to the MB.

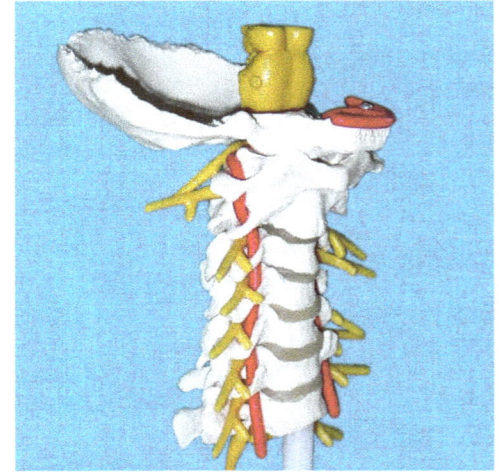

Fig. 3: Photograph showing the structures around the cervical spine.

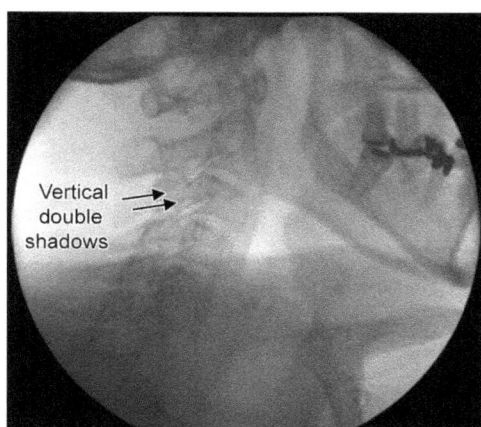

Fig. 4: Lateral image of cervical spine. The right and the left articular pillars are not superimposed. To get the correct image, observe the movement of the vertical lateral margins of the articular pillars (arrows at C3 level) with right or left C-arm rotation under continuous fluoroscopy to superimpose the articular pillars in the vertical direction. Then tilt the C-arm in the cephalic or caudal direction under continuous fluoroscopy to superimpose the facet joint lines to eliminate the oblique/horizantal double shadows (parallax) to obtain a true lateral view of the cervical spine where the right and the left articular pillars are superimposed.[1]

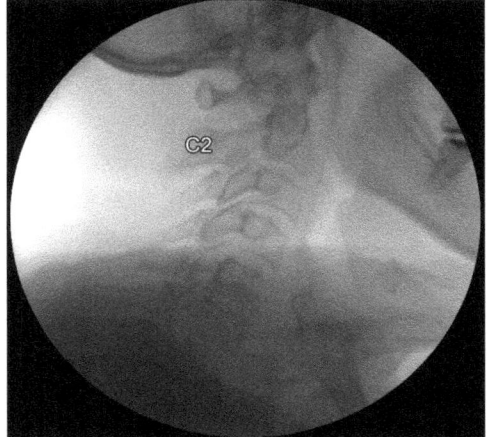

Fig. 5: After appropriate rotation of the C-arm to the right or left under continuous fluoroscopy and then tilting the C-arm in the cephalic or caudal direction, the right and the left articular pillars are superimposed. The facet joint lines appear crisp with the vertebral bodies and discs outlined. The pedicals appear in the upper and posterior aspects of the vertebral body. This image is good to identify the target point for C3 medial branch block (MBB). The C-arm will need to be adjusted again if other level MBBs are planned.

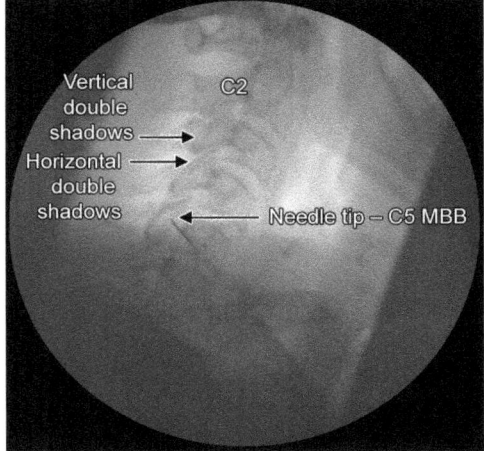

Fig. 6: Needle tip is at the target point to block the C5 MBB. Note that there are double shadows (parallax) at the C3 and C4 levels. The horizantal/oblique double shadows (parallax) as indicated by the arrows along the facet joint line at the C3/4 level should be eliminated by cephalic or caudal tilt and the vertical double shadows (parallax) at the C3 level should be eliminated by right or left rotation before doing C4 and C3 MBB, respectively.

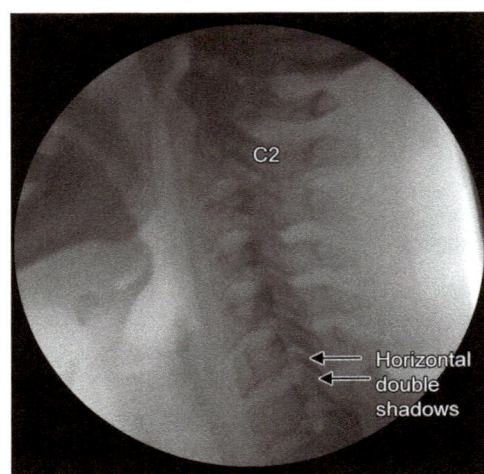

Fig. 7: In this image, there are double shadows (parallax) shown by arrows at the C5/6 and C6/7 levels. Tilting the C-arm in cephalic or caudal direction will eliminate the double shadows (parallax).

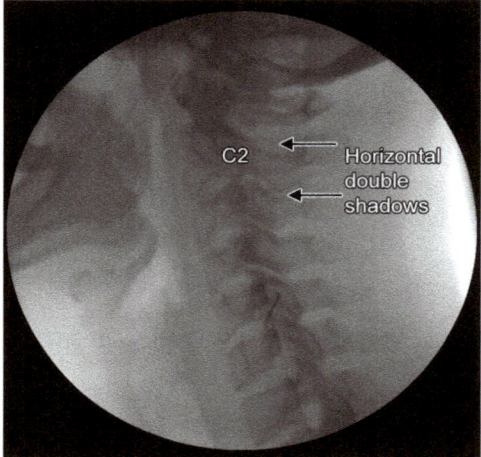

Fig. 8: Tilting the C-arm (compared with Figure 7) has eliminated the parallax at the C5 level. The needle tip is at the target point for C5 MBB. Observe the double shadows (parallax) at upper and lower borders of C2 and at C3 levels.

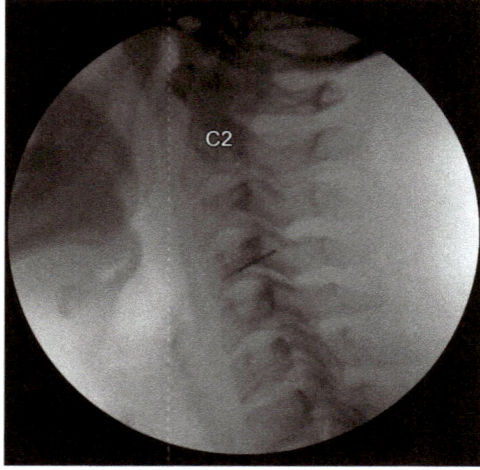

Fig. 9: Needle tip at the target point for C4 MBB.

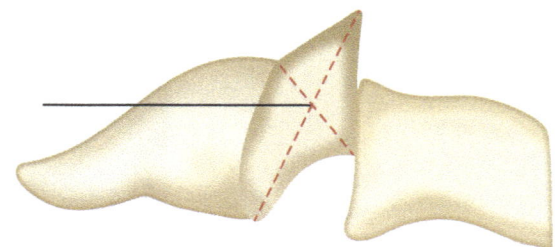

Fig. 10: Diagram showing the centroid of the articular pillar. The target area for medial branch block is the center of the rhomboid.

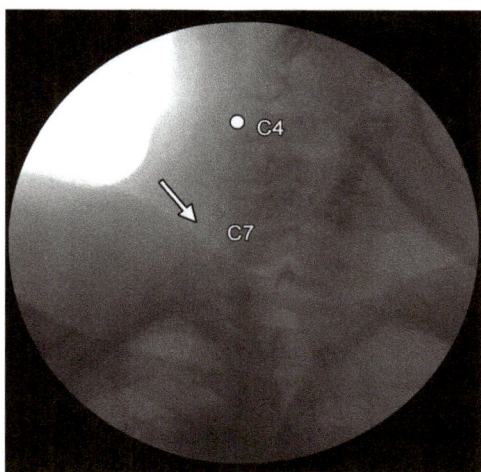

Fig. 11: *Prone position:* An antero-posterior (AP) view of the cervical spine. The target point for the MBB is the most medial aspect on the waist of the respective articular pillar. This image is appropriate for C4 MBB. The arrow points to the junction of the superior articular process and the transverse process of C7 which appears like a front of a "Ski boot."

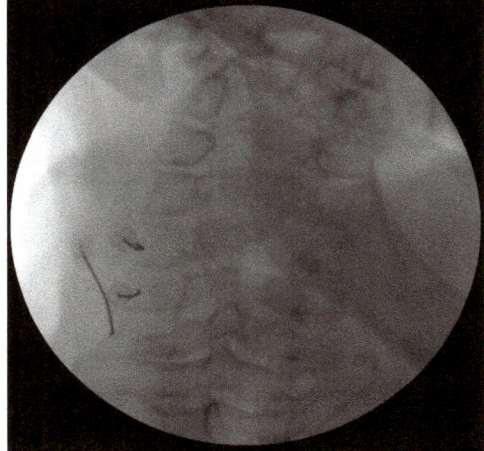

Fig. 12: *Prone position:* AP fluoroscopic image of cervical spine with needle tips in position for left C5, C6 and one of the target points for the C7 medial branch block.

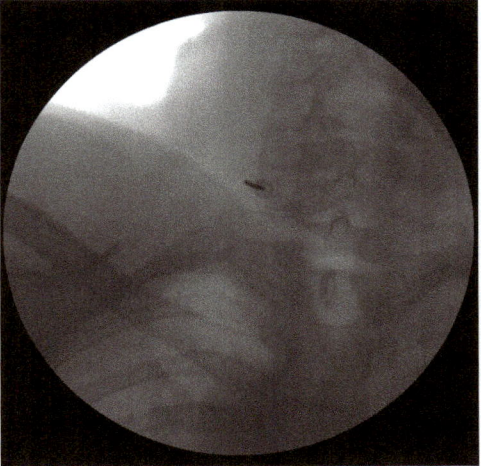

Fig. 13: *Prone position:* Needle tip at the base of the superior articular process at its junction with the transverse process, one of the target points for C7 medial branch block.

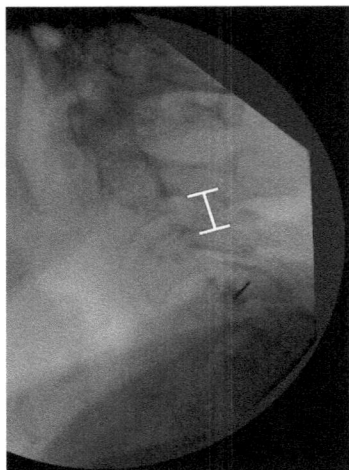

Fig. 14: *Lateral position:* Third occipital nerve block: Image shows the imaginary line bisecting the C2–3 facet joint line and the upper and the lower target points along the bisecting line.

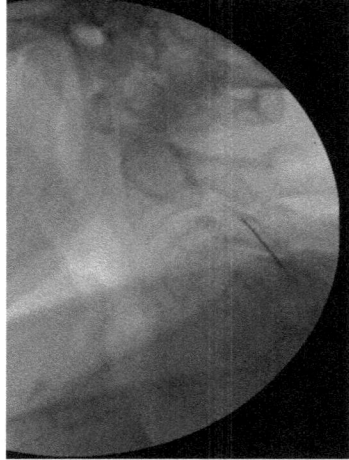

Fig. 15: *Lateral position:* Needle tip at the lower target area for the third occipital nerve block.

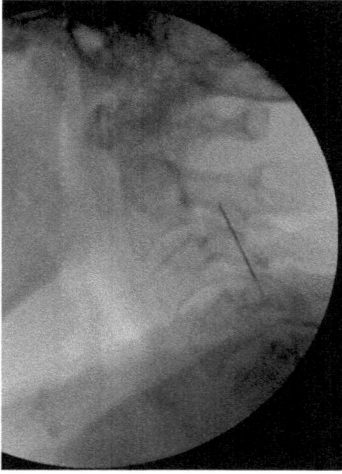

Fig. 16: *Lateral position:* Needle tip at the upper target area for third occipital nerve block.

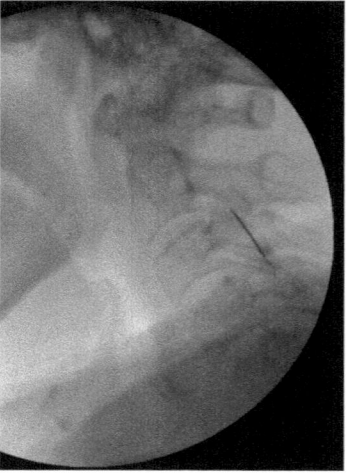

Fig. 17: *Lateral position:* Needle tip at the mid-target area for the third occipital nerve block. The needle tip should lie on the bone at the superior edge of the C3 articular process along the bisecting line.

Flowchart 1: Cervical facet joint pain algorithm for pain in the middle and lower area of the neck.

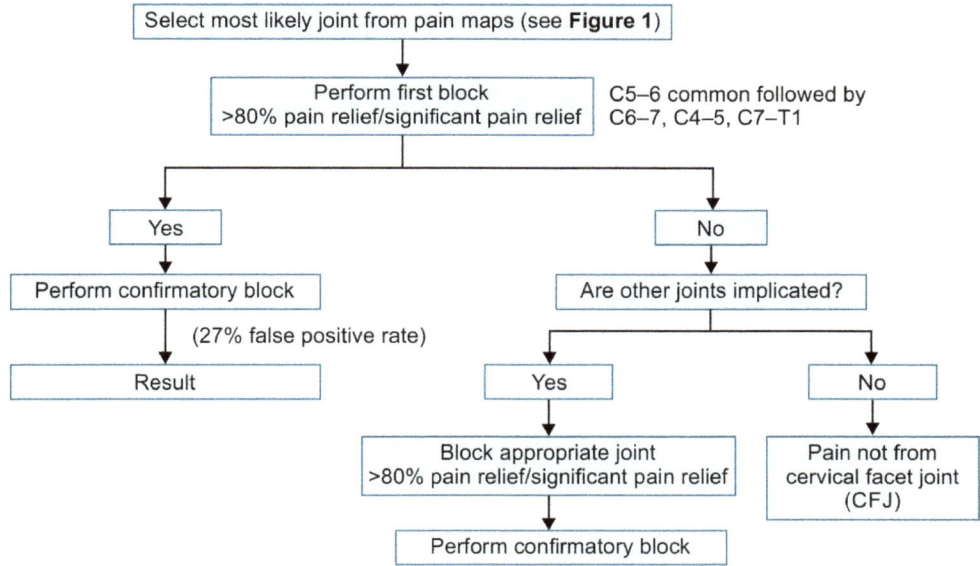

Flowchart 2: Cervical medial branch block algorithm for pain in the upper neck. Based on clinical assessment some patients may benefit from assessing the C2–3 and C3–4 facet together.

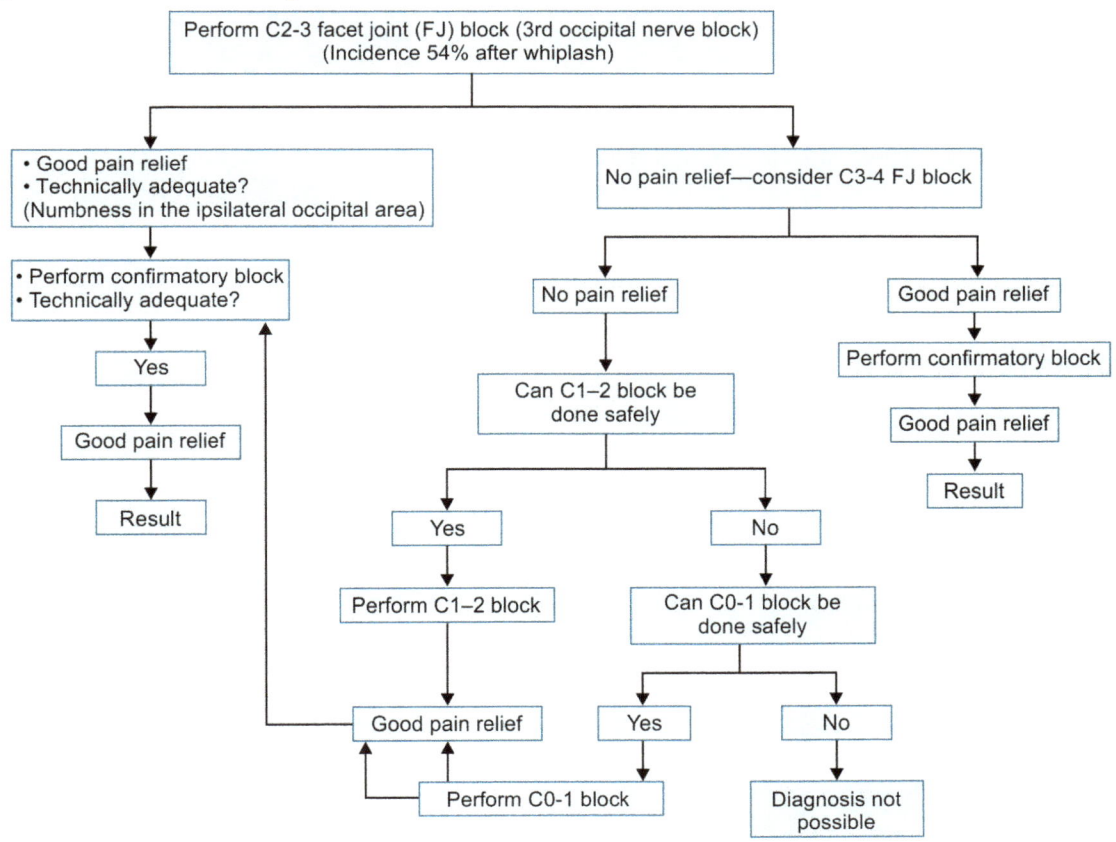

REFERENCE

1. Gupta S, Varma S. Cervical medial branch block. In: Baheti DK, Bakshi S, Gupta S, Singh RSP (Eds). Interventional Pain Management: A Practical Approach, 2nd edition. New Delhi: Jaypee Brothers Medical Publishers; 2016. pp. 220-9.

CHAPTER 14

Cervical Medial Branch Radiofrequency Ablation

Quyen Van Truong

BASIC INFORMATION

Indications
- Cervical spondylosis
- Cervical facet arthropathy
- Cervical facet-mediated pain after two successful diagnostic cervical medial branch blocks (>50–80% pain relief)

Contraindications
- Unwilling patient
- Bleeding disorders
- Presence of red flags

Radiofrequency Lesioning
- 0.5–1 cc of anesthetic is injected prior to radiofrequency lesioning
- The time and duration of lesioning vary with different practitioners.
- Consider one to two 90-second cycles at 80–85°C.

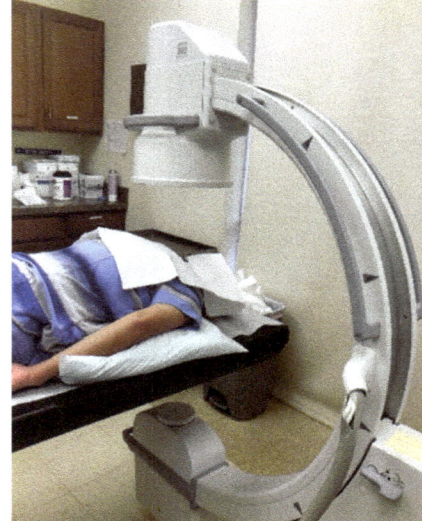

Fig. 2: *Step 2:* Fluoroscope anteroposterior position.

PROCEDURE DETAILS

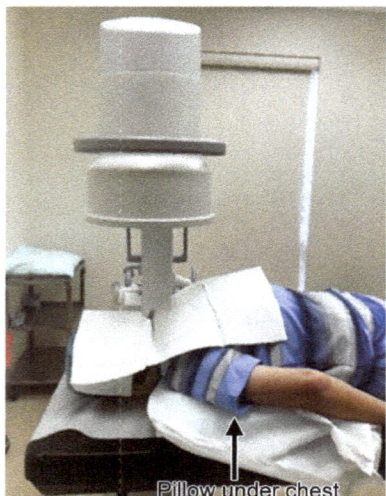

Fig. 1: *Step 1:* Position of patient.

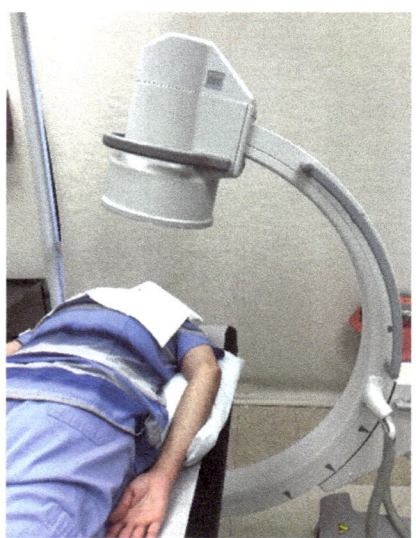

Fig. 3: *Step 3:* Fluoroscope ipsilateral oblique view 20–30°.

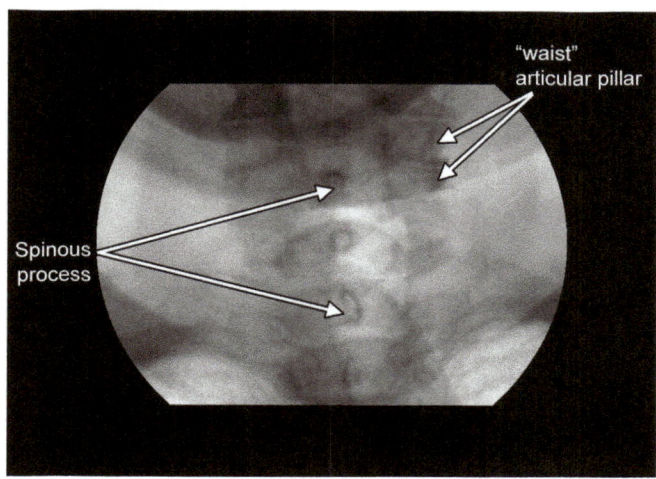

Fig. 4: *Step 4:* Parts of C spine. Optimize view of the "waist" of articular pillar (lateral groove).

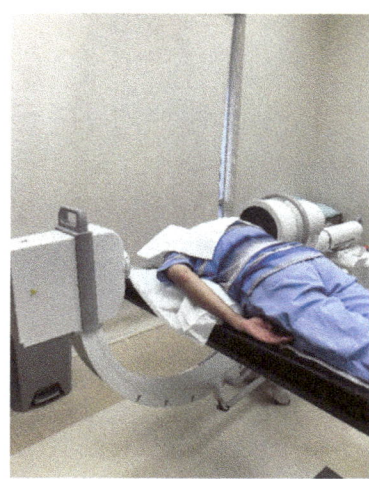

Fig. 5: *Step 5:* Fluoroscope lateral view.

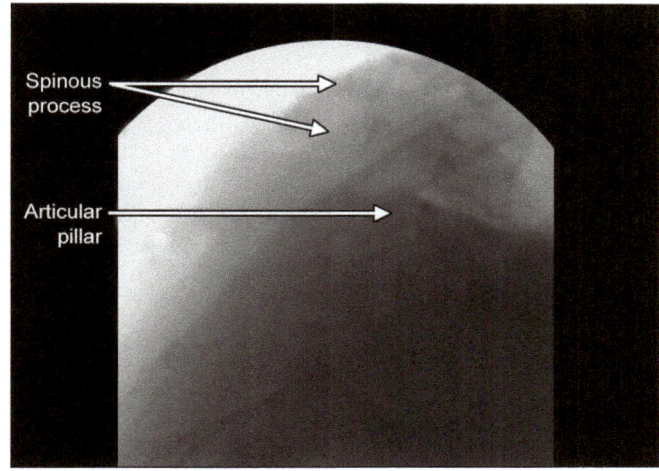

Fig. 6: *Step 6:* Parts of C spine. Lateral view to view center of articular pillar.

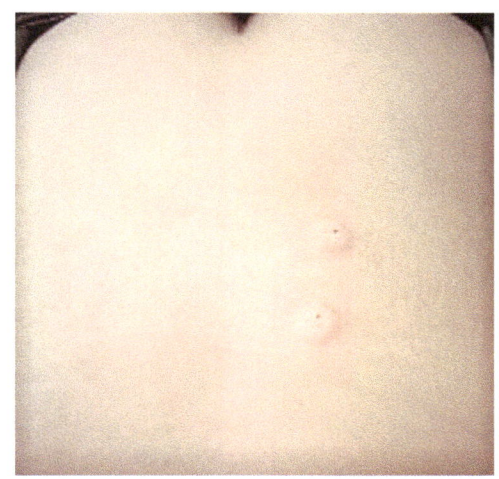

Fig. 7: Intradermal skin wheal.

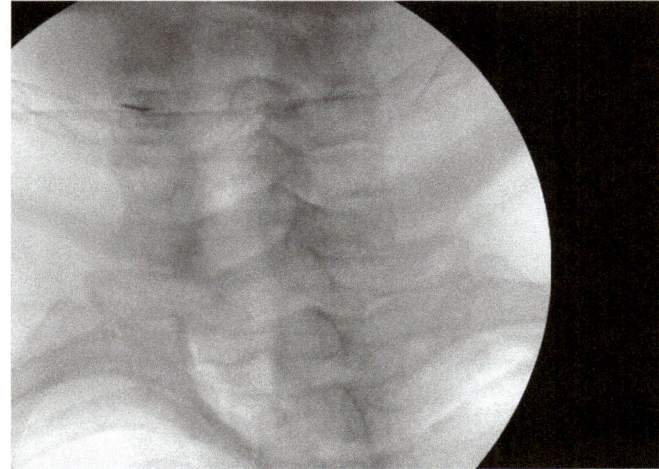

Fig. 8: Entry point—Electrode tip at "waist" of articular pillar in ipsilateral oblique view.

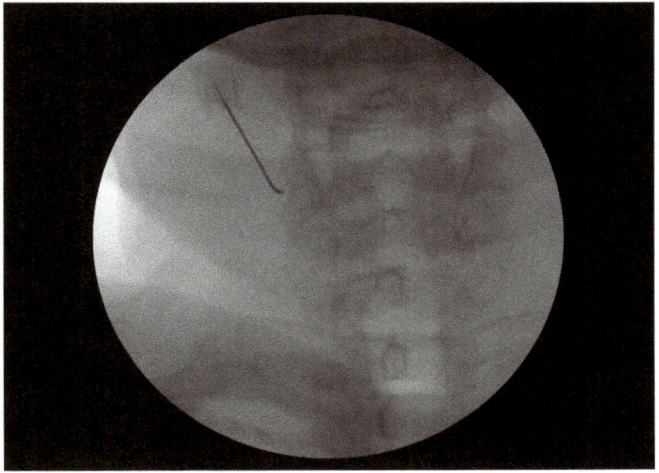

Fig. 9: *Step 7:* Electrode tip advanced to waist of articular pillar in AP view.

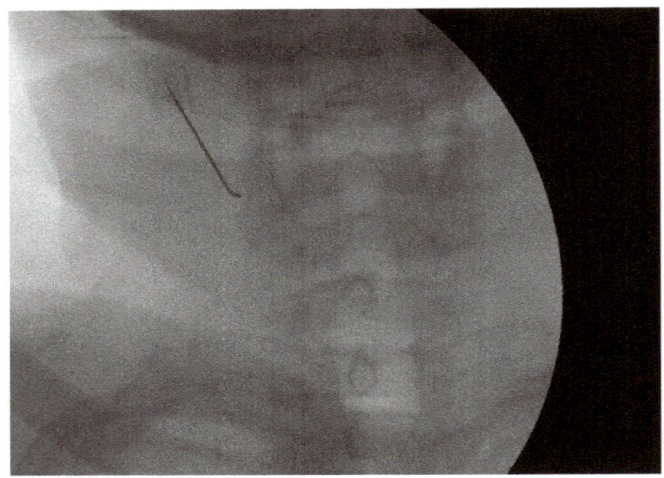

Fig. 10: *Step 8:* Electrode tip advanced to waist of articular pillar in AP view.

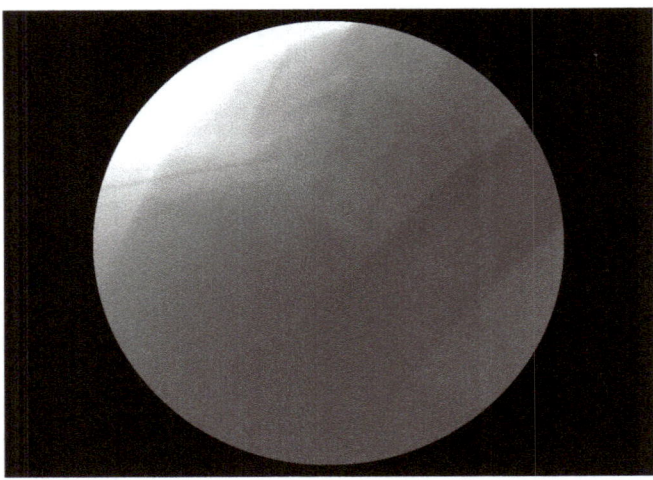

Fig. 11: *Step 9:* Electrode tip advanced to the center of the articular pillar in lateral view to check depth.

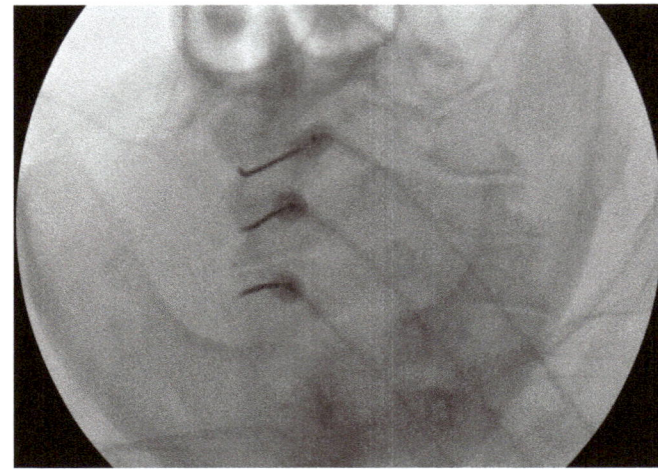

Fig. 12: *Step 10:* Radiofrequency electrodes properly positioned and connected for testing and lesioning (80–85°C for 90-second cycle).

CHAPTER 15

Cervical Radiofrequency Denervation in Lateral Patient Position

Sherdil Nath, Sanjeeva Gupta

INTRODUCTION

The lateral position is the preferred patient position of the authors for cervical facet joint radiofrequency (RF) denervaton and the technique is described with the help of some cases.

Note: To safely perform a cervical medial branch block (MBB) or MB radiofrequency denervation (RFD) procedure, a perfect lateral view is necessary, with the right and the left articular pillars aligned and double shadows eliminated. The continuous fluoroscopic screening to observe the direction in which the two (right and the left) articular pillars move can be very helpful in achieving this. (Refer to Chapter 13 on Cervical Medial Branch Blocks). It is also advisable to be proficient in lumbar procedures before attempting procedures in the neck.

We would also advise that one should attend relevant cadaver courses and also observe and/or initially work with a colleague and do procedures jointly with colleagues who perform cervical procedures regularly. It is also advisable to position the patient and obtain fluoroscopic views to confirm that the target areas are visible on fluoroscopy before scrubbing for the procedure. If the target areas are not visible, especially the lower cervical areas, then one option would be to do the upper cervical procedure in lateral position and the lower levels in prone position. If the neck is very short and the patient has significant cervical spondylosis, then the entire procedure may have to be performed in prone position if the target areas are visible. If completely impossible to identify anatomical skeletal structures, then the procedure should not be attempted.

This is a procedure than can cause serious complications. There is no place for foolhardiness.

The results of the RFD procedure depend on (apart from good patient selection), knowing the location and direction of target nerves, precise needle positioning, and adequate lesion size.

Figures 1A and B show the different sizes of egg white coagulation when RF cannulae of different gauges and active

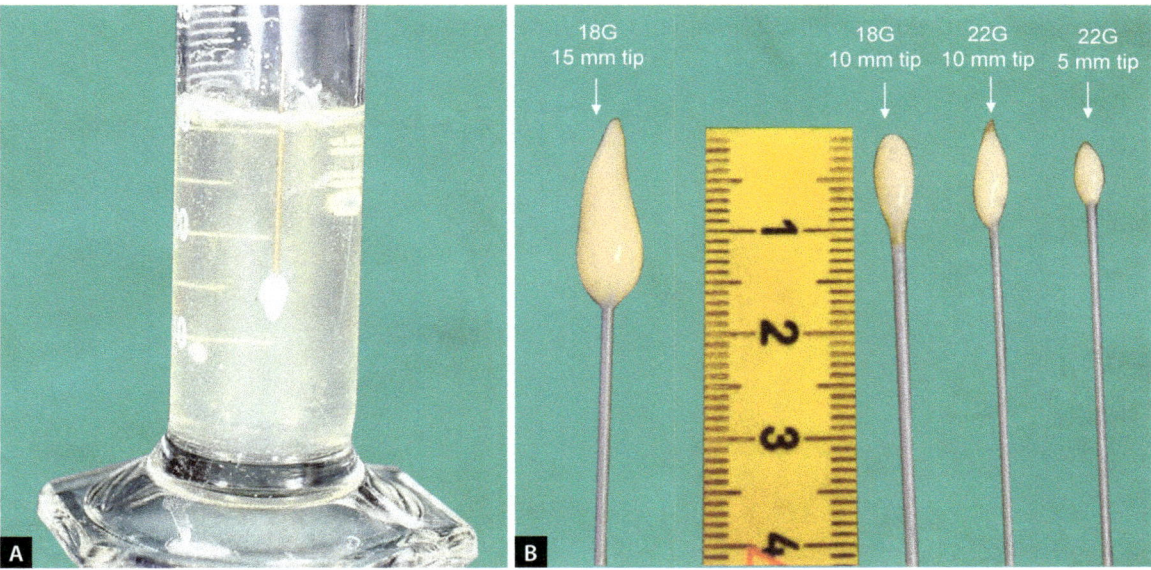

Figs. 1A and B: Different sizes of egg white coagulation with RF cannulae of different gauges and active tip sizes. The images in **Figure 1A** and **Figures 2A and B** were taken by Dr Sherdil Nath in 1986. To Dr Sanjeeva Gupta's knowlegde (who is a co-author of this chapter and also an editor), Dr Sherdil Nath was the first pain physician to describe the most appropriate placement of the RF cannula in relation to the nerves that are being denervated (parallel to the nerve as shown in **Figure 2B**), which has significantly improved the outcome of RFD procedures.

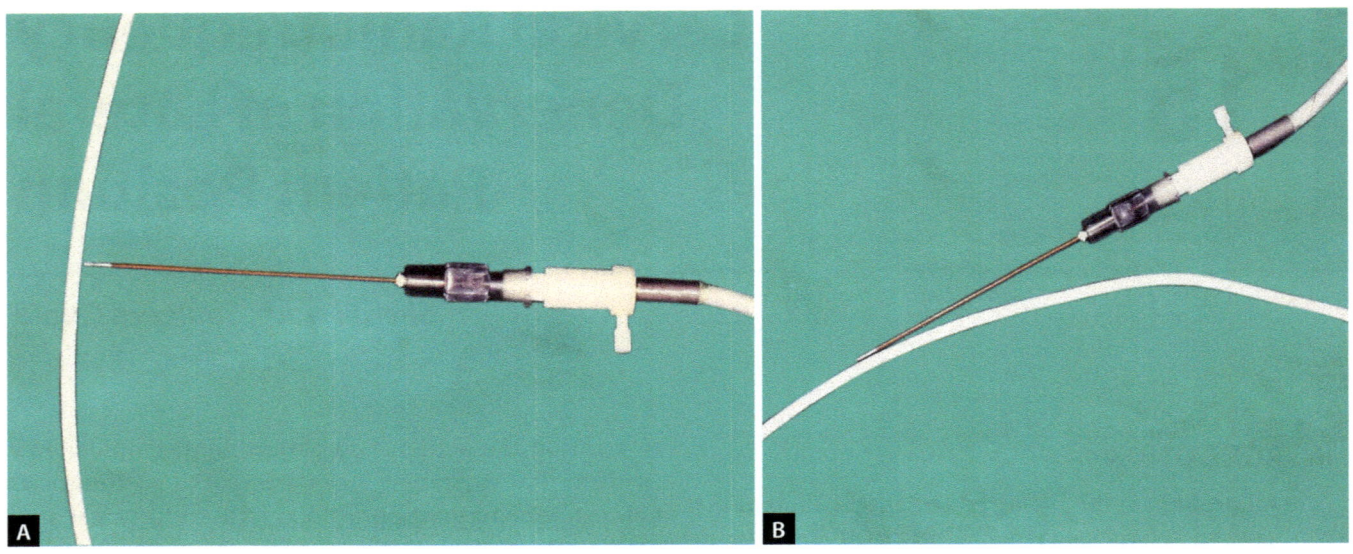

Figs. 2A and B: Position of RF cannulae tip should be parallel to the nerve as shown in Figure 2B.

tip sizes are placed in egg white and current passed through the electrodes, as in an RF procedure.

As indicated in **Figures 2A and B**, placing the RF cannula tip perpendicular to the nerve (A) that is being denervated does not create the desired lesion. The cannula needs to be aligned parallel to the nerve (B).

INTERESTING CASES

Case 1

Step 1: Positioning the patient **(Fig. 3)** is extremely important to visualize the cervical spine image on fluoroscopy (especially the lower levels). Pull the lower shoulder down and push a pillow or rolled sheet toward the dependent shoulder to maintain the position (long arrow). Ask the patient to flex the hips and knees (short arrow) as much as possible toward the chest and to hold their knees with their hands to maintain the position (as shown in the image, the knees and hips should be bent more toward the chest).

Step 2: After obtaining a perfect lateral view with the right and the left articular pillars superimposed (eliminate the double shadows (Refer to Chapter 13 on Cervical Medial Branch Blocks). You will see here that C3, C4, and C5 have no double shadows but C2 does), the skin insertion point is in line with the facet joints, the same distance behind the posterior margin of the articular pillar as the distance between the anterior and posterior borders of the articular pillar (long arrows) **(Fig. 4)**.

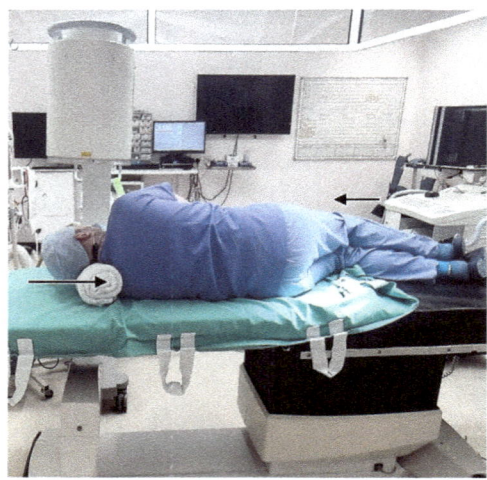

Fig. 3: Positioning the patient.

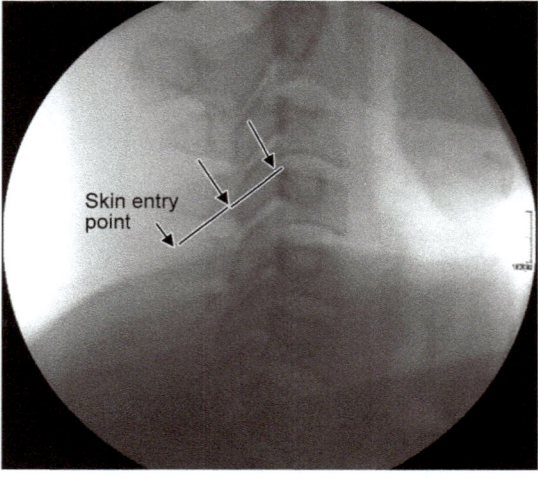

Fig. 4: After obtaining a perfect lateral view with the right and the left articular pillars superimposed the skin entry point is determined.

Step 3: *Making bone contact:* This is the first hazard that you need to be aware of. *Never* advance the cannula beyond the posterior border of the vertebral body. After injecting local anesthetic (LA) in the skin and muscles, advance the cannula carefully till you get to the posterior border of the vertebral body, monitoring the progress at all times with fluoroscopy. If no bone contact is made, then retract and advance again a little deeper. Inject more LA as required. Repeat till bone contact is made in the center of the articular pillar; you will need more LA when you touch bone. A curved tipped 18G 10-mm active tip RF cannula is used for this procedure. It is navigated parallel to the C3/4 and C4/5 facet joint lines to place the needle in the groove where your target nerve lies, in the middle of the articular pillar (arrows) and then advanced further to be as close to the anterior border of the articular pillar **(Fig. 5)** (also See Cases 2 to 4).

Step 4: Inferior oblique view **(Fig. 6)**. The C-arm in rotated anteriorly by about 30°–40° and tilted inferiorly to obtain this view. The optimal view is when the opposite pedicles appear in the dead center of the vertebral body (arrows) and the intervertebral disc appears well defined. No stimulation is necessary, neither sensory nor motor, as the tip of the electrode is clearly visible behind the posterior border of the foramen in this view. About 0.5-mL LA is injected and an RF lesion is performed at 80°C for 60 seconds and the RF needle pulled back by around 5 mm and the tip turned in the opposite direction and advanced by 5 mm and another lesion performed at each level.

Step 5: Lateral fluoroscopic view **(Fig. 7)**. An 18G cannula (or needle) with a curved 10-mm active tip RF needle is being placed for C6 MB RF. At the lower levels, the shadow due to

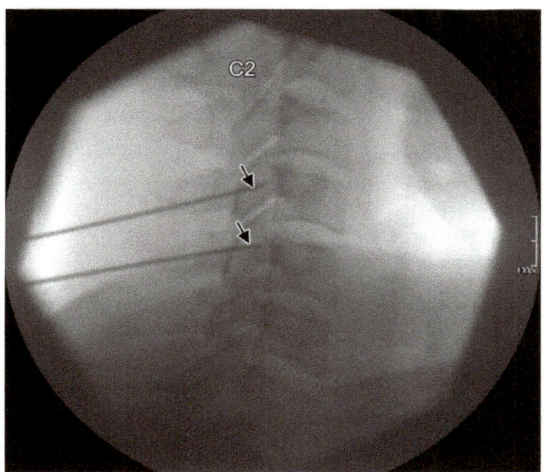

Fig. 5: Making bone contact in the center of the articular pillar.

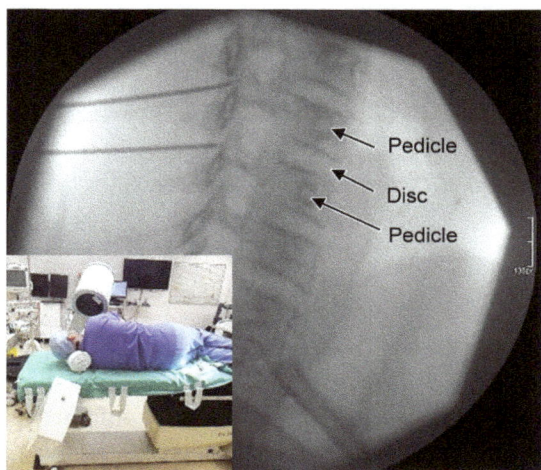

Fig. 6: Inferior oblique view. The opposite pedicle should be in the center of the vertebral body (arrows).

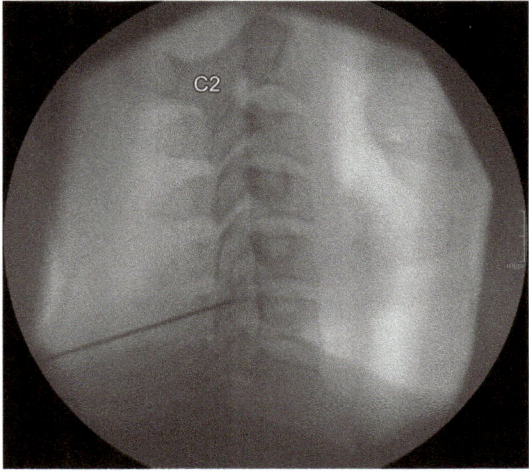

Fig. 7: *Lateral fluoroscopic view:* An 18G cannula (or needle) with a curved 10-mm active tip RF needle is being placed for C6 medial branch (MB) RF.

the shoulder can make it difficult to view the target areas. Appropriate positioning before commencing the procedure is important.

Step 6: It will be advisable to navigate the RF needle tip further by about 2 mm to be closer to the anterior margin of the respective superior articular process (SAP) **(Fig. 8)**.

Step 7: The needle is withdrawn by around 5 mm and the direction of the needle tip is rotated 180° so that it is pointing more cephalad, then advanced to within 2 mm of the posterior border of the foramen and another lesion performed. The entire procedure should be virtually pain free as plenty of LA is used **(Fig. 9)**.

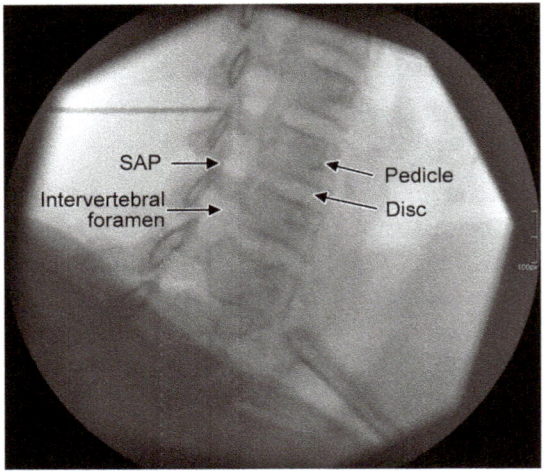

Fig. 8: Inferior oblique view showing the needle in being navigated for the first lesion. (SAP: superior articular process)

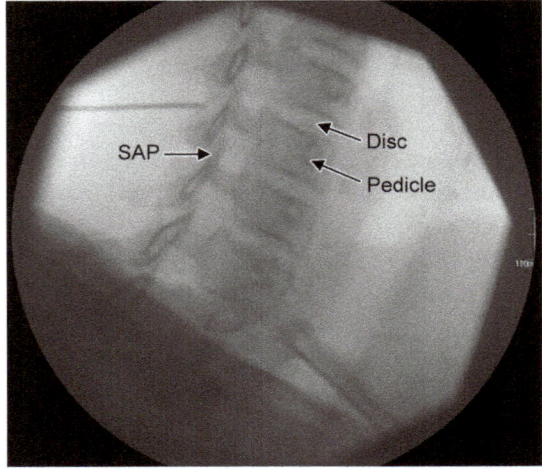

Fig. 9: Needle tip is rotated 180° and advanced within 2 mm of the posterior border of the foramen before a lesion is performed. (SAP: superior articular process)

Case 2

Step 1: A 45-year-old male patient had very good pain relief following MBB and was listed for RF. Lateral view showing an 18G cannula (or needle) with a curved 10-mm active tip RF cannula in position at C5 level. The needle tip is advanced up to the anterior border of the articular pillar. Note the double shadow at the C3 level (arrows). It is important to eliminate the double shadow at the level the procedure is being performed, and hence it is necessary to do the procedures one level at a time after readjusting the C-arm to get a perfect lateral view **(Fig. 10)**.

Step 2: Ipsilateral anterior inferior oblique view showing the position for the RF cannula tip close to the anterior border of the SAP and the intervertebral foramen (IVF) as seen in **Figure 11**, and hence the needle was withdrawn by about 2 mm before the first lesion was performed as shown in **Figure 12**.

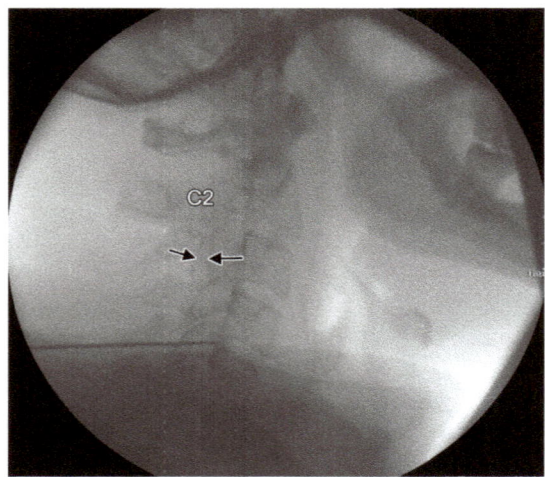

Fig. 10: Lateral view showing an 18G cannula (or needle) with a curved 10-mm active tip RF cannula in position at C5 level.

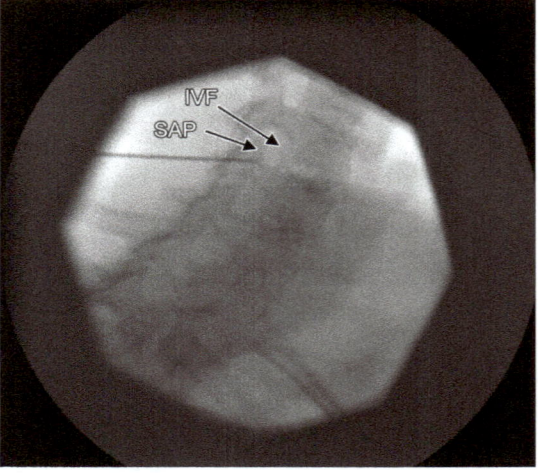

Fig. 11: Ipsilateral anterior inferior oblique view.

Step 3: Ipsilateral anterior oblique inferior view showing the position of the needle for the first lesion. About 0.5-mL LA is injected before lesioning. Note that in this case, the opposite pedicle at the level of the lesion is not exactly in the center of the vertebral body but the one above is. It may not always be possible to get a perfect image **(Fig. 12)**.

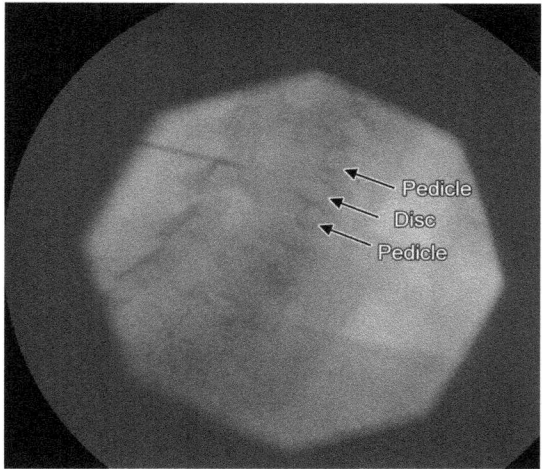

Fig. 12: Ipsilateral anterior oblique inferior view showing the position for the needle.

Step 4: Ipsilateral anterior oblique view showing that the RF cannula is pulled back by around 5 mm. The tip is now turned in the opposite direction and advanced by 5 mm and another lesion performed **(Fig. 13)**.

Step 5: Lateral view with the RF needle in place for C6 MB RF **(Fig. 14)**. At the C6 level, it is not always possible to navigate the RF cannula parallel to the facet joint lines as the shoulder can come in the way of the navigating hand and prevent us from getting the correct angle. If it is difficult to navigate the needle appropriately, then the C6 MB RFD procedure can be done in prone position. Alternatively, the entire procedure could be done in prone position if difficulty is anticipated on initial screening of the cervical spine before commencing the procedure. *Question:* Identify the double shadows in C3 to C5 levels.

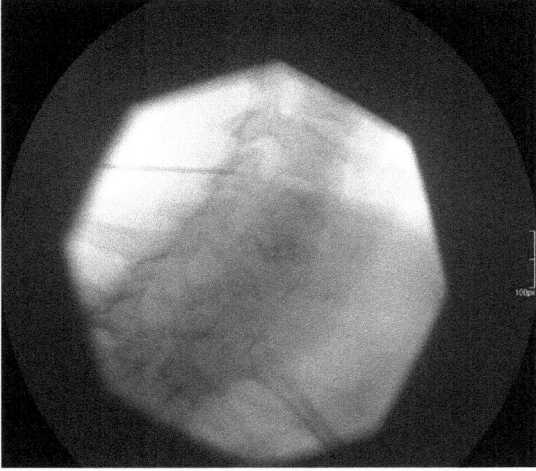

Fig. 13: Ipsilateral anterior oblique view showing the radiofrequency cannula.

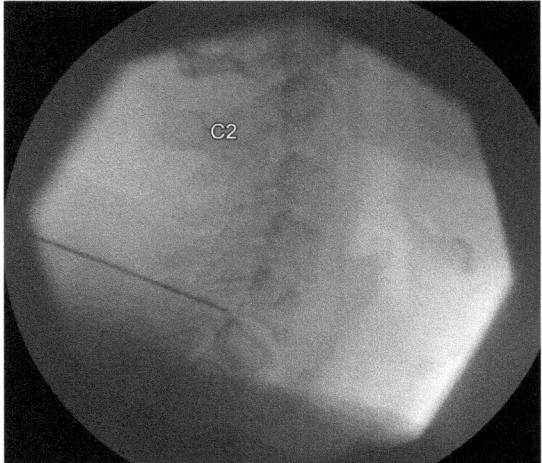

Fig. 14: Lateral view with the RF needle in place for C6 MB RF. (MBB: medial branch block; RF: radiofrequency)

Case 3

Step 1: A 71-year-old patient who presented with chronic pain in the lower part of the neck responded to C4 to C6 MBB and was listed for RF.

Lateral view: An 18G cannula (or needle) with a curved 10-mm active tip RF needle is being navigated for C6 MB RFD **(Fig. 15)**.

Step 2: Lateral view: RF needle in place for C6 MB RFD **(Fig. 16)**.

Step 3: Perfect lateral view (no double shadow, see Chapter 13) at C5 level. An 18G cannula (or needle) with a curved 10-mm active tip RF needle is being placed for C5 MB RFD. The needle tip is advanced parallel to the C4/5 and C5/6 facet joint lines and the tip is close to the anterior border of the articular pillar **(Fig. 17)**. The needle position is confirmed in the anterior inferior oblique view (always recommended).

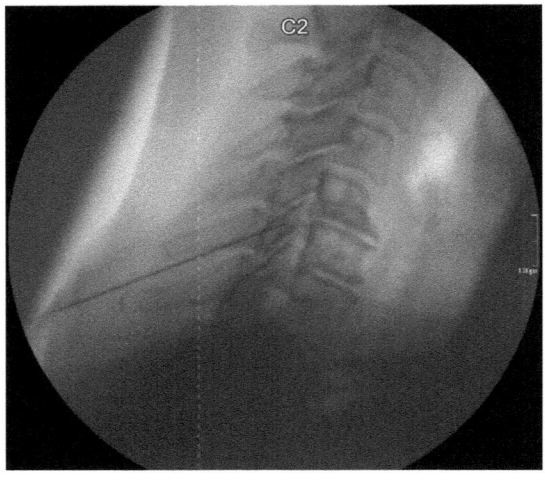

Fig. 15: Lateral view. An 18G cannula (or needle) with a curved 10-mm active tip RF needle is being navigated for C6 MB RFD.

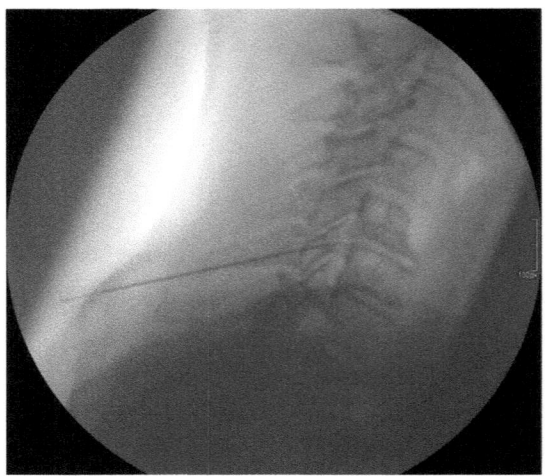

Fig. 16: Lateral view. RF needle in place for C6 MB RFD.

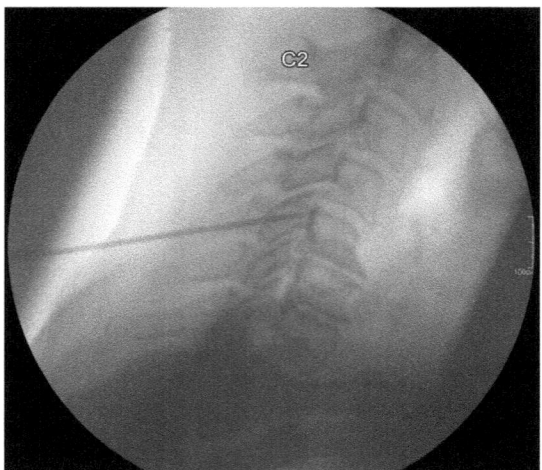

Fig. 17: Perfect lateral view. An 18G cannula (or needle) with a curved 10-mm active tip RF needle is being placed for C5 MB RFD.

Case 4

Step 1: A 63-year-old patient who had cervical spine surgery later developed neck pain. Patient responded with excellent pain relief following C4 to C6 MBB. This shows you that facet joint pain can occur/persist after fusion **(Fig. 18)**.

Step 2: An 18G cannula (or needle) with a curved 10-mm active tip RF needle is being navigated for C5 MB RFD. The needle tip is advanced parallel to the C4/5 and C5/6 facet joint lines to make bone contact in the middle of the articular pillar and then navigated to the anterior border of the articular pillar **(Fig. 19)**.

Step 3: Lateral view: An 18G cannula (or needle) with a curved 10-mm active tip RF needle is being navigated for C4 MB RFD **(Fig. 20)**. The needle tip is advanced parallel to the C3/4 and C4/5 facet joint lines to make bone contact in the middle of the articular pillar and then navigated to the anterior border of the articular pillar for C4 MB RFD. The needle position is confirmed in the anterior inferior oblique view before lesioning.

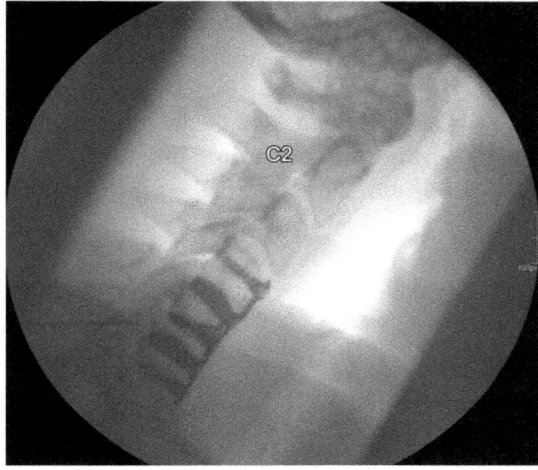

Fig. 18: Patient with cervical facet joint pain after surgery. This shows that facet joint pain can occur/persist after fusion.

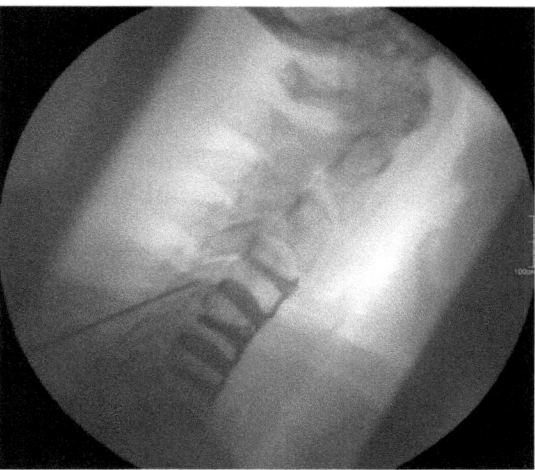

Fig. 19: An 18G cannula (or needle) with a curved 10-mm active tip RF needle being navigated for C5 medial branch (MB) radiofrequency denervation (RFD).

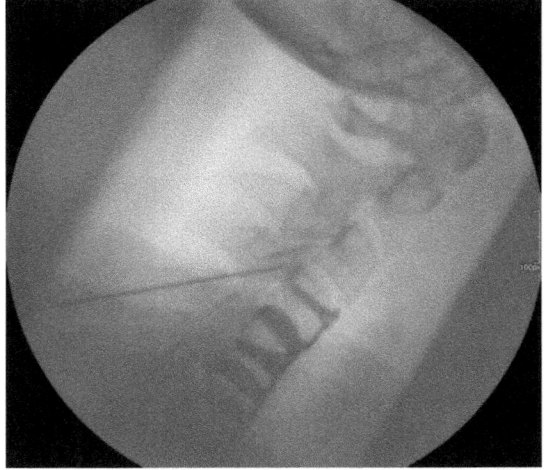

Fig. 20: An 18G cannula (or needle) with a curved 10-mm active tip RF needle is being navigated for C4 MB RFD.

Case 5

Third occipital nerve radiofrequency denervation is performed in patients who respond with excellent pain relief following third occipital nerve block (See Chapter 13). Only one side (right or the left) is performed at a given time. Performing bilateral third occipital nerve block or denervation can lead to ataxia.

Step 1: A perfect lateral view is obtained with the C2/3 facet joint line outlined and double shadow at the upper border of C2 eliminated (arrows) as in the **Figure 21**. (See **Fig. 10** and **Figs. 18** and **19** for double shadows at the upper border of C2).

Step 2: The skin entry points are in line with the C2/3 facet joint line, the same distance behind the posterior margin of the articular pillar as the distance between the anterior and the posterior borders of the articular pillar. Lesions are performed at three levels: just above and below the C2/3 facet joint line (long arrows) and the third at the level of the C2/3 facet joint line. An 18G cannula (or needle) with a curved 10-mm active tip RF needle is navigated parallel to the C2/3 facet joint line and the position of the needle confirmed in the anterior inferior oblique view. After injecting around 0.5 mL LA, two lesions are performed as described for MB RFD at each level. **Figure 22** shows the trajectory and position of the needles for the lesions above and below the C2/3 facet joint line.

Step 3: The skin entry point is in line with the C2/3 facet joint line, the same distance behind the posterior margin of the articular pillar as the distance between the anterior and the posterior borders of the articular pillar. **Figure 23** shows the trajectory and position of the needle for the lesion at the level of the C2/3 facet joint line. By performing lesions at three levels as described, a wide area of RF lesioning is covered taking into consideration the variability of the anatomic position and the course of the third occipital nerve.

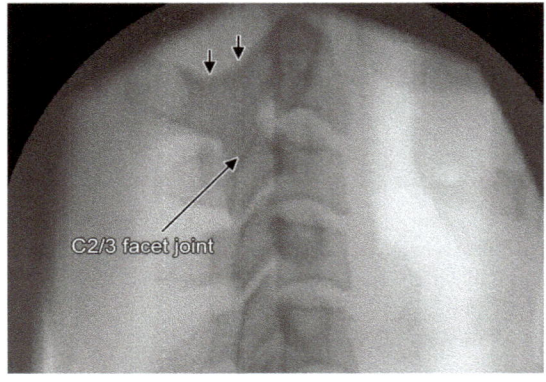

Fig. 21: *Third occipital nerve RFD:* A perfect lateral view is obtained with the C2/3 facet joint line outlined and double shadow at the upper border of C2 eliminated (arrows).

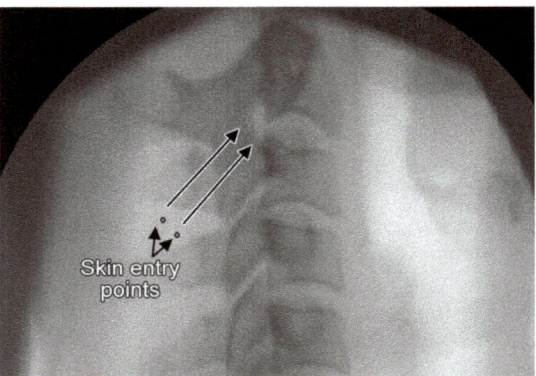

Fig. 22: *Third occipital nerve RFD:* Skin entry points and the trajectory and position of the needles for the lesions above and below the C2/3 facet joint line.

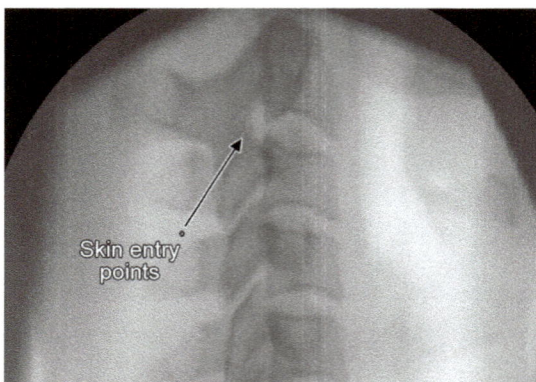

Fig. 23: *Third occipital nerve RFD:* Skin entry point and the trajectory and position of the needle for the lesions at the level of the C2/3 facet joint line.

FURTHER READING

1. Baker A, Baranidharan G, Toomey P, Nath S. Cervical spine interventions. In: Simpson K, Baranidharan G, Gupta S (Eds). Spinal Interventions in Pain Management (Oxford Specialist Handbooks in Pain Management). Oxford: Oxford University Press; 2012. pp. 71-91.
2. Gupta S, Dhandapani K. Applied anatomy and fluoroscopy for spinal interventions. In: Simpson K, Baranidharan G, Gupta S (Eds). Spinal Interventions in Pain Management (Oxford Specialist Handbooks in Pain Management). Oxford: Oxford University Press; 2012. pp. 1-10.
3. Gupta S, Varma S. Cervical medial branch block. In: Baheti DK, Bakshi S, Gupta S, Singh RSP (Eds). Interventional Pain Management: A Practical Approach, 2nd edition. New Delhi: Jaypee Brothers Medical Publishers; 2016. pp. 220-9.
4. Lord SM, Barnsley L, Wallis B, McDonald GJ, Bogduk N. Percutaneous radiofrequency neurotomy for chronic zygapophyseal joint pain. N Eng J Med. 1996;335:1721-6.
5. The British Pain Society and Faculty of Pain Medicine of the Royal College of Anaesthetists (2nd edition). (2020) (Working Party Chair: Dr Sanjeeva Gupta). Standards of good practice for spinal interventional procedures in pain medicine. [online] Available from https://www.britishpainsociety.org/static/uploads/resources/files/BPS_and_FPM_Spinal_Intervention_Guidelines_PDF_Final_May_2020_2_new_ISBN.pdf [Last accessed May, 2022].
6. Third occipital nerve blocks. In: Bogduk N (Ed). Practice Guidelines for Spinal Diagnostic and Treatment Procedures, 2nd edition. San Francisco, CA: International Spinal Intervention Society; 2013. pp. 141-63.

Section 4: Chest and Thorax

- **Intercostal Nerve Block**
  Dwarkadas K Baheti

- **Intrapleural Block**
  Dwarkadas K Baheti

CHAPTER 16

Intercostal Nerve Block

Dwarkadas K Baheti

BASIC INFORMATION

Indications
- Fractured ribs
- Sternotomy
- Thoracotomy
- Postherpetic neuralgia
- Postsurgical thoracic or abdominal nerve entrapment
- Upper abdominal surgeries
- Appendectomy

Contraindications
- Local infection
- Coagulopathy
- Unwilling patient

Equipment and Drugs
- 25G ¾ inch needle
- 22G 1½ inch needle
- 5 cm radiofrequency (RF) needle with 5-mm active tip
- 2, 3, and 5-mL syringe
- 1–2% lignocaine
- 0.25–0.5% bupivacaine
- Absolute alcohol
- Radiofrequency generator

Complications
- Pneumothorax
- Local anesthetic allergy or toxicity due to proximity to blood vessels
- Infection

Important Tip
Alcohol block should be avoided as it might cause post-procedure neuritis.

PROCEDURE DETAILS

Step 1: Position—Patient in prone position with both the arms to hang over the sides of the table **(Fig. 1)**. It will maximize anterior motion of the scapular and maximize surface of the upper ribs that is accessible from a posterior approach.

Step 2: Locate the angle of the rib approximately 8 cm lateral to the spine **(Fig. 2)**. This is the point at which most ribs make a sharp turn in direction from extending laterally to pointing anteriorly.

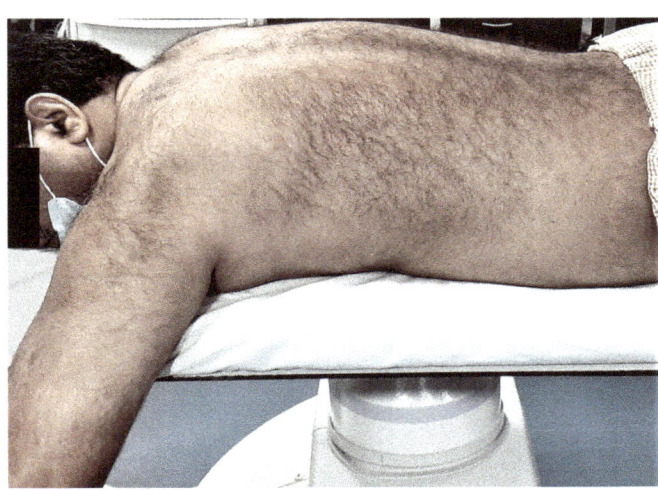

Fig. 1: Position of patient.

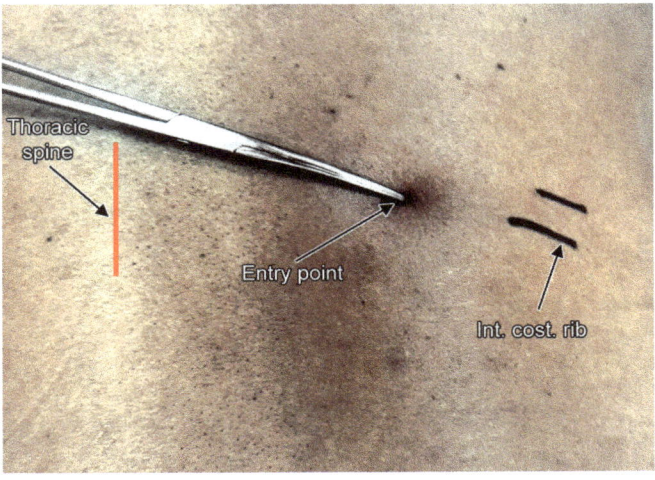

Fig. 2: Marker at needle entry point.

Step 3: Take a 22-gauge, spinal needle is pushed deep enough to contact the inferior portion of the rib. After contacting the rib as seen in **Figure 3**.

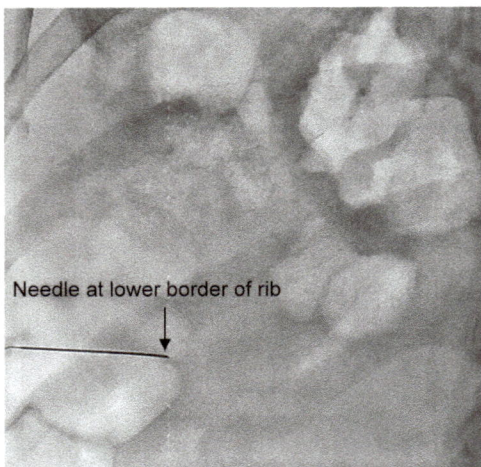

Fig. 3: Needle at lower border of rib.

Step 4: Now hold the needle firmly and try to redirect under the rib to "walk off" the inferior margin of the rib.

Step 5: Once this is done advance the needle approximately 3 mm deep to the lower margin as seen **(Fig. 4)**.

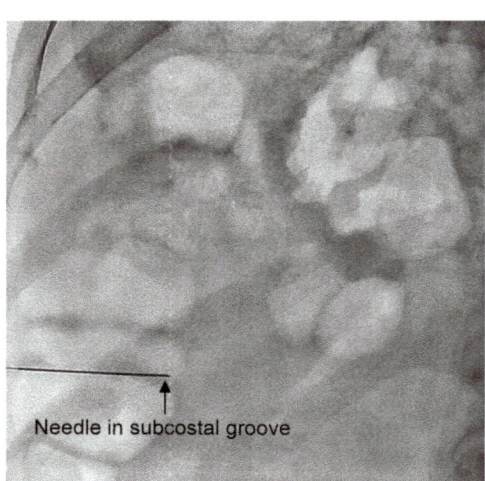

Fig. 4: Needle in the subcostal groove.

Step 6: Now confirm the negative aspiration for air or blood for inadvertent perforation of vessel or pleura.

Step 7: After repeated aspiration inject half-to-one cc of contrast to confirm the spread of dye along the inferior border of the rib as seen in **Figure 5**.

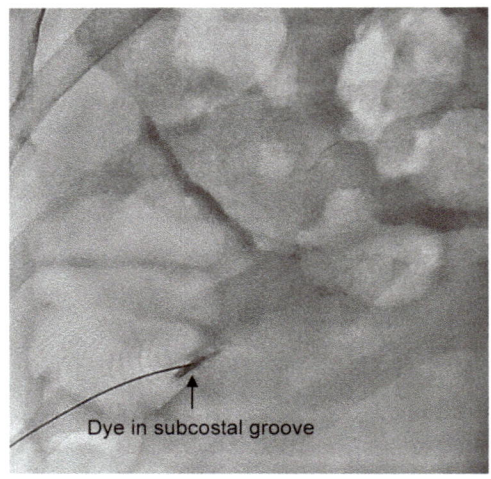

Fig. 5: Dye spread in the subcostal groove.

Step 8: Now inject the local anesthetic for pain relief or if for postoperative pain relief, the indwelling catheter can be used.

According to indication one can use mixture of local anesthetic with steroid OR radiofrequency ablation.

Many a times, one may need multiple level intercostal nerve blocks as per the indication.

Step 9: Now shift the patient to recovery room for observation.

Declaration

Part of the text and some images are taken with permission from M/s Jaypee Brothers Medical Publishers, New Delhi from the chapter "Intercostal Nerve Block" published in the book, *Interventional Pain Management: A Practical Approach* 2009 and 2018 edited by DK Baheti, Sanjay Bakshi, Sanjeeva Gupta, and RP Gehdoo.

CHAPTER 17

Intrapleural Block

Dwarkadas K Baheti

BASIC INFORMATION

Indications
- Carcinoma of lung
- Carcinoma of gallbladder
- Secondary in the lung
- Post-herpetic neuralgia
- Post-surgical thoracic or abdominal nerve entrapment
- Upper abdominal surgeries
- Post-thoracotomy pain

Contraindications
- Patient unable, unwilling to consent or uncooperative patient
- Known allergy to contrast
- Local or systemic infection
- Coagulopathy
- Pregnancy
- Concurrent use of anticoagulants
- Coexisting disease producing significant CVS or respiratory compromise
- Immunosuppression

Equipment/Types and Sizes of Needle
- C-arm fluoroscopy or CT scan along with monitoring and resuscitation facility.
- 26-gauge for skin infiltration and deep infiltration of local anesthetic.
- Epidural set (16-guage needle with epidural catheter and filter).

Drugs and Concentration
- Inj. lignocaine—2% (Xylocard—preservative free)
- Inj. iohexol (Omnipaque), a water-soluble contrast
- Inj. bupivacaine 0.25%
- Inj. phenol in glycerin—6–10% or Inj. tetracycline for pleurodesis

PROCEDURE DETAILS

Step 1: Explains the pleural anatomy (**Fig. 1**) how visceral pleura and visceral pleura are separated. Its vital to know about the placement of needle should be between these layers. As there is negative pressure between these layers so sucking of air or loss resistance technique is used.

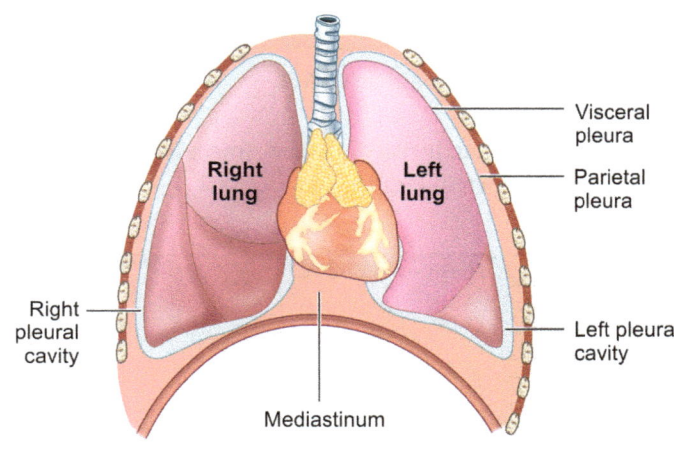

Fig. 1: Understanding of pleural anatomy.

Step 2: Patient is put in sitting position with hands supported on trolly with monitoring of vital signs and identify the 9th, 10th, and 11th intercostal space. The marking is done as seen in **Figure 2**.

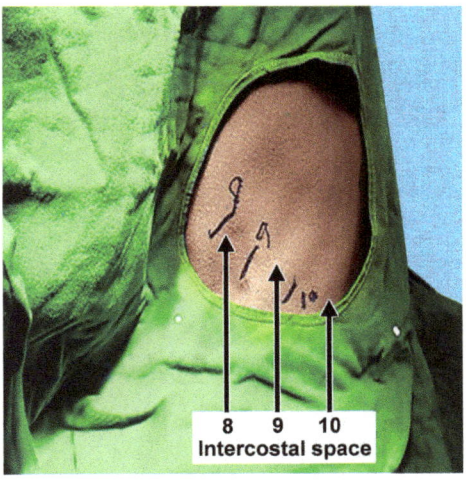

Fig. 2: Position for block and identifying and marking of Intercostal (IC) space.

Step 3: Now identify the 10th intercostal space and inject Inj. lignocaine 2% about 3–5 cc (**Fig. 3**).

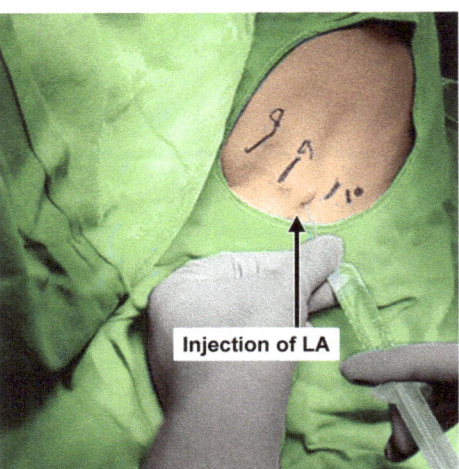

Fig. 3: Injecting of local anesthesia (LA).

Once position of needle is confirmed. Inject Inj. omnipaque 1–2 cc dye as shown in **Figure 5**.

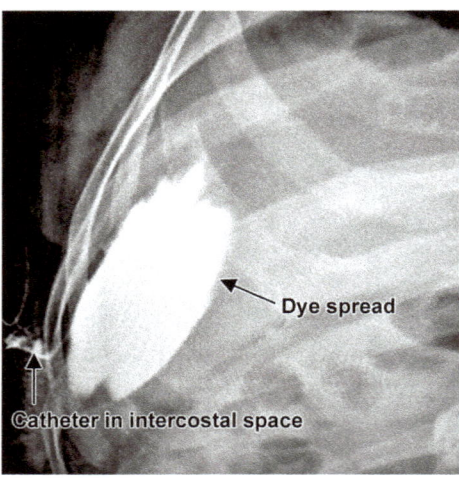

Fig. 5: Dye spread space confirming with hanging.

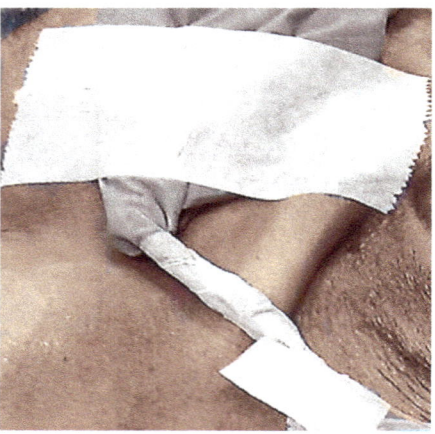

Fig. 7: Final dressing.

Step 4: Take Toughy needle and introduce into the space with hanging drop technique as shown in (**Refer Video No. 5**) **Figure 4**.

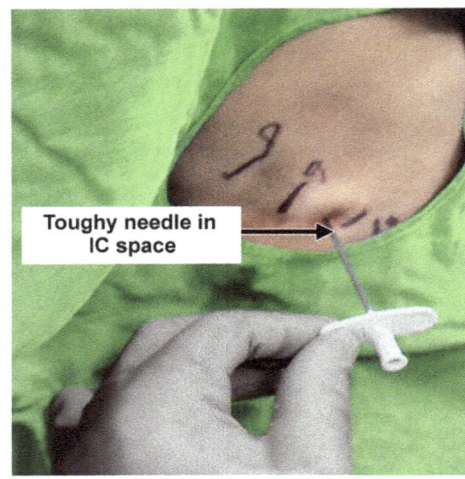

Fig. 4: Toughy needle in intercostal drop technique.

Step 5: Now inject 2–3 mL of local anesthetic and tunnel the catheter through epidural needle and fix it to the thoracic wall as shown in **Figure 6**.

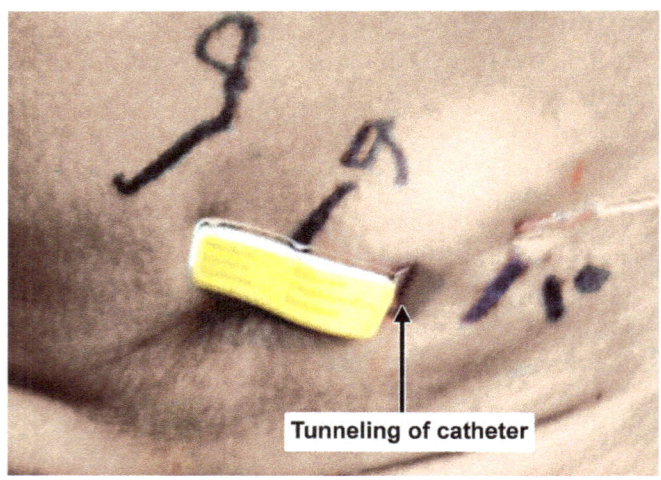

Fig. 6: Tunneling and fixation of epidural catheter.

Step 7: Do the dressing as shown in **Figure 7**.

Step 8: Shift the patient of recovery room for observation for few hours.

Declaration

Part of the text and some images are taken with permission from M/s Jaypee Brothers Medical Publishers, New Delhi, from the chapter "Intrapleural Block" published in the book, *Interventional Pain Management: Practical Approach* 2009 and 2018 edited by DK Baheti, Sanjay Bakshi, Sanjeeva Gupta, and RP Gehdoo.

SECTION 5

Lumbosacral Spine

- **Interlaminar Lumbar Epidural Block**
  Sanjay Bakshi

- **Transforaminal Lumbar Epidural Block**
  Dwarkadas K Baheti, Sanjeeva Gupta

- **Lumbar Transforaminal Epidural Steroid Injections: Technical Challenges**
  Sanjeeva Gupta, Dwarkadas K Baheti, Sanjay Bakshi

- **Lumbar Medial Branch Block and Radiofrequency Ablation**
  Anil Sharma, Sanjeeva Gupta

- **Caudal Epidural Block**
  Sanjay Bakshi

- **S1 Nerve Root Block and Technical Challenges**
  Sanjeeva Gupta, Manohar Sharma, Sanjay Bakshi

- **Sacroiliac Joint Block**
  Sanjeeva Gupta, Babita Ghai

- **Sacroiliac Joint Radiofrequency Denervation**
  Samir Ranjit Jani, Sanjeeva Gupta, Ganesan Baranidharan

- **Sacroiliac Joint Fusion: A Minimally Invasive Posterior Approach**
  Samir Ranjit Jani

- **Piriformis Tendon and Muscle Injection**
  Yashwant Laxman Nankar, Dwarkadas K Baheti

- **Pudendal Nerve Block and Pulsed Radiofrequency Procedure**
  Sanjeeva Gupta, Babita Ghai

- **Coccygeal Nerve Block**
  Yashwant Laxman Nankar, Dwarkadas K Baheti

CHAPTER 18

Interlaminar Lumbar Epidural Block

Sanjay Bakshi

INTERLAMINAR LUMBAR EPIDURAL STEROID INJECTION

Basic Information

Indications
- Lumbar radiculopathy
- Lumbar disc herniation
- Lumbar spinal stenosis

Contraindications
- Unwilling patient
- Untreated infection
- Pregnancy
- Bleeding problems or blood thinners
- Allergy to medications
- Severe cardiovascular or respiratory compromise
- Dye allergies use alternate dye or premedication

Equipment and Supplies
- C-arm
- Epidural tray with Tuohy needle and LOR syringe
- Connection tubing
- IV if sedation planned
- Appropriate monitors

Medications
- Contrast dye
- Steroid—dexamethasone or Kenalog
- Local anesthetic
- Preservative-free saline

PROCEDURE

Step 1: Patient in prone position. After skin preparation and draping, take the initial fluoroscopic anteroposterior (AP) view as shown in **Figure 1**.

Step 2: Mark skin entry point with marker as shown in **Figure 2**.

Step 3: Now advance 18-gauge Tuohy needle slowly toward lamina till the needle is in contact with lamina as shown in **Figure 3**. This avoids advancing the needle too far. Now walk off the lamina.

As soon as you walk off the lamina, use loss of resistance (LOR) technique to enter epidural space. Confirm needle position in lateral view under fluoroscopy as in **Figure 4**.

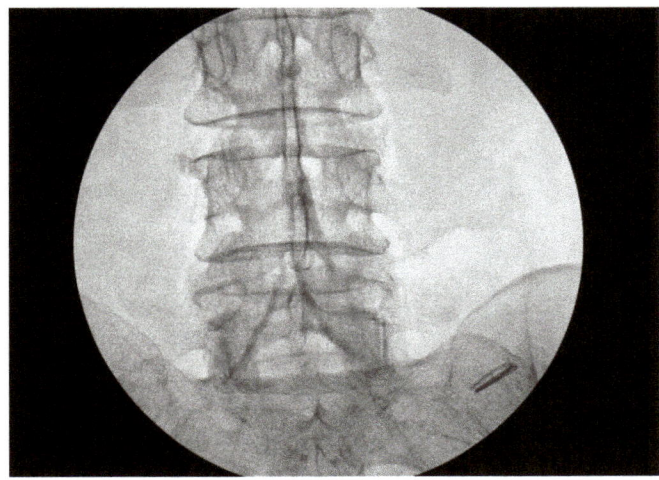

Fig. 1: Posteroanterior view—lumbosacral spine.

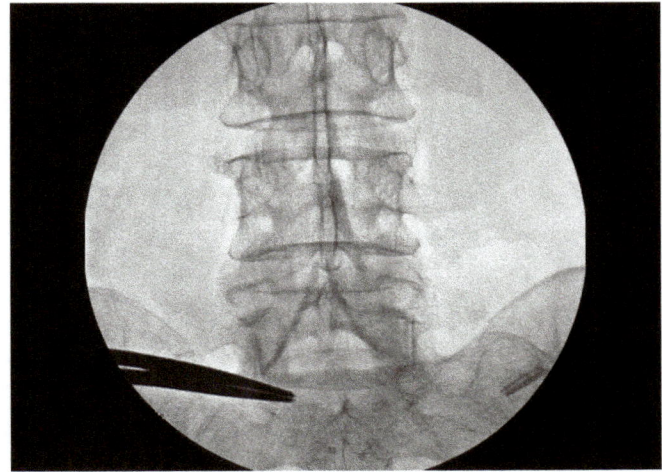

Fig. 2: Marker at entry point.

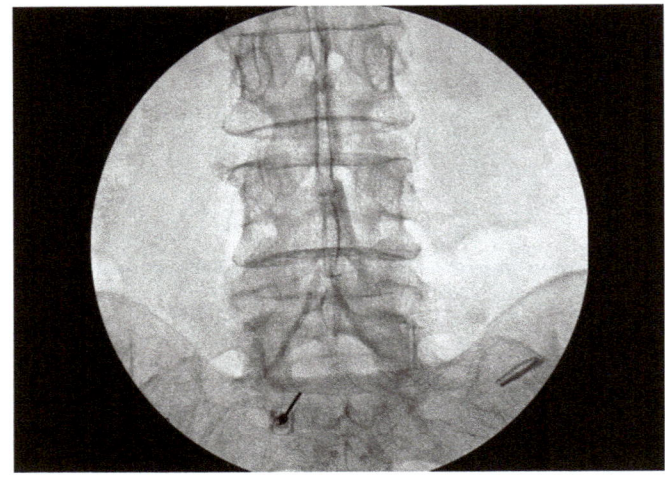

Fig. 3: Tuohy needle touching lamina anteroposterior view.

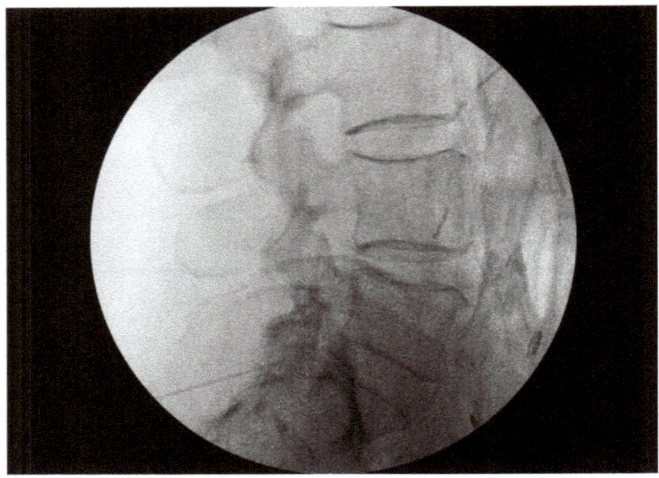

Fig. 4: Tuohy needle in lateral view.

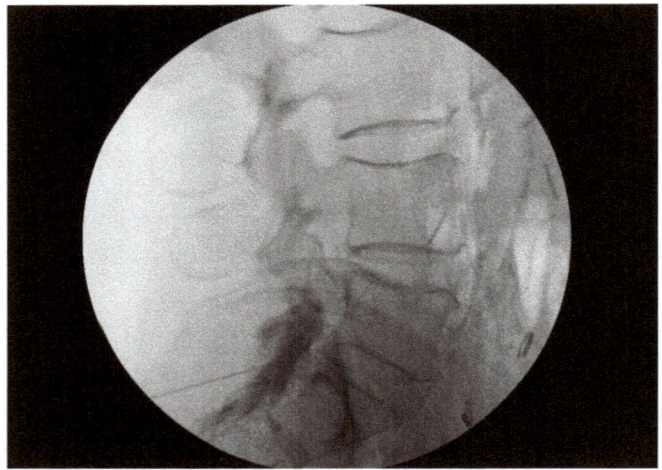

Fig. 5: Dye spread in lateral view.

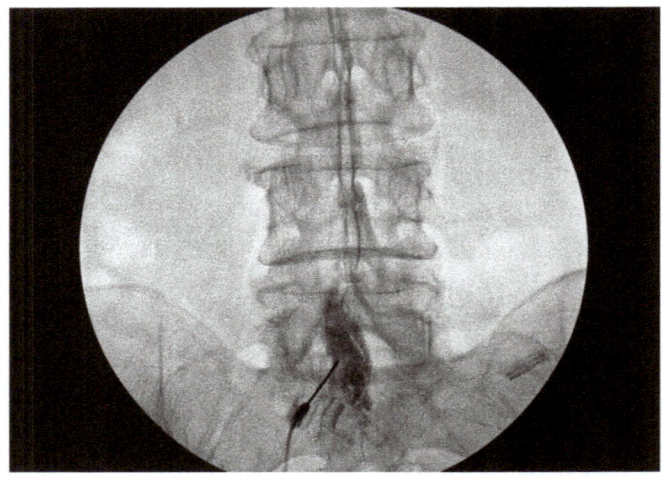

Fig. 6: Dye spread in anteroposterior view.

Step 4: Now inject 2-3 cc contrast under continuous fluoroscopy and confirm the spread of dye in lateral view as seen in **Figure 5** and in AP view as seen in **Figure 6**.

Step 5: Now inject the medication 4-6 cc, i.e., combination of steroid with local anesthetic or normal saline.

Step 6: Shift the patient for monitoring of vitals for few hours.

CHAPTER 19

Transforaminal Lumbar Epidural Block

Dwarkadas K Baheti, Sanjeeva Gupta

BASIC INFORMATION

Transforaminal lumbar epidural block (TFLEB) is one of the most common pain procedure performed by pain physician.

To understand and make easy the technical challenges one may face while performing these blocks few challenging cases are discussed in the Chapter 20.

TFLEB had high level evidence and some of references are listed at the end.

IMPORTANT TIPS

- As the procedure is done under local anesthesia and sedation try to be as gentle as possible while redirecting and navigating the needle in deeper plane towards the target area.
- Movement of the needle in the deeper planes should be gradual. Once the needle tip is near the intervertebral foramen the needle should be advacned by millimeters. Communicating with the patients regarding any symptoms in the lower limb during the procedure is very important to prevent nerve injury.
- Always confirm position of needle in antero-posterior (AP) and lateral views using the 3D principle discussed under Figure 2 in Chapter 1.
- Repeated negative aspiration at every step.

Indications

- Lumbar radiculopathy
- Lumbar disc herniation/prolapse
- Lumbar foraminal/spinal stenosis
- Post-laminectomy pain/failed back syndrome

Equipment

- C-arm preferably with digital subtraction imaging.
- Procedure tray with spinal needle preferably short bevel
- Leur lock syringes and extension tubing
- Appropriate monitors and resuscitation trolley

MORE INFORMATION

Author (DKB) routinely combines TFLEB with caudal epidural block in most of his patients. He has observed and as reported by patient's experienced better and prolonged pain relief than with *only* TFLEB in most of lumbar radiculopathy patients in more than thirty years of clinical practice.

The possible explanations are as follows:
- Most of his patients often complained of pain and tenderness in sacral area
- Caudal epidurogram (routinely done) often showed filling defect in sacral foramen on one or both sides.
- Due to practice style in India, he believes to provide maximum pain relief in one sitting (Due to poor follow-up, financial restriction and lack of insurance coverage).

Drugs

- Intravenous access is advisible for patients having TFLEB
- Water soluble neural safer contrast dye
- Steroid—Dexamethasone or Triamcinolone (Kenalog)
- Local anesthetic
- Preservative free saline

Contraindications

- Unwilling patient
- Untreated infection
- Pregnancy
- Bleeding problems or blood thinners
- Allergy to medications
- Presence of red flags

Complications
- Nerve root injury
- Paralysis/paraplegia
- Intrathecal injection
- Hematoma

ADDITIONAL TIPS
- Review latest MRI scan images and any fluoroscopic images of previous procedures.
- Obtain informed consent

TRANSFORAMINAL LUMBAR EPIDURAL BLOCK-STEPWISE APPROACH

CASE 1

Patient had pain in the right lower limb in the right L5 and S1 nerve distribution due to L5 and S1 nerve root irritation in the L4/5 and L5/S1 recess due to degenerative changes in the lumbar spine and disc bulges at L4/5 and L5/S1 levels respectively as shown in the MRI scan image (see **Figure 9A**). The patient was not responding adequately to conservative measures including pharmacotherapy. This patient was consented for right L5/S1 transforaminal epidural and right S1 nerve root injection.

Step 1: Patient in prone position with pillow under lower abdomen and pelvis as shown in **Figure 1**.

Step 2: Prepare and drape the patient for TFLEB—subpedicular technique.

Obtain a AP view with the spinous process in the middle of the two pedicles and then tilt the C-arm cephalic by few degrees to square the vertebral end plate closest to the target point **(Figs. 2A and B)**.

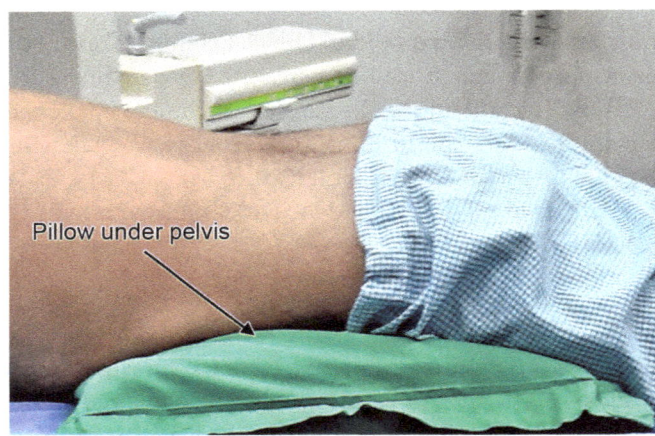

Fig. 1: *Position of patient:* Prone position with a pillow under the lower abdomen and pelvis to decrease the lumbar lordosis.

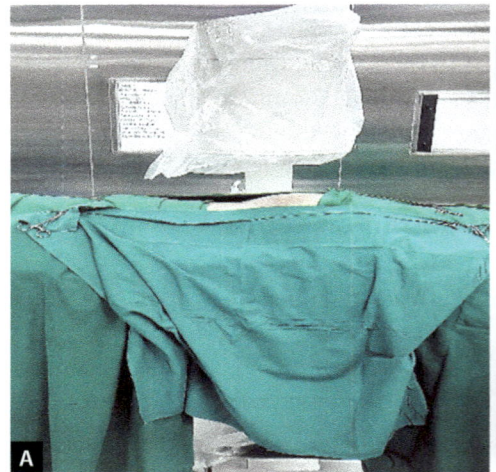
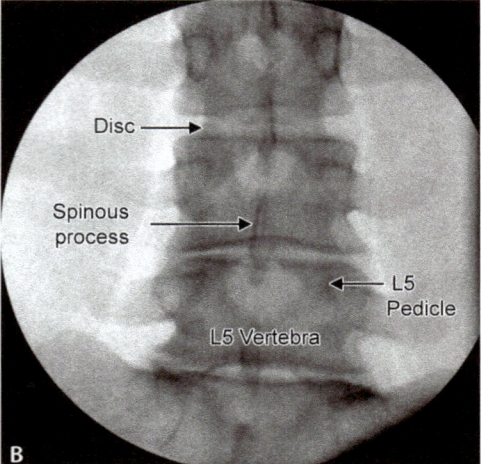

Figs. 2A and B: Fluoroscope in AP view.

Step 3: Once the AP view is obtained and the vertebral endplates are 'squared off' by around 5° to 10° cephalic tilt, identify the bony structures as shown in **Figure 3**.

Step 4: Rotate the C-arm in the right oblique direction to obtain a "scotty view" and identify the structures relevant to TFLEB as shown in **Figure 4**.

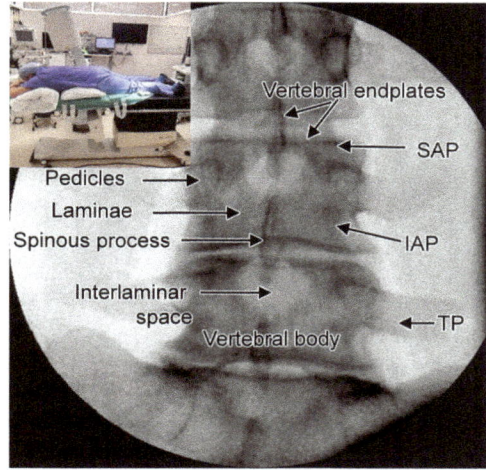

Fig. 3: Fluoroscopy in 5 to 10° cephalic tilt to square the vertebral endplates. (SAP: superior articular process; IAP: inferior articular process; TP: transverse process).

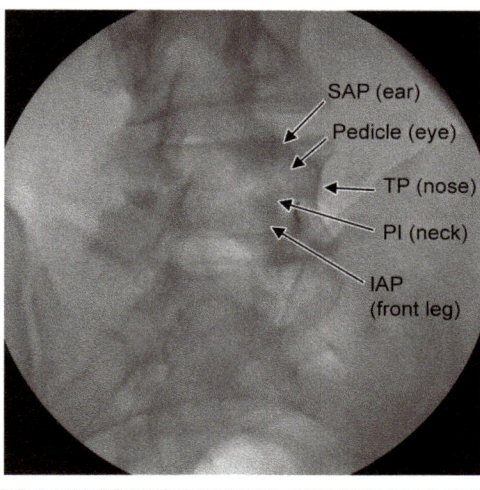

Fig. 4: *TFLEB fluoroscopy:* Identify the structures of the spine in oblique view. (SAP: superior articular process; IAP: inferior articular process; TP: transverse process; PI: pars interarticularis)

Step 5: Maintain the oblique position of fluoroscope and place a pointer at the skin entry point of needle as shown in **Figure 5A**. Take 22G spinal needle with curved tip as seen in **Figure 5B**.

Step 6: Raise the intradermal wheel with local anesthetic at the needle entry point.

Principles of navigation and perfect placement of needle are as follows:
- Follow Three "D" principle, i.e., Depth, Direction and Destination to reach the target as described in Figure 2 in Chapter 1.
- At regular intervals, check the depth and direction of needle under fluoroscope.
- Aim for end on view

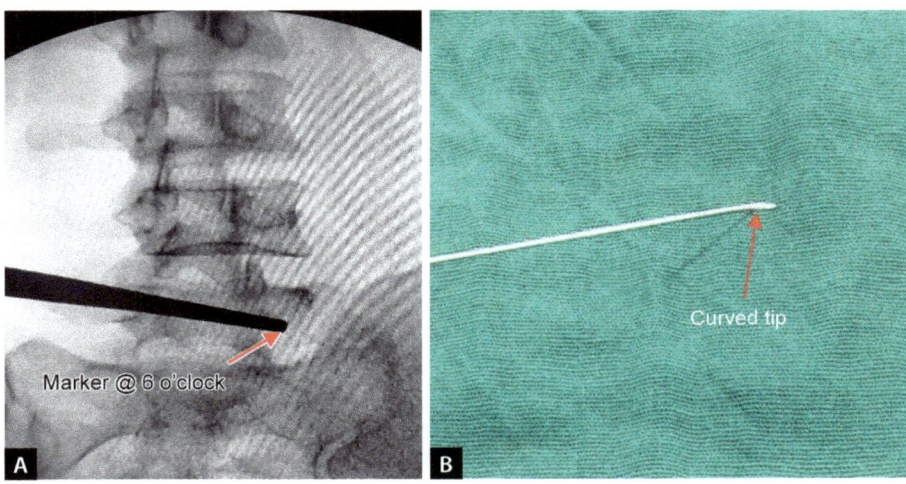

Figs. 5A and B: Marker at 6 o'clock position under pedicle in Scotty view, and curved tip needle.

Step 7: After obtaining AP view and rotating the C-arm to the right to obtain a "Scotty Dog" image a 22G or a 25G curved tipped spinal needle **(Figs. 5A and B)** is advanced.

Use a "Gun-barrel technique" to navigate to contact the lower end of the L5 pedicle (chin of the scotty dog) between the 5° clock and 6° clock position on the pedicle and then navigate by few millimeters (mm) just below the inferior margin of the pedicle (arrow) into the intervertebral foramen. End on view of the needle is seen in **Figures 6B**.

If the patient complains of radicular pain withdraw the needle a few mm and redirect.

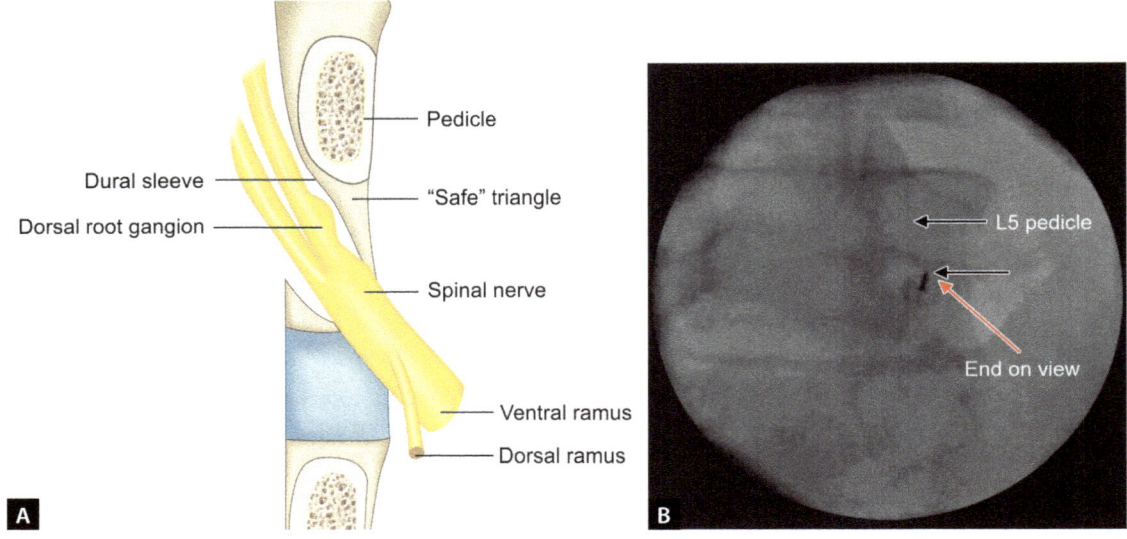

Figs. 6A and B: *Right TFLEB (subpedicular technique):* End on view of the needle.

Step 8: Confirm the depth of needle in lateral view as seen in **Figure 7**.

Step 9: In this patient, S1 nerve root block is also planned so a 22G spinal needle is directed following above principles of advancement into the S1 foramen as seen in the AP view in **Figure 8**.

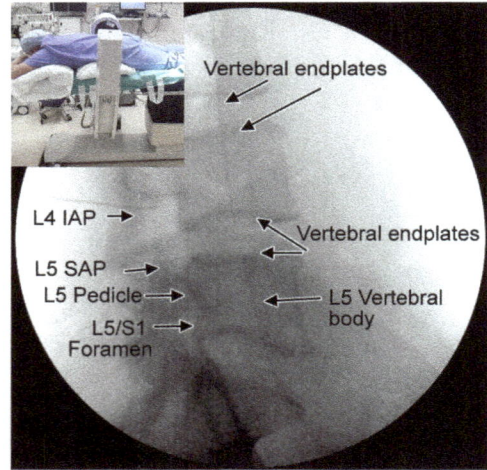

Fig. 7: TFLEB lateral view. This image is for illustration purpose only as it shows the needle at L4/5 level and not L5/S1 level. (SAP: superior articular process; IAP: inferior articular process). *Question:* Identify the needle tip in the L4/5 foramen.

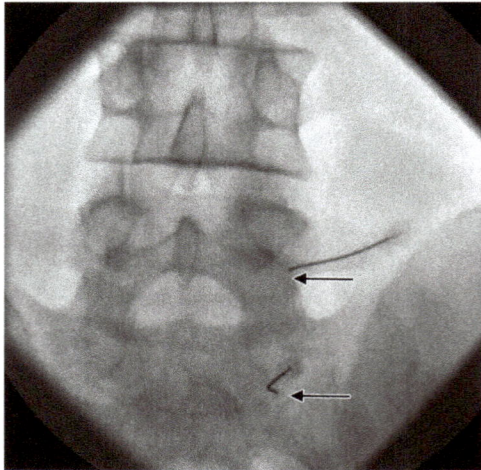

Fig. 8: *Right TFLEB:* AP view showing needles in positions at L5/S1 level and into the S1 foramen (arrows). Please also see Chapter 23—S1 root block for more details.

- Then obtain a lateral view and identify the structures relevant to TFLEB **(Figs. 9A and B)**.

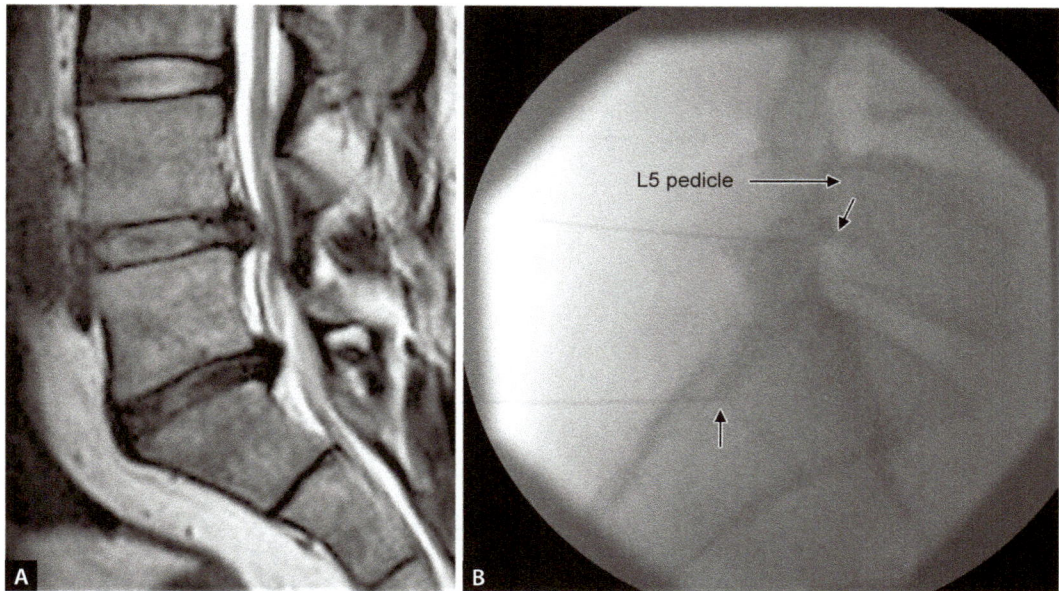

Figs. 9A and B: *Right TFLEB:* In lateral view, the needle tip can be seen in the L5/S1 intervertebral foramen just below the L5 pedicle and also in the S1 foramen (arrows). The sagittal T2 MRI scan image confirms that the procedure is being done at the correct levels (beware of transitional vertebra at L5/S1 levels).

Step 10: Now inject about 0.5 to 1.0 mL of water soluble nerual safe contrast in AP view under continuous fluoroscopy via an extention tubing attached to the spinal needle. Rule out vascular spread. The contrast can be seen spreading along the lower and inner border of the pedicle, into the epidural space and along the L5 nerve root **(Fig. 10)** but not in the area of the L5/S1 disc which is irritating the right S1 nerve root.

Step 11: Wait for some time and reconfirm that dye spread is not spreading towards the L5/S1 as seen in **Figure 11**.

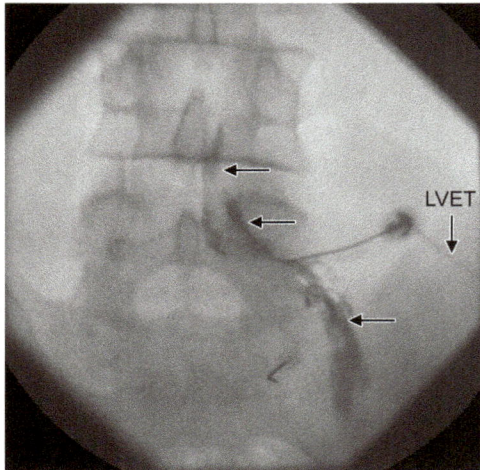

Fig. 10: *Right TFLEB:* Dye spread in AP view.

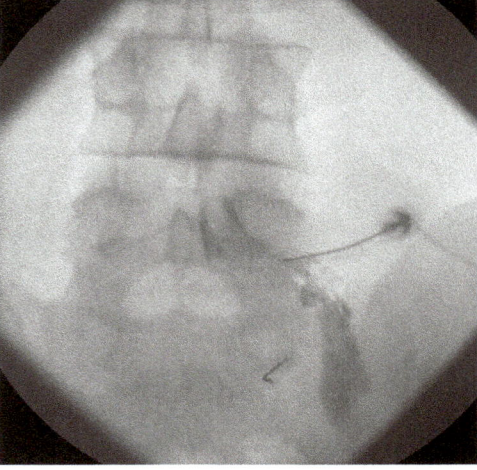

Fig. 11: *Right TFLEB:* Reconfirming that the contrast is not spreading towards the L5/S1 disc.

Step 12: Now inject contrast at the S1 level in AP view via an extention tubing attached to the spinal needle under continuous fluoroscopy. Rule out vascular spread. Confirm the contrast spread along the S1 nerve root as seen in **Figure 12**.

Step 13: Have a final look at the fluoroscopic view that the contrast spread at desired space and level before injecting the steroid. As seen in **Figure 13**.

Step 14: Now inject the mixture of steroid with normal saline OR steroid + local anesthetic **(Fig. 14)**. Some pain physicians use a particulate steroid such as methyl prednisolone or triamcinalone while some pain physicians prefer first using a non-particulate steroid such as dexamethasone.

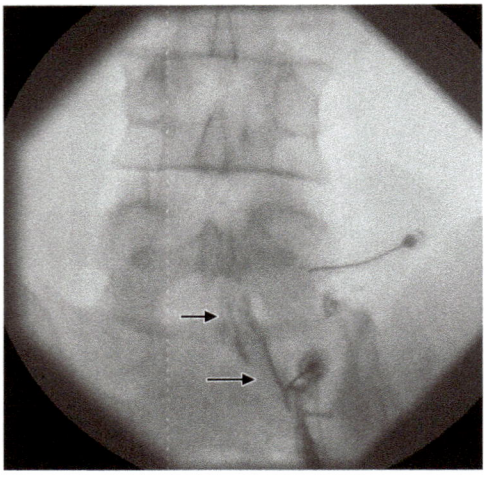

Fig. 12: Contrast spread at S1 level shows spreads along right S1 nerve root (arrows) and towards the area of the pathology at L5/S1 level.

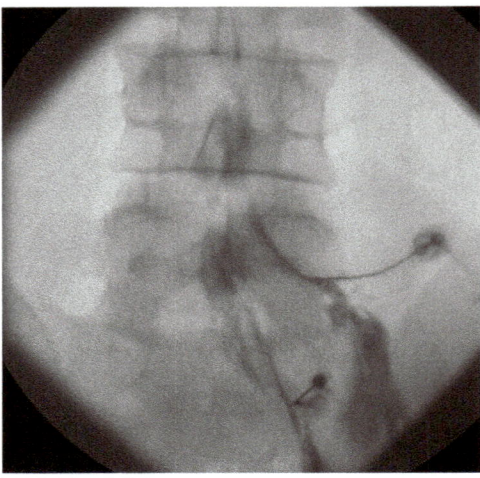

Fig. 13: *Right TFLEB:* Further contrast injection at S1 level shows good spread of contrast along the S1 nerve root and into the epidural space.

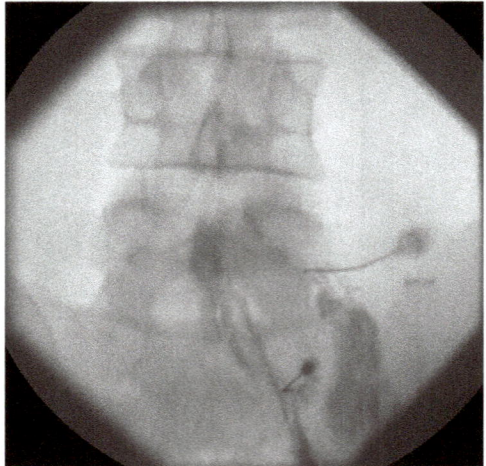

Fig. 14: *Right TFLEB:* Final AP image after injection of medications at L5/S1 and S1 level.

CASE 2

This patient had radicular pain in the left L5 distribution due to irritation of the left L5 nerve root in the L4/5 recess due to L4/5 disc bulge.

Step 1: First obtain a true AP view and then tilt the C-arm by 5–10° to "square off" the vertebral endplate closest to the target point and then rotate the C-arm to the left to obtain a left oblique "scotty view" and identify the structures relevant to left TFLEB **(Fig. 15)**.

Step 2: After injection of local anesthetic advance a 22G curved tip needle following steps described in Case 1 and obtain a end on view as in **Figure 16**.

Step 3: Now turn fluoroscope in lateral positions to visualize tip of needle just under pedicle in lateral view as seen in **Figure 17**.

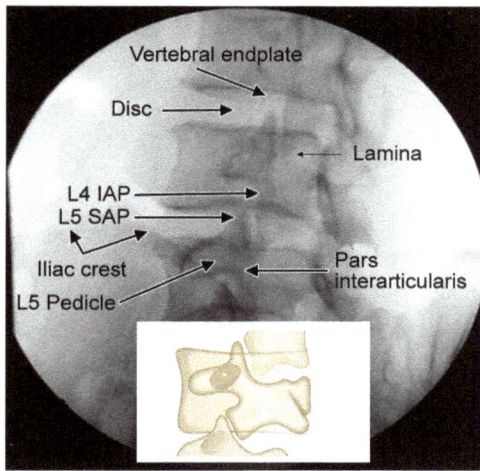

Fig. 15: Scotty dog view.

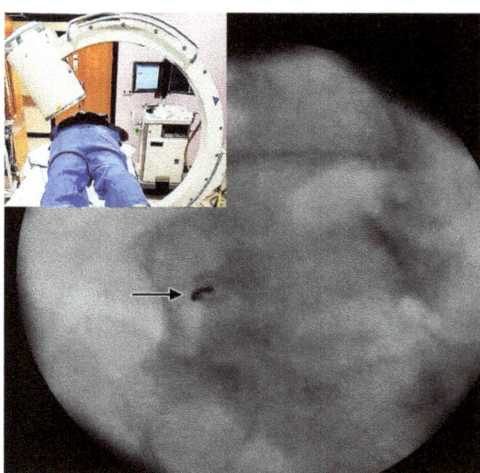

Fig. 16: *Left L5/S1 TFLEB:* Left oblique view with the needle tip (arrow) "End on view" at the lower end of the left L5 pedicle (chin of the scotty dog).

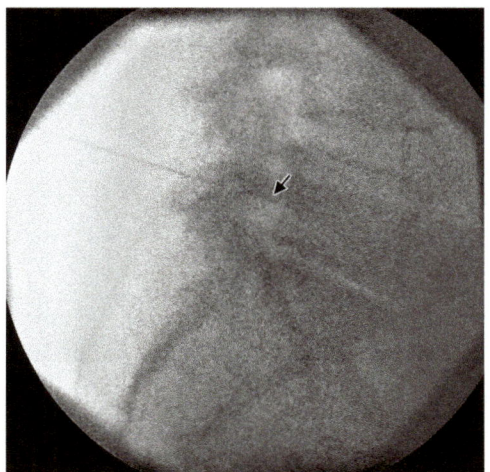

Fig. 17: Lateral view showing the needle tip in the L5/S1 intervertebral foramen (arrow).

Step 4: Rotate fluoroscope C-arm back to AP view to visualize the tip of needle under pedicle as seen in **Figure 18**.

Step 5: Now inject contrast in AP view via an extention tubing attached to the block needle under continuous fluoroscopy. Rule out vascular spread. Confirm contrast spread as in **Figure 19**.

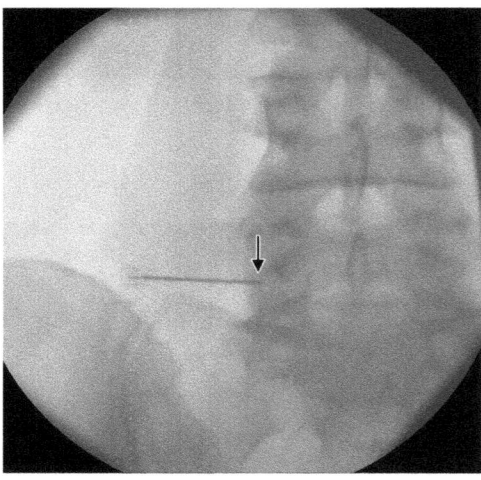

Fig. 18: True AP view (L5 spinous process in the center of two L5 pedicles) showing the tip of the needle at around 7 o'clock position of the left L5 pedicle (should be lateral 6 o'clock position to decrease the chances of dural sleeve puncture).

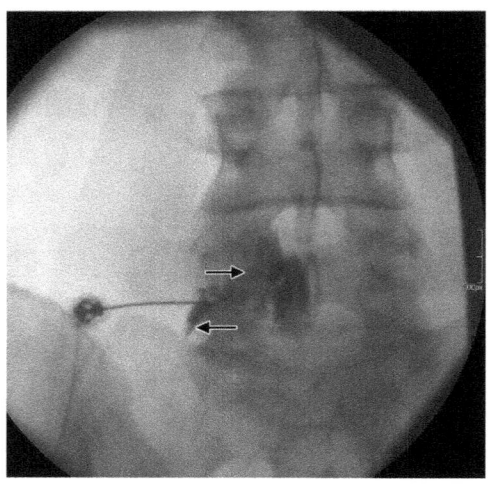

Fig. 19: Contrast injected in AP view shows contrast spread along the pedicle and left L5 nerve root (arrows).

Step 6: Final view after injection of medications as seen in **Figure 20**.

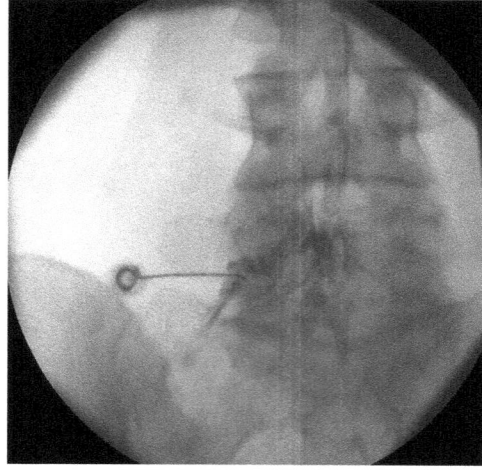

Fig. 20: Final AP view after injection of medications (L4/5 recess).

CASE 3

Patient had right L5 radicular pain due to irritation of right L5 nerve root in the L4/5 recess due to degenerative changes and disc bulge at L4/5 level. Although the patient also had disc bulge at L5/S1 level contacting the right S1 nerve root they did not have any neuropathic symptoms in the right S1 distribution, and hence S1 root block was not considered in this case. Some clinicians prefer to routinely do pre- and post- ganglionic TFLEB (reference 12) but in this case, it was decided to do only postganglionic TFLEB at L5/S1 level.

Step 1: Following the steps described in Case 1 advance the curved tip needle as seen in **Figure 21** in AP view.

Step 2: Rotate the fluoroscope laterally to confirm the tip of needle under pedicle as seen in **Figures 22B**.

Step 3: Inject the contrast and confirm spread in AP view as seen in **Figure 23**.

Step 4: Injection of medications **(Fig. 24)**.

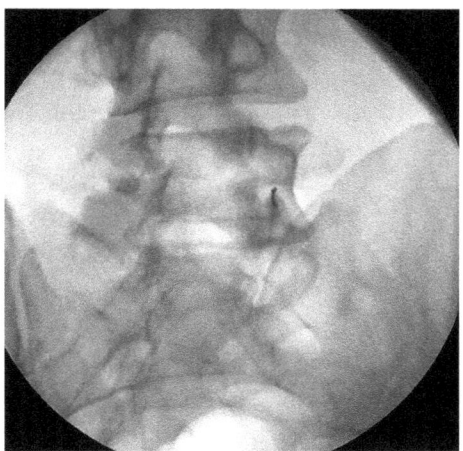

Fig. 21: Needle in position for right L5/S1 TFLEB (subpedicular technique).

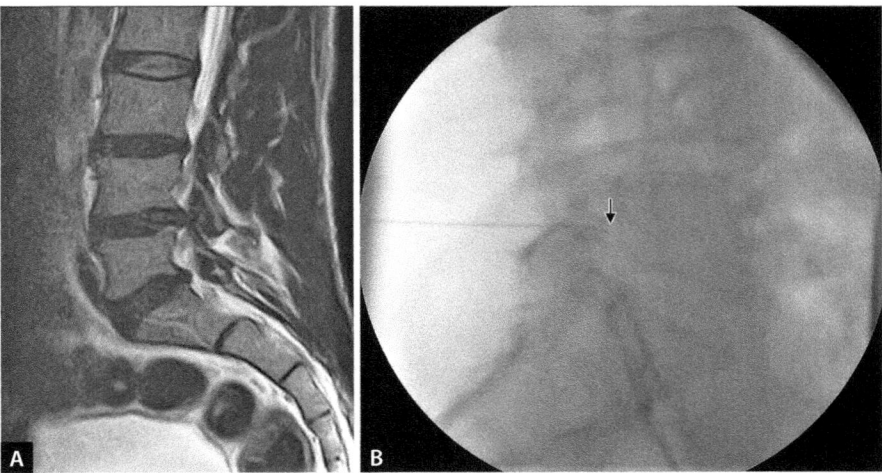

Figs. 22A and B: Lateral view showing the needle tip in the L5/S1 intervertebral foramen (arrow). Comparing the lateral fluoroscopic view with the sagittal T2 MRI scan image confirms that the procedure is being done at the correct level (beware of transitional vertebra at L5/S1 levels).

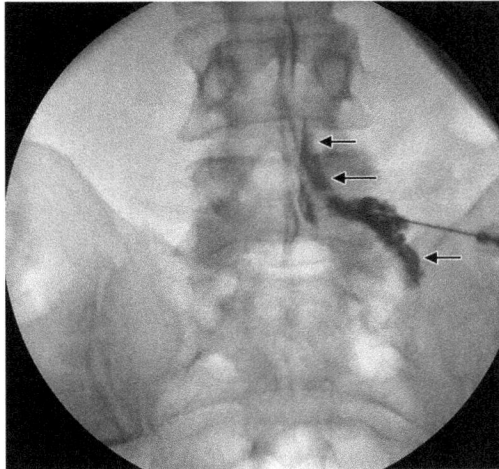

Fig. 23: Contrast spread in AP view along the pedicle, into the epidural space and along the right L5 nerve root (arrows).

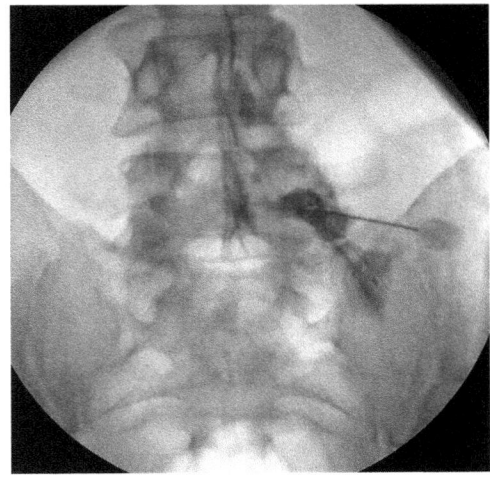

Fig. 24: Final AP view after injection of steroid.

FURTHER READING

1. Evran S, Kayhan A, Tahsin Saygi O, et al. The synergistic effect of combined transforaminal and caudal epidural steroid injection in recurrent lumbar disc herniations. Cureus. 2021;13(1): e12538.
2. Ghahreman A, Bogduk N. Predictors of a favorable response to transforaminal injection of steroids in patients with lumbar radicular pain due to disc herniation. Pain Med. 2011;12: 871-9.
3. Ghahreman A, Ferch R, Bogduk N. The efficacy of transforaminal injection of steroids for the treatment of lumbar radicular pain. Pain Med. 2010;11:1149-68.
4. Gupta S, Gupta H, Baranidharan G, Sharma M. Technical challenges of performing S1 root block: role for double needle and multilevel needle technique. British Journal of Pain. 2021;15(2):129-33. (doi:10.1177/2049463720960497)
5. Gupta S. Double needle technique: an alternative method for performing difficult sacroiliac joint injections. Pain Physician. 2011;14:281-4.
6. Gupta S. Pre-contrast injection multiple needle placement technique: an alternative method for performing challenging transforaminal epidural steroid injections for radicular pain. Pain Medicine Case Reports. 2020; 4(2):39-44.
7. Helm Ii S, Harmon PC, Neo C, et al. Transforaminal epidural steroid injections: a systematic review and meta-analysis of efficacy and safety. Pain Physician. 2021; 24 (S1): S209-32
8. Simpson K, Baranidharan G, Gupta S (Eds). Lumbar spine interventions. In: Spinal interventions in pain management: Oxford Specialist Handbook in Pain Medicine. Oxford University Press. 2012. pp. 46-51.
9. Lumbar Transforaminal Access. In: Practice guidelines for spinal diagnostic and treatment procedures. Bogduk N (Ed). International Spine Intervention Society, San Francisco, CA: 2013. pp. 459-538.
10. MacVicar J, King W, Landers MH, Bogduk N. Review Article: The effectiveness of lumbar transforaminal injection of steroids: a comprehensive review with systematic analysis of the published data. Pain Medicine. 2013;14:14-28.
11. Min Cheol C, Dong Gyu L. Outcome of transforaminal epidural steroid injection according to the severity of lumbar foraminal spinal stenosis. Pain Physician. 2018;21:67-72.
12. Pairuchvej S, Arirachakaran A, Keorochana G, et al. The short and midterm outcomes of lumbar transforaminal epidural injection with preganglionic and postganglionic approach in lumbosacral radiculopathy: a systematic review and meta-analysis. Neurosurg Rev. 2018; 41(4):909-16.
13. Wilby MJ, et al. Surgical microdiscectomy versus transforaminal epidural steroid injection in patients with sciatica secondary to herniated lumbar disc (NERVES): a phase 3, multicentre, open-label, randomised controlled trial and economic evaluation. Lancet Rheumatol. 2021;3:e347-56.
14. WJ Kim, HY Shin, SH Yoo, HS Park. Comparison of epidural spreading patterns and clinical outcomes of transforaminal epidural steroid injection with high-volume injectate via the subpedicular versus the retrodiscal approach. Pain Physician. 2018;21:269-78.

CHAPTER 20

Lumbar Transforaminal Epidural Steroid Injections: Technical Challenges

Sanjeeva Gupta, Dwarkadas K Baheti, Sanjay Bakshi

TECHNICALLY CHALLENGING CASE 1 (FIGS. 1 TO 8)

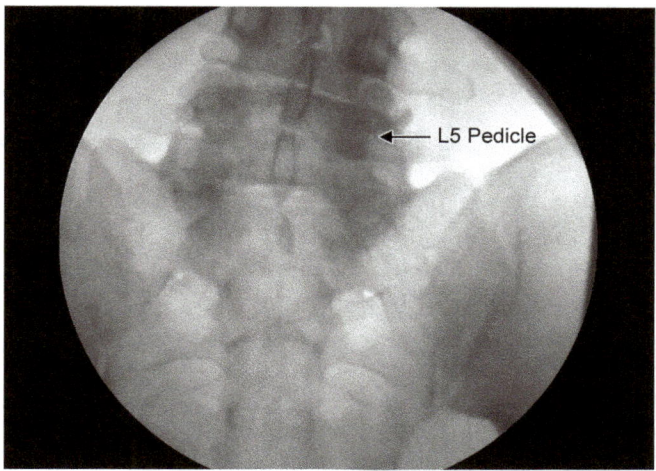

Fig. 1: Antero-posterior (AP) view of the lumbosacral spine. Patient presented with radicular pain in the right L5 distribution due to irritation of the nerve in the right L4/5 recess. MRI showed that the patient had significant degenerative changes of the lower lumbar spine including osteophytes that could make the transforaminal epidural injection technically challenging. The MRI images were discussed with the musculoskeletal radiologist to facilitate planning.

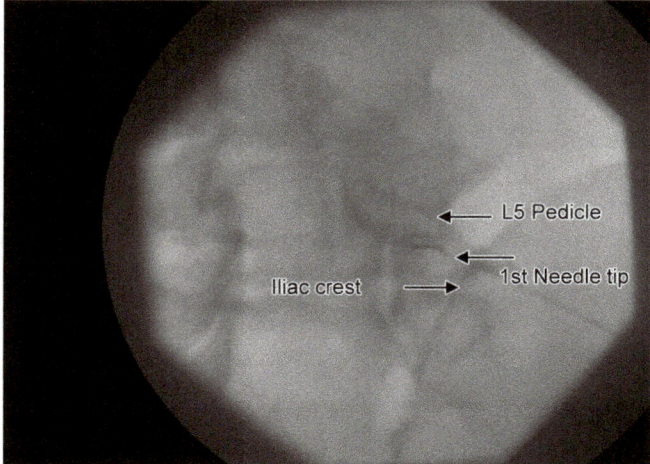

Fig. 2: Right oblique view. A curved tip 22G spinal needle was placed at the L5/S1 level using the subpedicular technique but due to degenerative changes in the target area, the needle could not be placed more medially as shown in the image.

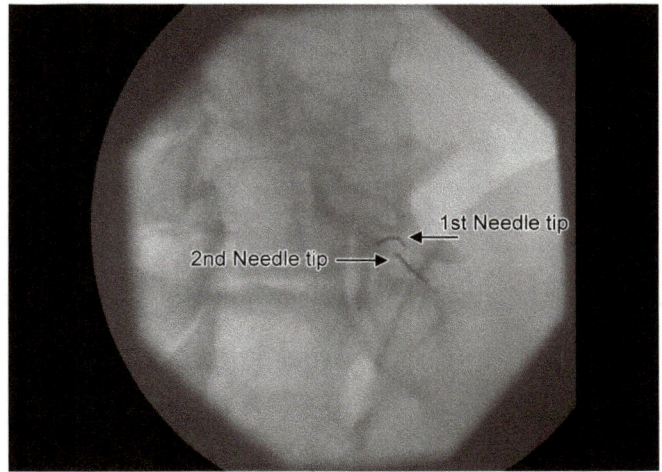

Fig. 3: Right oblique view. As the tip of the first needle was not in a satisfactory position, it was decided to insert a second needle using a different trajectory, the skin entry site being lateral to the first needle (not using along the X-ray beam—gun barrel technique). The tip of the 2nd needle is below and medial to the 1st needle.

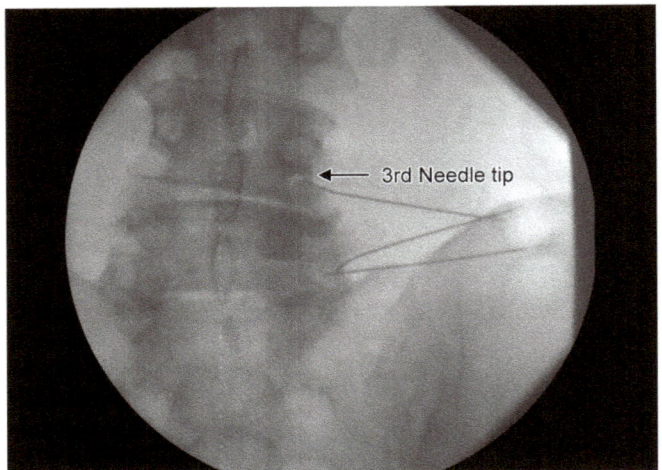

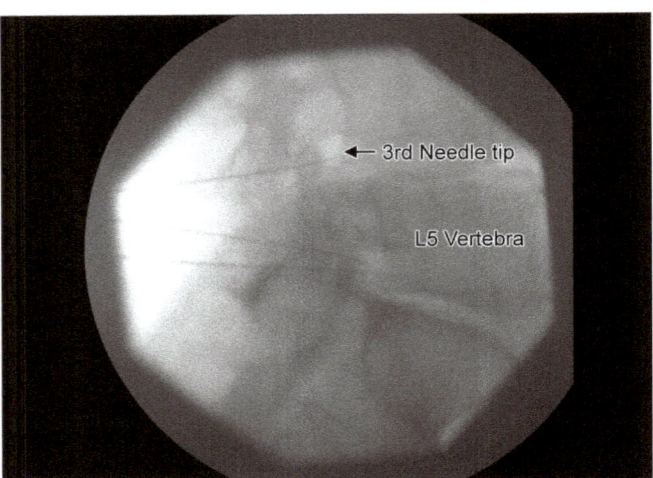

Fig. 4: Antero-posterior view with the third needle in place at the L4/5 level. As there was difficulty in placing the two needles at the L5/S1 level as osteophytes were encountered during the procedure, it was decided to place a third needle at the L4/5 level by the retrodiscal/infraneural technique (nearer the site of the pathology compared to L4/5 subpedicular technique).
Source: Reproduced from Gupta S. Pre-contrast injection multiple needle placement technique: an alternative method for performing challenging transforaminal epidural steroid injections for radicular pain. Pain Med Case Rep. 2020;4(2):39-44.

Fig. 5: Lateral view with the three needles in place. Please note that the tip of the third needle is just behind the L4/5 disc and nearer the site of the pathology (compared to if the needle was placed by the subpedicular technique at the L4/5 level).
Source: Reproduced from Gupta S. Pre-contrast injection multiple needle placement technique: an alternative method for performing challenging transforaminal epidural steroid injections for radicular pain. Pain Med Case Rep. 2020;4(2):39-44.

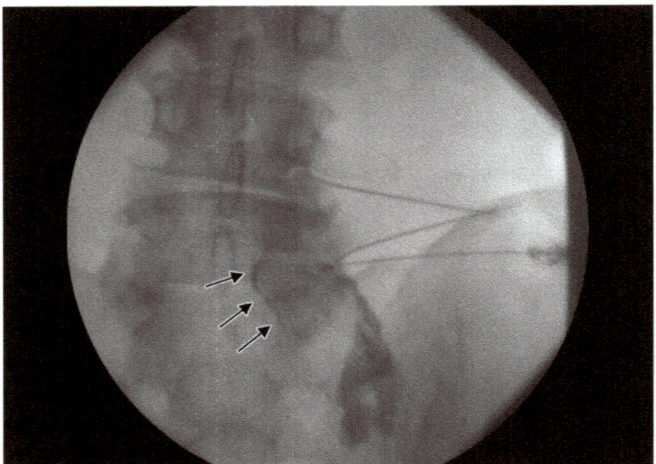

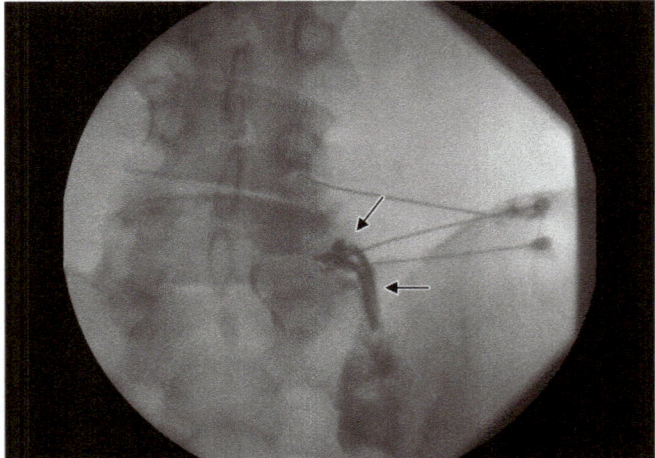

Fig. 6: Antero-posterior (AP) view. When contrast was injected under continuous fluoroscopy in AP view through an extension tubing attached to the second needle (tip medial to the first needle at the L5/S1 level), the contrast spread was at the lower margin of the L5 pedicle and below (arrows) but not into the L4/5 recess, the site of the pathology.

Fig. 7: Antero-posterior (AP) view after injecting the contrast via the first needle with the tip lateral to the second needle showing the contrast spread laterally along the distal L5 nerve root (arrows) but not into the L4/5 recess, the site of the pathology.
Source: Reproduced from Gupta S. Pre-contrast injection multiple needle placement technique: an alternative method for performing challenging transforaminal epidural steroid injections for radicular pain. Pain Med Case Rep. 2020; 4(2):39-44.

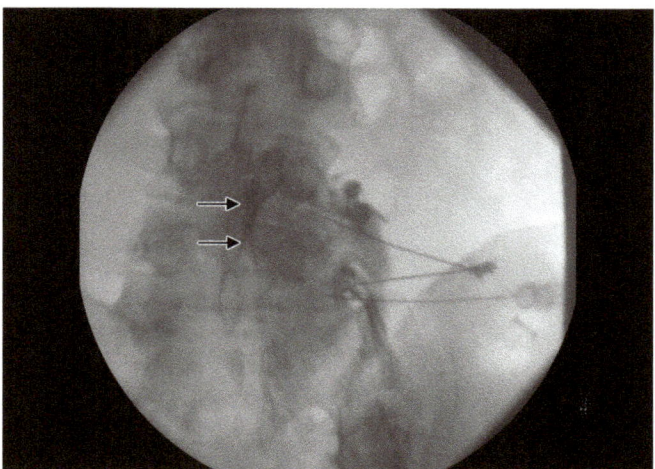

Fig. 8: Antero-posterior (AP) view after contrast injection under continuous fluoroscopy in AP view through an extension tubing attached to the third needle placed at the L4/5 level (infraneural/retrodiscal technique). Contrast is seen spreading into the L4/5 recess, the site of the pathology.
Source: Reproduced from Gupta S. Pre-contrast injection multiple needle placement technique: an alternative method for performing challenging transforaminal epidural steroid injections for radicular pain. Pain Med Case Rep. 2020;4(2):39-44.

TECHNICALLY CHALLENGING CASE 2 (FIGS. 9 TO 11)

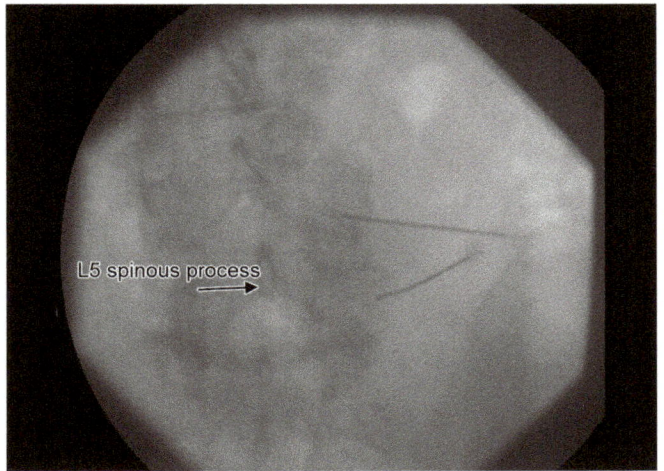

Fig. 9: Elderly patient with significant lumbar spondylosis. Difficulty was encountered in placing the needle at the L5/S1 level using the subpedicular technique and hence another needle was placed in the L4/5 infraneural/retrodiscal area.
Source: Reproduced from Gupta S. Pre-contrast injection multiple needle placement technique: an alternative method for performing challenging transforaminal epidural steroid injections for radicular pain. Pain Med Case Rep. 2020;4(2):39-44.

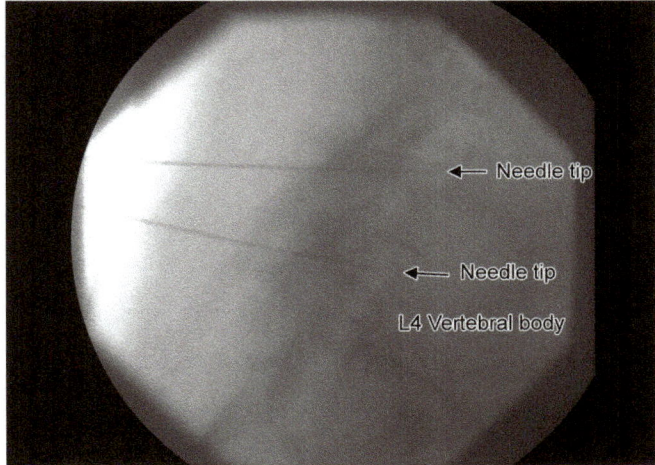

Fig. 10: Lateral view showing the needle tips in the intervertebral foramen. Subpedicular technique at the L5/S1 level with the needle tip in the upper half of the intervertebral foramen and infraneural/retrodiscal needle at the L4/5 level with the needle tip at the lower half of the intervertebral foramen.
Source: Reproduced from Gupta S. Pre-contrast injection multiple needle placement technique: an alternative method for performing challenging transforaminal epidural steroid injections for radicular pain. Pain Med Case Rep. 2020;4(2):39-44.

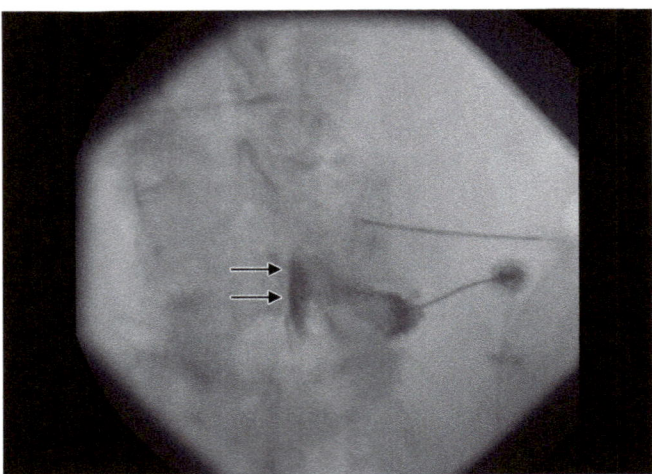

Fig. 11: On injecting contrast at the L5/S1 level in the antero-posterior view under continuous fluoroscopy through an extension tubing the contrast spread into the L4/5 recess (arrows), the site of pathology. The needle at L4/5 was removed without injecting anything.
Source: Reproduced from Gupta S. Pre-contrast injection multiple needle placement technique: an alternative method for performing challenging transforaminal epidural steroid injections for radicular pain. Pain Med Case Rep. 2020;4(2):39-44.

TECHNICALLY CHALLENGING CASE 3 (FIGS. 12 TO 15)

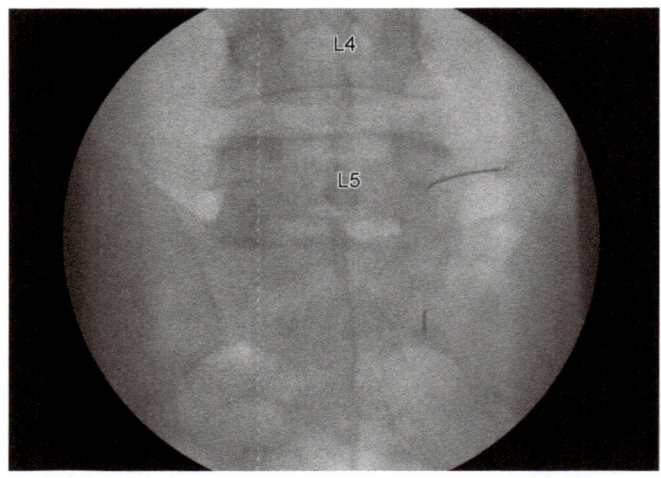

Fig. 12: Patient had radicular pain in the right L5 and S1 distributions. Antero-posterior view showing needle placed at the right L5/S1 level (subpedicular technique) and at S1 level.
Source: Reproduced from Gupta S. Pre-contrast injection multiple needle placement technique: an alternative method for performing challenging transforaminal epidural steroid injections for radicular pain. Pain Med Case Rep. 2020;4(2):39-44.

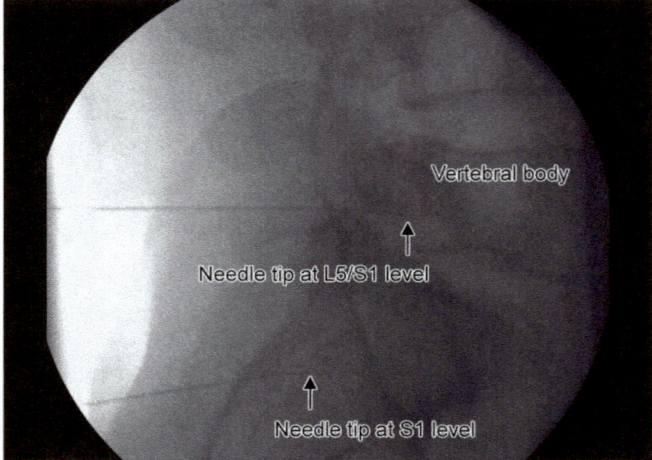

Fig. 13: Lateral view with needle tips in the L5/S1 and S1 foramen.
Source: Reproduced from Gupta S. Pre-contrast injection multiple needle placement technique: an alternative method for performing challenging transforaminal epidural steroid injections for radicular pain. Pain Med Case Rep. 2020;4(2):39-44.

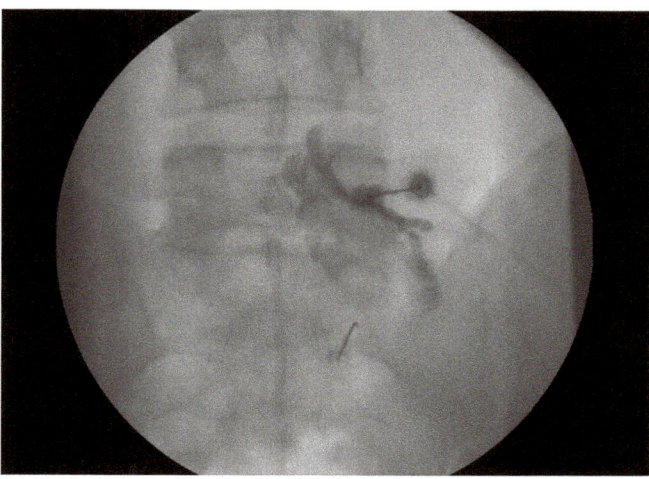

Fig. 14: Contrast injected through the needle at the right L5/S1 level covers the L5 nerve root but not the S1 root. If on contrast injection at the L5/S1 level, there was contrast spread along the S1 nerve root also then the needle at the S1 level would be removed decreasing the risks to the patient compared to if steroid is injected through this needle. It can also be argued that the needle at S1 could be placed if necessary only after contrast was injected through the needle at the L5/S1 level and if the contrast did not spread along the S1 nerve, thus decreasing the risk further.
Source: Reproduced from Gupta S. Pre-contrast injection multiple needle placement technique: an alternative method for performing challenging transforaminal epidural steroid injections for radicular pain. Pain Med Case Rep. 2020;4(2):39-44.

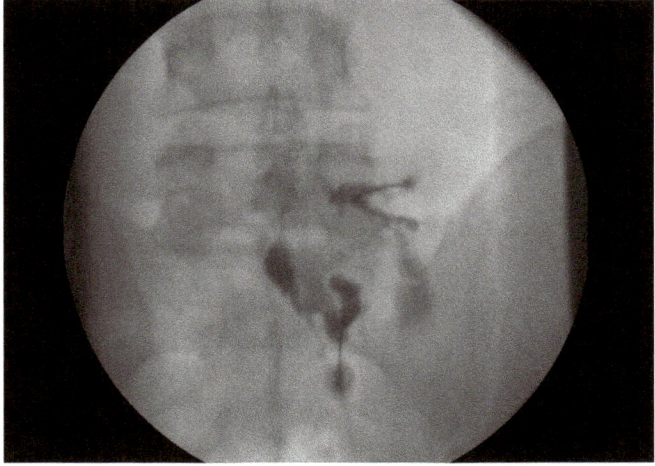

Fig. 15: Contrast injected through the needle at the right S1 level covers the area of S1 nerve root.
Source: Reproduced from Gupta S. Pre-contrast injection multiple needle placement technique: an alternative method for performing challenging transforaminal epidural steroid injections for radicular pain. Pain Med Case Rep. 2020;4(2):39-44.

TECHNICALLY CHALLENGING CASE 4 (FIGS. 16 TO 19)

A 65-year-old patient presents with low back pain and left lower limb pain in left L5 distribution. MRI scan showed L4/5 disc prolapse compressing left L5 nerve root in the L4/5 recess. The patient was on optimal pharmacotherapy but continued to be troubled with pain in the left lower limb.

Options considered were:
- L5/S1 transforaminal lumbar epidural steroid injection (TFESI)
- L4/5 TFESI
- Both L5/S1 and L4/5 TFESI (pre- and postganglionic)
- Interlaminar epidural at the L4/5 level directing to left
- Caudal epidural was considered, but it was felt that the site of pathology far away from the site of injection and the steroid may not reach the pathology.
- It was decided to start with left L5/S1 TFESI.

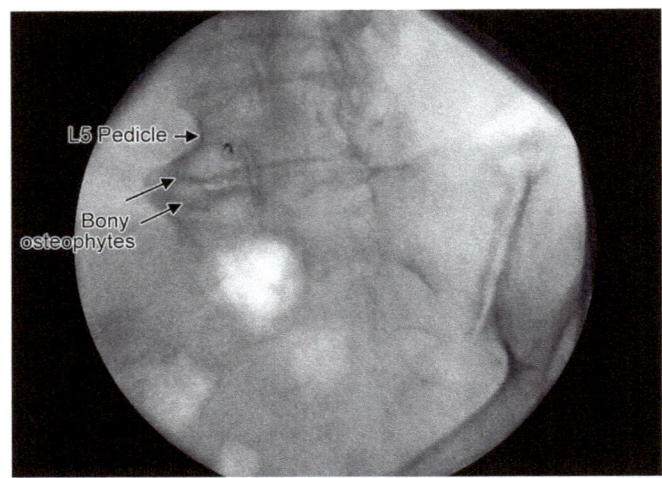

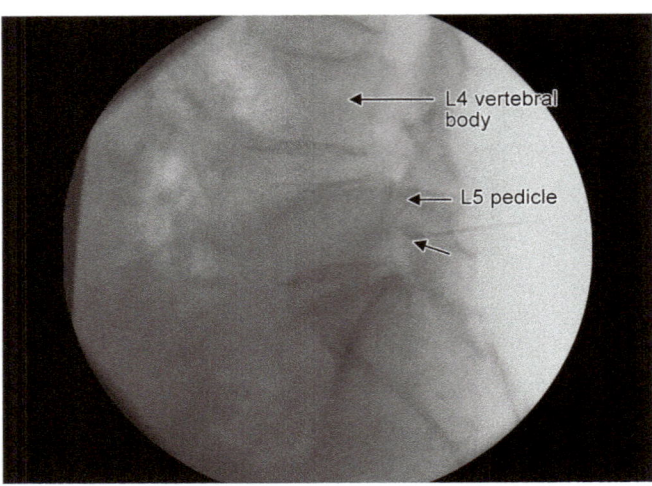

Fig. 16: *Left L5/S1 TFESI:* Left oblique view. Osteophytes from the vertebral body can been seen in the target site area (see Chapter 1 also). A curved tip needle is seen in the L5 subpedicular area and is being navigated into the L5/S1 foramen. As we are aware that the vertebral body is anterior to the target site and not in our way to the intervertebral foramen, the needle was easily navigated into the L5/S1 foramen.

Fig. 17: *Left L5/S1 TFESI:* Lateral view. Needle tip can be seen in the L5/S1 intervertebral foramen (arrow).

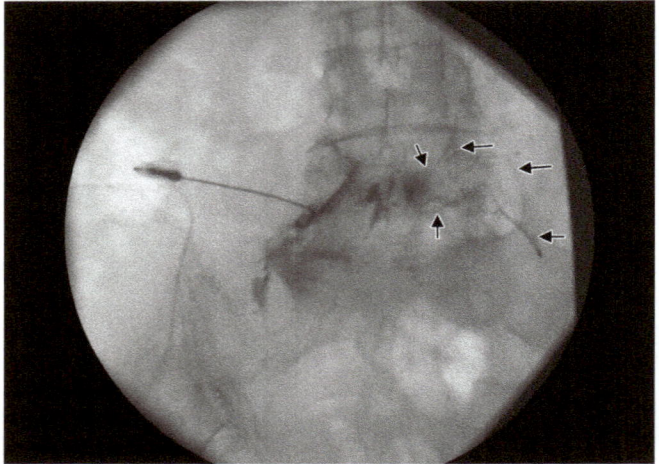

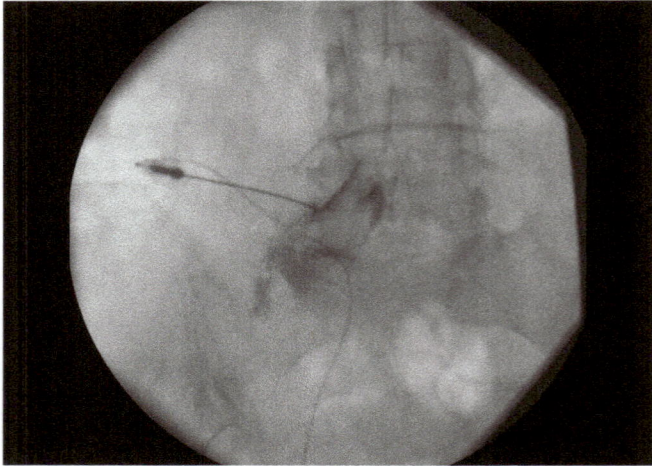

Fig. 18: When contrast was injected via a low-volume extension tubing in antero-posterior (AP) view under continuous fluoroscopy, vascular spread to the opposite side (arrows) was identified in addition to the contrast outlining the nerve root and spreading into the epidural space along the left L5 pedicle. It is important to note that the contrast should be injected in the AP view under continuous fluoroscopy to rule out vascular spread. **Figure 19** shows a static image in which the vascular spread cannot be seen as the contrast has run off/disappeared by the time the static image was obtained. Digital subtraction imagining, if available, would be better to rule out vascular spread.

Fig. 19: Same patient as in Figure 18—postcontrast injection static image. Vascular spread cannot be seen. What are the choices? In this case, an interlaminar epidural steroid injection was done directing the needle to the left.

TECHNICALLY CHALLENGING CASE 5 (FIGS. 20 TO 23)

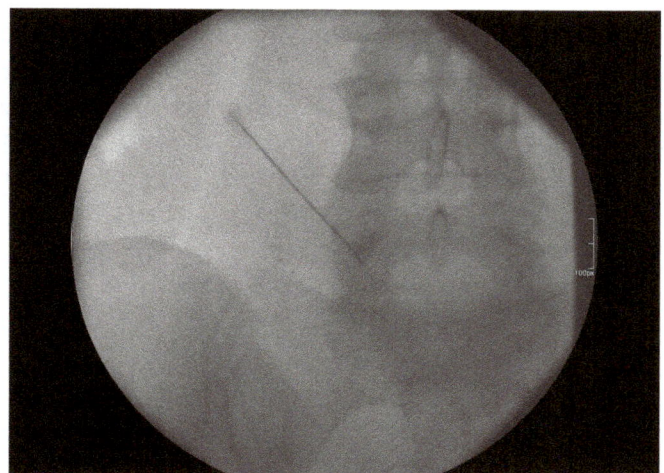

Fig. 20: After placing a 22G spinal needle in left oblique view and checking the depth of the needle tip in lateral view, a antero-posterior (AP) view was obtained. The needle tip is seen below the L5 pedicle and just lateral to the 6°clock position of the left L5 pedicle.

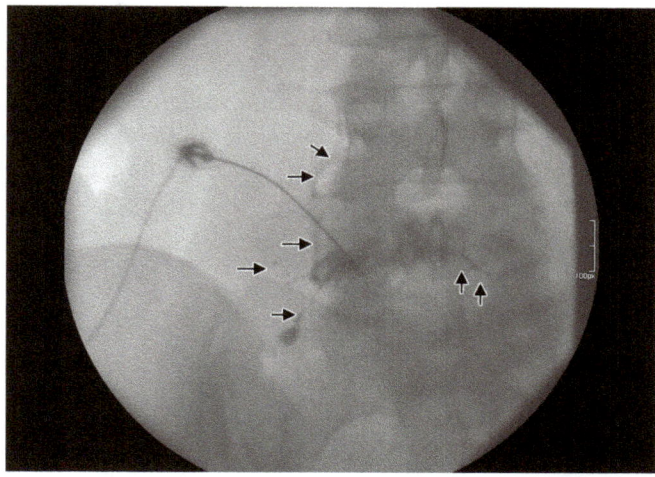

Fig. 21: When contrast was injected in antero-posterior (AP) view under continuous fluoroscopy, vascular spread was seen (arrows). This patient was consented for injection of local anesthetic and triamcinolone (particulate steroid). Options considered were: (1) Abandon the procedure and relist for another day; (2) Interlaminar epidural at the L5/S1 level directing the needle tip to the left; (3) Caudal epidural injection; (4) Withdraw the needle by around 5 mm and reinject the contrast. Option (4) was selected in this patient.

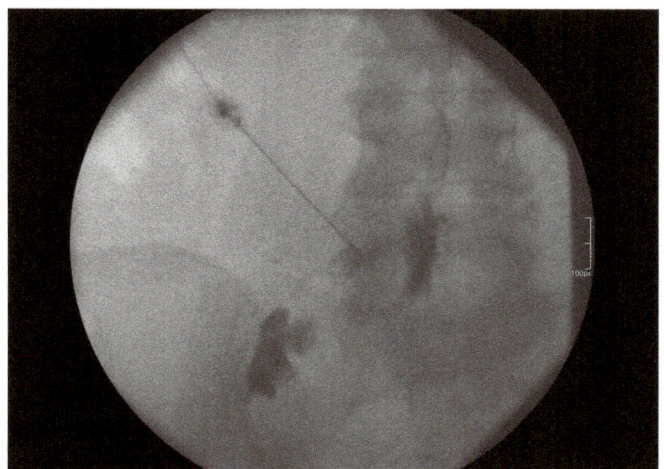

Fig. 22: *Left L5/S1 transforaminal epidural injection:* When the contrast was injected in antero-posterior view under continuous fluoroscopy after withdrawing the needle by around 5 mm, the contrast spread was satisfactory into the epidural space and along the L5 nerve root with no vascular spread seen. As there was vascular spread during the procedure after discussion with the patient (not sedated), local anesthetic and dexamethasone (non-particulate) were injected.

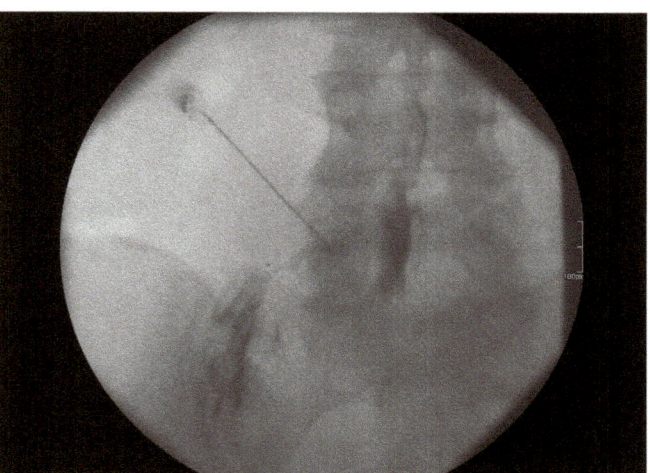

Fig. 23: *Left L5/S1 transforaminal epidural injection:* Final image after injection of local anesthetic and dexamethasone shows good spread of the contrast/medication.

TECHNICALLY CHALLENGING CASE 6 (FIGS. 24 TO 28)

DESCRIPTION

This patient had right L5 radicular pain due to irritation of the L5 nerve root in the L4/5 recess due to significant lumbar spondylosis. It was decided to do a pre- and postganglionic TFESI in this patient. When navigating the needle at the L5/S1 level (subpedicular technique), the author (SG) encountered challenges and was not sure if the contrast spread would be satisfactory and hence another needle was placed at the L4/5 level by the infraneural/retrodiscal technique so that the needle tip would be closer to the site of the pathology compared to if the subpedicular technique was used at the L4/L5 level.

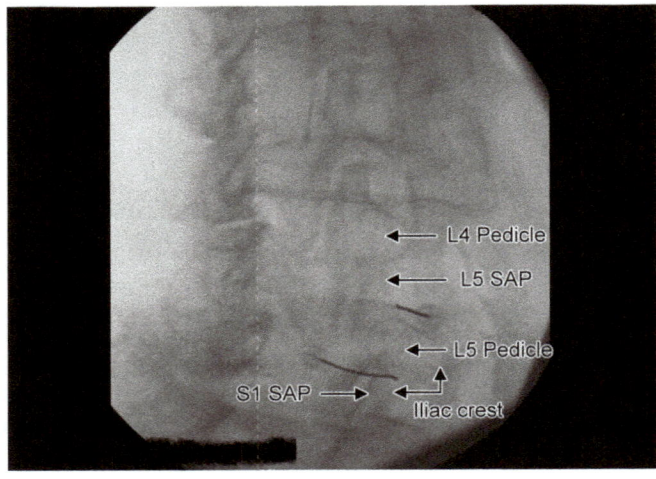

Fig. 24: Right oblique view with needles in place at the right L5/S1 (subpedicular technique) and the right L4/5 (infraneural/retrodiscal) levels for TFESI. For the L4/5 infraneural/retrodiscal technique, the needle tip is directed to the lower part of the lateral margin of the L5 superior articular process (SAP) using the "gun-barrel technique"—lateral view is used to judge the depth of the needle as there is a risk of entering the disc.

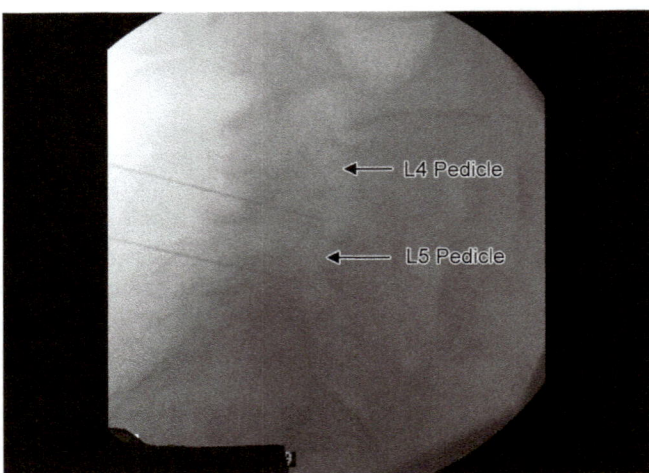

Fig. 25: Lateral view showing the needle tips just below the L5 pedicle (L5/S1 subpedicular technique) and above the L5 pedicle (infraneural/retrodiscal technique) in the lower half of the L4/5 intervertebral foramen.

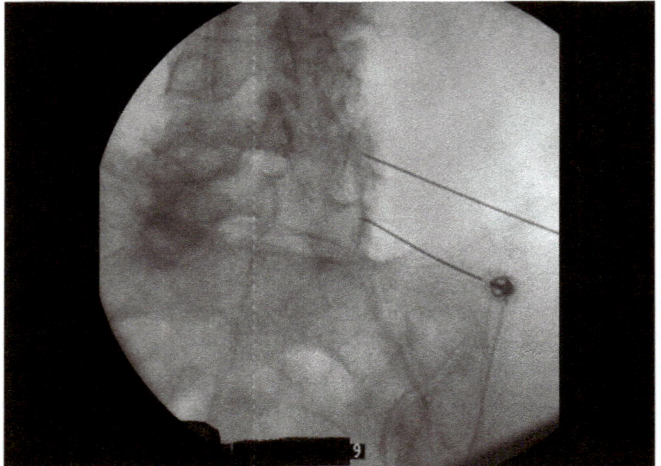

Fig. 26: Antero-posterior view with the two needles in place and connected to a low-volume extension tubing in preparation for injecting contrast under continuous fluoroscopy to ascertain satisfactory spread of contrast and to rule out vascular spread (if available, digital subtraction imaging would be better to rule out vascular spread).

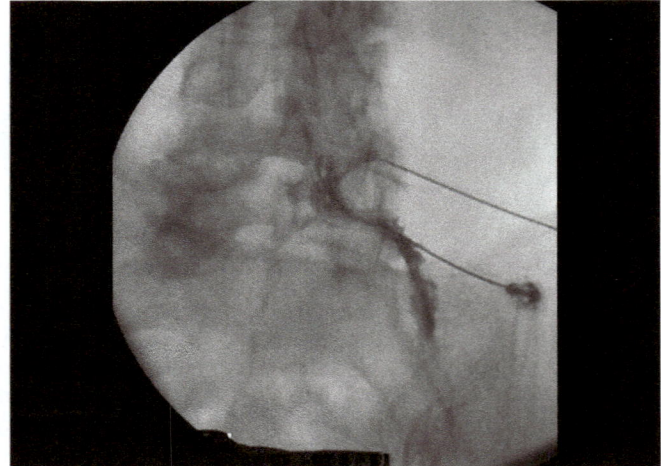

Fig. 27: *Antero-posterior view:* Contrast injection revels good spread of contrast along the L5 nerve root, the pedicle, and into the epidural space.

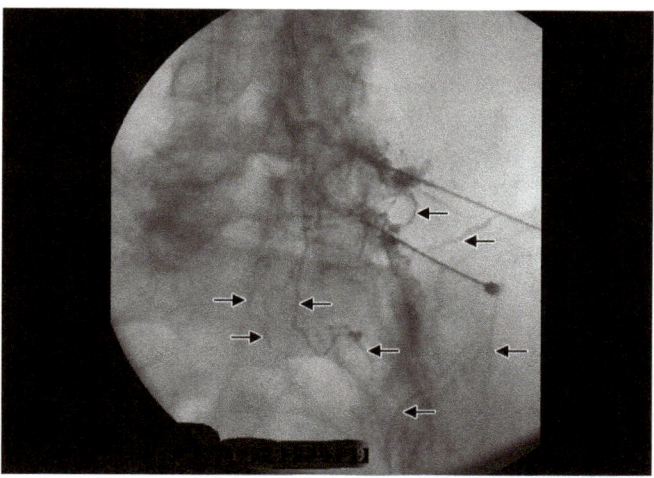

Fig. 28: On injecting contrast through the needle at the L4/5 infraneural/retrodiscal level, there was further improvement in the contrast spread but there was also vascular spread (arrows), and hence this needle was withdrawn without injecting anything more through the needle. The entire dose of the steroid was injected at L5/S1 level.

TECHNICALLY CHALLENGING CASE 7 (FIGS. 29 TO 35)

DESCRIPTION

One of the authors (SG) has been managing this patient for over 20 years. The patient had lumbar spine surgery over 20 years ago and initially had persistent never root irritation and pain down the left lower limbs in L5 distribution. This was managed by left L5/S1 TFESI on multiple occasions with good pain relief for around 6 months each time. The patient subsequently developed neuropathic pain in bilateral L5 distribution and a bilateral L5/S1 TFESI was planned as interlaminar epidural was considered not appropriate as lumbar spine surgery had been performed at this level and there was a high risk of dural puncture. When the left L5/S1 transforaminal epidural was attempted on this occasion,

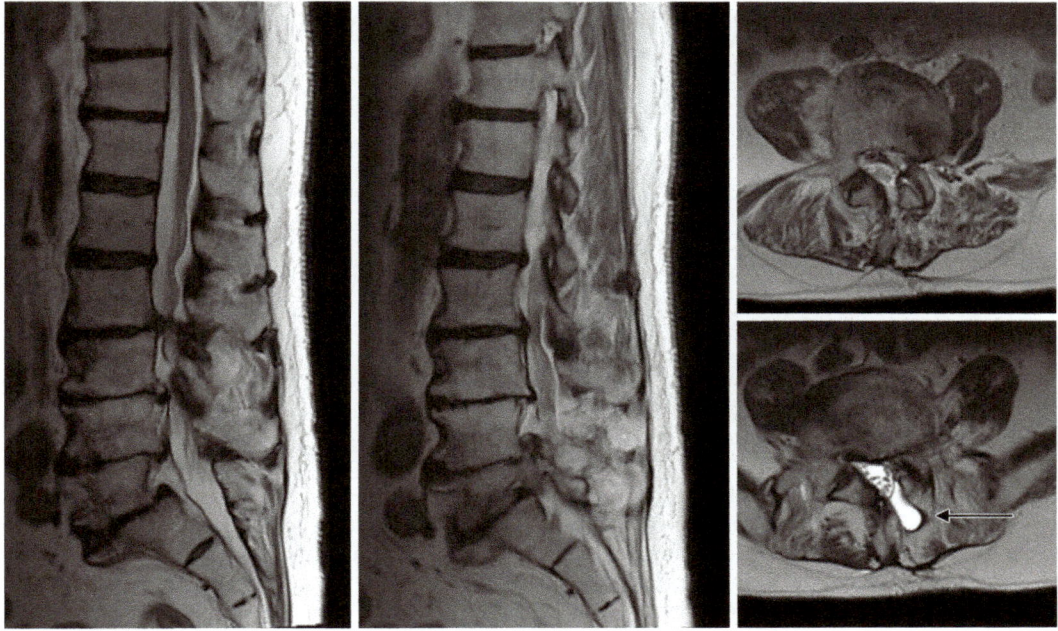

Fig. 29: T2 sagittal and axial MRI scan images of the patient. Scoliosis of the lumbar spine convex toward left. Grade 2 retrolisthesis of L4 on L5 and anterolisthesis of L5 on S1. Sever loss of disc height. Moderate-to-severe spinal stenosis at the L2/3 level. Moderate-to-severe exit foraminal and recess stenosis at multiple levels on both sides. Pseudomeningocele in the left paraspinal location through laminectomy (arrow in the lower axial image).

the patient had shooting pain down the left lower limb in L5 distribution and continued to have such symptoms despite reinserting the needle in a different trajectory. The procedure was abandoned and in consultation with the patient, a caudal epidural was planned as interlaminar epidural was not considered safe. When contrast was injected during the caudal epidural procedure, a filling defect was identified as shown in **Figure 31**, and hence Racz catheter was navigated to the site of the pathology for targeted steroid injection. In this case, Racz catheter was used only to navigate the tip to the site of the pathology (Racz procedure including hypertonic saline injection was not done). If Racz catheter is not available, an epidural catheter could be used instead but this will have to be handled very carefully so that the catheter is not sheered/cut by the tip of the epidural needle. The patient responded with excellent pain relief for 6–9 months each time. This patient was offered spinal cord stimulator earlier on during management but he declined.

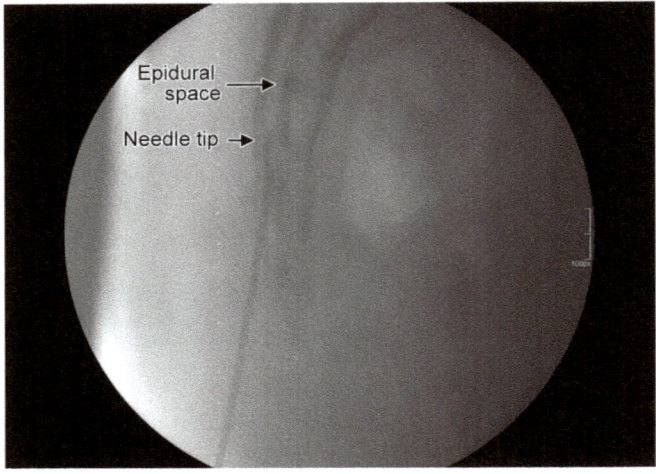

Fig. 30: *Lateral view:* Epidural needle in the caudal epidural space.

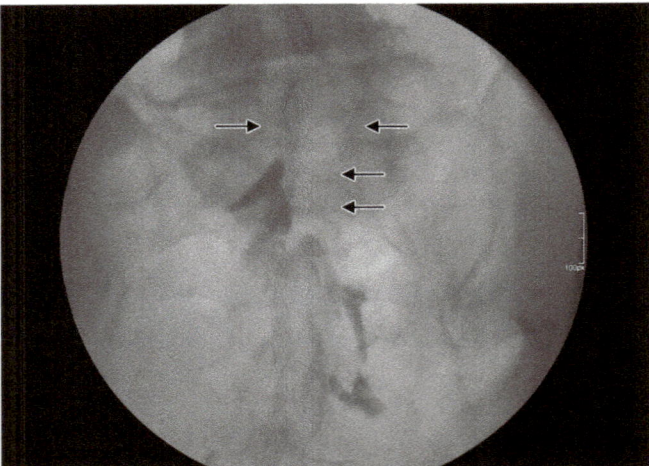

Fig. 31: When contrast was injected, a filling defect was identified (arrows) and the contrast did not reach the site of the pathology (L5/S1 level) and hence a targeted steroid injection at around the L5 nerve root area with Racz catheter was considered appropriate.

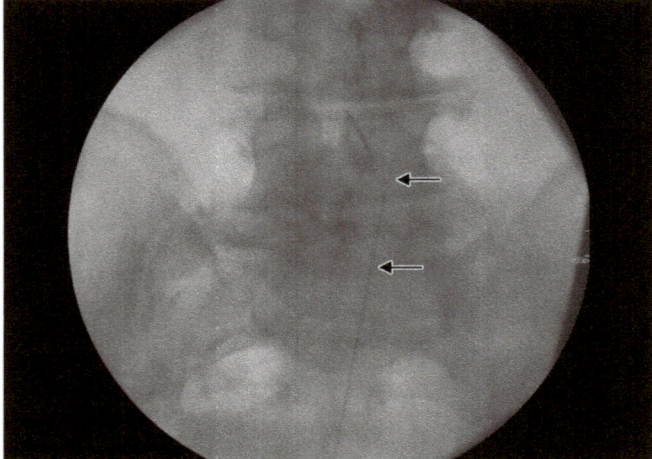

Fig. 32: Racz catheter was navigated via the caudal route to the site of the pathology on the right side. The tip of Racz catheter can be seen in the area of the right L5 pedicle at the L5/S1 level on the right side (arrow). In this case, Racz catheter was used only to navigate the tip to the site of the pathology (Racz procedure including hypertonic saline injection was not done). If Racz catheter is not available, an epidural catheter could be used instead but this will have to be handled very carefully so that the catheter is not sheered/cut by the tip of the epidural needle.

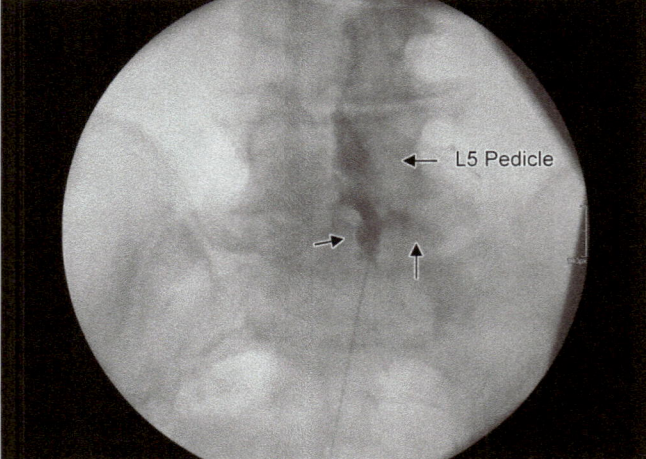

Fig. 33: Contrast was injected under continuous fluoroscopy in antero-posterior view and the contrast can be seen spreading in the right L5/S1 area and along the right L5 nerve root (arrows).

CHAPTER 20 | Lumbar Transforaminal Epidural Steroid Injections: Technical Challenges

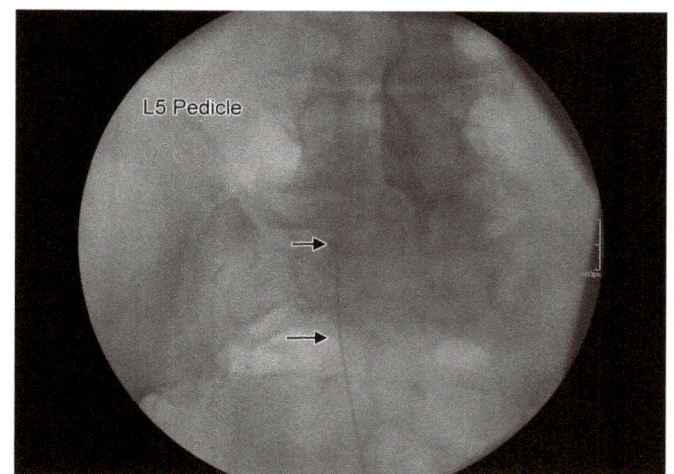

Fig. 34: Racz catheter placed via the caudal root and redirected toward the left L5 nerve root area (arrow).

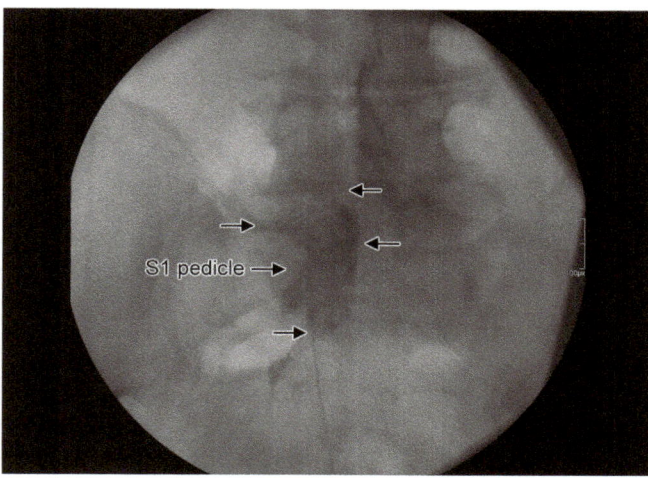

Fig. 35: Contrast was injected via Racz catheter under continuous fluoroscopy in antero-posterior view and can be seen spreading in the area of the L5/S1 disc on the right side (arrows). The contrast spread was not optimal but on injecting local anesthetic and steroid, the spread was toward the left L5 nerve root and the patient had good pain relief for around 6 months with improved quality of life.

Chapter 21

Lumbar Medial Branch Block and Radiofrequency Ablation

Anil Sharma, Sanjeeva Gupta

LUMBAR MEDIAN BRANCH BLOCK AND RADIOFREQUENCY ABLATION

Basic Information

Indications

To obtain long-term pain relief from pain originating from facet joints which is confirmed by 80% pain relief by two separate diagnostic medial branch blocks.

Contraindications

Absolute:
- An active systemic infection or a localized infection within the procedural field
- Uncooperative patient
- Allergy to medication(s) that cannot be safely mitigated by pretreatment
- Pregnancy

Relative:
- Concurrent treatment with anticoagulants constitutes a relative contraindication for lumbar medial branch radiofrequency neurotomy. The risks of continuing or discontinuing anticoagulants should be discussed with the patient, possibly involving the patient's cardiologist and/or primary care provider, if indicated.
- Spinal hardware is not a contraindication to medial branch radiofrequency neurotomy, but its presence may complicate needle placement. The risk of heating spinal hardware exists as well. Tissue temperature and impedance should be continuously monitored, and patients should be able to communicate pain or other adverse sensations.
- Caution is advised in patients who have cardiac pacemakers and defibrillators. If a decision is made to proceed with radiofrequency neurotomy in these patients, physicians should consider the following recommendations to maximize safety and minimize complications:
  - Educate the patient on the potential hazards and risks of radiofrequency neurotomy in the setting of a pacemaker or defibrillator.
  - Ensure the patient is followed by a cardiologist/electrophysiologist and obtain prior approval from the provider, which should be documented in the patient's medical record.
  - If recommended by a cardiologist or electrophysiologist, consider coordination of the radiofrequency neurotomy procedure with the cardiac device manufacturer to have on-site support for interrogation of the cardiac device during the procedure in the event that reprogramming of the device is required. Placement of a magnet over the device during the procedure may be necessary to prevent triggering the device by radiofrequency energy. Removal of the magnet or use of external defibrillator/pacing electrodes may be necessary in case of occurrence of cardiac arrhythmias during the radiofrequency neurotomy.
- Other implantable devices, such as spinal cord stimulators and deep brain stimulators, should be turned off during the procedure. A neurologic examination should be performed before and after the procedure as well, and the stimulator should be restarted after the procedure to ensure proper functioning. The grounding pad should be placed such that the path for the electrical current is as far as possible from the device. The procedure should be abandoned, if the risk of stimulator electrode heating during the neurotomy cannot be eliminated.
- Immunosuppression

STEP-WISE PROCEDURE

Step 1: The patient is placed in a prone position with a pillow under the abdomen to reduce lumbar lordosis. Endplates are lined up at the L4–5 level **(Fig. 1)**.

Step 2: Slight oblique view is obtained around 10–15° **(Fig. 2)**.

Step 3: A slightly more oblique view is obtained to identify the junction of the transverse process, pedicle and superior articular process (SAP; **Fig. 3**).

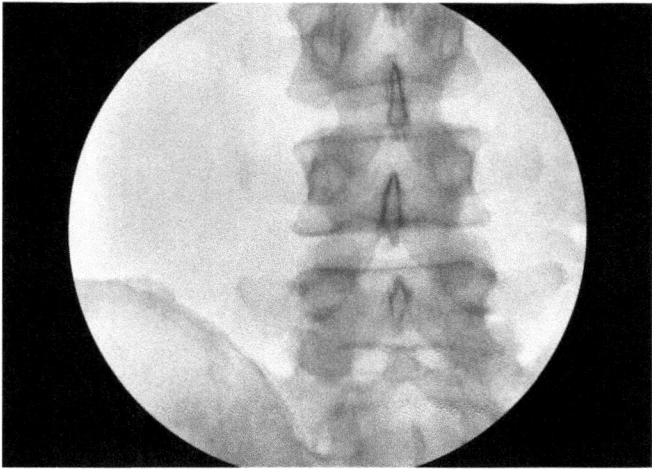

Fig. 1: Endplates are lined up at the L4-5 level.

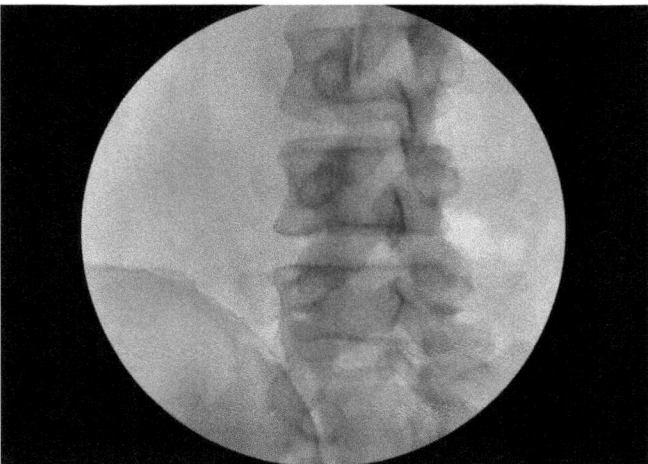

Fig. 2: Slight oblique view is obtained around 10–15°.

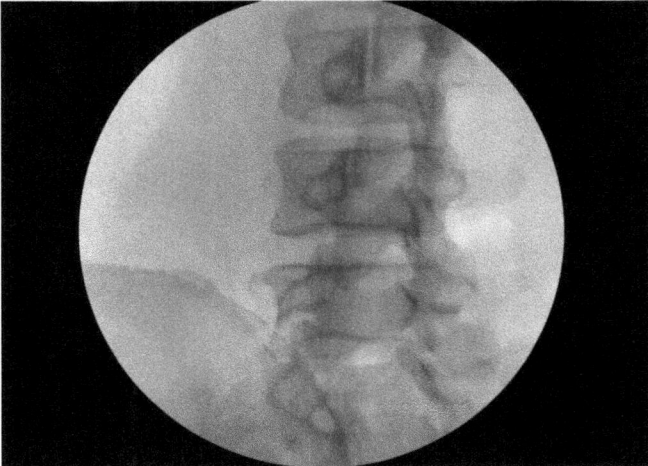

Fig. 3: Identify the junction of transverse process, pedicle and superior articular process.

Step 4: The caudal tilt of the C-arm is done (**Fig. 4**).

Step 5: More caudal tilt and Conning are done to reduce radiation (**Fig. 5**).

Step 6: Skin is injected with 1% lidocaine, a 25-gauge spinal needle is introduced, and a bony contact is made at the junction of the superior transverse process and pedicle and 0.5 mL of 2% lidocaine is injected (**Fig. 6**).

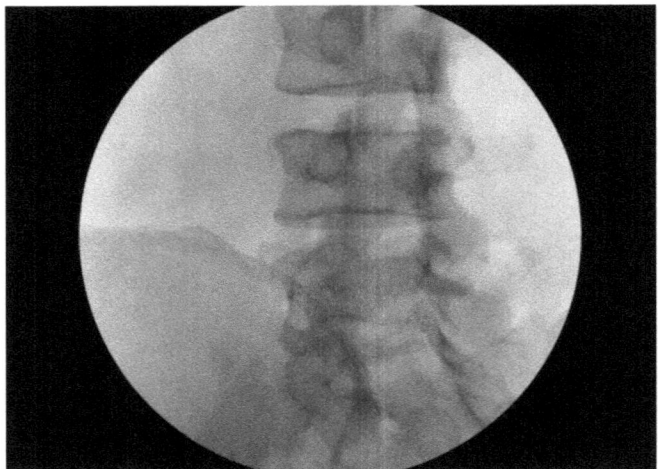

Fig. 4: The caudal tilt of the C-arm is done.

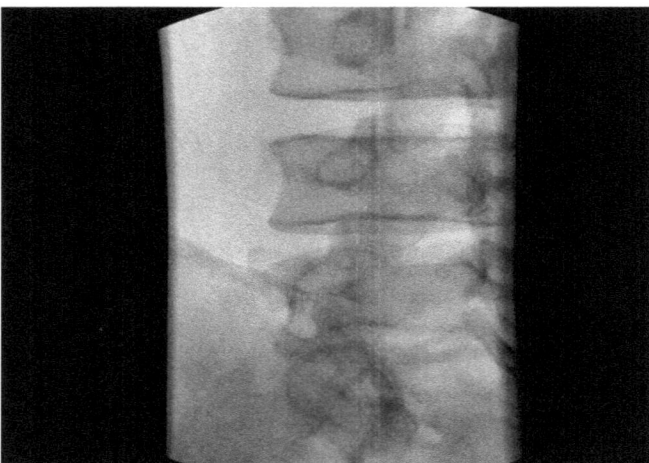

Fig. 5: More caudal tilt and conning are done to reduce radiation.

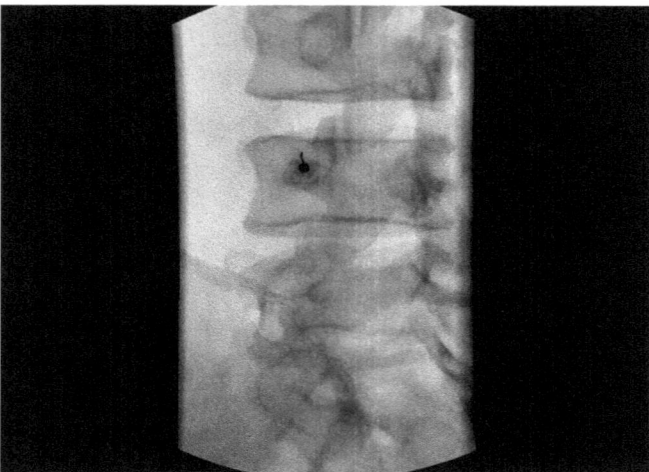

Fig. 6: Needle at the junction of the superior transverse process and pedicle.

Step 7: A similar procedure is done at the L4 medial branch (**Fig. 7**).

Step 8: A radiofrequency (RF) needle with a 10-mm curved active tip is introduced at the L3 medial branch (**Fig. 8**).

Step 9: Needle placed at L4 medial branch (**Fig. 9**).

Step 10: Anteroposterior (AP) view of the RF needles at the junction of transverse process and SAP (**Fig. 10**).

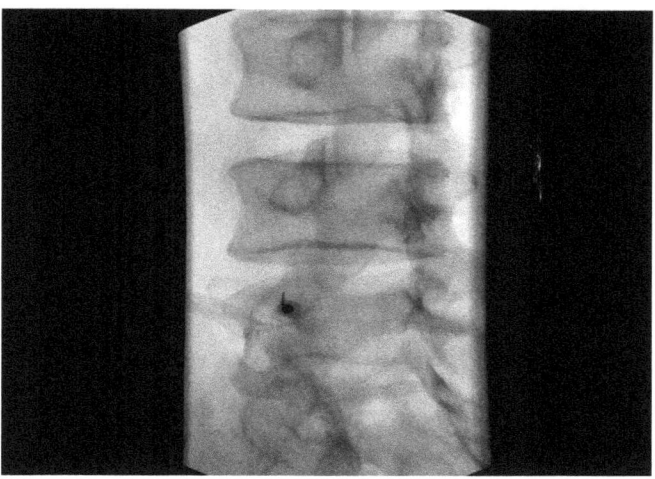

Fig. 7: A similar procedure is done at the L4 medial branch.

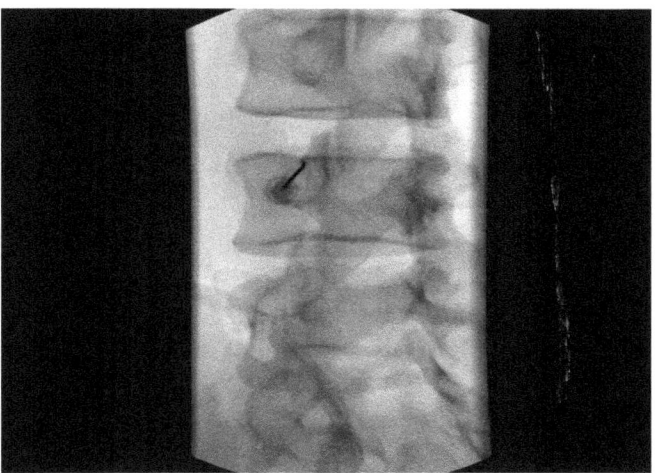

Fig. 8: A radiofrequency needle with a 10-mm curved active tip at the L3 medial branch.

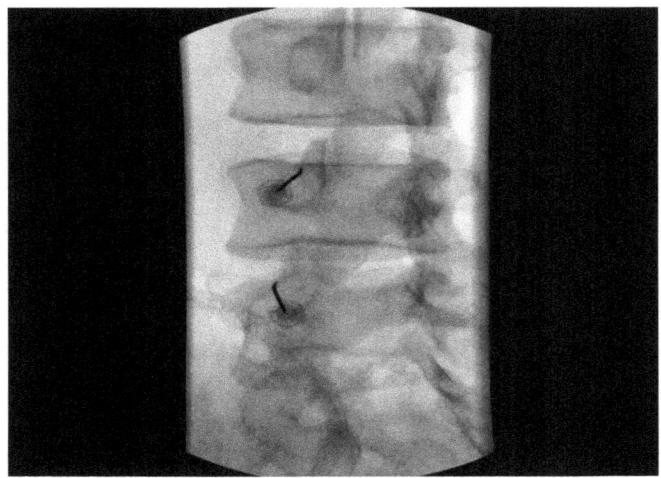

Fig. 9: A radiofrequency needle placed at L4 medial branch.

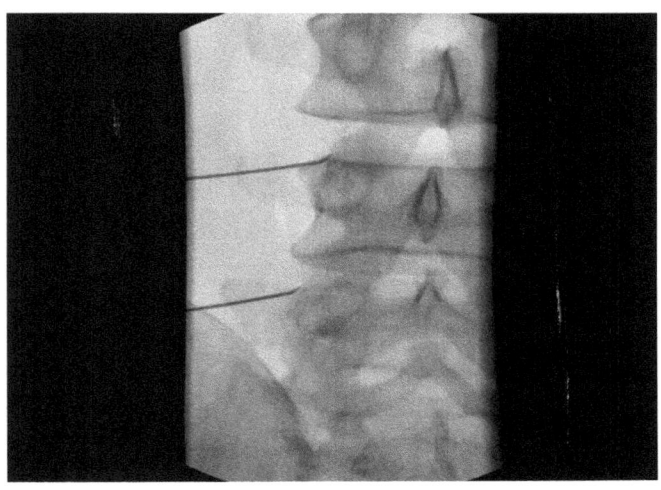

Fig. 10: Anteroposterior view—radiofrequency needles at the junction of transverse process and superior articular process.

Step 11: Needle active tip parallel to the medial branch **(Fig. 11)**.

Step 12: L5 medial branch blocked with 25-gauge spinal needle **(Fig. 12)**.

Step 13: 10-mm active tip curved needle placed at L5 medial branch **(Fig. 13)**.

Step 14: L5 needle placed parallelly **(Fig. 14)**.

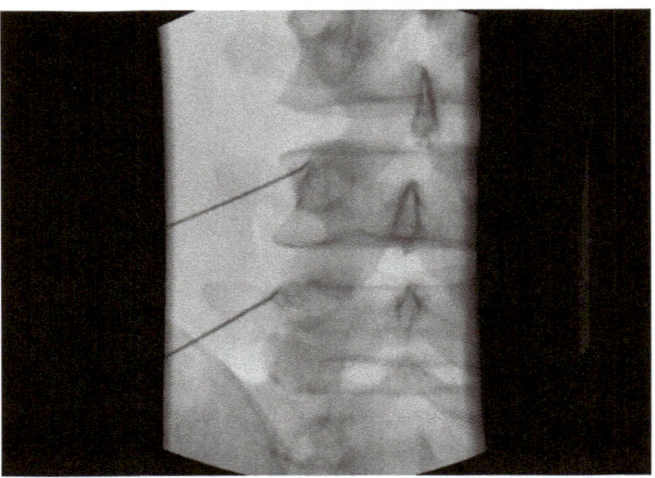

Fig. 11: Radiofrequency needle active tip parallel to the medial branch.

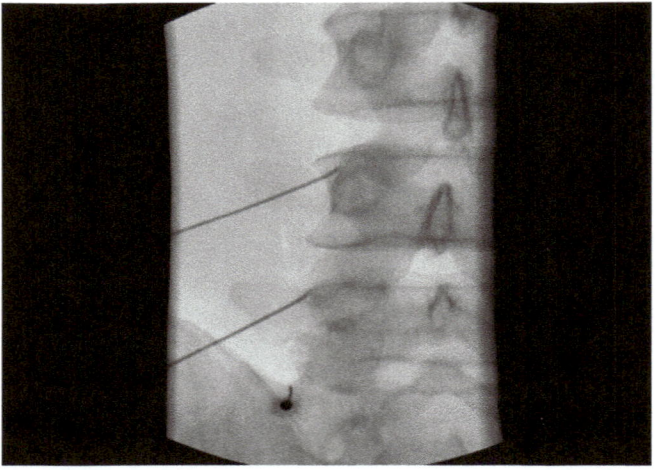

Fig. 12: L5 medial branch blocked with 25-gauge spinal needle.

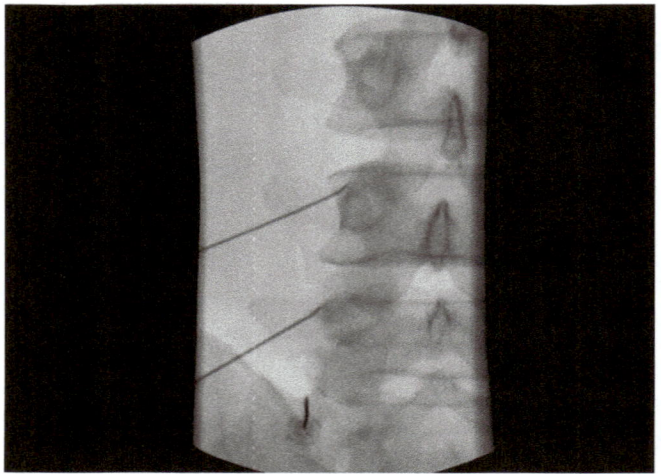

Fig. 13: 10-mm active tip curved RF needle placed at L5 medial branch.

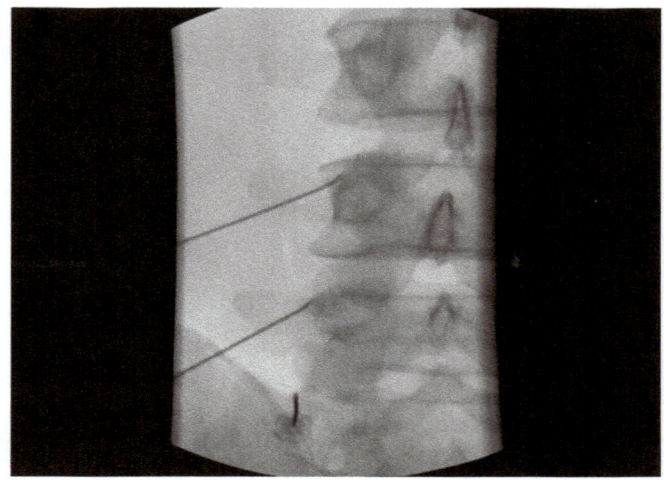

Fig. 14: The RF needle in placed parallel to the L5 medial branch.

Step 15: Lateral view, confirming that the needle tip is away from the neural foramen **(Fig. 15)**.

Step 16: Lateral view with endplates lined up **(Fig. 16)**.

Step 17: Final AP view. The active tip is placed parallel to the medial branch **(Fig. 17)**.

Step 18: Slight adjustment is made **(Fig. 18)**.

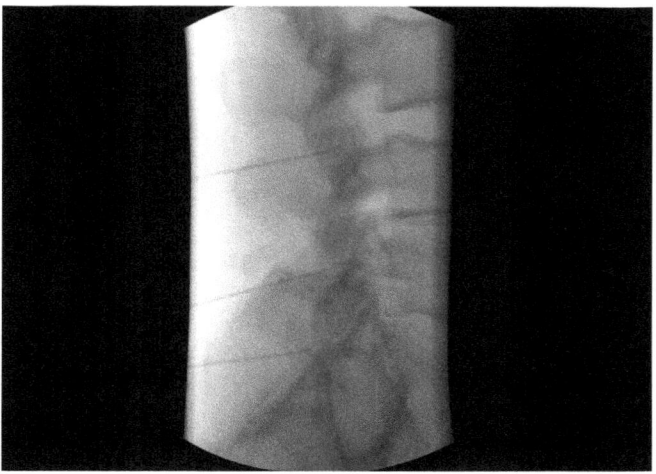

Fig. 15: Lateral view, confirming that the needle tip is away from the neural foramen.

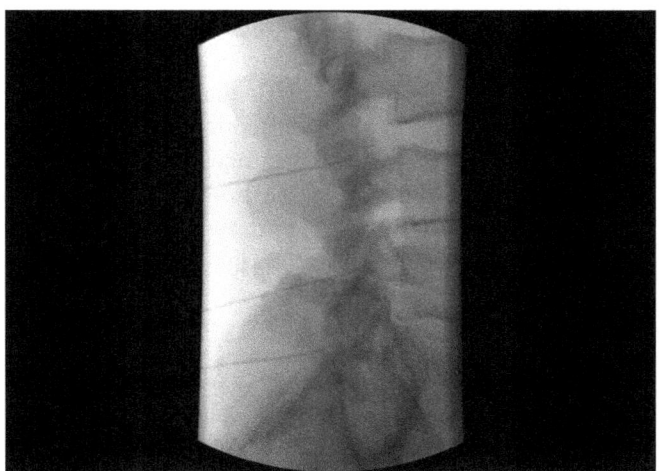

Fig. 16: Lateral view with endplates lined up.

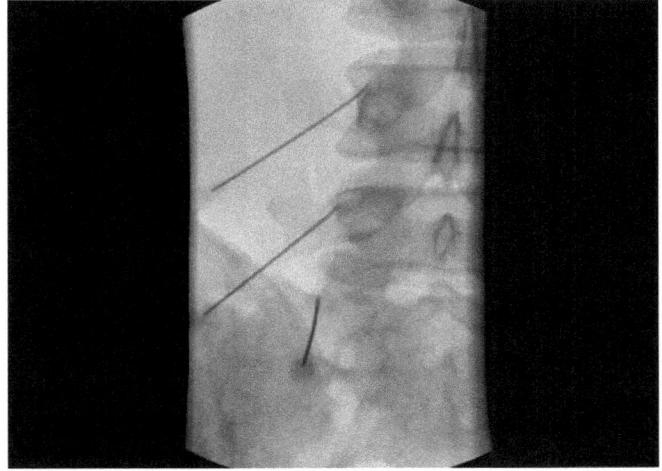

Fig. 17: Final anteroposterior view. The active tip is placed parallel to the medial branch.

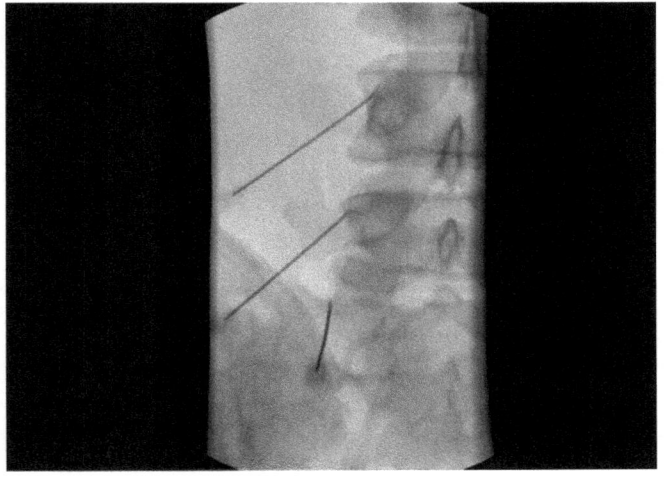

Fig. 18: Slight adjustment made.

Step 19: Radiofrequency lesion is performed at 80° for 90 seconds and repeated after rotating the needle 180° (**Fig. 19**).

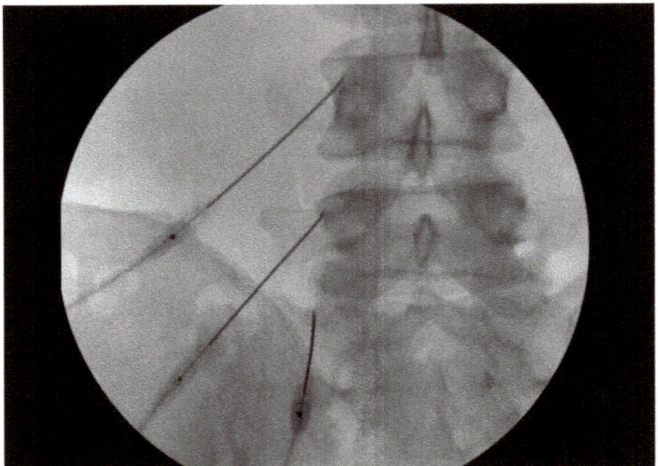

Fig. 19: Radiofrequency lesion being performed at 80° for 90 seconds and repeated after rotating the needle 180°.

Alternative Technique of Performing Lumbar Medial Branch Radiofrequency Denervation (Described by Dr Sherdil Nath)

It is always important to know multiple techniques of preforming the same procedure or to confirm that the radiofrequency denervation (RFD) cannula is in the correct position when in doubt, and hence we describe additional technique of performing lumbar RFD.

10 easy steps for lumbar radiofrequency denervation (RFD) as described by Dr Sherdil Nath:
1. Identify the L5-S1 disc
2. Identify the L5 vertebral body
3. Rotate the C-arm laterally to see the curvature formed by the superior articular process (SAP) and transverse process
4. Tilt inferiorly keeping the curvature in view
5. View curvature as medially and inferiorly as possible
6. Skin entry point is below curvature at lower border transverse process, use plenty of LA
7. Make bone contact below curvature, inject LA
8. Advance in the posterolateral view (needle at 4 o'clock for Left side or 8 o'clock for right side)
9. Inferior tunnel view to confirm needle on bone in middle of curvature
10. Cephalad or superior view with needle at 6 o'clock to see depth of needle tip on the upper surface of the transverse process

Make two adjacent lesions for 60 seconds each at 80° by withdrawing and re-inserting the needle using the curved tip to navigate to a position 2–3 mm beside the first lesion.

CASE 1

Step 1: Obtain a True AP view with the spinous process in the middle of the two pedicles (*See* Chapter 1). Identify the L5-S1 disc by tilting the C-arm by 5° to 10° in the cephalic direction

Step 2: Identify the L5 vertebral body (**Fig. 20**).

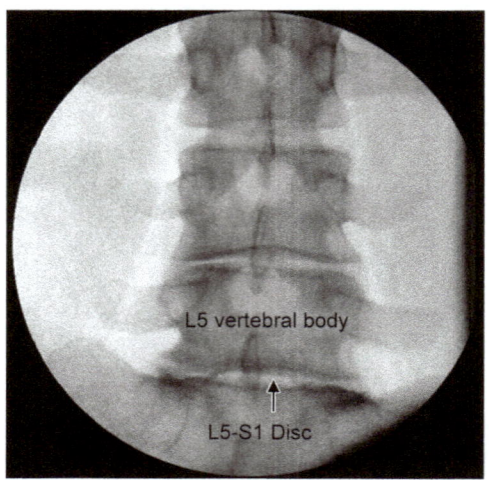

Fig. 20: Identify L5 vertebral body and the L5/S1 disc space.

Step 3: Rotate the C-arm laterally till you see the curvature formed by the transverse process (TP) and the superior articular process (SAP) (arrow) **(Fig. 21)**.

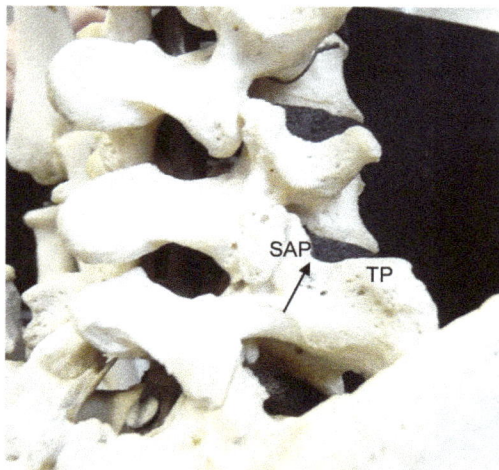

Fig. 21: Arrow points to the curvature at junction of the superior articular process (SAP) and the transverse process (TP).

Step 4: Tilt the C-arm inferiorly keeping the curvature in view.

Step 5: Gradually rotate the C-arm as medially and as inferiorly as possible keeping in view the curvature. If the SAP is hypertrophied the curvature will be lost sooner than expected and if this occurs rotate the C-arm laterally until the curvature is visible again. Arrows are pointing to the curvatures at L4 level **(Figs. 22A and B)**.

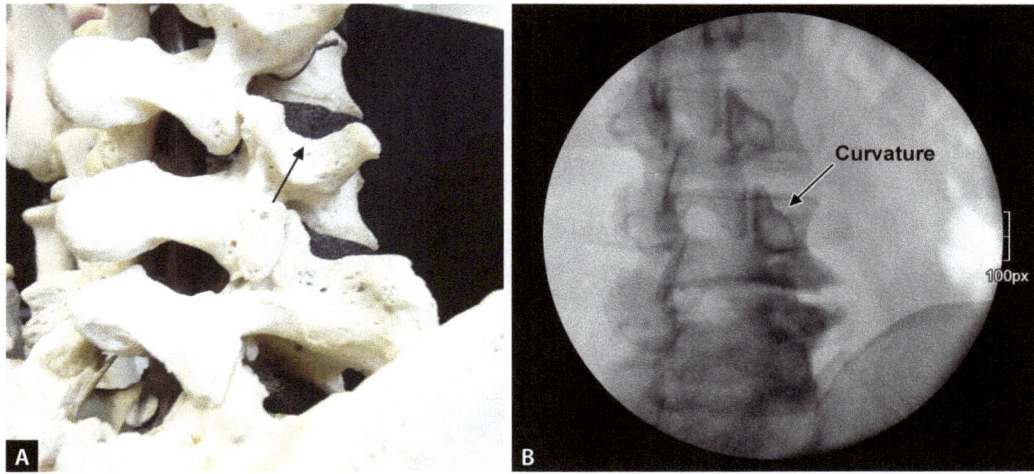

Figs. 22A and B: Curvature formed by the superior articular process and the transverse process.

Step 6: Skin entry point **(Fig. 23A)** is below the curvature at lower border of the transverse process, use plenty of LA.

Step 7: Make bone contact below the curvature in the middle of the pedicle **(Fig. 23B)**. Inject local anesthesia.

In Figures **23A to C**, an 18G 10-mm curved active tip RF cannula is being navigated at the right L4 level. It has been advanced further and is close to the margin of the junction of the SAP, pedicle and the transverse process, maintaining bone contact as it is advanced.

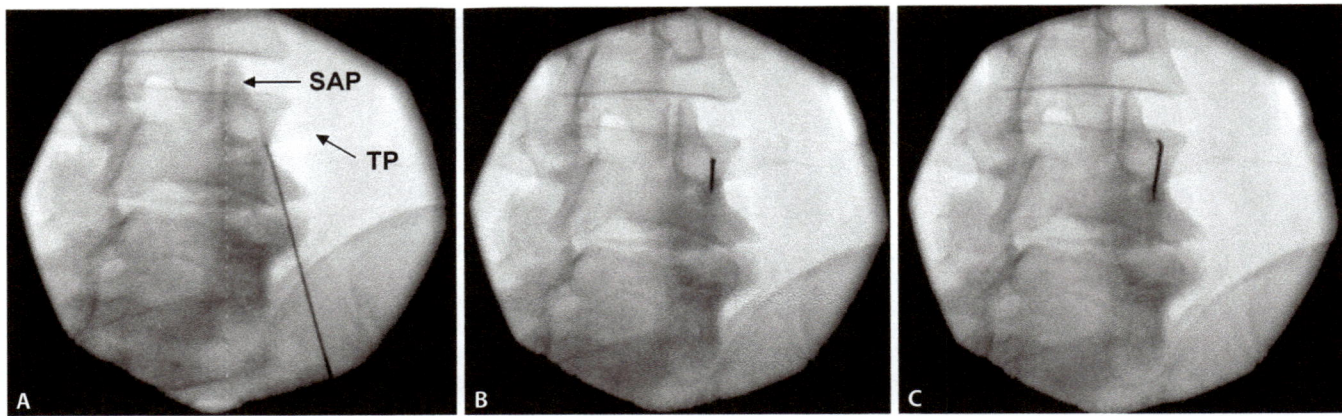

Figs. 23A to C: (A) Skin entry point at the inferior border of the transverse process (TP); (B) RF cannula contacting the bone; (C) RF cannula navigated to the junction of the superior articular process (SAP) and transverse process (TP).

Step 8: Posterolateral view with the RF cannula at 8 o'clock position to confirm tip is just short of the upper edge of the junction of the SAP and transverse process (4 o'clock position when doing left side).

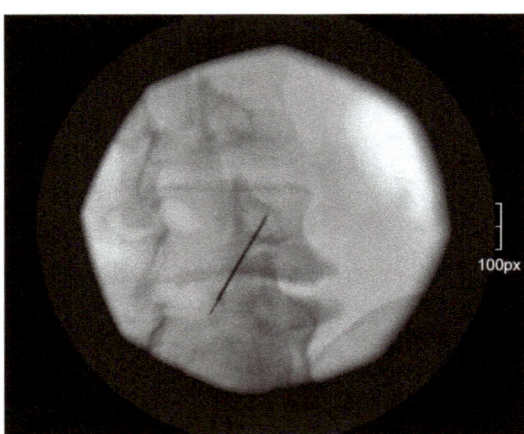

Fig. 24: Posterolateral view with the RF cannula at around 8 o'clock position.

Step 9: C-arm in inferior/lower tunnel view.

C-arm view: A—from the side; B—from the head end.

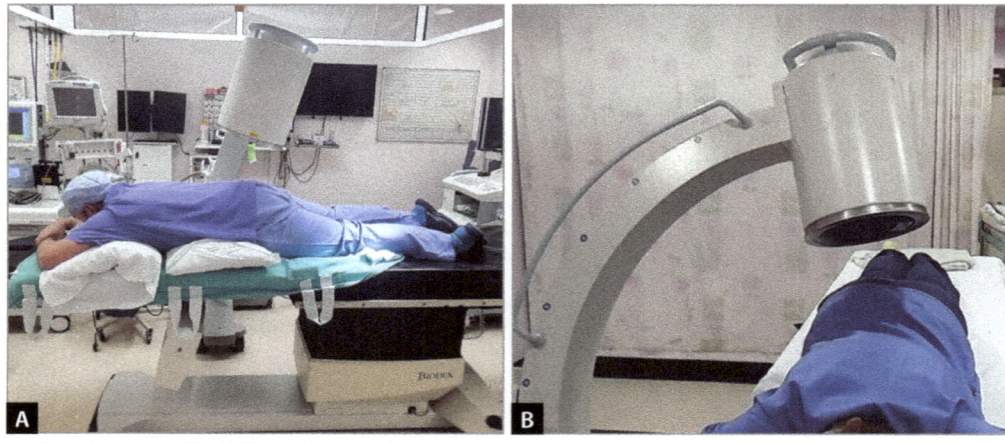

Figs. 25A and B: C-arm—inferior/lower tunnel view. (A) View from the side; (B) View from the head end.

Step 9: Inferior/lower tunnel view: The C-arm in tilted caudally to see the RF cannula from below to confirm bone contact.

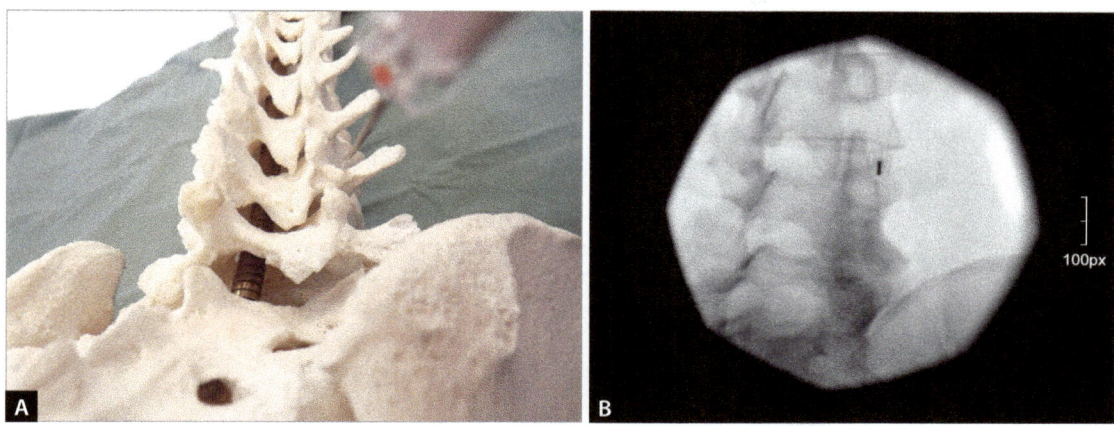

Figs. 26A and B: *Inferior/lower tunnel view:* The C-arm in tilted caudally to see the RF cannula from below to confirm bone contact.

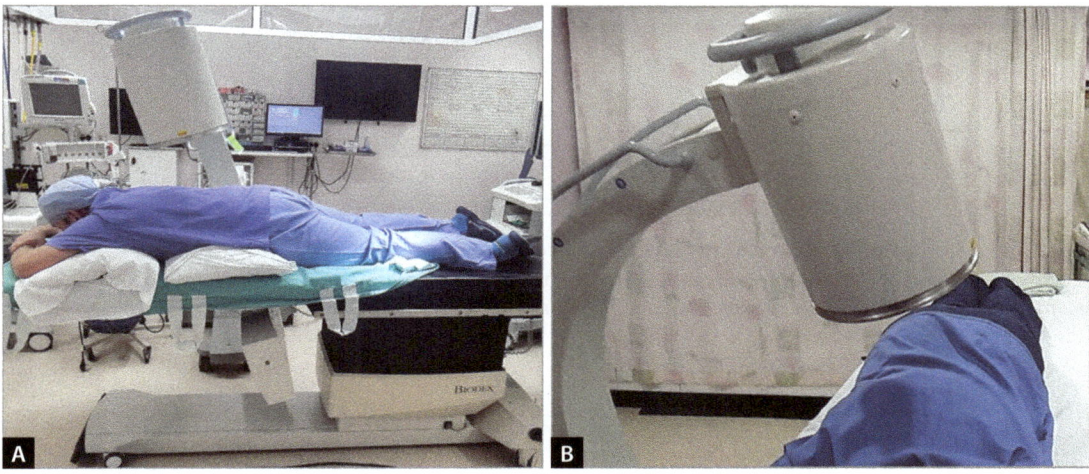

Figs. 27A and B: *C-arm superior view:* (A) View from the side; (B) View from the front.

Step 10: C-arm in superior view.

C-arm view: A—from the side; B—from the head end

Adjust the rotation to get the needle to the 6 o'clock position (*See* **Figure 27**)

Step 10: Cephalic/superior view: The C-arm is moved in the cephalic direction maintaining the RF cannula in 6 o'clock position to see the superior surface of the transverse process. The tip of the RF cannula should stop short of the anterior edge (arrow) of the junction of the SAP, pedicle and the transverse process (TP) **(Figs. 28A and B)**.

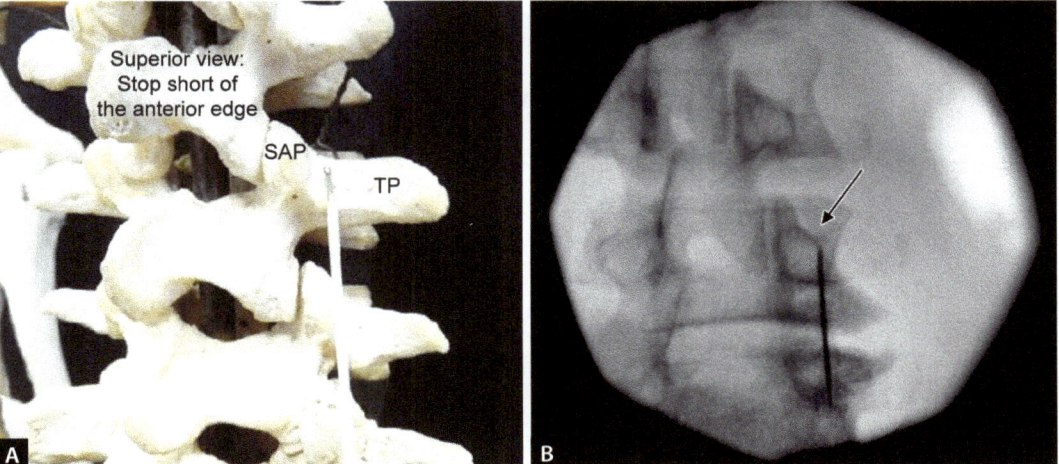

Figs. 28A and B: *Cephalic/superior view:* The C-arm is moved in the cephalic direction maintaining the RF cannula in 6 o'clock position. The tip of the RF cannula should stop short of the anterior edge (arrow) of the junction of the SAP, pedicle and the transverse process (TP).

Some steps from other cases will be described in the following figures.

CASE 2

After steps 1 to 5 have been followed:

Step 6: Skin entry point: Lower border of transverse process under the curvature **(Fig. 29)**.

Step 7: Posterolateral view with the RF cannula at 8 o'clock position to confirm tip just short of the upper edge of the junction of the SAP and transverse process **(Figs. 30A and B)** (4 o'clock position when doing left side).

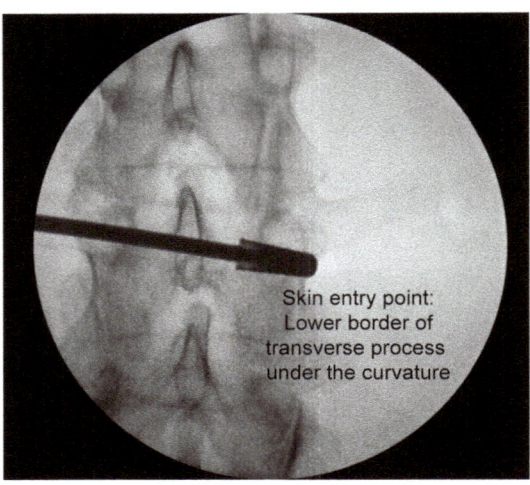

Fig. 29: Skin entry point lower border of transverse process under the curvature.
Source: Reproduced by Permission of Oxford University Press. Nath S. Lumbar Facet Radiofrequency Denervation, pages 56-62 (Page 61, Figure 4.10(a)). In: Spinal Interventions in Pain Management. Simpson K, Baranidharan G, Gupta S (Eds), 2012.

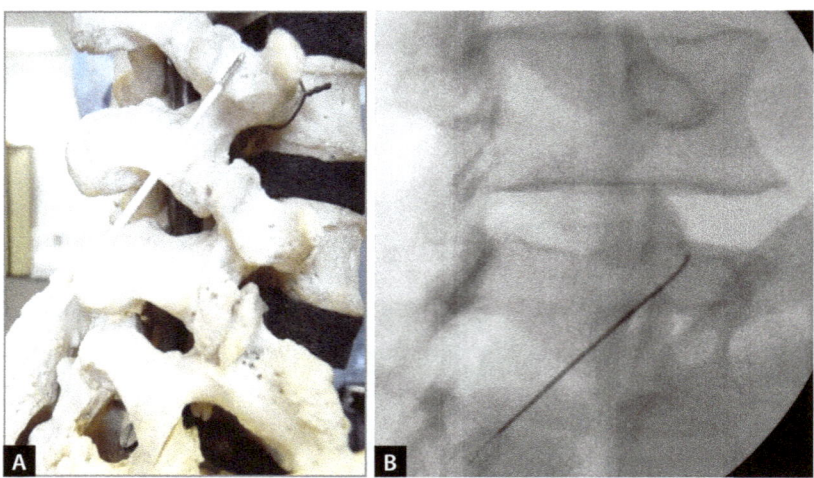

Figs. 30A and B: Posterolateral view with the RF cannula at 8 o'clock.

Step 8: Inferior/lower tunnel view confirms bone contact **(Fig. 31)**.

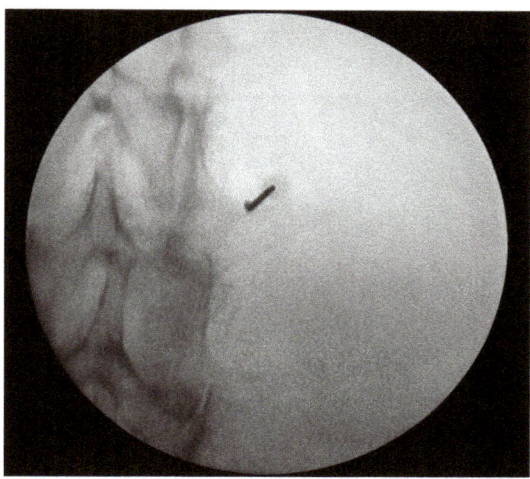

Fig. 31: Inferior/lower tunnel view confirms bone contact.
Source: Reproduced by Permission of Oxford University Press. Nath S. Lumbar Facet Radiofrequency Denervation, pages 56-62 (Page 61, Figure 4.11(a)). In: Spinal Interventions in Pain Management. Simpson K, Baranidharan G, Gupta S (Eds), 2012.

Step 9: Cephalic/superior view: The C-arm is moved in the cephalic direction maintaining the RF cannula in 6 o'clock position to see the superior surface of the transverse process. The RF cannula is not far enough in this image **(Fig. 32)**.

Step 10: Cephalic/superior view: The RF cannula has been advanced by around 2 mm and is now in place **(Fig. 33)**.

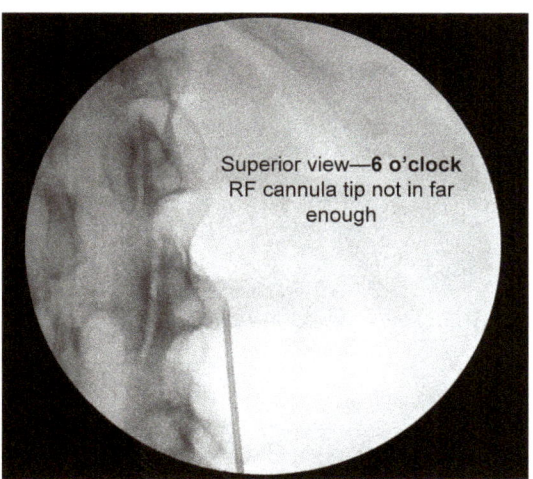

Fig. 32: Cephalic/superior view with RF cannula in 6 o'clock position.

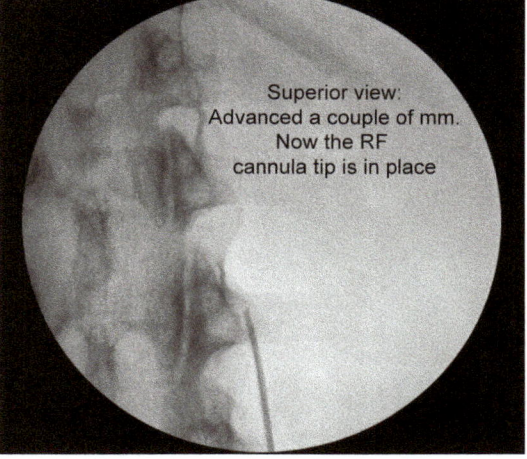

Fig. 33: Superior view of cannula.
Source: Reproduced by Permission of Oxford University Press. Nath S. Lumbar Facet Radiofrequency Denervation, pages 56-62 (Page 61, Figure 4.10(b)). In: Spinal Interventions in Pain Management. Simpson K, Baranidharan G, Gupta S (Eds), 2012.

L5 dorsal ramus radiofrequency denervation: After Steps 1 to 5 have been followed and visualizing the curvature as inferiorly as possible.

Step 6: Skin entry point for L5 DR RFD is below the curvature formed by the junction of the superior articular process (SAP) of S1 and the ala of the sacrum **(Fig. 34)**.

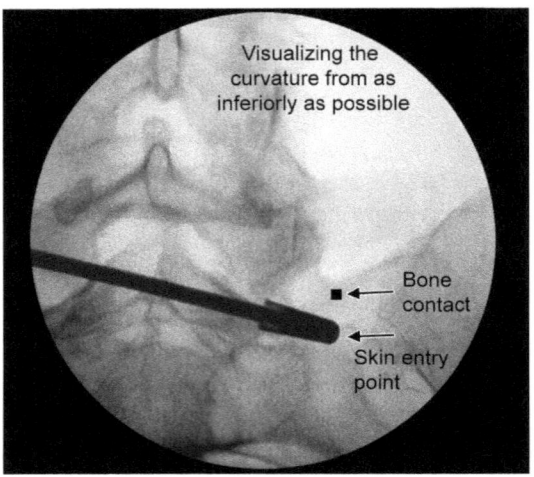

Fig. 34: Skin entry point for L5 DR RFD.
Source: Reproduced by permission of Oxford University Press. Nath S. Lumbar Facet Radiofrequency Denervation, pages 56-62 (Page 61, Figure 4.12(a)). In: Spinal Interventions in Pain Management. Simpson K, Baranidharan G, Gupta S (Eds), 2012.

Step 8: Posterolateral view with the RF cannula at 8 o'clock position to confirm tip is just short of the upper edge of the junction of the SAP and transverse process **(Fig. 35)** (4 o'clock position when doing left side).

Step 9: Inferior view to confirm that the RF cannula is in contact with bone at the 'V' shaped junction of the superior articula process (SAP) of S1 and ala of sacrum **(Fig. 36)**.

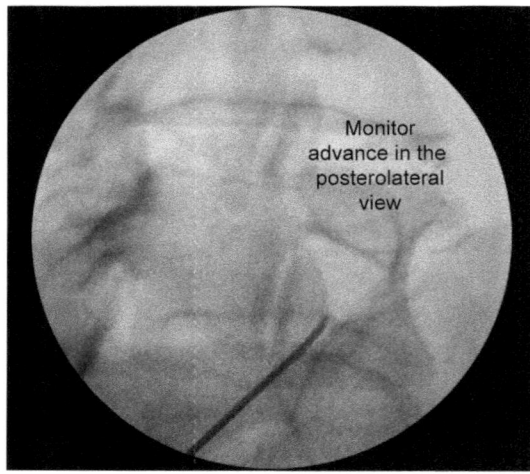

Fig. 35: Cannula in posteriolateral view.
Source: Reproduced by permission of Oxford University Press. Nath S. Lumbar Facet Radiofrequency Denervation, pages 56-62 (Page 61, Figure 4.12(d)). In: Spinal Interventions in Pain Management. Simpson K, Baranidharan G, Gupta S (Eds), 2012.

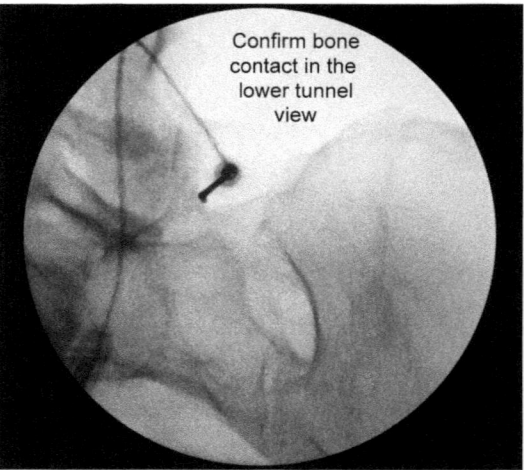

Fig. 36: Inferior view to confirm that the RF cannula is in contact with bone.
Source: Reproduced by permission of Oxford University Press. Nath S. Lumbar Facet Radiofrequency Denervation, pages 56-62 (Page 61, Figure 4.12(b)). In: Spinal Interventions in Pain Management. Simpson K, Baranidharan G, Gupta S (Eds), 2012.

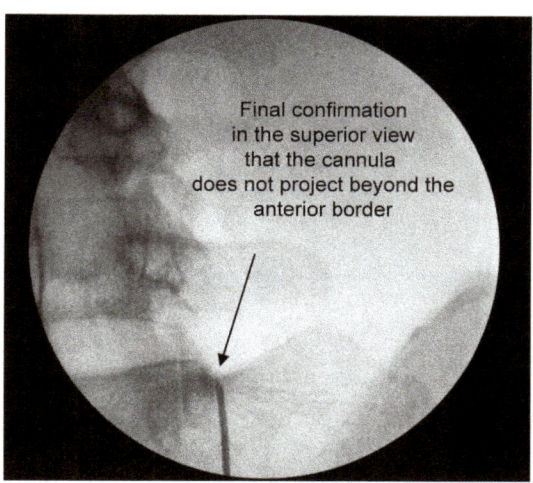

Fig. 37: Cannula in superior view.
Source: Reproduced by Permission of Oxford University Press. Nath S. Lumbar Facet Radiofrequency Denervation, pages 56-62 (Page 61, Figure 4.12(c)). In: Spinal Interventions in Pain Management. K Simpson K, Baranidharan G, Gupta S (Eds), 2012.

Step 10: Superior view (cephalad) view: The fluoroscopy C-arm is tilted cephalic by about 20–25° in oblique view looking from above to confirm the RF cannula tip is just short of anterior border of the junction of the SAP of S1 and the ala of sacrum **(Fig. 37)**.

Please also see Chapter 25 on sacroiliac joint RFD, case 1, Figures 18 to 25, for another technique of performing L5 dorsal rami radiofrequency denervation.

ACKNOWLEDGMENTS

We thank Dr Sherdil Nath, Consultant in Pain Medicine, Sweden and Dr G Baranidharan, Consultant in Pain Medicine, Leeds Teaching Hospital NHS Trust, UK, for providing and allowing us to use some of their images in this chapter.

FURTHER READING

1. Navani AH, Melnik I, Derby R, Lee JE. Lumbar facet join, medial branch and radiofrequency procedures. In: Baheti DK, Bakshi S, Gupta S, Singh RSP (Eds). Interventional pain management: a practical approach, 2nd edition. New Delhi: Jaypee Brothers Medical Publishers; 2016. pp. 241-53.
2. Baranidharan G, Raphael JH, Menon R, Nath S, Gupta S, Evans N. Lumbar Spine Interventions. In: Spinal Interventions in Pain Management: Oxford Specialist Handbooks in pain management. Simpson K, Baranidharan G, Gupta S (Eds). Oxford University Press 2012, pp. 37-70.
3. Nath S, Nath CA, Pettersson K. Percutaneous lumbar zygapophysial (facet) joint neurotomy using radiofrequency current, in the management of chronic low back pain: a randomized double-blind trial. Spine. 2008;33(12): 1291-7.

CHAPTER 22

Caudal Epidural Block

Sanjay Bakshi

BASIC INFORMATION

Indications
- Lumbar radiculopathy
- Lumbar disc herniation
- Lumbar spinal stenosis

Contraindications
- Unwilling patient
- Untreated infection
- Pregnancy
- Bleeding problems or blood thinners
- Allergy to medications
- Severe cardiovascular or respiratory compromise
- Dye allergy. Use alternate dye or premedication

Equipement and Supplies
- C-arm
- Procedure tray with spinal needle
- Connection tubing
- IV if sedation planned
- Appropriate monitors

Medications
- Contrast dye
- Steroid—dexamethasone or Kenalog
- Local anesthetic
- Preservative-free saline

PROCEDURE DETAILS

Step 1: Position as shown in **Figures 1 and 2**.

Step 2: Prone position with initial lateral view of C-arm. Procedure is always started in lateral view **(Fig. 3)**.

Step 3: Confirm and feel the sacrococcygeal ligament.

Step 4: Now inject local anesthetic for sacrococcygeal ligament. Push a 21-gauge spinal needle into the caudal epidural space. Confirm under fluoroscopy as shown in **Figures 3 and 4**.

Step 5: Inject contrast Inj. Omnipaque 2–3 cc and confirm spread of dye in lateral and anteroposterior views as shown in **Figures 5 and 6**.

Fig. 1: Pillow under pelvis.

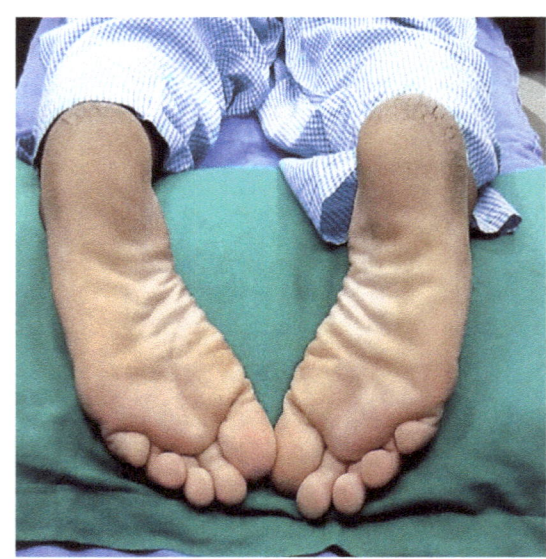

Fig. 2: Toes rotated inward.

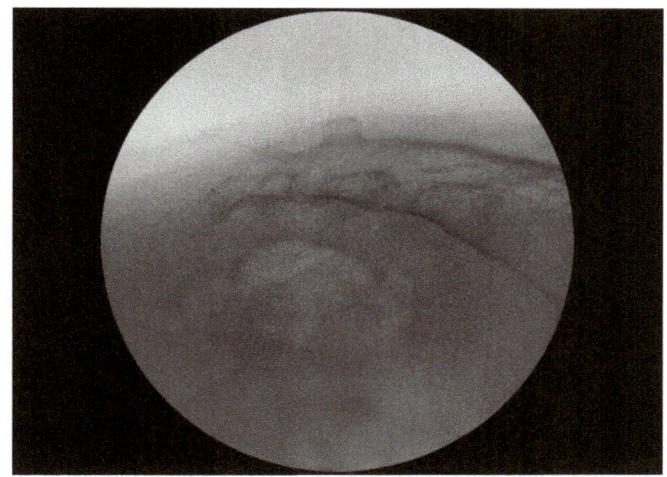

Fig. 3: Needle at the entrance of caudal epidural space.

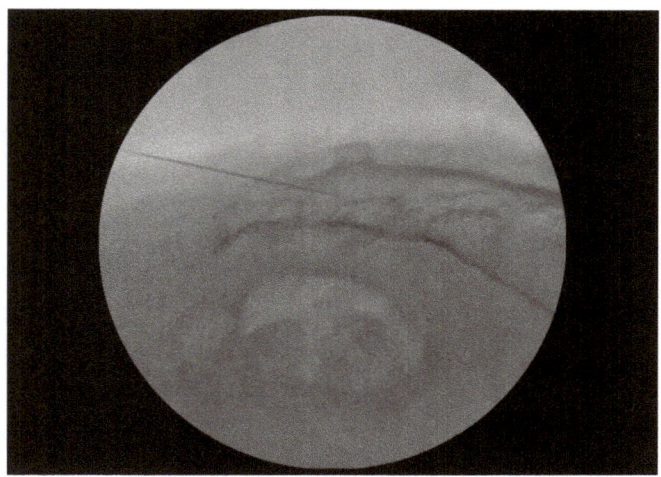

Fig. 4: Needle in caudal space.

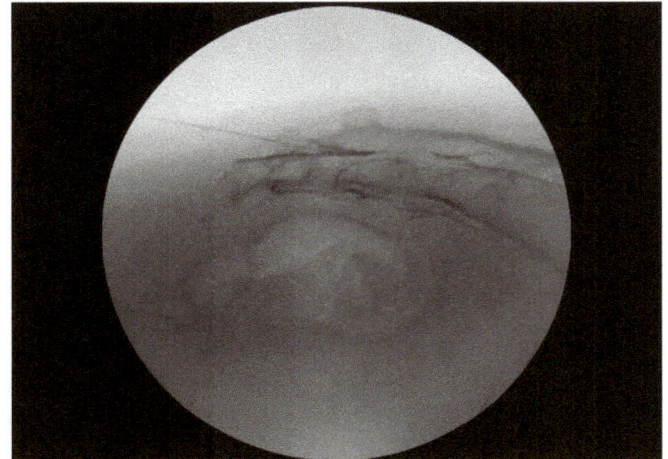

Fig. 5: Dye spread in lateral view.

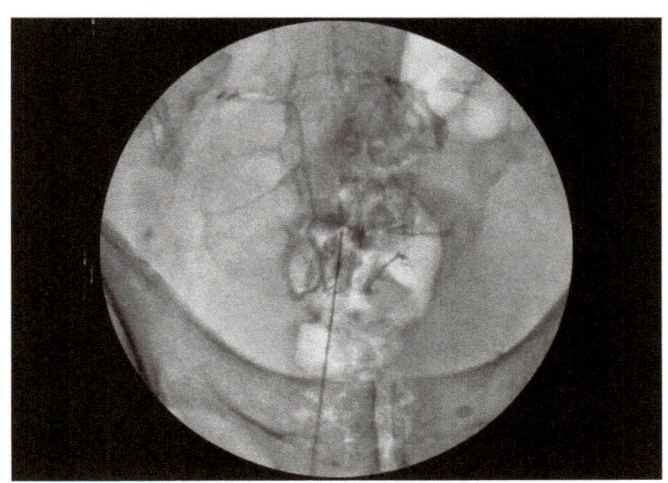

Fig. 6: Dye spread in anteroposterior view.

Step 6: Once dye spread is confirmed, inject the selected steroid in caudal epidural space.

Step 7: Shift the patient to the recovery room for monitoring of vital signs for few hours.

CHAPTER 23

S1 Nerve Root Block and Technical Challenges

Sanjeeva Gupta, Manohar Sharma, Sanjay Bakshi

CASE 1

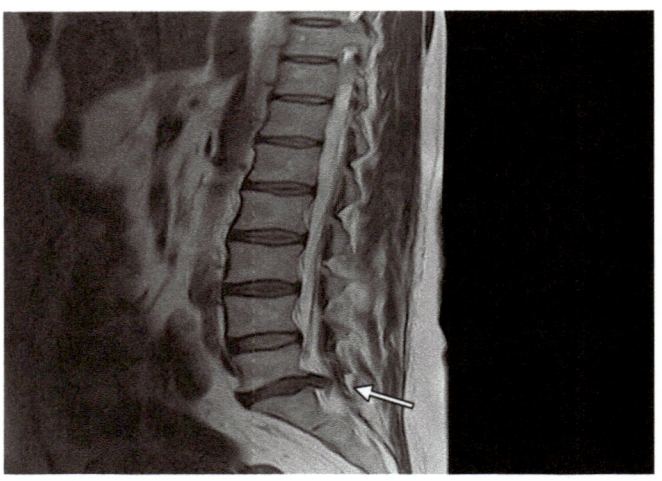

Fig. 1: The sagittal T2 MRI scan image showing moderate-sized posterior central and left paracentral disc protrusion at L5/S1 level displacing and compressing the left transiting S1 nerve root in the lateral recess (arrow).

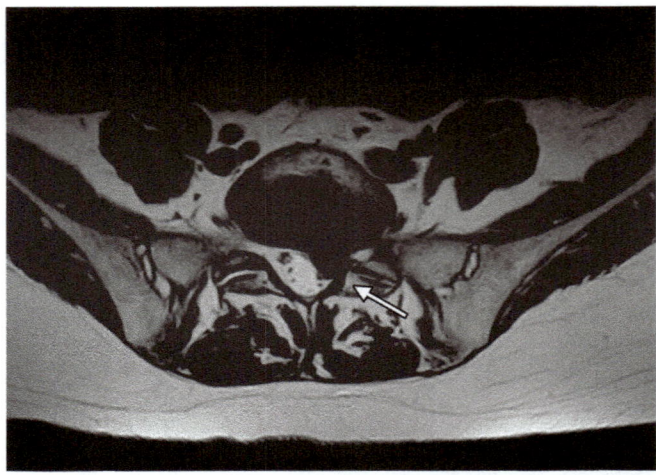

Fig. 2: The axial T2 MRI scan image showing a moderate-sized posterior central and left paracentral disc protrusion at L5/S1 displacing and compressing the left transiting S1 nerve root in the lateral recess (arrow).

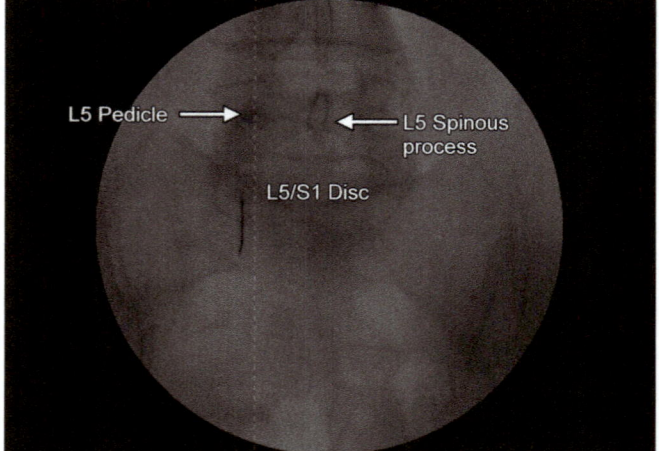

Fig. 3: Patient in prone position with a pillow under the lower abdomen and pelvis. Antero-posterior (AP) view with cephalic tilt in an attempt to square the L5/S1 disc helps identify the S1 foramen. If you are having difficulty in identifying the S1 foramen, consider identifying the ipsilateral L5 pedicle and try to identify the S1 foramen just below the likely area of the S1 pedicle for the S1 subpedicular block.

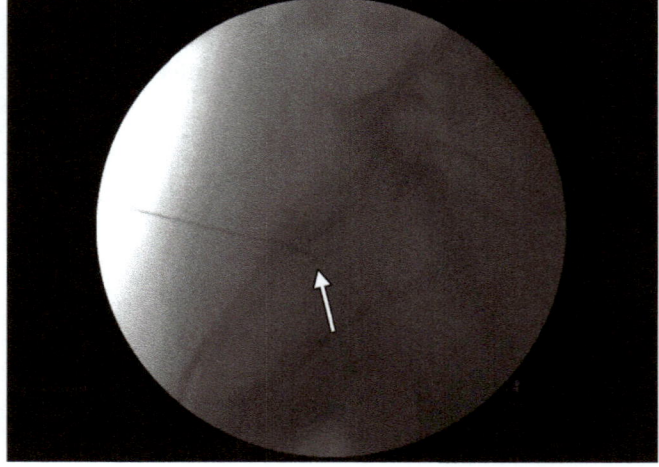

Fig. 4: Lateral fluoroscopic view showing the needle tip advanced into the left S1 foramen. The arrow points to the tip of the needle.

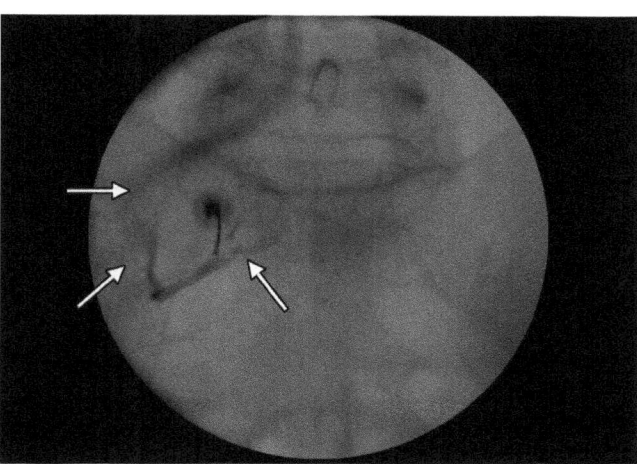

Fig. 5: AP fluoroscopic view showing vascular spread (arrows) when contrast was injected under *continuous fluoroscopy* during a transforaminal S1 root block. Note that the contrast must be injected in AP view under continuous fluoroscopy to rule out vascular spread. The incidence of vascular spread is less likely if the needle tip is placed in the medial and superior quadrant of the S1 foramen. On digital subtraction imaging, the incidence of vascular uptake was 4.9% when the needle was placed in the medial half of the sacral foraminal area as compared to 38.6% when the needle tip was in the lateral half of the sacral foraminal area. Digital subtraction imaging is more likely to pick up vascular spread compared to continuous fluoroscopy.

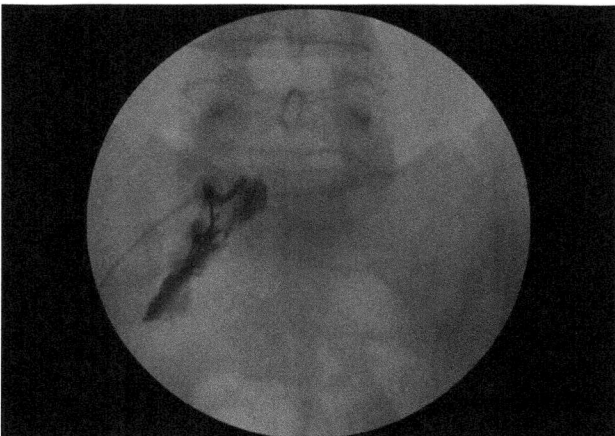

Fig. 6: AP fluoroscopic view showing appropriate spread of the contrast toward the L5/S1 disc on advancing the needle by around 3 mm after vascular spread was encountered as shown in **Figure 5**. In most cases, advancing or retracting the needle by millimeters is enough to facilitate appropriate contrast spread toward the site of the pathology. However, if the vascular spread continued despite moving the needle, then either a second needle could be placed at the S1 level (see Case 2) or the procedure could be carried out using the L5/S1 infraneural/retrodiscal technique.

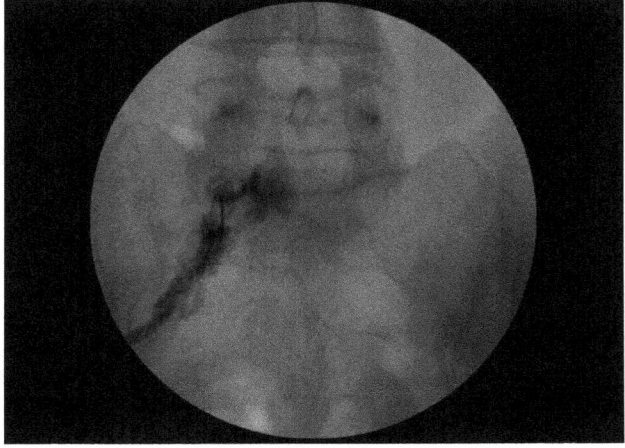

Fig. 7: Final AP fluoroscopic image showing appropriate spread of the contrast and a mixture of local anesthetic and dexamethasone toward the L5/S1 disc, the site of the pathology.

SECTION 5 | Lumbosacral Spine

CASE 2

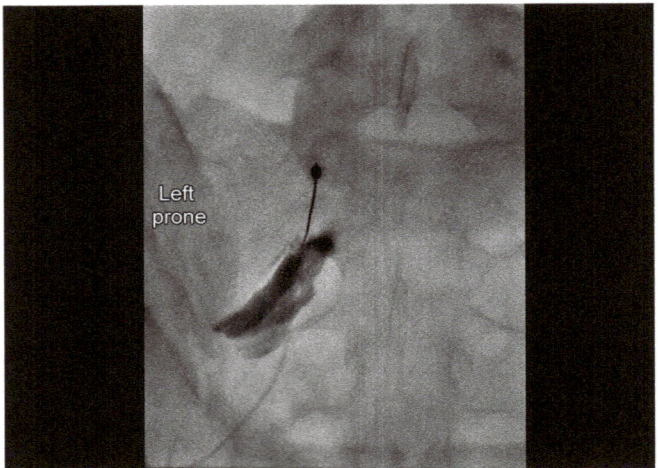

Fig. 8: AP fluoroscopic view showing the contrast spread away from the L5/S1 disc.
Source: Reproduced from Gupta S, Gupta H, Baranidharan G, Sharma M. Technical challenges of performing S1 root block: role for double needle and multilevel needle technique. British J Pain. 2021;15(2):129-33.

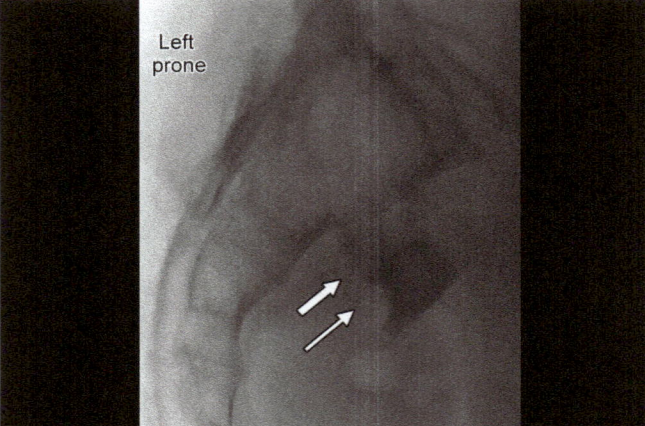

Fig. 9: Lateral fluoroscopic view showing the contrast spread anteriorly (white arrows) and away from the L5/S1 disc and not toward the L5/S1 disc, the site of the pathology. The contrast continued to spread anteriorly despite withdrawing the needle, and hence a second needle was inserted, medial to the first needle, as shown in **Figure 10**.
Source: Reproduced from Gupta S, Gupta H, Baranidharan G, Sharma M. Technical challenges of performing S1 root block: role for double needle and multilevel needle technique. British J Pain. 2021;15(2):129-33.

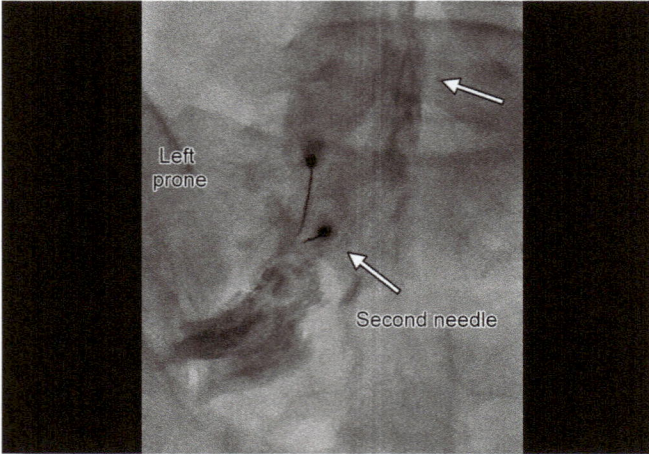

Fig. 10: (Double needle technique) AP fluoroscopic view with the *second needle* (medial to the first) in place. The contrast was seen spreading toward the L5/S1 disc, the site of the pathology. This is the final image after a mixture of local anesthetic and dexamethasone was injected. The contrast can be seen spreading upward toward the L5 vertebral body.
Source: Reproduced from Gupta S, Gupta H, Baranidharan G, Sharma M. Technical challenges of performing S1 root block: role for double needle and multilevel needle technique. British J Pain. 2021;15(2):129-33.

CASE 3

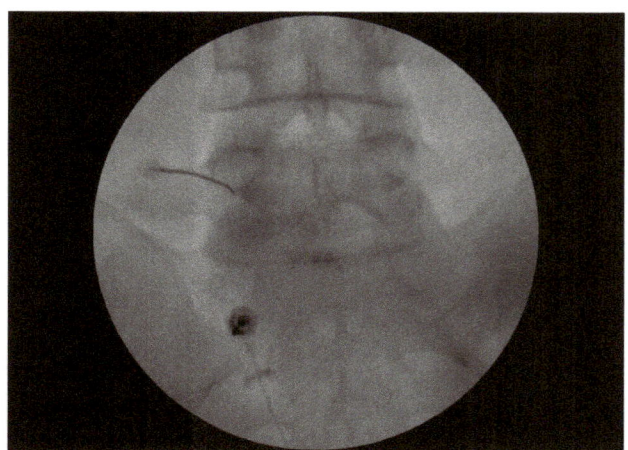

Fig. 11: AP fluoroscopic view showing the *Direction* (Also see Figure 2 in Chapter 1 regarding 3D principle) of the needle placement at S1 and L5/S1 levels (subpedicular technique). Some clinicians prefer to do a pre- and a postganglionic block for pain in S1 distribution due to pathology at the L5/S1 disc level.

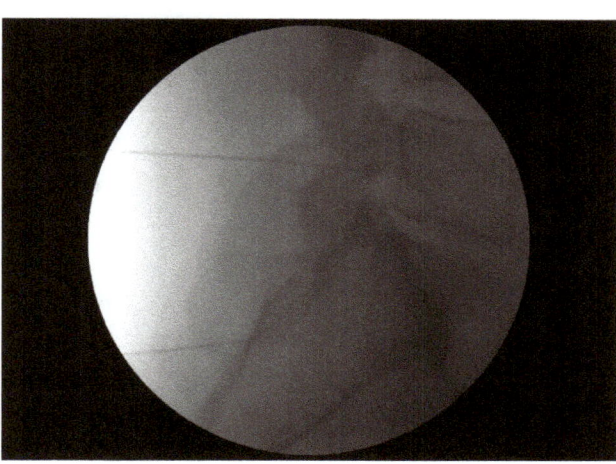

Fig. 12: In lateral fluoroscopic view, the *Depth* (Also see Figure 2 in Chapter 1 regarding 3D principle) of the needle is assessed and if necessary advanced further. The image shows placement of needles at the S1 and L5/S1 foramen levels (subpedicular technique).

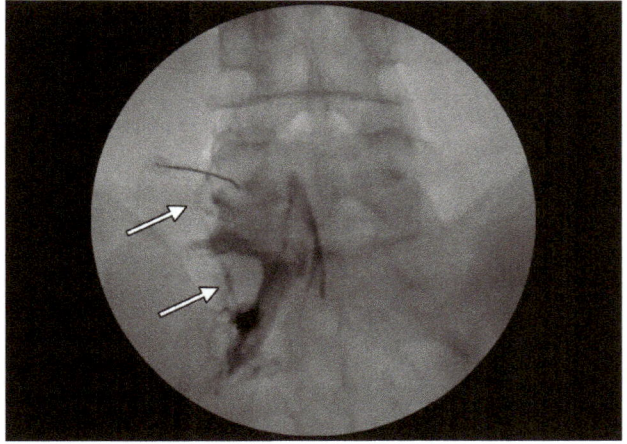

Fig. 13: AP fluoroscopic view on injecting contrast via a low volume extension tubing attached to the needle under *continuous fluoroscopy* showing contrast spread along the left S1 nerve root as well as vascular spread (arrows). In this case, the needle was withdrawn by around 5 mm and contrast injected again as shown in **Figure 14**.

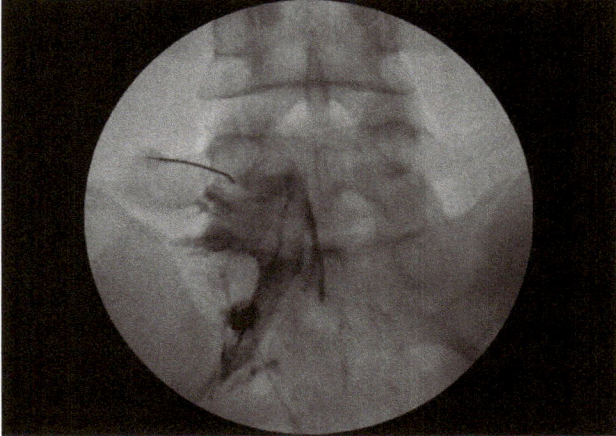

Fig. 14: AP fluoroscopic view on injecting contrast under continuous fluoroscopy after withdrawing the needle by around 5 mm shows contrast spread along the left S1 nerve root and toward the L5/S1 disc but no vascular spread.

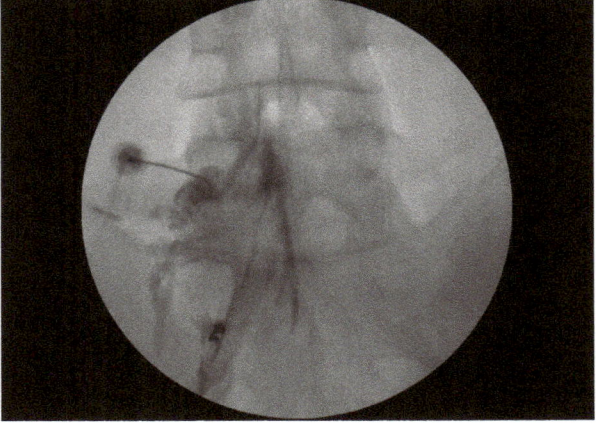

Fig. 15: AP fluoroscopic view on injecting contrast via a low volume extension tubing attached to the needle under continuous fluoroscopy at the L5/S1 level (subpedicular technique). Some clinicians prefer to do a pre- and a postganglionic block for pain in S1 distribution due to pathology at the L5/S1 disc level.

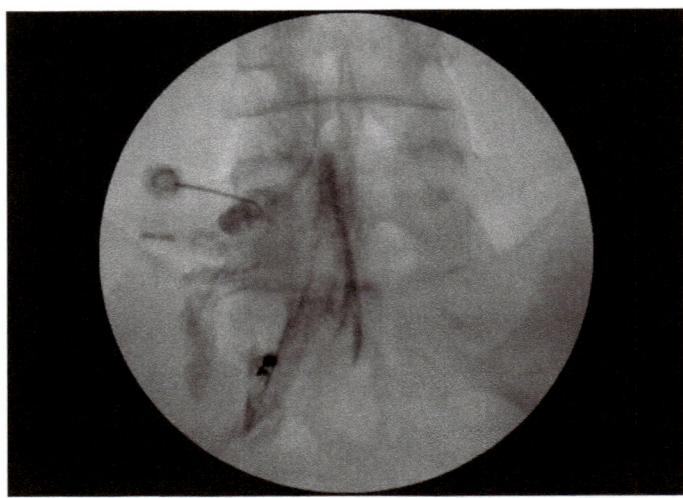

Fig. 16: The final image after injection of a mixture of local anesthetic and dexamethasone at both the S1 and the L5/S1 level.

Flowchart 1: A step-wise plan when performing S1 root block.

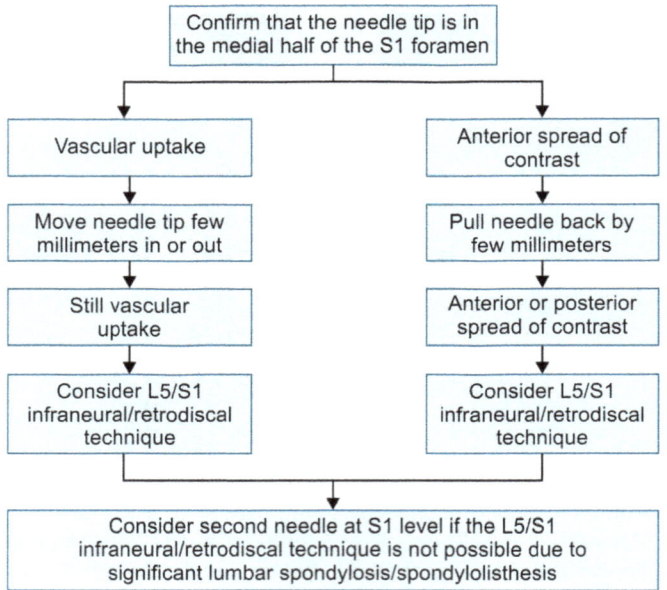

Note: If at any stage in this plan, there is no vascular uptake and satisfactory spread of contrast, then accept that needle tip position to complete the injection.
Source: Reproduced from Gupta S, Gupta H, Baranidharan G, Sharma M. Technical challenges of performing S1 root block: role for double needle and multilevel needle technique. British J Pain. 2021;15(2):129-33.

FURTHER READING

1. Gupta S, Gupta H, Baranidharan G, Sharma M. Technical challenges of performing S1 root block: role for double needle and multilevel needle technique. British J Pain. 2021;15(2):129-33.
2. Gupta S. Pre-contrast injection multiple needle placement technique: an alternative method for performing challenging transforaminal epidural steroid injections for radicular pain. Pain Med Case Rep. 2020;4(2):39-44.
3. Kim WJ, Shin HY, Yoo SH, Park HS. Comparison of epidural spreading patterns and clinical outcomes of transforaminal epidural steroid injection with high-volume injectate via the subpedicular versus the retrodiscal approach. Pain Phys. 2018;21:269-78.
4. Park SJ, Kim SH, Kim SJ, Yoon DM, Yoon KB. Comparison of incidences of intravascular injection between medial and lateral side approaches during traditional S1 transforaminal epidural steroid injection. Pain Res Manag. 2017;2017:6426802.

Chapter 24: Sacroiliac Joint Block

Sanjeeva Gupta, Babita Ghai

INTRODUCTION

Sacroiliac joint (SIJ) pain is more common in women. A female patient with maximum pain below L5 level with tenderness over the SIJ suggests that the patient may have pain originating from the SIJ. Injection of local anesthetic into the sacroiliac joint (SIJ) is a diagnostic procedure. However, adding steroid with the local anesthetic into the SIJ can often provide good pain relief in some patients. Some pain physicians prefer to block the nerves that supply the sacroiliac joint with local anesthetic instead of injection local anesthesia into the SIJ.

Note: **Figures 1 to 9** have been taken from S Gupta, J Richardson. Sacroiliac joint block. In: Baheti DK, Bakshi S, Gupta S, Gehdoo RP (Eds). Interventional Pain Management: A Practical Approach, 1st edition. New Delhi. Jaypee Brothers Medical Publishers; 2009. pp. 198-203.

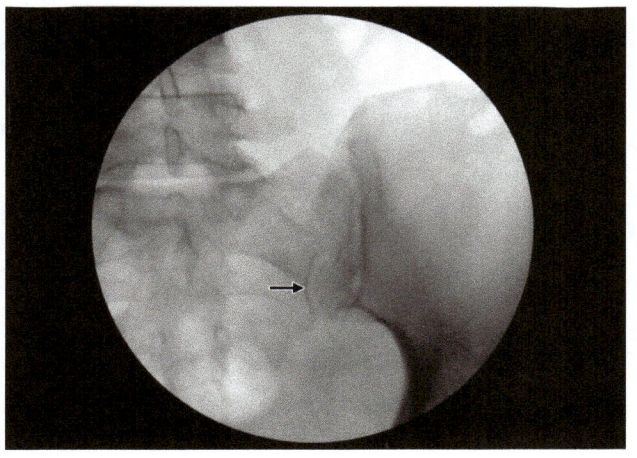

Fig. 1: Posteroanterior view of the right sacroiliac joint. Normally, the medial joint lines are the posterior joint lines (arrow).

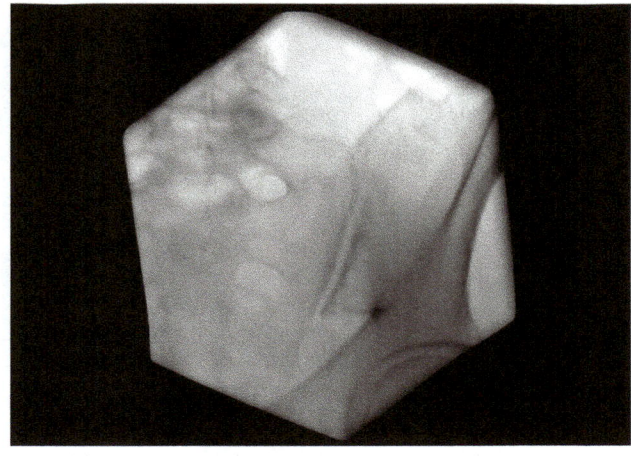

Fig. 2: The anterior and the posterior joint lines of the right SIJ have been superimposed by contralateral oblique rotation of the C-arm.

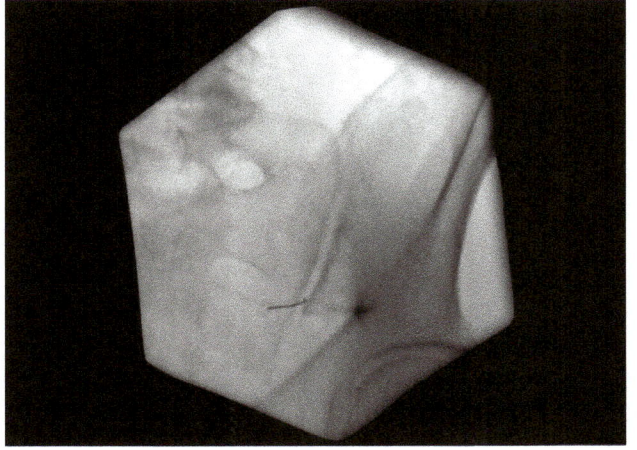

Fig. 3: A 22-G needle with a curved tip is seen entering the inferior part of the right sacroiliac joint.

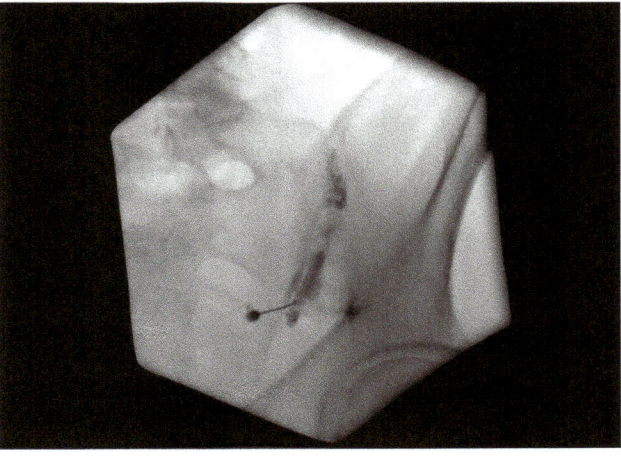

Fig. 4: Contrast medium spread along the right sacroiliac joint (contralateral oblique view).

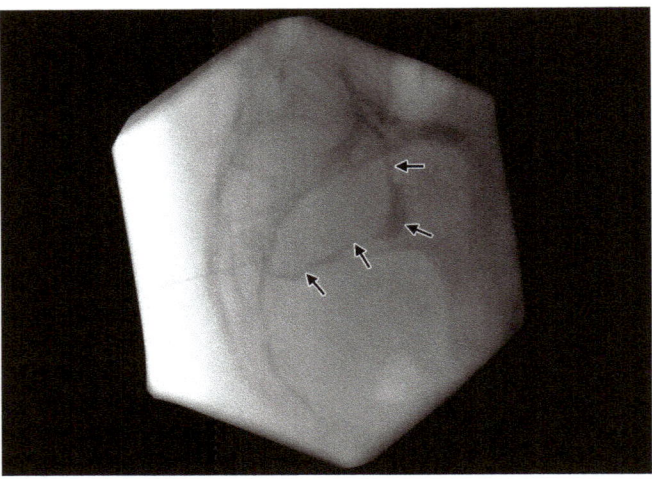

Fig. 5: Contrast medium spread can be seen along the perimeter of the joint line in lateral view as indicated by the arrows (A lateral view is normally not necessary as this will increase the X-ray exposure unless you are suspecting that the needle has gone too far).

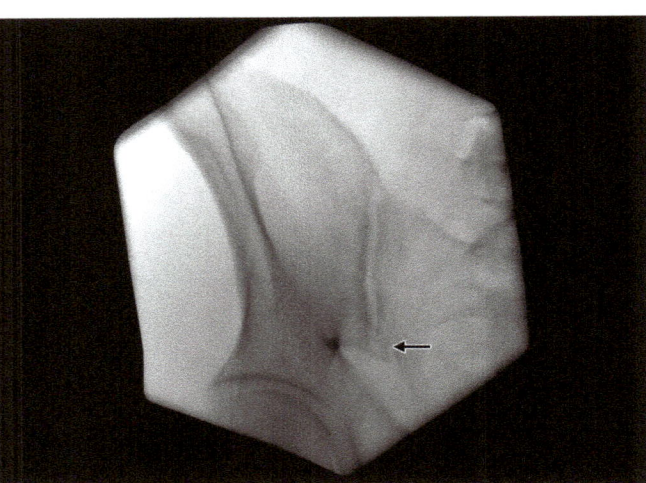

Fig. 6: *Left sacroiliac joint block*: The medial joint lines are the margins of the posterior SIJ (arrow).

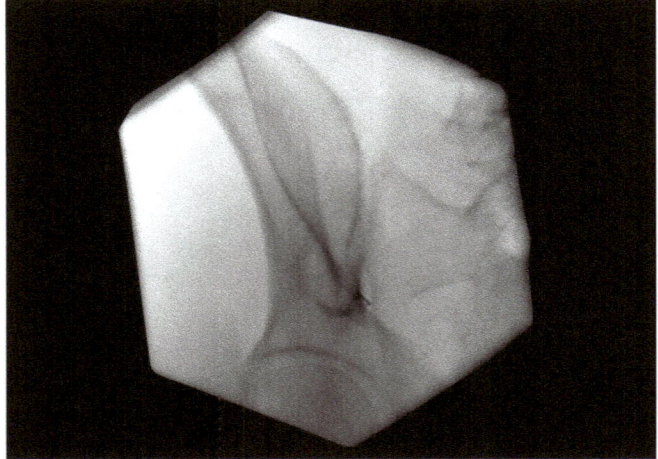

Fig. 7: With slight contralateral oblique rotation, the posterior joint lines have become crisp and a curved tip needle is seen entering the joint (in this case the anterior and posterior joint lines have not been superimposed).

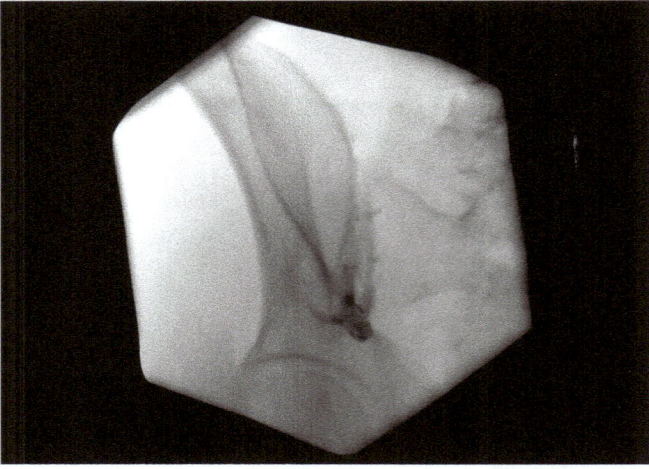

Fig. 8: Contrast medium spread in the left sacroiliac joint.

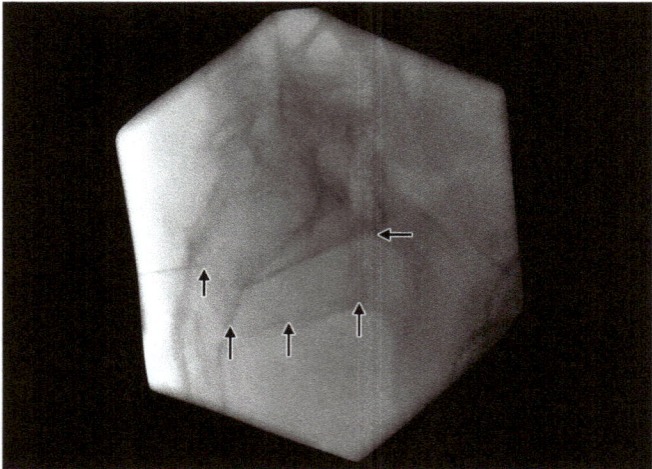

Fig. 9: Lateral view showing the tip of the needle and the perimeter of the joint line as shown by the arrows (A lateral view is normally not necessary as this will increase the X-ray exposure unless you are suspecting that the needle has gone too far).

SACROILIAC JOINT BLOCK: DOUBLE NEEDLE TECHNIQUE

(See Reference 2 for more details)

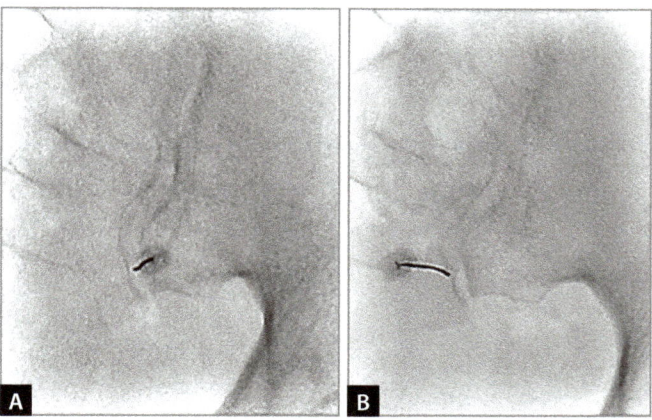

Figs. 10A and B: (A) A curved tipped spinal needle is advanced into the right sacroiliac joint; (B) On continuous fluoroscopy in the contralateral oblique direction, the tip of the needle appears to be on the bone.

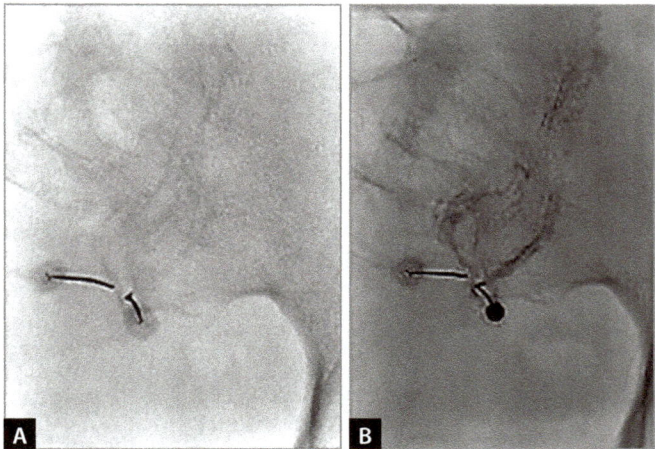

Figs. 11A and B: (A) On continuous fluoroscopy (it could be ipsilateral or contralateral rotation), another translucent joint area is identified and a second needle is advanced into the joint; (B) Contrast is injected through the second needle and the sacroiliac joint is outlined. If on injecting contrast the needle tip is suspected not to be in the joint, then inject the contrast through the already placed other needle to evaluate if this is in the joint. The double needle technique increases the chances of the needle tip being in the SIJ before injecting medications into the joint.

FURTHER READING

1. Gupta S. Double needle technique: an alternative method for performing difficult SIJ injections. Pain Phys. 2011;14(3): 281-4.
2. Gupta S, Richardson J. Sacroiliac joint block. In: Baheti DK, Bakshi S, Gupta S, Gehdoo RP (Eds). Interventional pain management: a practical approach, 1st edition. New Delhi: Jaypee Brothers Medical Publishers; 2009. pp. 198-203.
3. Sacroiliac joint access. In: Bogduk N (Ed). Practice guidelines for spinal diagnosis and treatment procedures, 2nd edition. International Spin Intervention Society; 2013.
4. Schwarzer AC, Aprill CN, Bogduk N. The sacroiliac joint in chronic low back pain. Spine. 1995;20(1):31-7.

CHAPTER 25

Sacroiliac Joint Radiofrequency Denervation

Samir Ranjit Jani, Sanjeeva Gupta, Ganesan Baranidharan

BASIC INFORMATION

Neuroanatomy of SI joint: Predominantly L5, S1, S2, S3. Variable supply individual to individual (L4 and S4 innervation may occur).

Overview

- SI joint pathology is estimated to be 20% of all low back pain.
- True diarthrodial synovial joint produced by the junction of the sacrum and iliac wings bilaterally.
- Lock and key mechanism to limit movement; grooves on each surface confer stability.
- Posterior aspect of SI is further supported by strong ligaments (SI, sacrotuberous).
- *Common risk factors for SI pain:* Leg-length disparity, scoliosis, pregnancy, gait abnormalities, motor vehicle accidents, falls, and lumbosacral fusion.

Diagnosis

- Sharp "knife"-like pain located inferior to belt line/pelvic crest
- Radicular component into posterior thigh; rarely extends beyond knee
- Difficulty from getting from a seated position such as getting off toilet
- *Physical examination:* Tenderness on PSIS; Thigh Thrust, FABER, Fortin finger test
- *Imaging:* Limited value; X-ray/CT/MRI may show degeneration but can appear normal and still be pain generator.
- *Dual-diagnostic fluoroscopic-guided local anesthesia blocks gold standard:*
  - Rotate image intensifier 10–15° contralateral to target joint
  - Add 5° cephalad tilt to open inferior one-third of joint
  - Place needle parallel to fluoroscopic imaging into the inferior one-third of the joint
  - Low-volume contrast to confirm intra-articular placement
  - Triamcinolone 80 mg + 3–5 mL
  - *Place both intra- and extra-articular (go in and out of joint while injecting):*
    – Studies have shown extra-articular injections provide equal relief to intra-articular.
    – Evidence pain is from tendon insertions (enthesopathy) not degenerative joint disease.
  - >50% relief after each injection for duration of local anesthesia is diagnostic of sacroiliac pathology.

PROCEDURE

Step 1: Patient should be placed in prone position as shown in **Figure 1**.

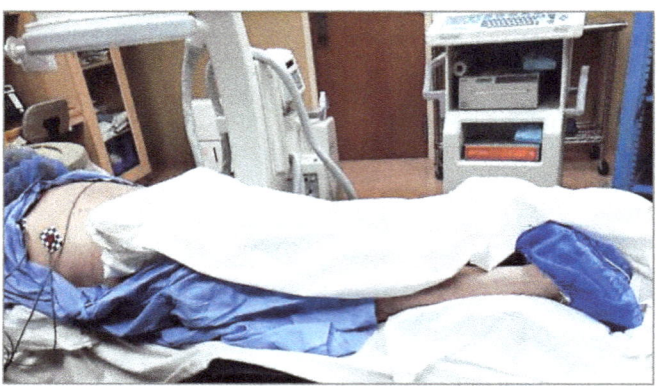

Fig. 1: Patient prone position.

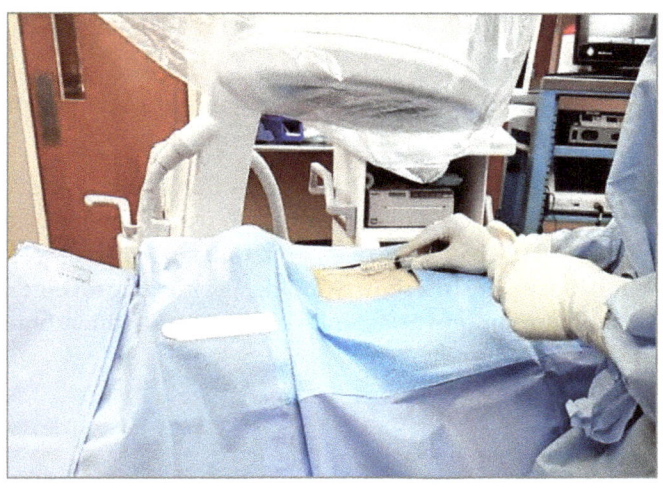

Fig. 2: C-arm position of sacrum.

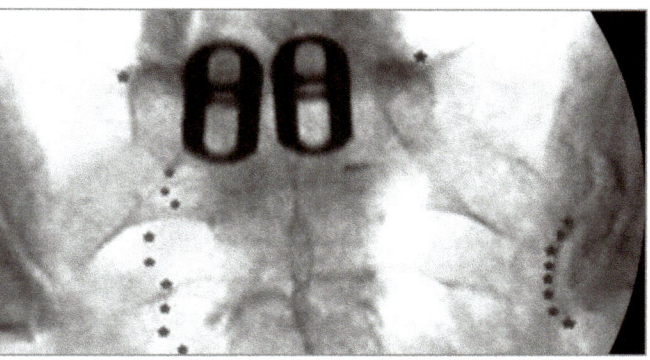

Fig. 3: Initial fluoroscopy image and injection of lidocaine 1% 1 mL. (Stars indicate target sites for radiofrequency ablation. Left side shows the L5 dorsal rami as well targeting the lateral branches of S1-3 in close proximity to foramen; Right side shows L5 dorsal rami and target for "leap-frog" technique).

The C-arm may be kept in an anteroposterior (AP) orientation or with slight cephalad angulation of the image intensifier **(Fig. 2)**.

Step 2: There are two options to ablate the nerves; lateral to the foramen as it exits or medial to the joint **(Fig. 3)**.

Step 3: Insert the radiofrequency needle to target the L5 dorsal rami first. A large bore RF needle (16/18G) should be used. The cannula is inserted and under direct fluoroscopy advanced until the desired position until bone is contacted. The needle tip should be perpendicular and flat against the course of the nerve. Target the L5 dorsal rami by tilting the fluoroscope cephalad 10-15° to allow needle to lay across nerve. Place the needle just lateral to the L5/S1 facet joint at the junction with the sacral ala. On lateral imaging, the needle should be away from the L5/S1 foramen. Once in adequate location, check on AP and lateral imaging, perform sensory/motor testing, and proceed with the first ablation.

Step 4: Insert other 2 RFA cannulas targeting S2 and S3; retarget initial cannula targeting L5 dorsal rami to target S1; prior to ablation confirm needle placement in AP and lateral imaging **(Fig. 5)**.

Three cannula and probes inserted for quicker operative time. Each one targeting the lateral branch of the corresponding sacral nerve. Previous L5 cannula was retracted and placed more caudal to target S1 nerve. 1st new cannula was inserted 1-2 cm inferior from S3 foramen and targeting cephalad to lay across S3 nerve. Lastly, 2nd new cannula was inserted lateral to S1 foramen and steered laterally to lay across the S2 nerve. Bipolar lesioning can be done between the S2 and S3 probes, if desired.

Alternative option is to perform "Leapfrogging" technique. Insert cannula in close proximity to another one; perform monopolar or bipolar lesioning. Continue to manipulate the RF cannula along the medial border of the joint "leapfrogging" the cannulas performing lesions

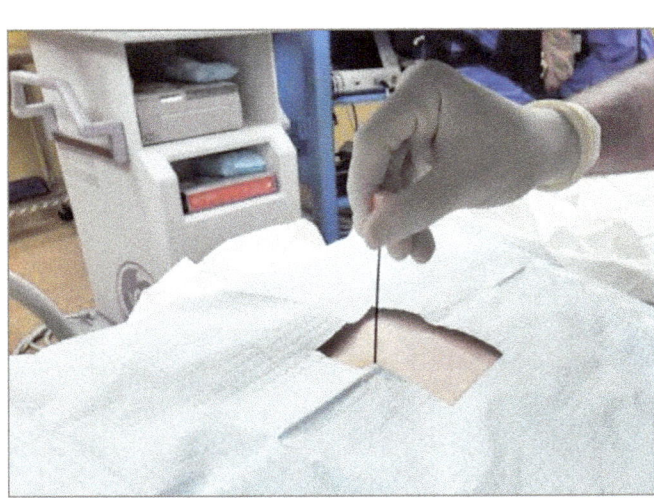

Fig. 4: Insertion of 18G cannula to target the L5 dorsal rami as the first location to target.

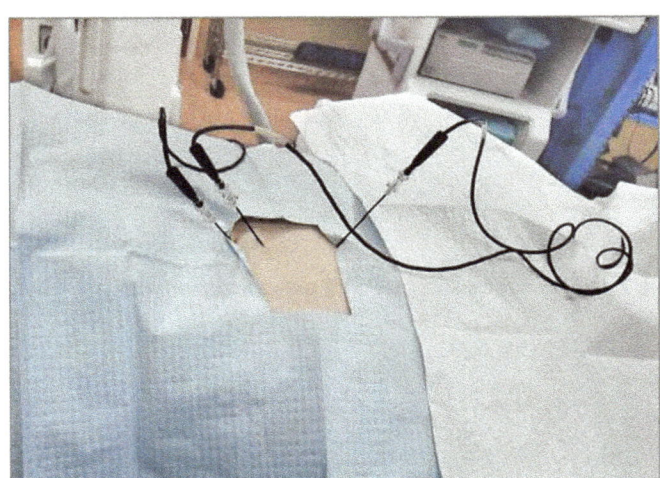

Fig. 5: Three cannulas inserted redirected to target the lateral border of S1/S2/S3. Probes are inserted and lesioning is under process.

along the joint line as shown in **Figure 6**. It is called leapfrogging as each needle is withdrawn and placed cephalad to the previous needle "jumping" over the previous needle entry.

Step 5: Sensory stimulation (less than 0.6 volts at 50 hertz) and motor testing (negative up to 2 volts at 2 hertz) should take place prior to administering 0.5 mL lidocaine 2% **(Fig. 7)**.

Step 6: Perform thermal lesions. Can be performed as monopolar and/or a combination of bipolar burns. Typical settings are: 80°C for 90 seconds. Note resistance should be 200-400 ohms.

Step 7: Shift patient to recovery for monitoring of vital signs and neurological examination prior to discharge.

Patient may have procedural pain for 2-3 days postoperative. Advise to place ice. Follow up in 2-3 weeks, majority of patients will see benefit at that point. Can take up to 6 weeks for full nerve destruction. Should provide improvement in pain by minimum 50% for 6-12 months at which point procedure can be repeated.

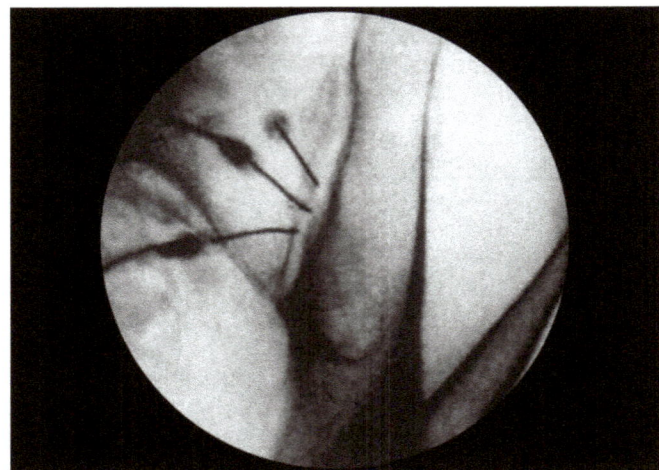

Fig. 6: Multiple radiofrequency cannula performing a "leapfrog" technique over medial border of SI joint.

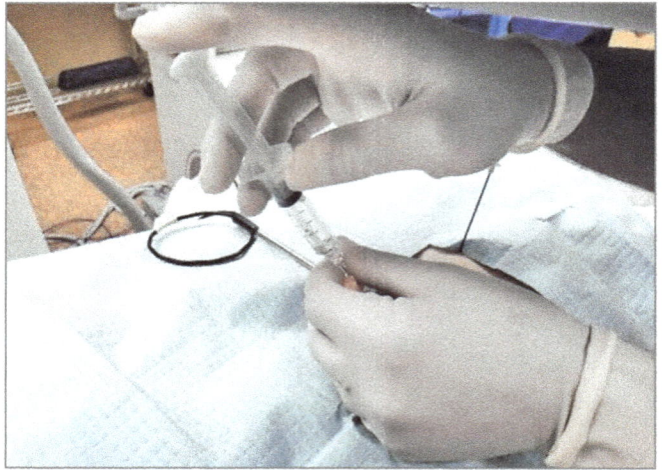

Fig. 7: Injecting local anesthesia for patient comfort and larger burn area prior to lesion.

SACROILIAC JOINT RADIOFREQUENCY DENERVATION WITH SIMPLICITY 3 PROBE

ADDITIONAL INFORMATION (BY SANJEEVA GUPTA AND GANESAN BARANIDHARAN)

Case 1

Step 1: Patient in prone position with pillows under the pelvis and lower lumbar area to slant the pelvis slightly downwards towards the lumber spine.

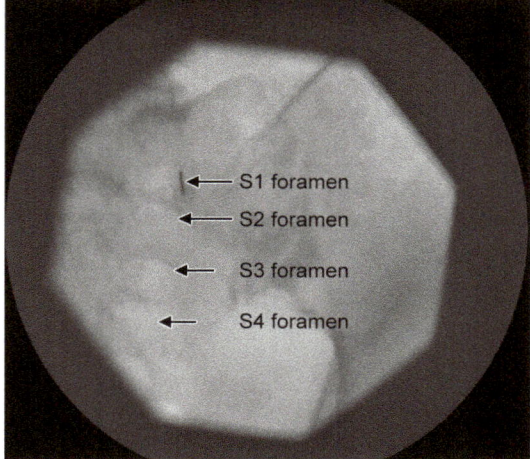

Fig. 8: AP view of the right hemipelvis showing the right sacroiliac joint (SIJ) and the S1 to S4 sacral foramen. Tip of the spinal needle is lateral to right S1 foramen to inject local anesthetic.

Step 2: **(Fig. 9)**

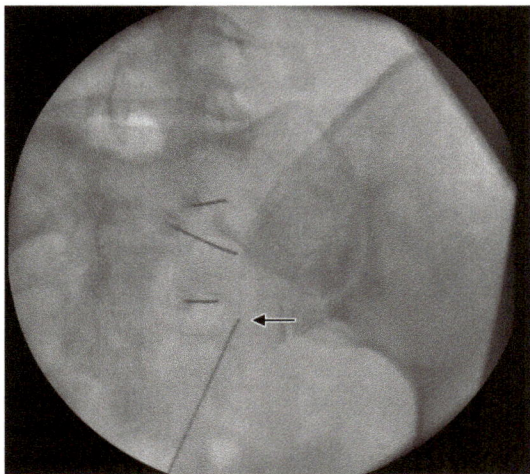

Fig. 9: *AP view:* 22G spinal needles placed lateral to S1 to S3 foramens to inject local anaesthetic to block the S1 to S3 lateral branches supplying the right SIJ. Another spinal needle is advanced to contact the lower end of the posterior sacral plate at or just below the S4 foramen (arrow) and lateral view is then obtained to confirm the depth of this needle.

Step 3: **(Fig. 10)**

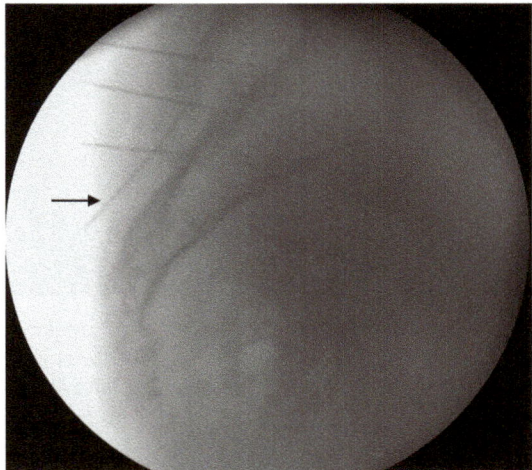

Fig. 10: Lateral view of the sacrum. Observe that the three spinal needle at S1 to S3 foramen levels are contacting the posterior sacral plate and the 4th needle (arrow) is seen sliding posterior to the sacrum and not in the pelvic cavity. The size of the sacrum and its curvature is observed to plan the procedure and decide the skin entry point for inserting the simplicity 3 probe. Local anesthesia is injected along the curvature of the sacrum to facilitate the procedure under local anaesthesia and if necessary mild sedation under appropriate monitoring.

Step 4: (**Fig. 11**)

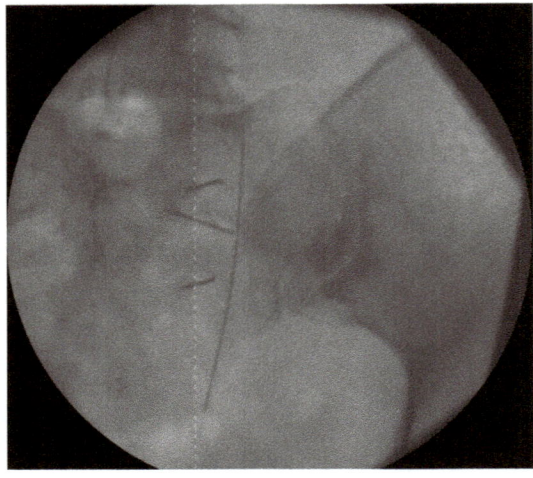

Fig. 11: AP showing the spinal needles in position to anesthetize the area where the simplicity 3 probe is planned to be navigated.

Step 5: (**Fig. 12**)

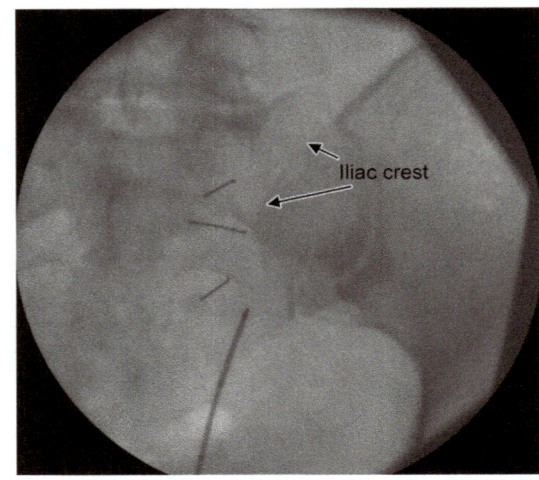

Fig. 12: Simplicity 3 probe is seen contacting the posterior sacral plate at around the S4 foramen level and lateral to the sacral foramens but medial to the iliac crest. The skin entry point for the simplicity 3 probe is at around the upper end of the ipsilateral hip joint area or slightly above.

Step 6: (**Fig. 13**)

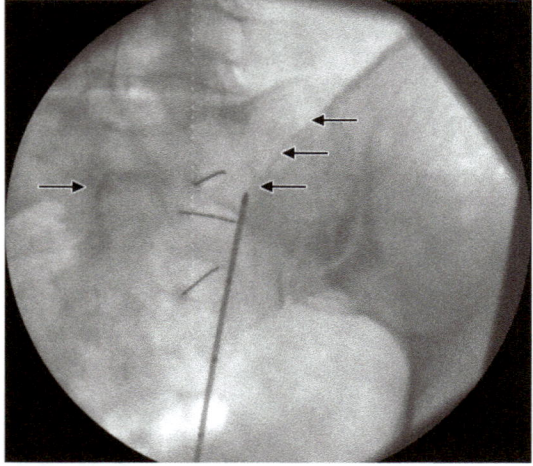

Fig. 13: Simplicity 3 probe being advanced gradually making contact with the posterior sacral plate as it is advanced and keeping it lateral to the sacral foramen but medial to the iliac crest (arrows).

Step 7: (**Fig. 14**)

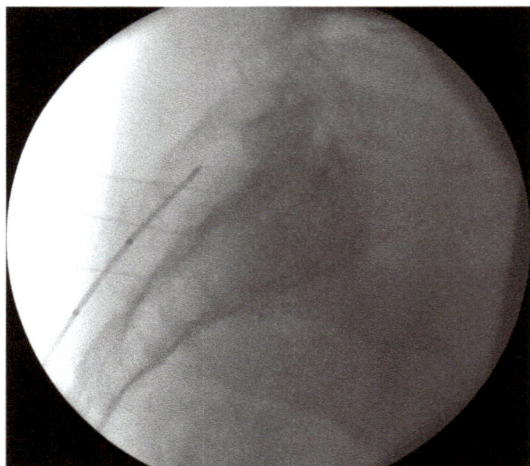

Fig. 14: Frequent lateral view is obtained to judge the trajectory of the Simplicity 3 probe.

Step 8: (**Fig. 15**)

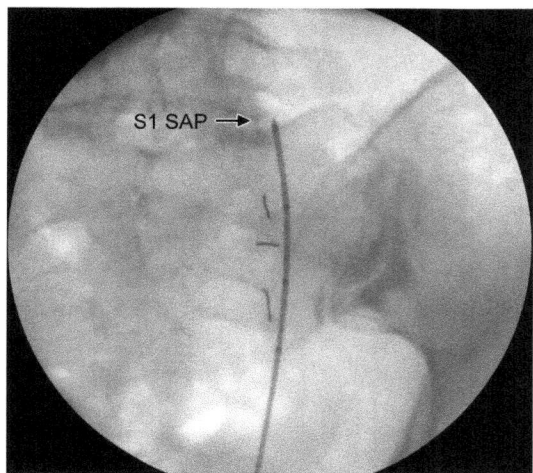

Fig. 15: AP view showing that the tip of the simplicity 3 probe has reached the level of the junction of the superior articular process (SAP) of S1 and the ala of the sacrum (L5 dorsal rami and lateral branches).

Step 9: (**Fig. 16**)

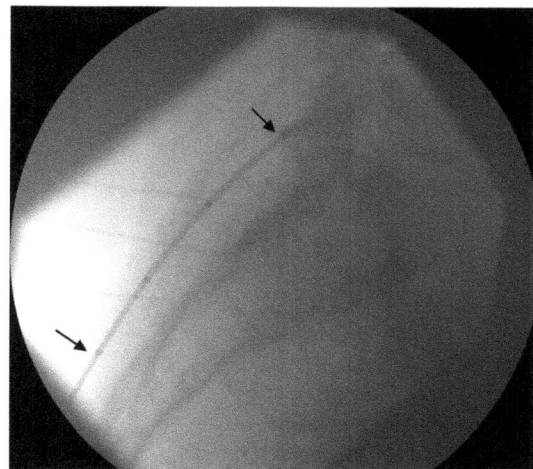

Fig. 16: Lateral view with the simplicity 3 probe in position. The probe appears a little away from the posterior sacral plate but the size of the lesion created by the probe should cover the areas of the sacral lateral branches supplying the SIJ. Varying positions of the probe in relation the posterior sacral plate is shown later on in this chapter. The area between the two arrows will be lesioned by the probe.

Step 10: (**Fig. 17**)

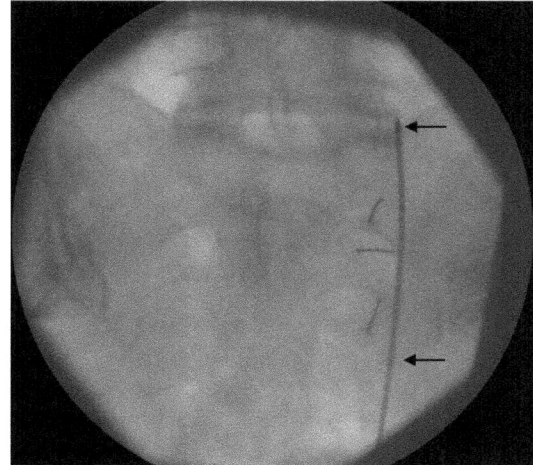

Fig. 17: Final AP view. Radiofrequency lesioning is performed using the simplicity 3 protocol for 5 to 7.5 minutes at 80°C under continues monitoring. Please remove the spinal needle before the RF lesioning is started. If the needles are in place and are contacting the simplicity 3 probe, then this can lead to subcutaneous tissue and skin burn. The area between the two arrows will be lesioned by the probe.

Step 11: (**Fig. 18**)

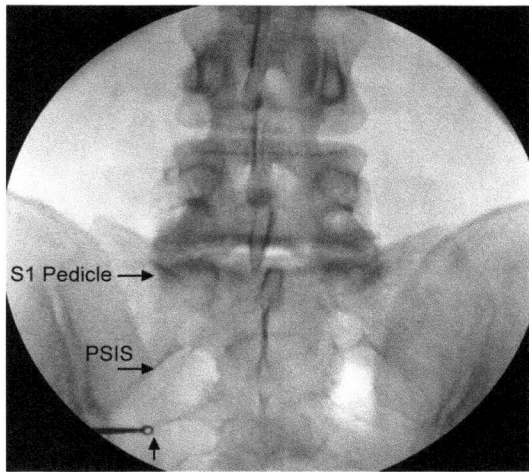

Fig. 18: *L5 Dorsal Rami (DR) RF:* In some cases when the operator is unable to navigate the simplicity 3 probe to the L5 DR area or if the tip of the probe is further away from the bone at the level of L5 DR area, then a L5 DR RF is also conducted. To place the needle tip parallel to the L5 DR, it is advisable to puncture the skin (pointer) between the S2 and S3 foramen and then navigate the RF cannula tip towards the L5 DR. Watch for posterior superior iliac spine (PSIS) and the S1 pedicle as they can come in the way when navigating the RF cannula. (Please also see the Chapter 21 on Lumbar Radiofrequency denervation regarding alternate techniques of performing L5 dorsal rami RF)

Step 12: (**Fig. 19**)

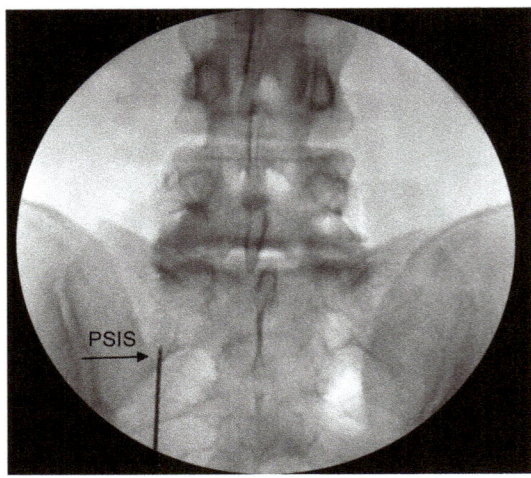

Fig. 19: *L5 Dorsal Rami RF (DR RF):* The RF cannula is being navigated slowly towards the L5 DR and the tip is medial to the posterior superior iliac spine (PSIS) in this image.

Step 13: (**Fig. 20**)

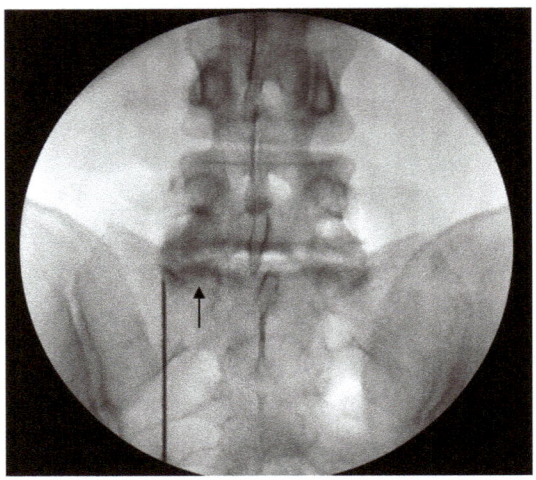

Fig. 20: *L5 Dorsal Rami RF (DR RF):* When the tip of the RF cannula is at the S1 pedicle area the curve of the RF cannula tip is turned laterally to navigate past the S1 pedicle. Once past the S1 pedicle (arrow), the tip is turned medially and navigated further.

Step 14: (**Fig. 21**)

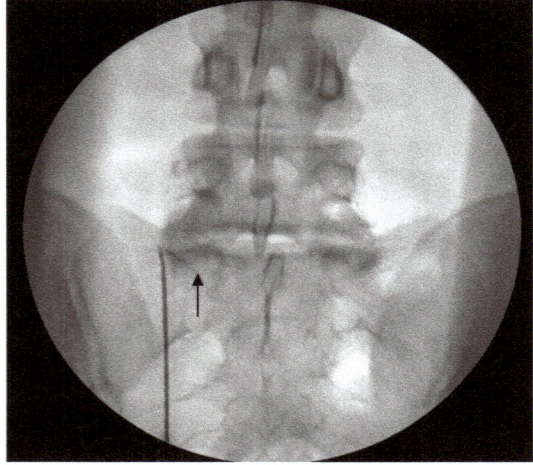

Fig. 21: *L5 Dorsal Rami RF (DR RF):* The curved tip of the RF cannula is turned laterally to get past the S1 pedicle (arrow).

Step 15: (**Fig. 22**)

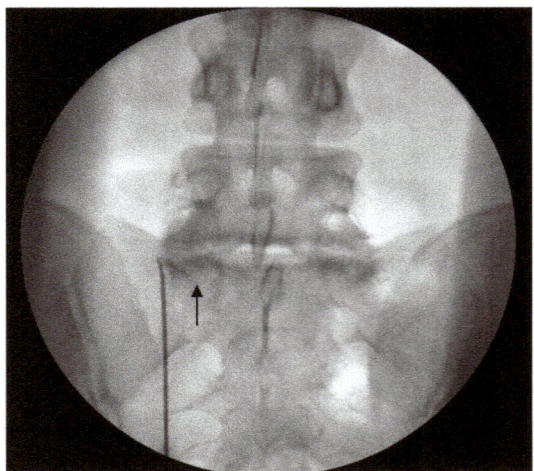

Fig. 22: *L5 Dorsal Rami RF (DR RF):* Once the RF cannula tip is past the S1 pedicle the curved tip is turned medially to navigate further towards the junction of the superior articular process (SAP) of S1 and the ala of the sacrum.

Step 16: **(Fig. 23)**

Step 17: **(Fig. 24)**

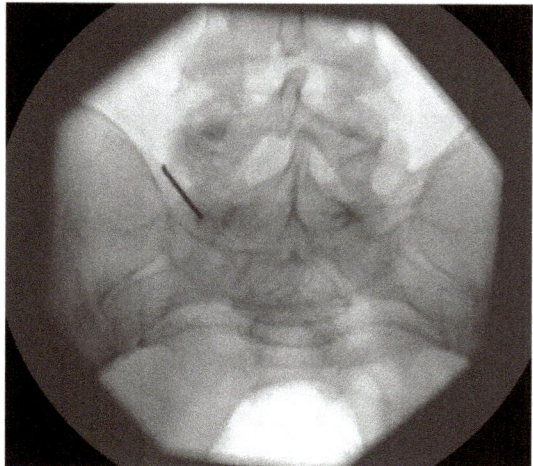

Fig. 23: *L5 Dorsal Rami RF (DRRF):* Posterolateral view.

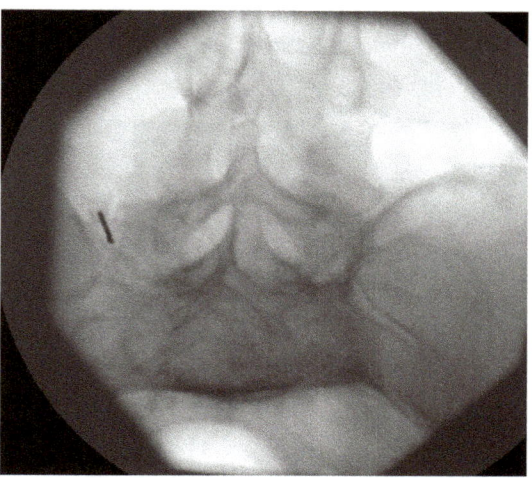

Fig. 24: *L5 Dorsal Rami RF (DRRF):* Inferior oblique tunnel view. Tilt the C-arm caudally until the gun-barrel view of the RF cannula is obtained. From the gun-barrel view, tilt the C-arm caudally by about 5° to 10° to obtain the inferior tunnel view. The RF cannula is in the groove formed by the SAP of S1 and the ala of the sacrum and parallel to the L5 DR. Confirm bone contact in the inferior tunnel view. Some clinicians will obtain a lateral view also to confirm that the needle tip is not in the L5/S1 intervertebral foramen.

Step 18: **(Fig. 25)**

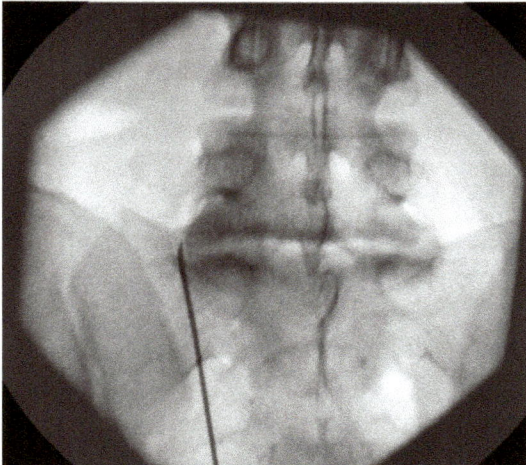

Fig. 25: *L5 Dorsal Rami RF (DR RF):* Final confirmation in the superior view that the RF cannula tip does not project beyond the anterior border. This image is obtained by tilting the C-arm cranially by about 5° to 10°. RF lesion is performed at 80°C for 90 seconds with the curved tip turned medially and another RF lesion performed with the curved tip turned laterally.

Case 2

Patients have different sacral anatomy and the final position of the simplicity 3 probe may vary between patients. Some images of 2 more cases will demonstrate this.

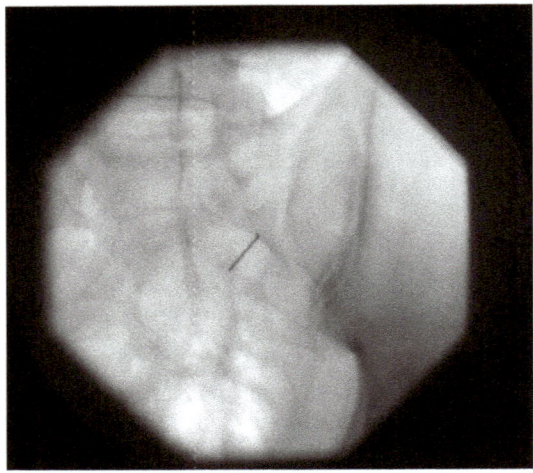

Fig. 26: AP view of the right hemipelvis. Needle tip lateral to S2 foramen for injecting local anesthetic.

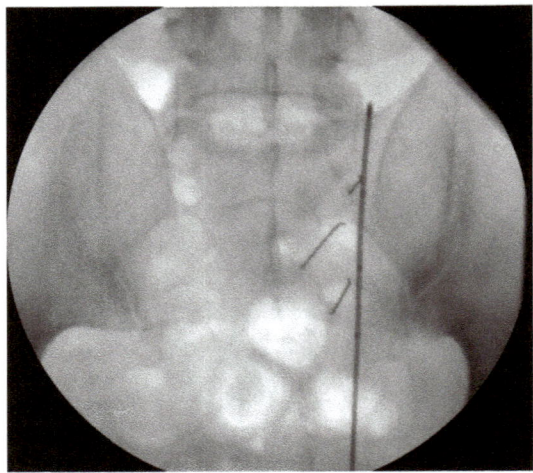

Fig. 27: AP view. The simplicity 3 probe is in place. The three spinal needle that were used to inject local anesthetic can also be seen.

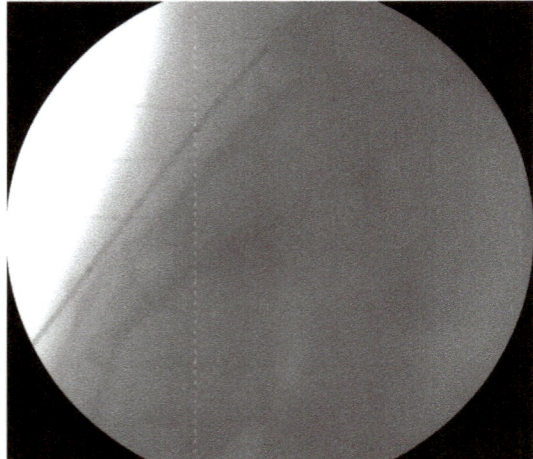

Fig. 28: Lateral view shows the simplicity 3 probe in place. Observe that the sacral anatomy/curvature is different in this case compared to Case 1 and the simplicity 3 probe is closer to the posterior sacral plate compared to in Case 1. A lateral view before inserting the simplicity 3 probe can help decide the skin entry point of the probe taking into consideration the curvature/anatomy of the sacrum.

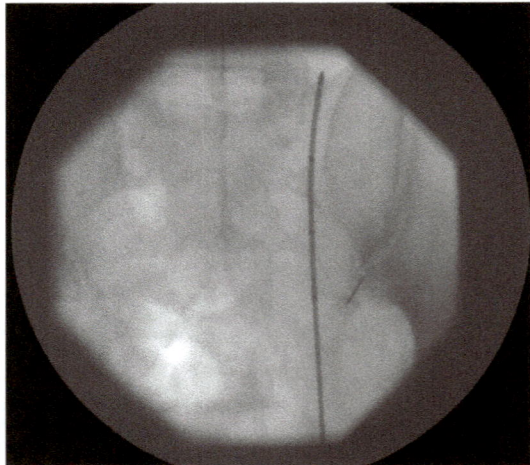

Fig. 29: Final AP view with the simplicity 3 probe in place. RF lesioning is performed for 5 to 7.5 minutes at 80°C using the simplicity 3 protocol while constantly monitoring the patient for any adverse effects. Please remove the spinal needles used to inject local anesthesia before the RF lesioning is started. If the needles are in place and are contacting the simplicity 3 probe, then this can lead to subcutaneous tissue and skin burn.

Case 3

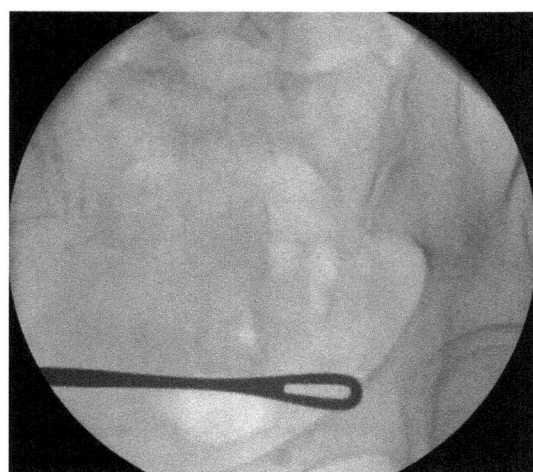

Fig. 30: Approximate skin puncture point for SIJ RFD with simplicity 3 probe. Medial to the ipsilateral hip joint image or higher depending on the weight of the patient, size and curvature of the sacrum. The probe may contact the posterior sacral plate between the S3 and S4 foramen. This may vary depending on patients' weight, size and curvature of the sacrum (Image from Further Reading No. 2).

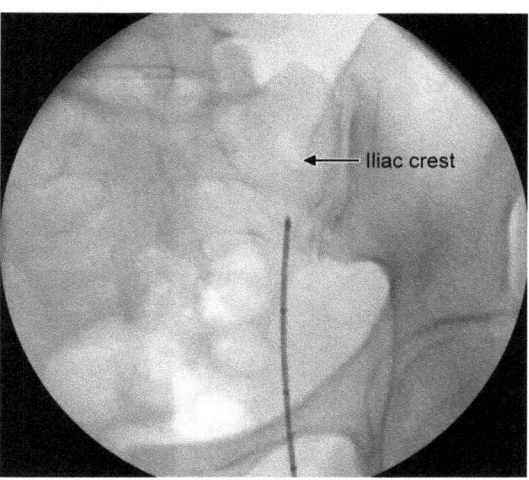

Fig. 31: Simplicity 3 probe being advanced in AP view lateral to sacral foramen and medial the sacroiliac joint and right iliac crest. Note the image of the iliac crest which can overhang on the SIJ. The tip of the probe is just medial to the iliac crest (arrow) (Image from Further Reading No. 2).

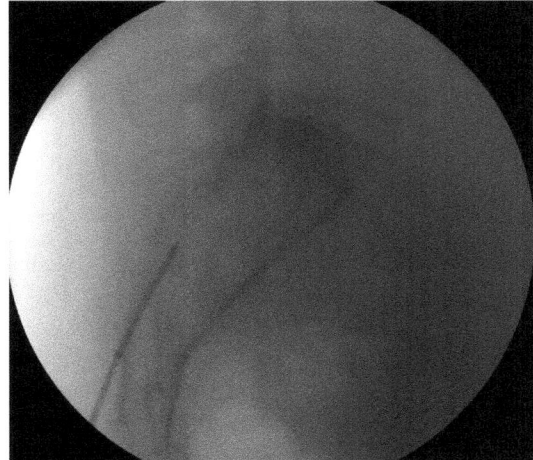

Fig. 32: Lateral view showing the simplicity probe. (Further Reading No. 2). Frequent checking in lateral view is important to confirm the depth of the probe. However, the probe is normally advanced in AP view (*See* Chapter 1, Figure 2 for 3D principles during fluoroscopic assisted procedures – Direction, Depth, Direction).

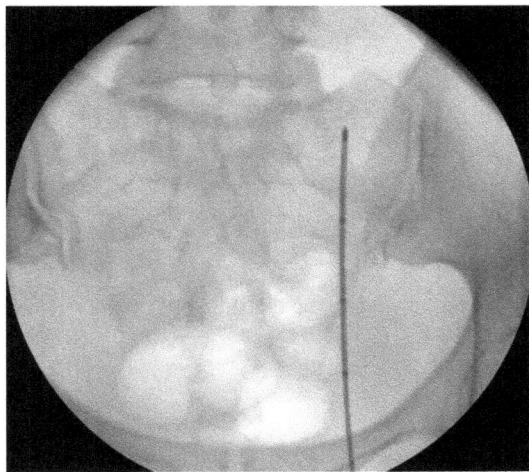

Fig. 33: The simplicity probe has been advanced further in AP view (Image from Further Reading No. 2).

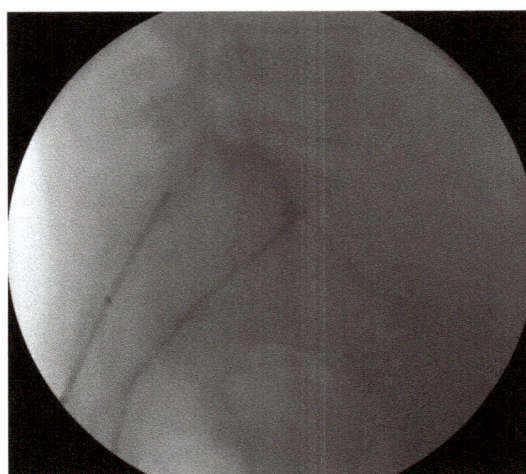

Fig. 34: Lateral view showing the simplicity 3 probe (Image from Further Reading No. 2).

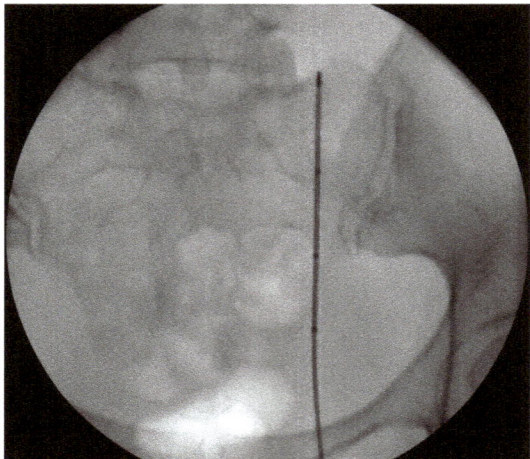

Fig. 35: AP view showing the final position of simplicity probe (Image from Further Reading No. 2).

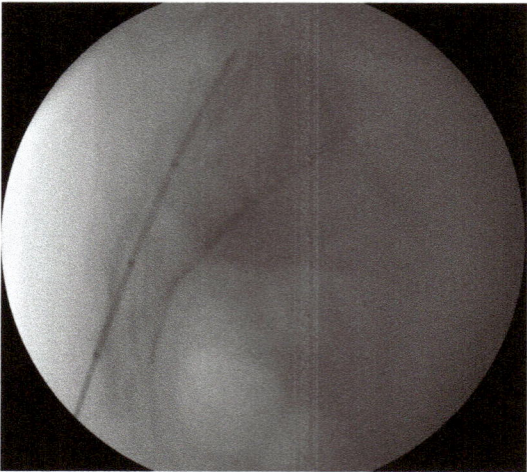

Fig. 36: Lateral view showing the final positing of the simplicity 3 probe. (Image from Further Reading No. 2).

Case 4

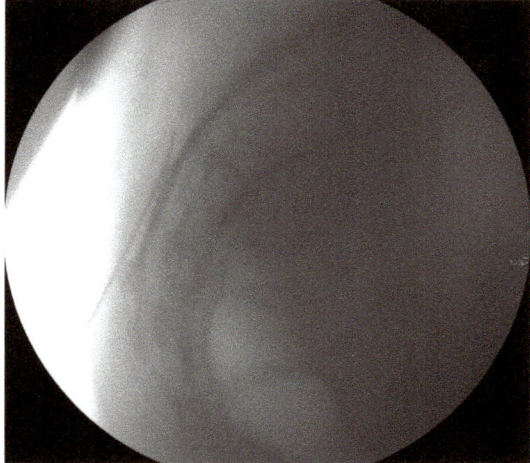

Fig. 37: A 22G spinal needle has been inserted in AP view and a lateral view obtained to gauge the depth of the needle (not in pelvic cavity) and also the curvature/anatomy of the sacrum.

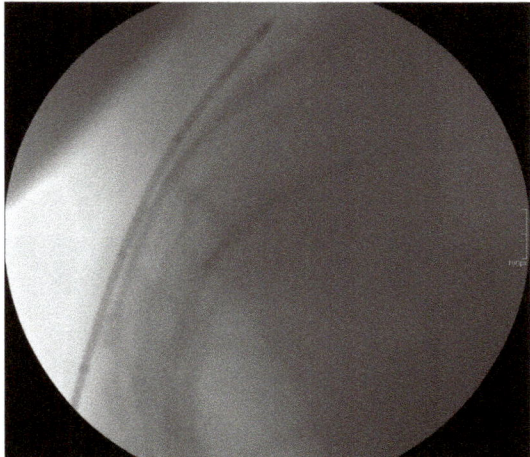

Fig. 38: Lateral view of the final position of the simplicity 3 probe.

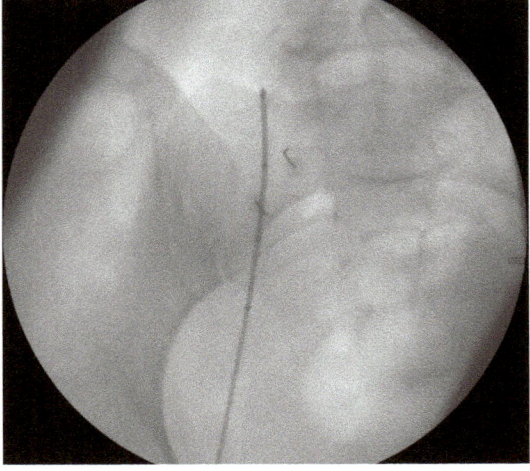

Fig. 39: Final AP view of the simplicity 3 probe. Remove the spinal needles used to inject local anesthetic before RF lesioning is commenced.

Case 5

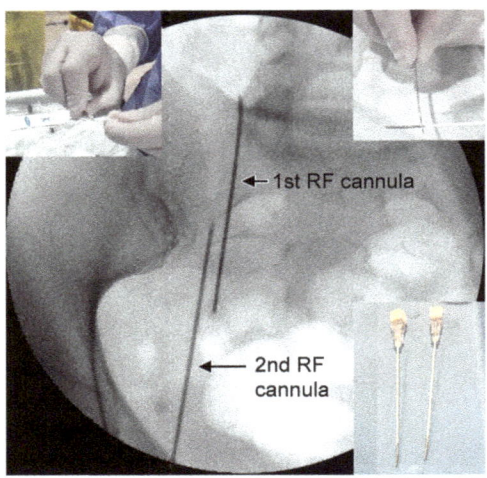

Fig. 40: 18G RF cannula technique (used by Dr GB). A strip lesion is performed from the L5 dorsal rami area to the lower end of the S3 foramen). About one inch of the distal tip of the 18G or 16G RF cannula is shaved off the insulation (as shown in the 3 images in the inset). AP view of the pelvis is obtained and the C-arm is tilted cephalic so that the sacral foramens are identifiable. The first RF cannula is inserted from around the S3 foramen level and directed to the L5 DR area as shown in the image and as described in Case 1 **Figure 18 to Figure 25**. In this case two RF cannulas are used as this shortens the operating time. The distal one inch of the second RF cannula is lateral to the S3 foramen area. Two unipolar RF lesions are performed at 80°C for 90 seconds.

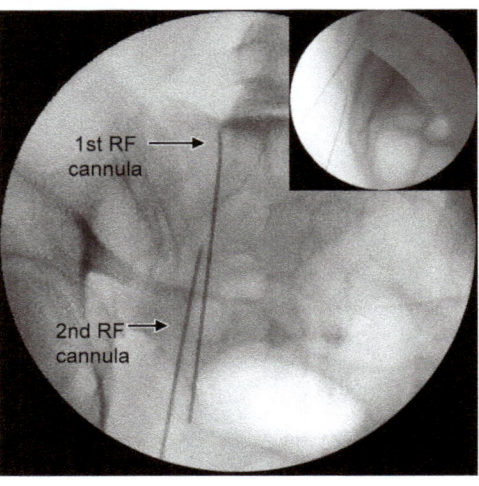

Fig. 41: After performing lesions at L5 DR area and lateral to the S3 foramen the 1st RF cannula is pulled back by a few mm and the second RF cannula is reinserted so that the distal one inch is lateral to the S2 foramen area. Unipolar RF lesions are performed at 80°C for 90 seconds. The image in the inset shows the depth of the RF cannula in the lateral view. Note the different trajectory and depth of both the RF cannula. They are not touching each other.

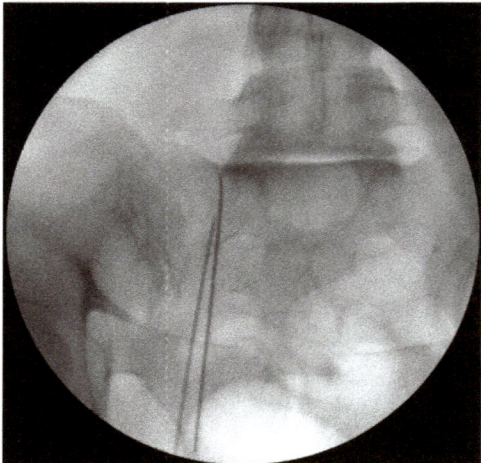

Fig. 42: The second RF cannula has been advanced further so that the distal one inch is lateral to the S1 foramen. RF lesions are performed at 80°C for 90 seconds.

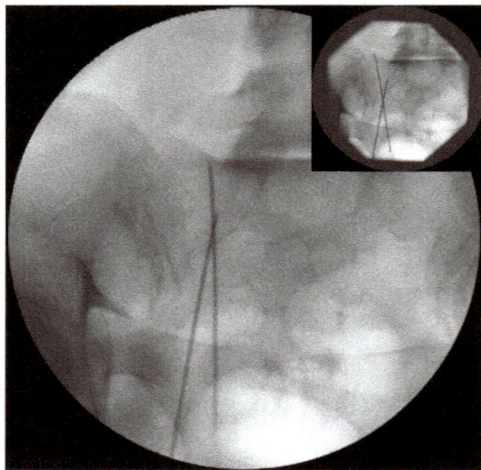

Fig. 43: After performing a lesion at L5 DR area and slightly below the distal tip of the 1st RF cannula is gradually navigated laterally as shown in this figure (and the inset) and RF lesions are performed at 80°C for 90 seconds.

FURTHER READING

1. Bayerl SH, Finger T, Heidan P, et al. Radiofrequency denervation for treatment of sacroiliac joint pain-comparison of two different ablation techniques. Neurosurg Rev. 2020;43(1):101-7.
2. Gupta S. Sacroiliac joint radiofrequency denervation. In: Interventional Pain Management: A Practical Approach. Baheti DK, Bakshi S, Gupta S, Gehdoo RSP (Eds). New Delhi: Jaypee Brothers Medical Publishers, New Delhi 2016; p. 265-70.
3. Gupta S. Technical Report: Double needle technique: an alternative method for performing difficult sacroiliac joint injections. Pain Physician. 2011;14:281-4.
4. Hansen H, Manchikanti L, Simopoulous T, Christo PJ, Gupta S, et al. A systematic evaluation of the therapeutic effectiveness of sacroiliac joint interventions. Pain Physician. 2012:15; E247-78.
5. Ikeda R. Innervation of the sacroiliac joint: macroscopic and histologic studies. J Nippon Med School. 1991;58:587-96.
6. Katz V. The sacroiliac joint: a potential cause of pain after lumbar fusion to the sacrum. J Spinal Disord Tech. 2003:16; 96-9.
7. Patel N. Twelve-month follow-up of a randomized trial assessng cooled radiofrequency denervtion as a treatment for sacroiliac region pain. Pain Pract. 2016;16(2):154-67.
8. Sacroiliac Joint Block. In: Practice guidelines for spinal diagnosis and treatment procedures. Bogduk N (Ed). International Spin Intervention Society. 2004. pp. 66-85.
9. Schwarzer AC, Aprill CN, Bogduk N. The sacroiliac joint in chronic low back pain. Spine. 1995;20:31-7.

CHAPTER 26

Sacroiliac Joint Fusion: A Minimally Invasive Posterior Approach

Samir Ranjit Jani

SACROILIAC JOINT FUSION

Basic Information

Indications
- Severe SIJ pain that impacts quality of life or significantly limits activities of daily living (ADLs)
- SIJ pain confirmed with at least three physical examination maneuvers that stress the SIJ and reproduce the patient's typical pain:
  - FABER test
  - Thigh thrust test
  - Distraction test
  - Compression test
  - Gaenslen test
- Confirmation of the SIJ as a pain generator with ≥50% acute decrease in pain upon fluoroscopically guided diagnostic intra-articular SIJ block with local anesthetic.
- Continued significant SIJ pain and/or limited ADLs after at least 6 months of nonsurgical treatment such as medication management, physical therapy, and/or injection therapy.
- X-ray and CT/MRI of the pelvis and sacrum should be done prior to proceeding with SIJ fusion to rule out alternative diagnoses that could cause a patient's pain or disability.

Contraindications
- Less than 6 months of SIJ pain and/or functional impairment
- Failure to pursue conservative treatment of the SIJ
- Pain not confirmed with a diagnostic SIJ block
- Presence of other pathology that would substantially prevent the patient from benefitting from SIJ fusion

Types of sacroiliac joint fusions:
- Posterior approach
- Lateral transarticular approach

Step 1: Position the patient prone on the operating table with contoured gel pad underneath the hips **(Fig. 1)**.

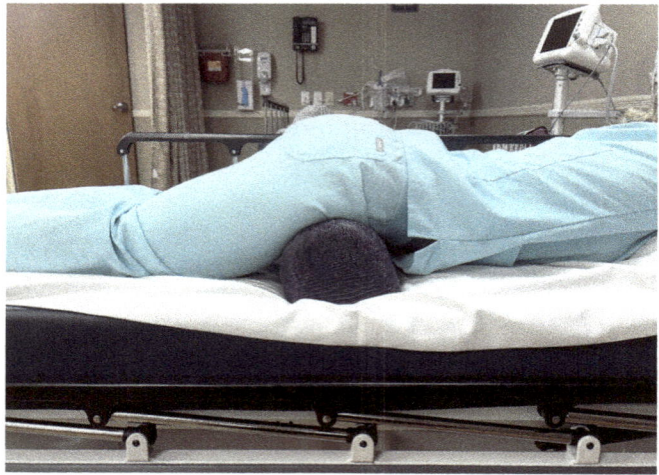

Fig. 1: *Step 1:* Prone position.

Step 2: In anteroposterior (AP) view, use a guide pin to enter inferior and medial to the posterior superior iliac spine (PSIS) and lateral to the S2 and S3 foramina. The ideal entry point is inferior to S2, superior to S3, medial to the PSIS, and lateral to the foramen **(Fig. 2)**.

Now, Step 3 will have **Figure 3**, i.e., point of entry for pin. We need a fluoroscopy image with marker here.

Step 3: Find the contralateral oblique angle that places the dorsal aspect of the joint superimposed over the anterior aspect of the joint, often referred to as the "river" view. The ideal position for the guidepin is where these two lines cross **(Fig. 4)**.

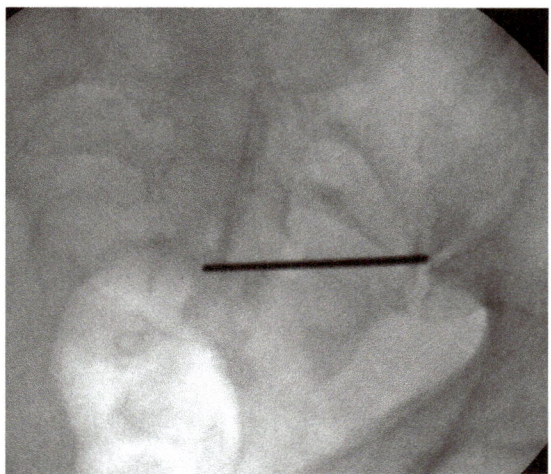

Fig. 2: Initial entry point to perform a right sacroiliac fusion in an AP view. Guide pin enters lower 1/3 of joint. Start lateral to where S2 and S3 meet; aim for the overlap of the anterior and posterior joint lines.

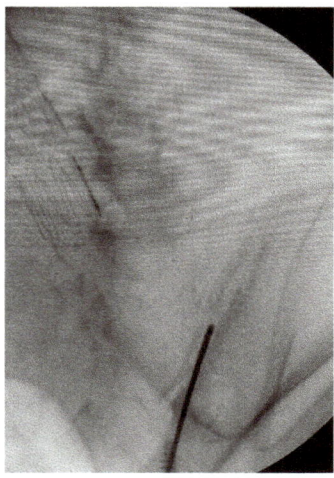

Fig. 3: Guide pin to lateral wall of sacrum.

Step 4: Once the joint has been entered, switch to a lateral view and advance the guide pin until the tip is stopped by the lateral wall of the sacrum making sure not to extend past the anterior cortical wall of the sacrum **(Fig. 4)**.

Step 5: After the guide pin is advanced to appropriate depth, make a 2–3-cm incision along the superior and inferior aspects of the pin.

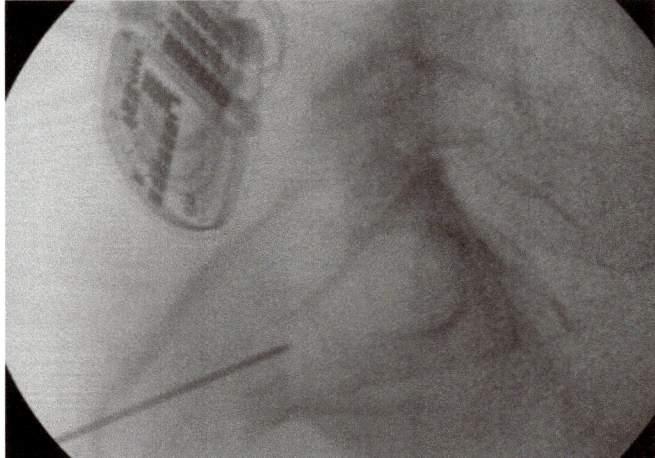

Fig. 4: Marker.

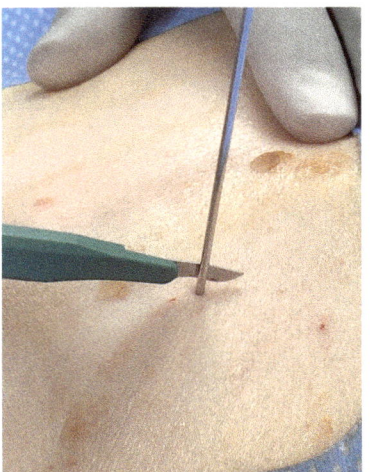

Fig. 5: Skin incision at inferior aspect of pin.

Step 6: Return to AP view and advance the joint finder over the guide pin and confirm that the angle of the joint finder matches the angle of the posterior aspect of the joint in anteroposterior and contralateral oblique views **(Fig. 6)**.

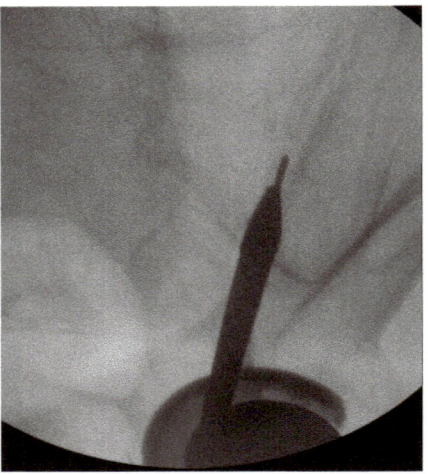

Fig. 6: Pin in joint—AP view.

Step 7: Go back to lateral view and advance the joint finder until it enters the joint.

Step 8: Return to anteroposterior view and slide the cannula over the joint finder and guide pin **(Fig. 8)**.

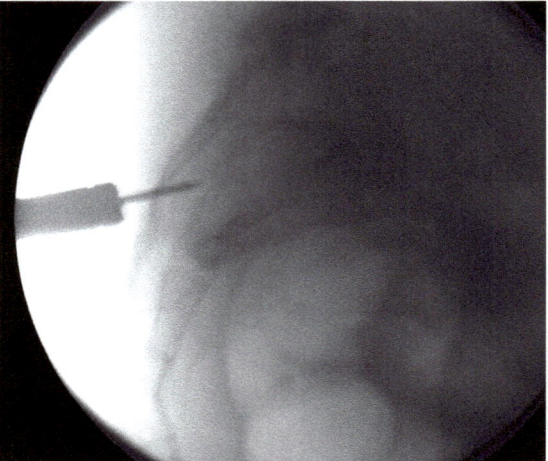

Fig. 7: Pin in lateral view.

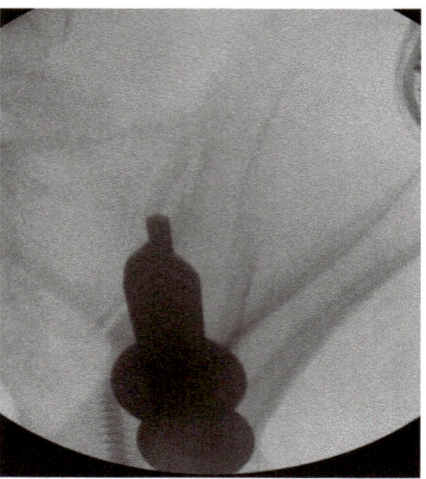

Fig. 8: Cannula over the joint finder and guide pin—AP view.

Step 9: Return to lateral view to advance the cannula until both tangs of the cannula are seated against the ilium and sacrum **(Fig. 9)**.

Step 10: Remove the joint finder and pin, leaving the cannula in the joint. In lateral view, advance the power drill, using live fluoroscopy, through the ilium into the sacrum until the drill is about 15 mm past the ventral tangs of the cannula **(Fig. 10)**.

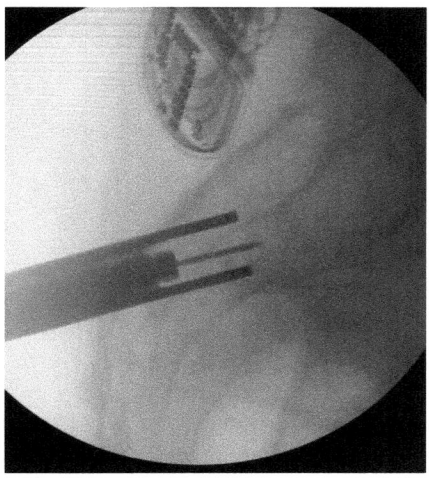

Fig. 9: Cannula until both tangs of the cannula are seated against the ilium and sacrum.

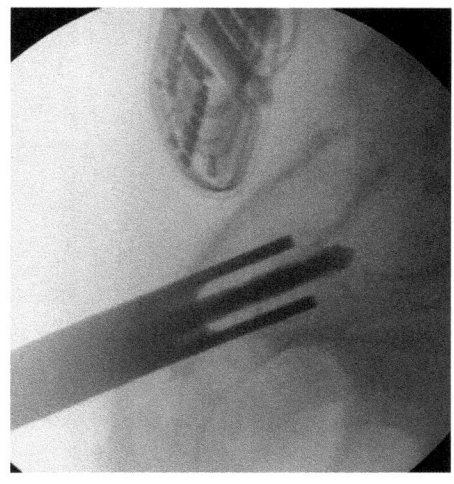

Fig. 10: Power drill through the ilium into the sacrum—lateral view.

Step 11: Remove the drill and then again in lateral view advance the decorticator about 15 mm past the ventral tangs of the cannula **(Fig. 11)**.

Step 12: Remove the decorticator and in lateral view, advance the implant with an inserter about 15 mm past the ventral tangs of the cannula **(Fig. 12)**.

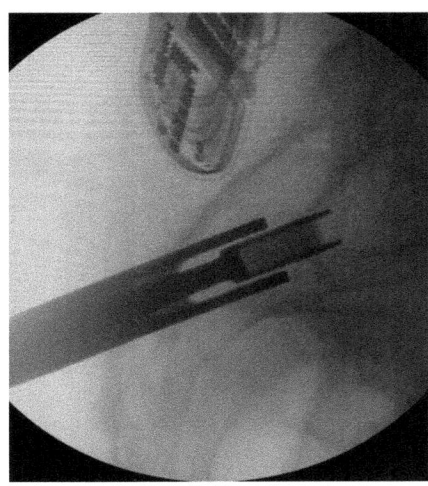

Fig. 11: *Step 11:* Decorticator in lateral view.

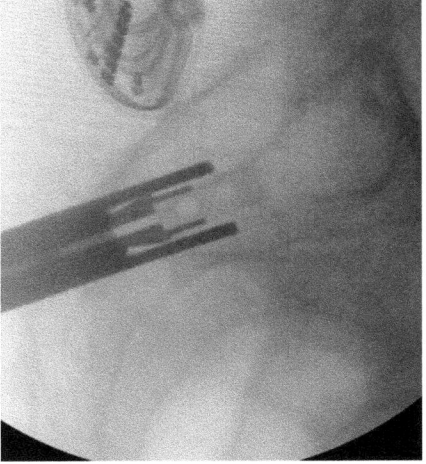

Fig. 12: Decorticator removed and implanted with inserter—lateral view.

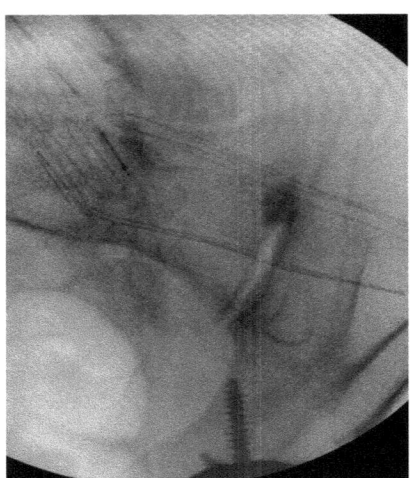

Fig. 13: In lateral view, the implant should sit between the ventral and dorsal cortical lines.

Step 13: Deploy the implant and remove the inserter **(Fig. 13)**. In lateral view, the implant should sit between the ventral and dorsal cortical lines and in AP view, the implant should be positioned medial to the anterior joint line and lateral to the posterior joint line.

Step 14: Following irrigation, suture the incision with the preferred technique of deep dermal and subcutaneous skin closure.

FURTHER READING

1. Lorio M. ISASS Policy 2016 Update: Minimally invasive sacroiliac joint fusion. Int J Spine Surgery. 2016;10:26.

27. Piriformis Tendon and Muscle Injection

Yashwant Laxman Nankar, Dwarkadas K Baheti

BASIC INFORMATION

Indications
- Patient with lower extremity radicular pain
- Patient refractory to conservative regimen

Contraindications
- Unwilling patient
- Local infection
- Caoagulopathies

Investigations
- Hemogram
- *X-ray:* Hip, sacroiliac joint (SI) joint, lumbosacral (LS) spine
- Magnetic resonance imaging (MRI) of LS spine
- Computed tomography
- Ultrasonography (USG) of pelvis
- Electromyograph

Equipment
- C-arm compatible surgical table
- C-arm with radiation safety devices
- Stimuplex set
- Nerve stimulator with needle 22-gauge 4 inch or longer
- Marker pen, metal marker
- 26-gauge, 1½ inch and 18-gauge, 1½ inch needle
- 2-, 5-, and 10-mL syringes

Medications
- Injection Iohexol (Omnipaque)
- Injection Normal Saline (0.9%)
- Injection Lidocaine (2%)
- Injection Bupivacaine or Ropivacaine (0.5%), preservative free
- Injection Aurocort (preservative-free Triamcinolone Acetonide), Methylprednisolone
- Injection Botulinum Toxin

Complications
Inadvertent direct injection of the Sciatic nerve, which usually results in a nondisabling and temporary sciatic Mononeuropathy

PROCEDURE DETAILS

Step 1: It is vital to understand the anatomy of piriformis muscle and tendon as seen in **Figure 1**.

Step 2: Put patient in prone position **(Fig. 2)** and rotate fluoroscope to identify the corresponding and acetabular region.

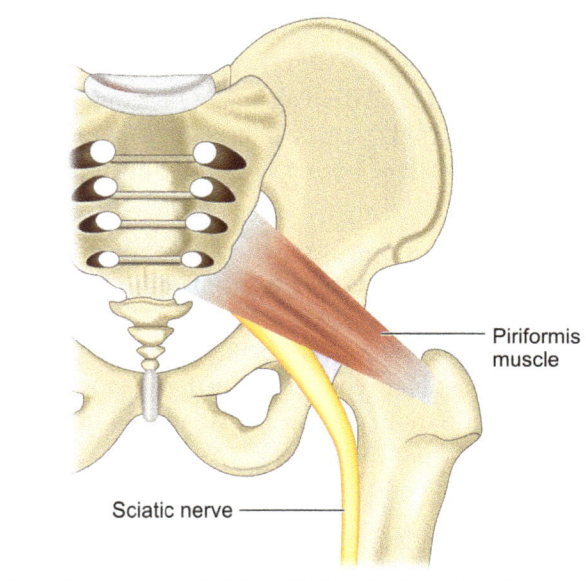

Fig. 1: Anatomy of piriformis muscle in relation to sciatic nerve.

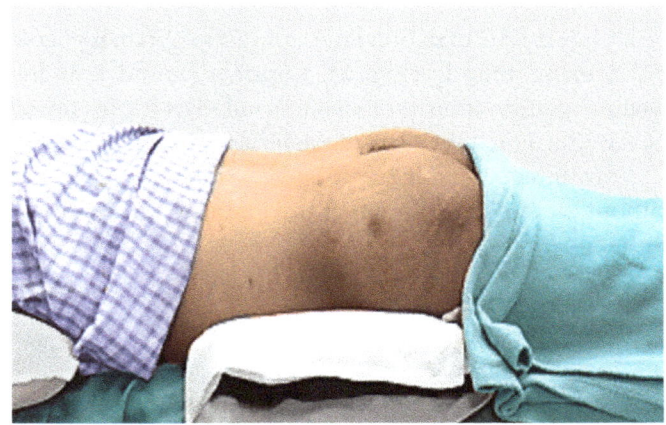

Fig. 2: Prone position.

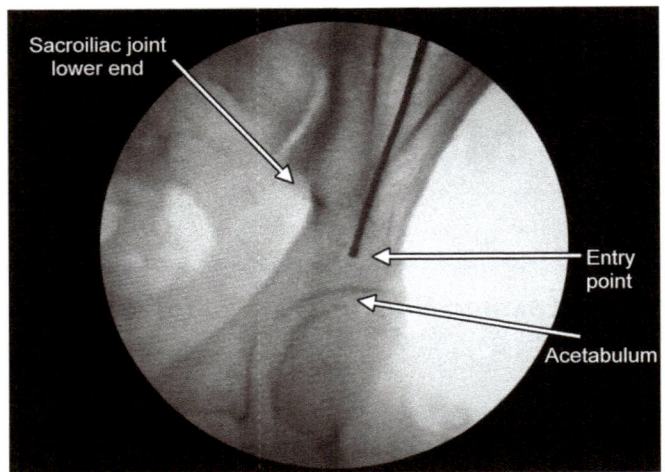

Fig. 3: Marker on the line joining most at needle entry point.

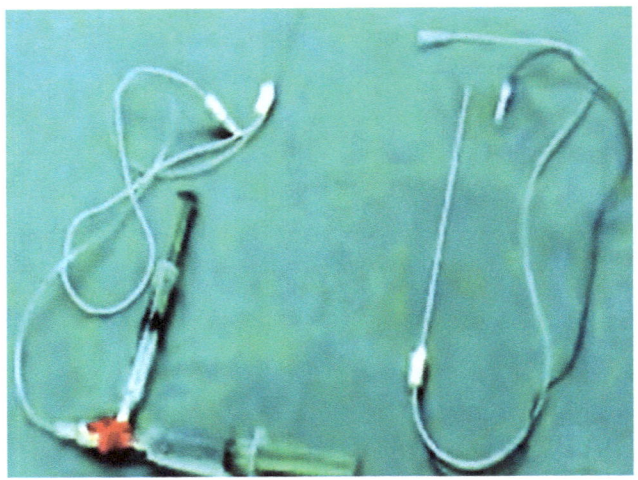

Fig. 4: Stimuplex needle.

Step 3: Now place the metal marker on the line joining most inferior aspect of the SI joint and the most superior-lateral aspect of the acetabulum. On this line, about one-third of the way medial from the acetabular landmark is the needle entry point **(Fig. 3)**.

Step 4: After painting and draping, inject 1% lignocaine; care must be taken to avoid the deeper structures to prevent loss of stimulating ability of the nerve stimulator by the local anesthetic.

Step 5 (Needle Placement): A 4-inch Stimuplex insulated needle **(Fig. 4)** is inserted and advanced under fluoroscopic guidance.

Now, stimulation output is obtained at 1.5–2.0 mA and 2-Hz frequency to obtain contraction of the gluteus maximus muscle. Then, the stimulator output is reduced until only a moderate gluteal twitch is observed.

Step 6: Now, advance needle until contraction of the gluteus is markedly diminished. The output is reduced to <0.6 mA and the needle tip is adjusted until there is just a discernible twitch noted at the needle hub and at the hip, which identifies the piriformis muscle **(Refer Video No. 13)**.

Step 7: Inject 1 mL of radiopaque contrast to obtain myogram of piriformis muscle **(Fig. 5)**. Contrast should flow in a diagonal pattern from cephalad to caudad as it goes toward the femoral attachment site of the piriformis muscle.

Now, inject 3 cc mixture of 0.25% bupivacaine with or without steroid into the piriformis muscle after negative aspiration for blood.

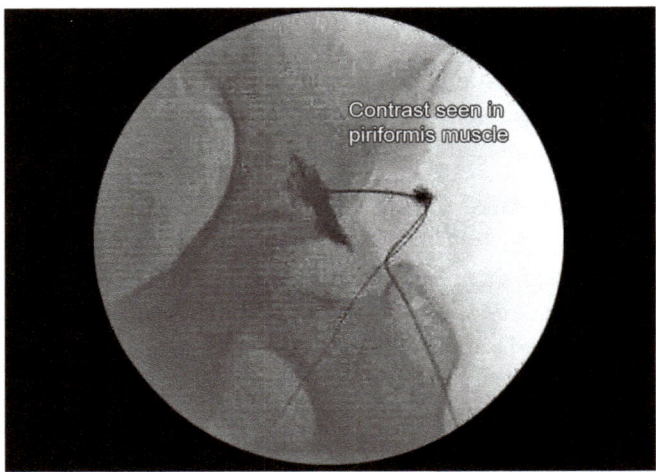

Fig. 5: Contrast in piriformis muscle.

In patients who are refractory to local and/or steroid medication, injection botulinum toxin 100 intrauterine (IU) is beneficial.

Precautionary Tips

- In case the dorsal aspect of the ileum is encountered, the needle should be pulled back 1–2 mm. The output is then adjusted until a slight twitch is obtained.
- In case paresthesias or contractions of the calf or foot muscles are seen, it indicates close proximity to the sciatic nerve.
- Never inject if the patient is feeling sharp pain shooting down his/her leg as the needle tip may be inside the sciatic nerve. Move the needle and retry.

CHAPTER 28

Pudendal Nerve Block and Pulsed Radiofrequency Procedure

Sanjeeva Gupta, Babita Ghai

BASIC INFORMATION

Indications
Diagnosis and treatment of chronic neuropathic pelvic pain due to pudendal neuralgia (PN)

Causes of Pudendal Neuralgia
- Injury to pudendal nerve or its blood supply during childbirth or during pelvic surgical interventions
- Traumatic injury due to fracture of the ischial spine
- Entrapment of the PN as it travels around the ischial spine between the sacrotuberous and sacrococcygeal ligaments or its courses through Alcock's canal
- Pelvic infection causing injury or dysfunction of the PN

Clinical Presentation
Neuropathic pain symptoms in the distribution of PN

Procedure Details
Pudendal nerve block (indication: PN)

Step 1: Patient in prone position (**Fig. 1**).

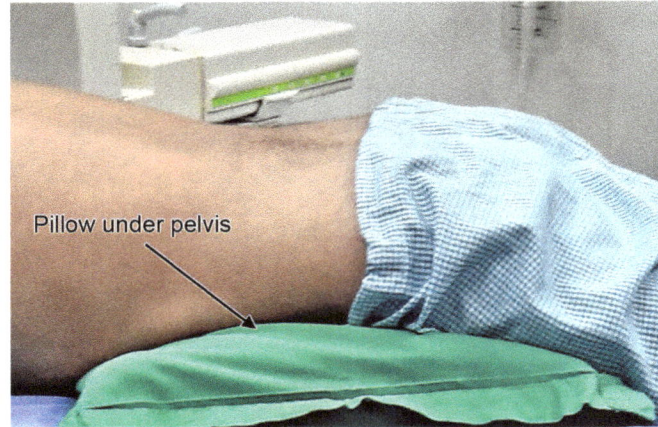

Fig. 1: Patient in prone position.

Step 2: Obtain a antero-posterior (AP) view fluoroscopic image at the level of the femoral heads to visualize the pelvic inlet.

The ischial spine is then identified by rotating the C-arm in the ipsilateral oblique direction by about 5–15°.

Navigate a curved tip 22G or a 25G spinal needle to contact the ischial spine and then direct the needle tip to the tip of the ischial spine (arrow in **Figure 2**). Up to 2 mL of local anesthesia may be injected around this area. The patient should be assessed within an hour after the procedure to find out the amount of pain relief obtained after the injection compared to the pain the patient had before the procedures during activities of daily living (ADL) (e.g., my pain is 50% better compared to what it was before the procedure during ADL).

If pulsed radiofrequency procedure (PRF) is planned please follow steps 3 and 4 (do not inject local anesthesia around the ischeal spine before PRF is performed).

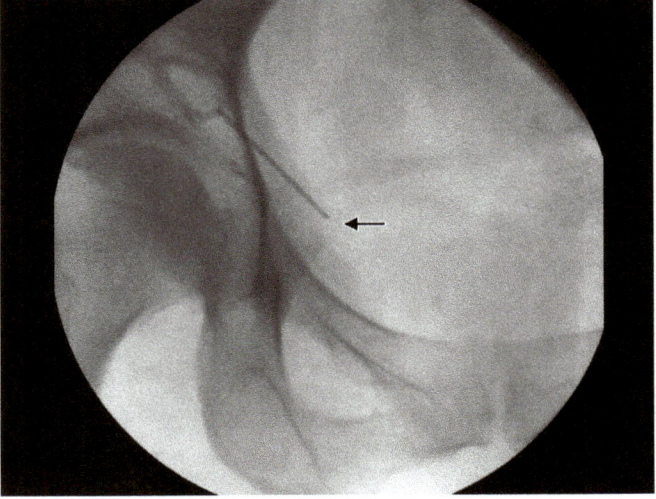

Fig. 2: A 22G curved tip spinal needle is being navigated to contact the left ischial spine (arrow).

Step 3: Direct a curved tip 20G 5-mm active tip radiofrequency (RF) needle to the tip of the left ischeal spine as described earlier and shown in **Figure 3**.

Step 4: Pudendal nerve pulsed radiofrequency (PRF) procedure. End on view of a 20G radiofrequency (RF) needle at the tip of the left ischial spine for PRF procedure for PN **(Fig. 4)**. Sensory stimulation at 50 Hz should reproduce patients' symptoms or tingling sensation in the symptomatic area. The position of the needle tip may have to be changed (slightly up or down or laterally), if symptoms are not reproduced on sensory stimulation.

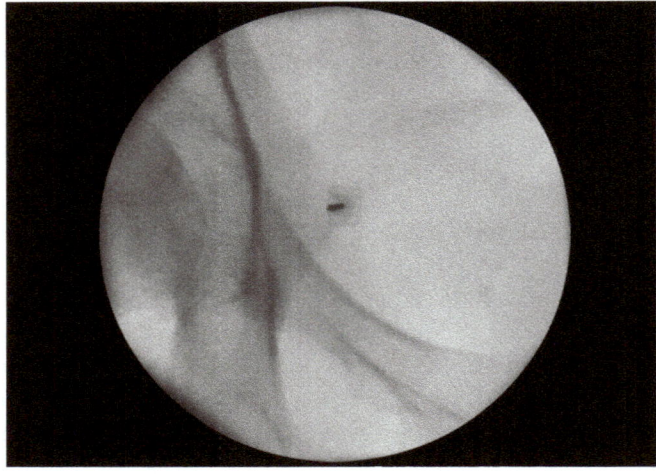

Fig. 3: Curved tip 20G 5-mm active tip RF needle is being navigated towards the tip of the left ischial spine.

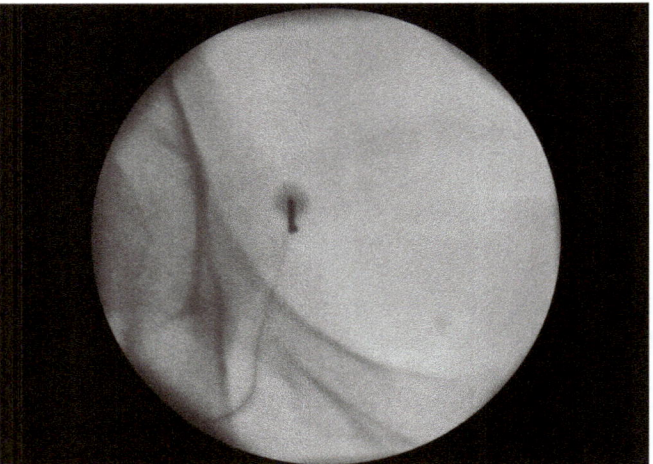

Fig. 4: Pudendal nerve pulsed radiofrequency procedure (PRF). The tip of the radiofrequency (RF) needle has been moved down slightly compared to **Figure 3** and sensory stimulation at 50 Hz reproduced tingling sensation around the patient's symptomatic areas. Three cycles of PRF procedure may be performed. Each 3 minutes' cycle is of 45 V with temperature not exceeding 42°C.

Step 5: The PRF procedure as performed on the left side may carried out on the right side if appropriate **(Fig. 5)**.

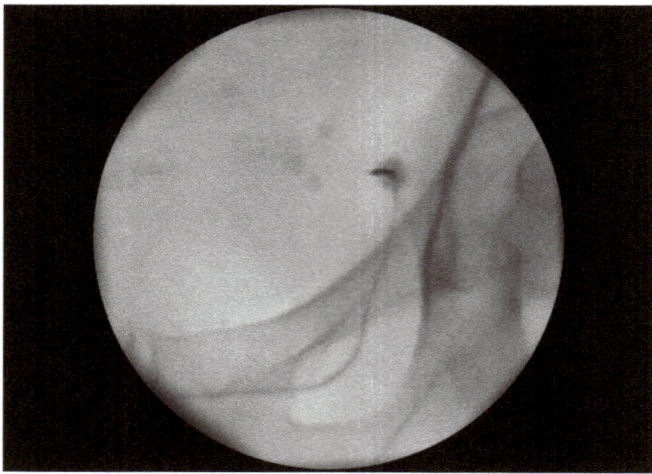

Fig. 5: Pudendal nerve pulsed radiofrequency procedure (PRF) on the right side.

FURTHER READING

1. Abdi S, Shenouda P, Patel N, Saini B, Bharat Y, Calvillo O. Technical report. Novel technique for pudendal nerve block. Pain Physician. 2004;7(3):319-22.
2. Pisani R, Stubinsky R, Datti R. Entrapment neuropathy of the internal pudendal nerve. Report of two cases. Scand J Urol Nephrol. 1997;31(4):407-10.
3. Snooks SJ, Swash M, Henry MM. Risk factors in childbirth causing damage to the pelvic floor innervation. Int J Colorectal Dis. 1986;1(1):20-4.

CHAPTER 29

Coccygeal Nerve Block

Yashwant Laxman Nankar, Dwarkadas K Baheti

BASIC INFORMATION

Coccygodynia has multiple elements apart from excruciating pain; it is embarrassing and psychologically disturbing.

Coccygeal nerve block is a useful tool in the armamentarium of pain physician in management of coccygodynia or coccygeal pain. The advantages of this nerve block are that both bowel and bladder functions are not affected.

Indications
- Coccygodynia or coccydynia
- Chronic pain after anus, rectum, and perineal surgery

Equipment
- C-arm compatible surgical table
- Radiation safety devices for all
- Marker pen, metal marker
- Needles 26- and 18G, 1½ inches
- Luer lock syringes 2, 5, and 10 mL and extension line

Medications
- *Nonionic contrast:* Iohexol (Omnipaque)
- Normal saline (0.9%)
- Lidocaine 2%; bupivacaine or ropivacaine 0.5%, preservative-free
- Depot steroid (preservative-free) such as Aurocort, methylprednisolone, and triamcinolone
- Botulinum toxin

Complications
- Infection
- Bleeding
- Tingling or numbness in the extremities
- Nerve damage that may occur due to a needle puncture

OTHER TREATMENT OPTIONS
- Radiofrequency (RFA) treatment of the sacral roots
- Coccygectomy

Advanced Options

Endoscopic Radiofrequency Ablation
The endoscopic RFA of the coccygeal nerves is being practiced at some canters in United States. It involves using an endoscope through which the coccyx and its nerve supply can be directly visualized.

Injection of Alcohol
Neurolytic such as alcohol, phenol, or glycerine to destroy the nerves was used earlier.

PROCEDURE DETAILS

Step 1: Patient in prone position with pillow under pelvis as shown in **Figure 1**.

Step 2: First, understand the anatomy of sacrum and coccyx in lateral view as seen in **Figure 2**.

Now identify the site and after preparation and draping of area, direct C-arm toward the sacrococcygeal junction in the anteroposterior (AP) view of the transverse process of coccyx. Put a metal marker on the most inferior aspect of the sacral hiatus as seen in **Figure 3**.

Step 3: The needle entry point is about 1 cm lateral to the lateral border of coccyx.

Inject 1% lignocaine and with a 22- or 25G spinal needle with slightly bending the tip (20–30°) **(Fig. 4)** and advance under fluoroscopic guidance.

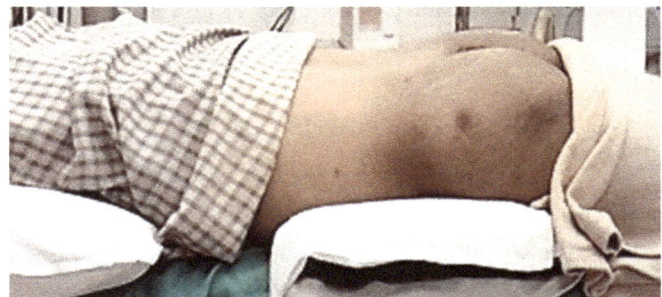

Fig. 1: Position of patient with pillow under pelvis.

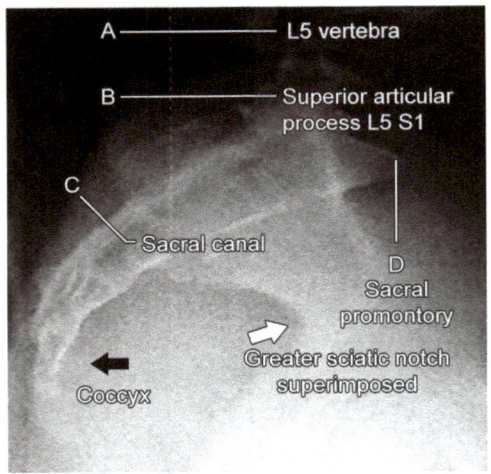

Fig. 2: Anatomy of sacrum and coccyx in lateral view.

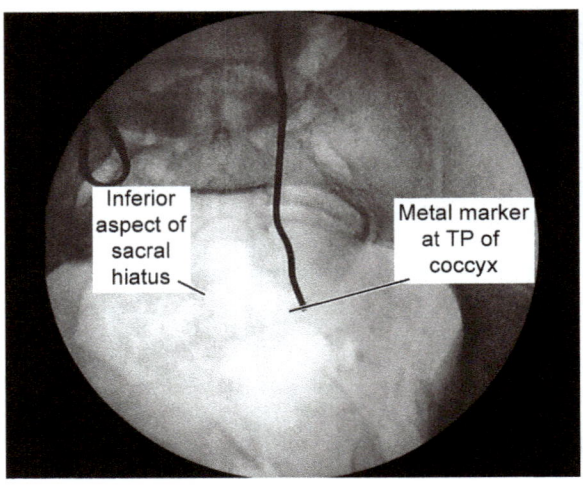

Fig. 3: Marker at tip of coccyx—anteroposterior view.

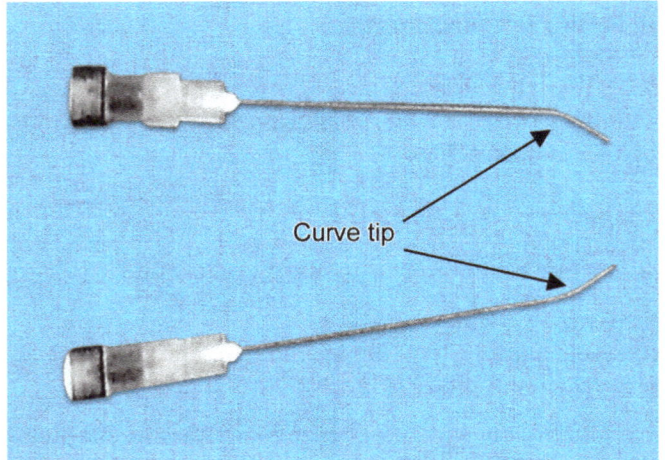

Fig. 4: Curve tip needle.

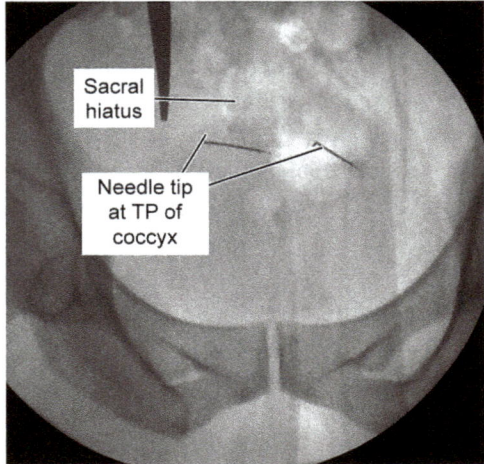

Fig. 5: Needle at the anterior margin of coccyx in anteroposterior view.

The needle trajectory is angled to directly contact the lateral aspect of coccyx, thus giving tactile sensation (**Fig. 5**).

The needle is then carefully advanced in lateral view with the tip just anterior margin of coccyx (**Fig. 6**).

Step 4: Now after repeated negative aspiration, inject 1 mL of Omnipaque and confirm in AP (**Fig. 7**) and lateral (**Fig. 8**) views.

Step 5: Again after negative aspiration, inject 0.25% bupivacaine with or without steroid about 3 cc.

Step 6: While withdrawing needle, inject 1% lignocaine in the needle track to prevent needle pain.

Step 7: Shift the patient to the recovery room for monitoring of vital signs.

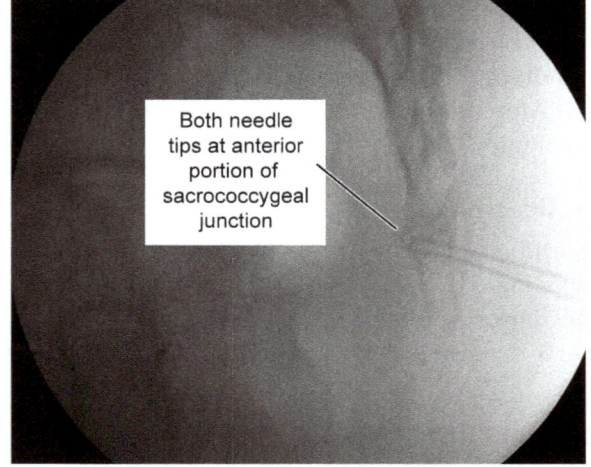

Fig. 6: Needle in lateral view.

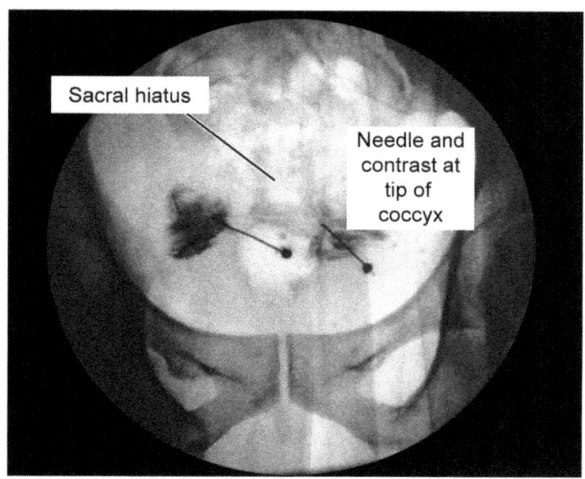

Fig. 7: Dye spread—anteroposterior view.

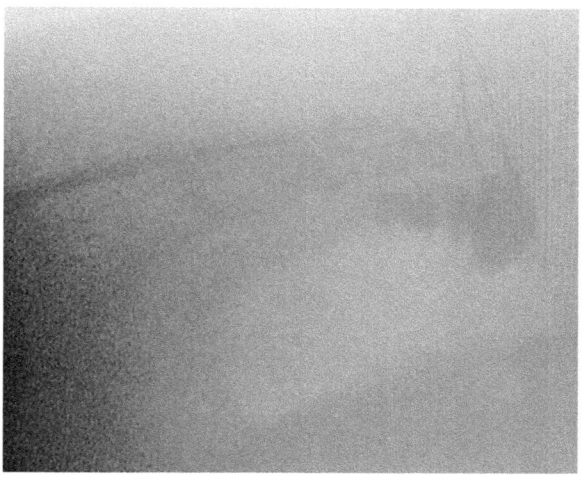

Fig. 8: Dye spread—lateral view.

Declaration

Part of the text and some images are taken with permission from M/s Jaypee Brothers Medical Publishers, New Delhi, from the book, *Interventional Pain Management: A Practical Approach* (2018) edited by DK Baheti, Sanjay Bakshi, Sanjeeva Gupta, and RP Gehdoo.

SECTION 6

Neuromodulation

- **Sacral Nerve Stimulation**
  Hemkumar Pushparaj, Manohar Sharma

CHAPTER 30

Sacral Nerve Stimulation

Hemkumar Pushparaj, Manohar Sharma

CLINICAL PEARLS

- S3 foramen can usually be identified in anteroposterior (AP) view. Bowel gas might obscure the view making identification difficult. Step 4 will be handy in such instances.
- Ipsilateral feet and anal opening is exposed during testing. The authors use a transparent drape around the anus. Stimulation of the lead should produce flexion of toes and/or anal motor response-bellowing (inward movement) of the pelvic floor. A strong response is often elicited at ≤2 mA on appropriately placed needles.
- The trajectory of needle should be in the most superior part of S3 foramen. The needle is inserted at an angle and someway cephalad (Step 5) to the intersecting lines in Step 4 for the same reason. Medial orientation in the AP view is also aimed for.
- If there is a poor response to stimulation:
  - Recheck the equipment. Usually, higher amplitude distorts anesthesia electrocardiogram (ECG) monitoring. This confirms equipment integrity.
  - Make sure that the radiological position is satisfactory. Parallax in lateral image may overestimate or underestimate the depth of the needle.
  - Other side might need to be targeted or rarely S4 is accessed if there is no response to bilateral S3 stimulation.
- In case of abnormal motor response such as foot rotation (S2 stimulation), radiology should be rechecked and needle reinserted.

PROCEDURE DETAILS

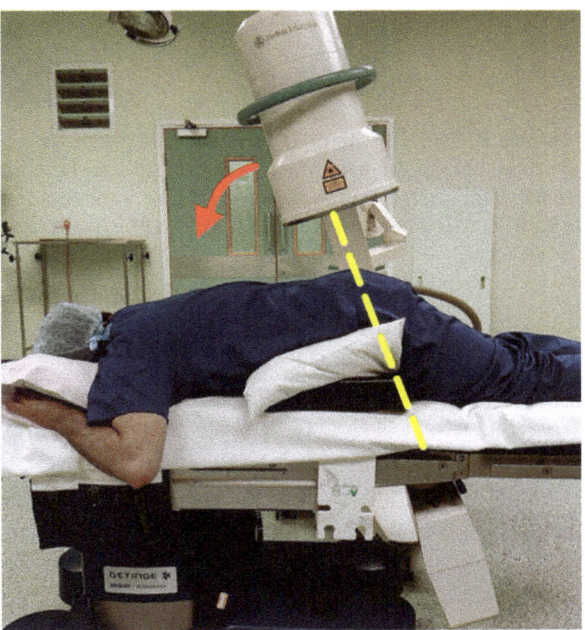

Figs. 1A and B: *Step 1:* Position the patient prone with pillow under abdomen to decrease lumbar lordosis. Also support patient's head, thorax, and hips. Feet should be lifted off the table with pillows under the shin.

Fig. 2: *Step 2:* Squaring the endplate of S1 by cephalad tilt of fluoroscopy.

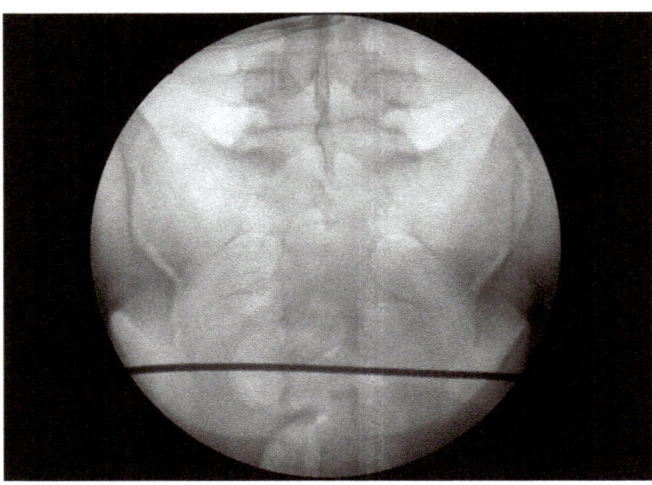

Fig. 3: *Step 3:* Adequately squared image of sacrum should be attained by adjusting fluoroscopy as shown in Steps 1 and 2.

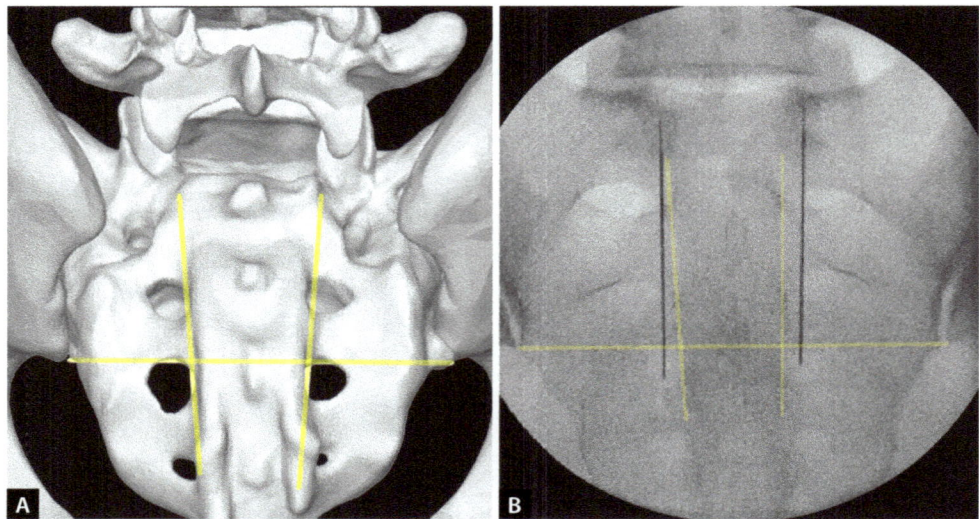

Figs. 4A and B: *Step 4:* Bilateral S3 foramen is targeted. In case of difficulty to locate the foramen, two parallel lines are drawn along the medial borders of the sacral foramen on either side, and the horizontal line running perpendicular to the vertical line from the lower border of sacroiliac joint intersecting these lines will locate the foramen and entry point.
Source: BodyParts3D is made by DBCLS, CC BY-SA 2.1 JP *https://creative commons.org/licenses/by-sa/2.1/jp/deed.en*.

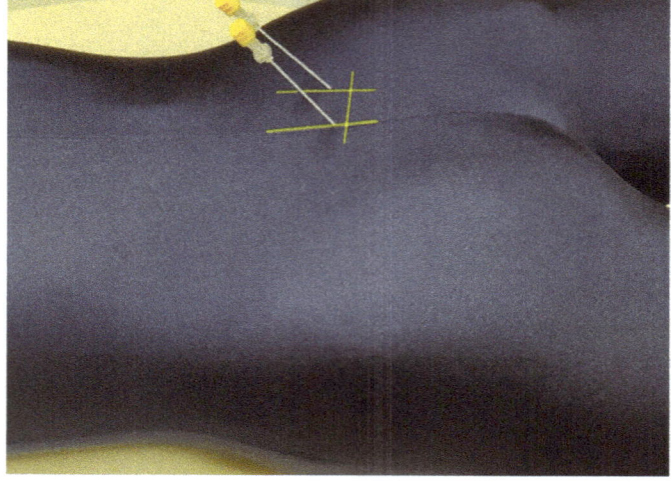

Fig. 5: *Step 5:* Needle is inserted in a slightly caudal trajectory so that the final position will be parallel to S3 nerve root. The point of entry into S3 foramen is denoted by the intersection of lines rather than the skin entry.

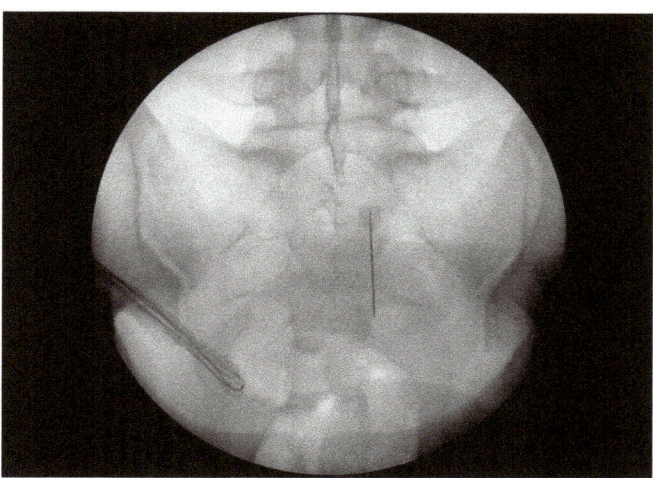

Fig. 6: *Step 6:* The needle is inserted in the medial and superior quadrant of the foramen. Lateral entry might miss the target nerve.

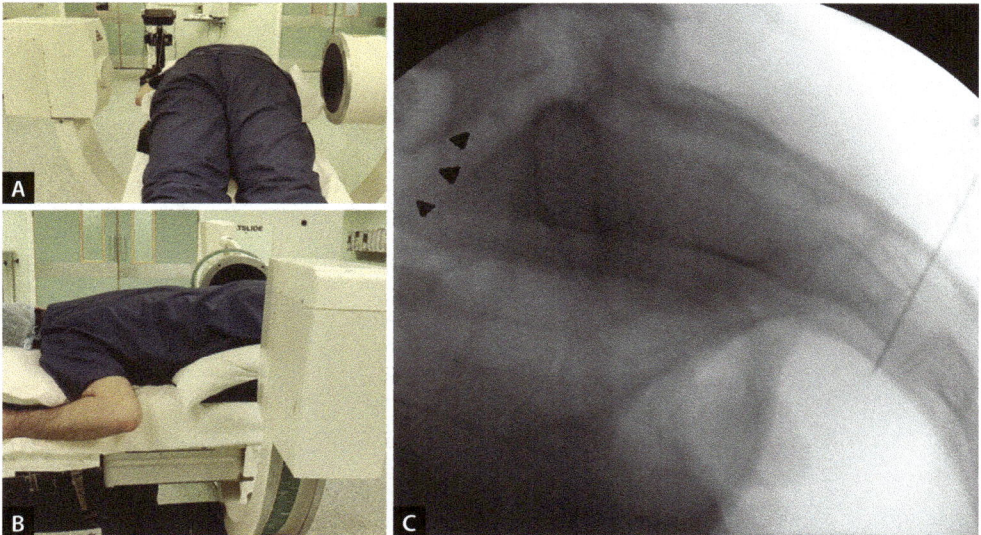

Figs. 7A to C: *Step 7:* Once foramen is accessed, the fluoroscopy is rotated by 90° to obtain a lateral image of the sacrum. Note that both iliac crests (black pointer) on either side should be overlapping without any parallax to get a true lateral image.

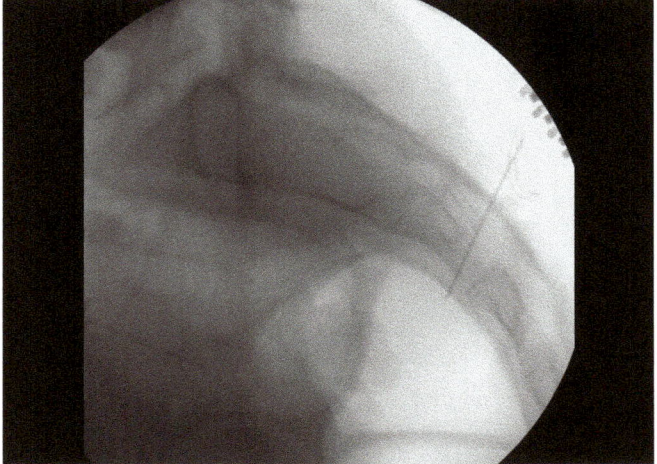

Fig. 8: *Step 8:* The needle is advanced just ventral the anterior S3 foramen. Care must be taken not to advance further as damage to rectum may occur. Appropriate stimulation is passed via the needle. The stimulation is increased in amplitude till good flexion of toes/bellowing of the pelvic muscles is seen in the perineum.

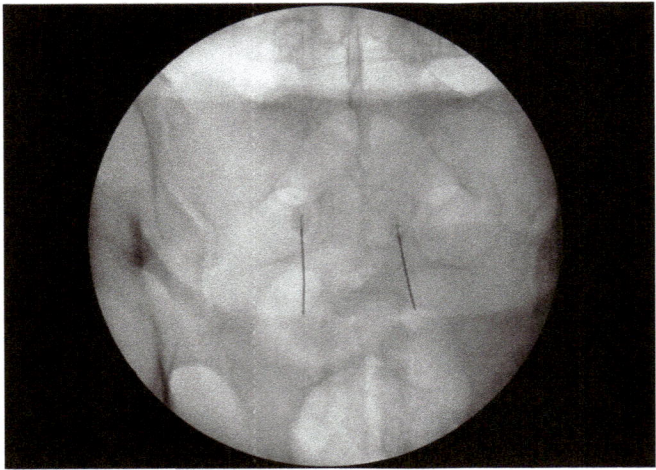

Fig. 9: *Step 9:* The same steps are repeated on the other side. Both sides are targeted for the trial phase of the treatment.

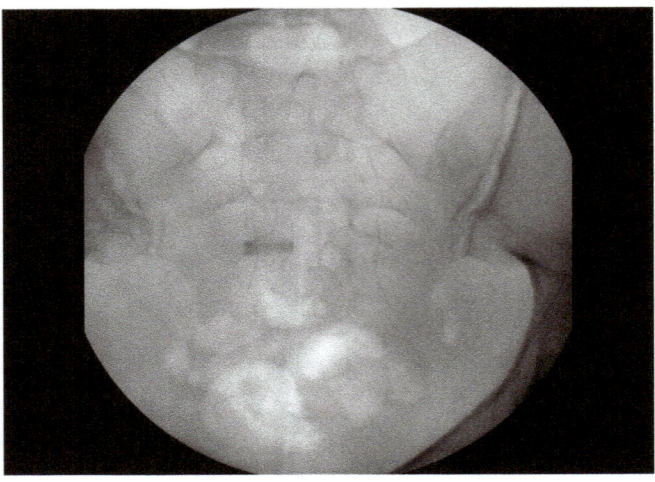

Fig. 10: *Step 10:* The trial lead is passed via both the needles and secured to the skin with adhesives. In our center, the trial usually lasts for 2 weeks, with one lead being stimulated for 1 week each. Some centers use a single lead trial as well.

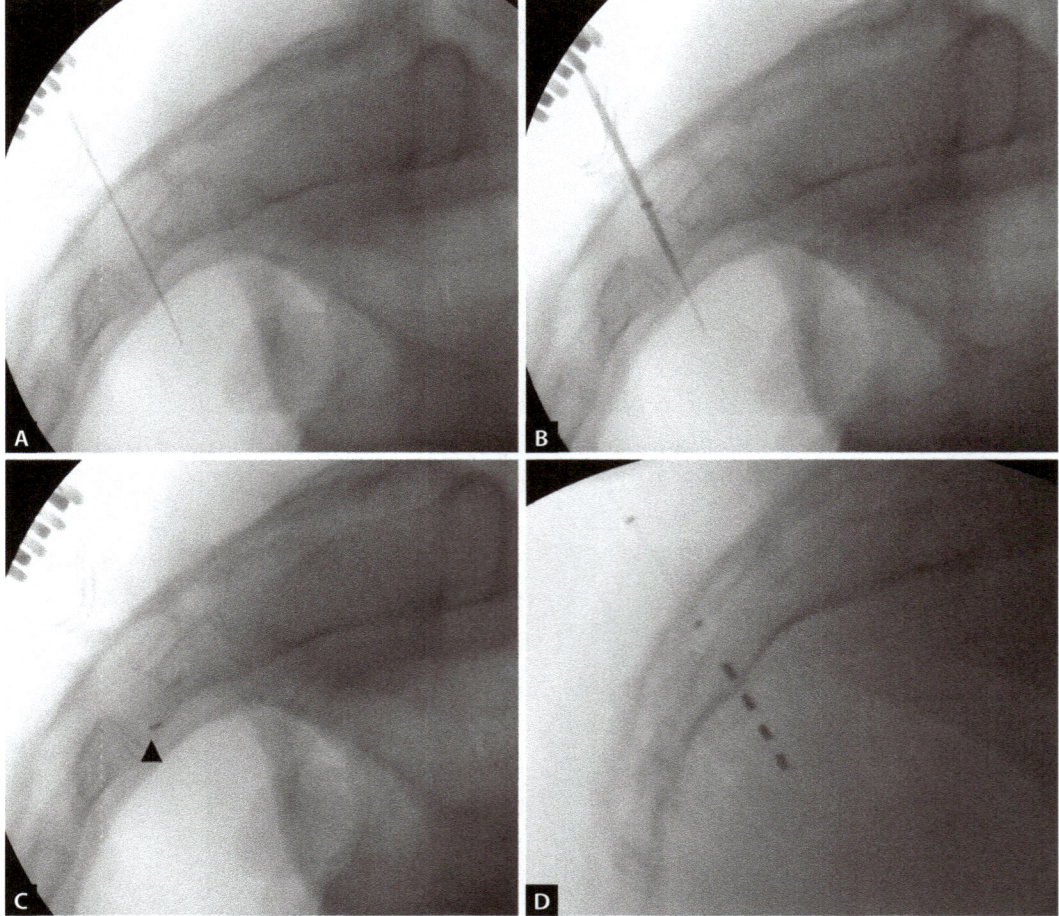

Figs. 11A to D: *Step 11:* Based on the outcome of the trial, a permanent implant is planned and performed with the same technique. Note that the side with maximal benefit is chosen to be implanted with a permanent lead. (A) S3 foramen is accessed with the needle as in Steps 1–8 and a guidewire is passed through it; (B) The needle is replaced by a sheath with radiopaque marking; (C) Guidewire is removed with the radiopaque marking on the sheath at the anterior S3 foramen (black pointer); (D) A permanent quadripolar electrode is placed through the sheath with electrodes 1, 2, and 3 ventral to and electrode 4 within the S3 foramen.

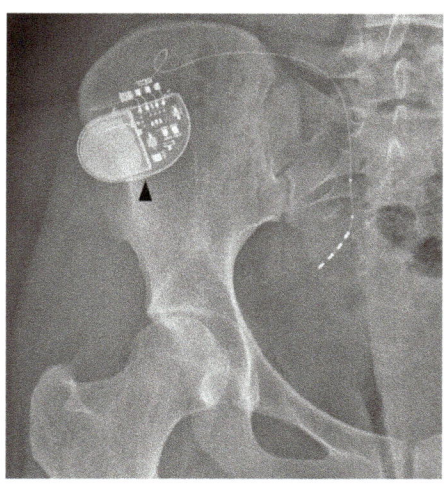

Fig. 12: *Step 12:* Implanted pulse generator (IPG) (black pointer) pocket is created at least 2 cm deep below the skin away from the sacroiliac joint. The lead is then tunneled to the IPG site and attached to IPG. The final position of quadripolar lead and IPG is shown in the figure. Note that the lead tip turns laterally along the direction of the nerve. IPG is placed away from any bony edges and the sacroiliac joint.

FURTHER READING

1. Brazzelli M, Murray A, Fraser C, Grant A. Systematic review of the efficacy and safety of sacral nerve stimulation for urinary urge incontinence and urgency frequency. Aberdeen: Review Body for Interventional Procedures; 2003. Commissioned by the National Institute for Clinical Excellence. [online] Available from http://www.nice.org.uk/nicemedia/live/11063/30825/30825.pdf. [Last accessed January, 2022].
2. Hull T, Giese C, Wexner SD, Devroede G, Madoff RD, Stormberg G, et al. Long-term durability of sacral nerve stimulation therapy for chronic fecal incontinence. Dis Colon Rectum. 2013;56(2):234-45.
3. Leong RK, de Wachter SG, Joore MA, van Kerrebroeck PE. Cost-effectiveness analysis of sacral neuromodulation and botulinum toxin A treatment for patients with idiopathic overactive bladder. BJU Int. 2011;108(4):558-64.
4. Matzel KE, Chartier-Kastler E, Knowles CH, Lehur PA, Munöz-Duyos A, Ratto C, et al. Sacral neuromodulation: standardized electrode placement technique. Neuromodulation. 2017;20(8):816-24.
5. Siegel S, Noblett K, Mangel J, Bennett J, Griebling TL, Sutherland SE, et al. Five-year follow up results of a prospective, multicenter study of patients with overactive bladder treated with sacral neuromodulation. J Urol. 2018;199(1):229-36.

SECTION 7

Peripheral Blocks

- **Radiofrequency Neurotomy of Suprascapular Nerve for Refractory Shoulder Joint Pain**
  Nick Plunkett, Allen Pinto

- **Tennis or Golfer's Elbow**
  Dwarkadas K Baheti

- **Hip Joint Injection**
  Yehia Kamel

- **Greater Trochanteric Bursa Injection**
  Yehia Kamel

- **Popliteal Nerve Block**
  Yashwant Laxman Nankar, Dwarkadas K Baheti

- **Calcaneal Spur Injection**
  Dwarkadas K Baheti

CHAPTER 31

Radiofrequency Neurotomy of Suprascapular Nerve for Refractory Shoulder Joint Pain

Nick Plunkett, Allen Pinto

TYPES OF TECHNIQUE

There are two sections:
- *Section 1:* Landmark technique
- *Section 2:* X-ray technique

Section 1: Landmark Technique

Step 1: Aim—to target the suprascapular nerve in its notch at tip of white arrow. **(Fig. 1)**.

Step 2: Put the patient in a sitting position. Prepare the radiofrequency (RF) machine and apply earth plate **(Fig. 2)**. Draw a line across the top edge of the spine of the scapula.

Step 3: Bisect that line with a line parallel to the longitudinal axis of the patient **(Fig. 3)**.

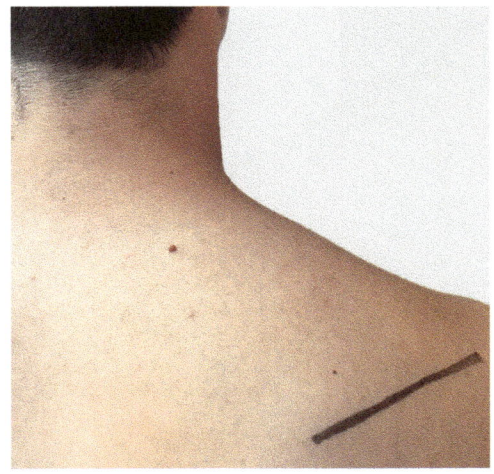

Fig. 2: Line across the top edge of the spine of scapula.

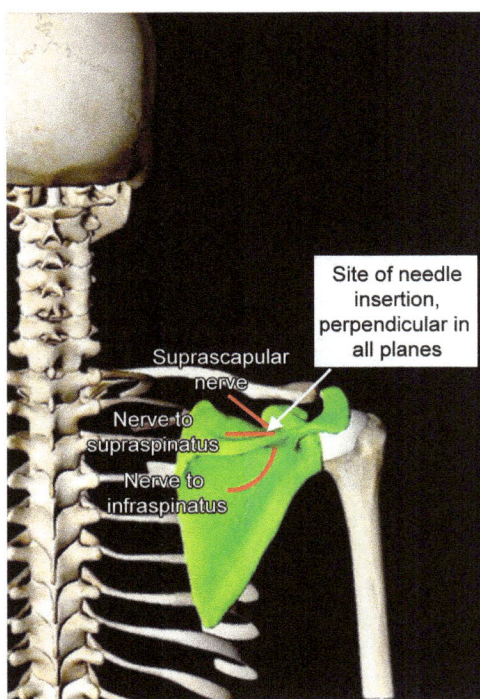

Fig. 1: Anatomy on skeleton.

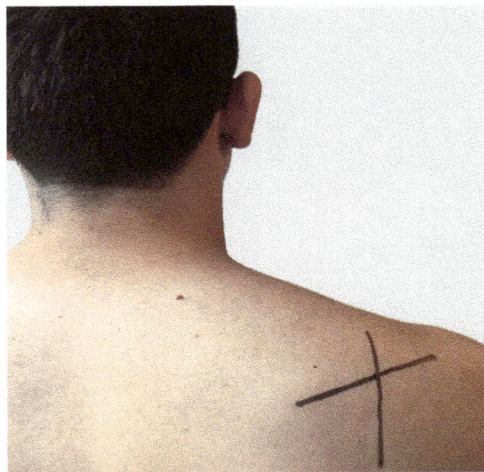

Fig. 3: Bisect line parallel to the longitudinal axis of the patient.

Step 4: Bisect the angle in the upper outer quadrant formed by the two previous lines **(Fig. 4)**. Mark an "X" 2.5 cm along this line. Clean skin, inject local anesthesia (LA) to 2 cm, and insert a 10-cm 18G RF needle perpendicular in all planes, aiming to enter scapular notch (see step 1—anatomy).

Technique: Aim to "slip" into the notch—some additional needle manipulation may be required. Needle depth should be maximally 5–6 cm. Stimulate (motor) aiming for twitch at 0.3–0.5 V threshold in supraspinatus and infraspinatus, and after LA instillation, lesion at 80°C for 90–120 seconds.

Pitfall—if too much LA is used, the nerve may become anesthetised and not responsive to stimulation.

Section 2: X-ray Technique

Step 1: Position the X-ray C-arm to obtain an anteroposterior (AP) view of the scapula **(Fig. 5)**.

Step 2: Apply the dispersive pad to the opposite shoulder **(Fig. 6)**.

Step 3: Clean the operative shoulder with surgical preparation.

Step 4: Apply a sterile drape to isolate the surgical field **(Fig. 7)**.

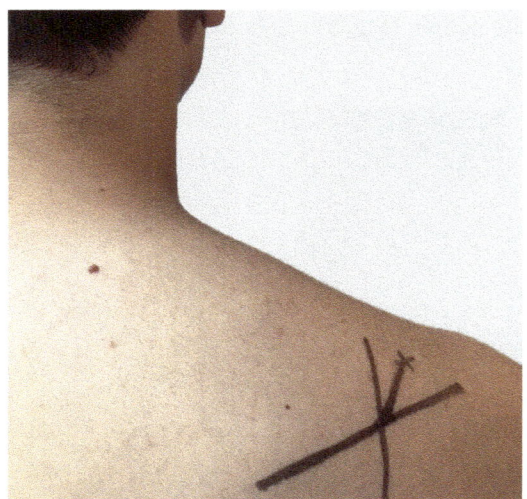

Fig. 4: Mark "X" 2.5 cm along line.

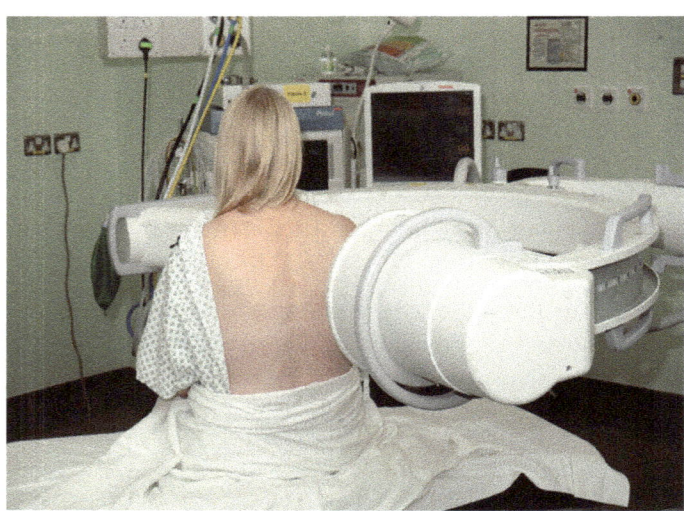

Fig. 5: Position the X-ray C-arm.

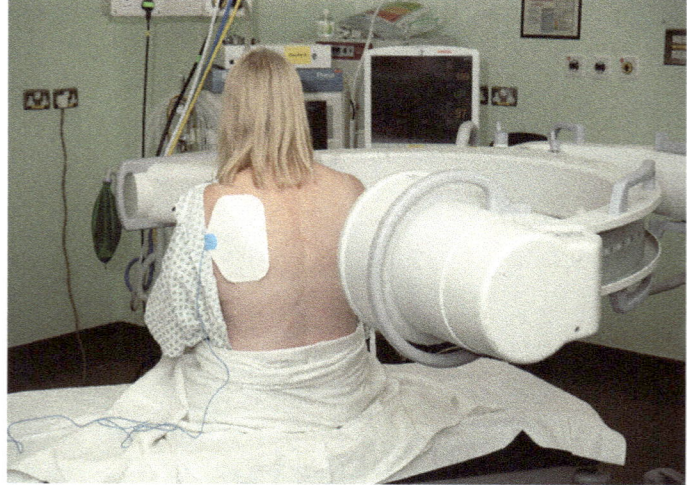

Fig. 6: Adhesive pad on the opposite side to obtain an anteroposterior view.

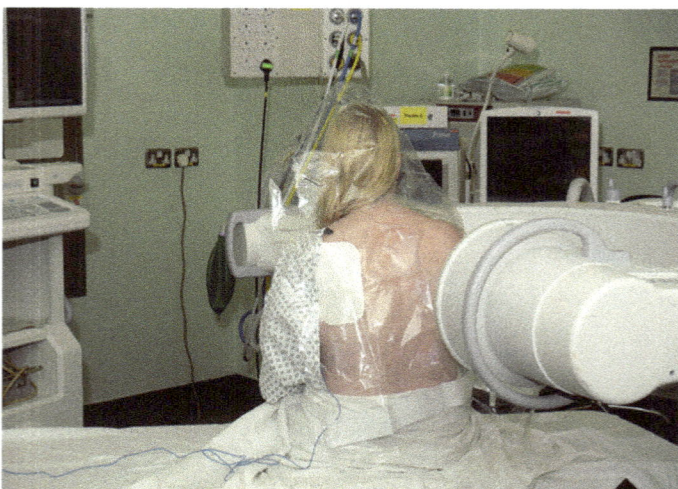

Fig. 7: Surgical preparation.

Step 5: Obtain an anteroposterior view of the scapula (**Fig. 8**).

Step 6: Identify the suprascapular notch (arrow) located at the medial end of the base of the coracoid process (**Fig. 9**).

Step 7: Angulate the C-arm to move the scapular spine out of the way (**Fig. 10**).

Step 8: Place the pointer above the scapular spine, in line with the suprascapular notch (**Fig. 11**).

Step 9: Infiltrate only the superficial tissues (skin and subcutaneous fat) with local anesthetic (**Fig. 12**).

Step 10: Introduce the RF cannula into the suprascapular notch, from above the scapular spine (**Fig. 13**).

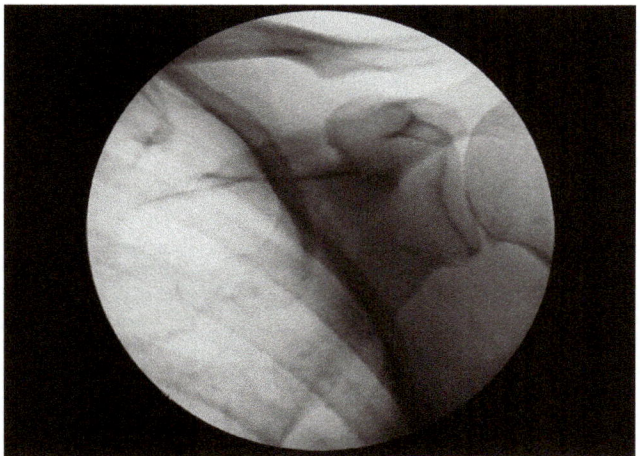

Fig. 8: Anteroposterior view of scapula.

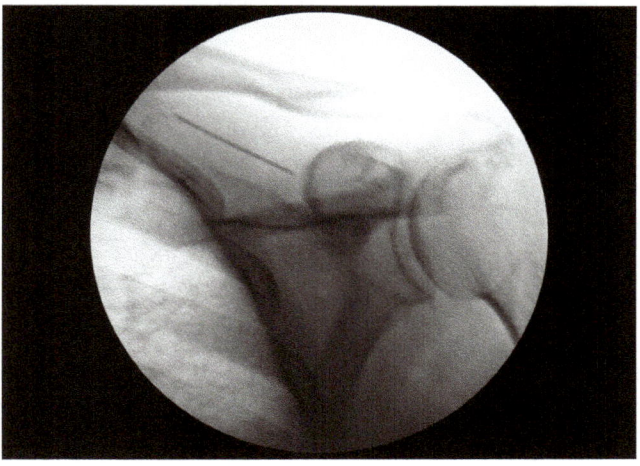

Fig. 11: Pointer above the scapular spine, in line with the suprascapular notch.

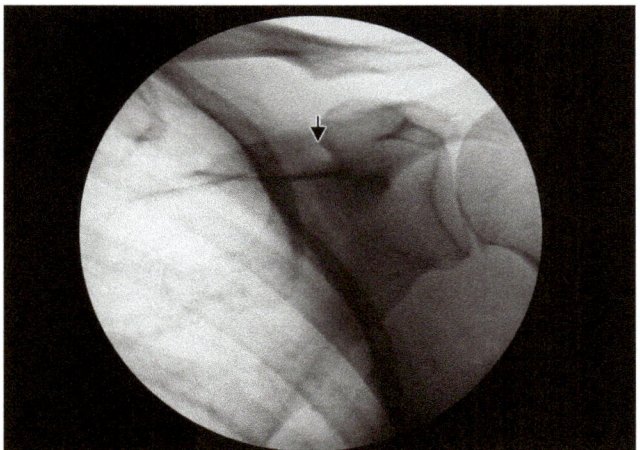

Fig. 9: Arrow at suprascapular notch.

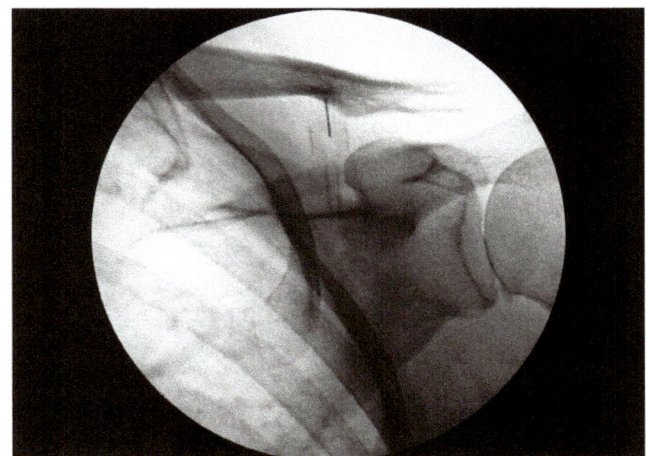

Fig. 12: Infiltration of local anesthetic.

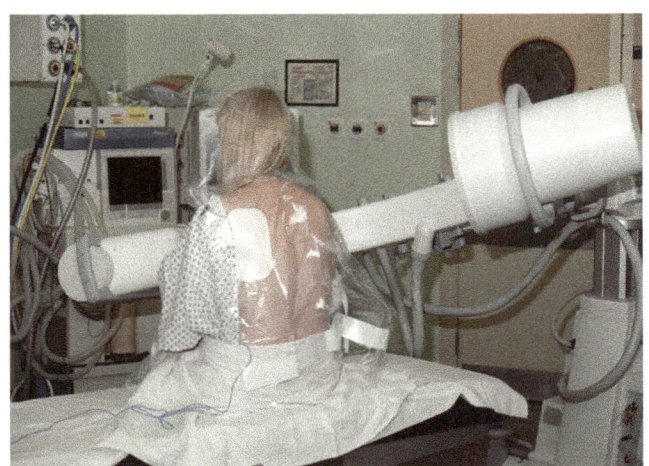

Fig. 10: Angulate the C-arm to move the scapular spine out of the way.

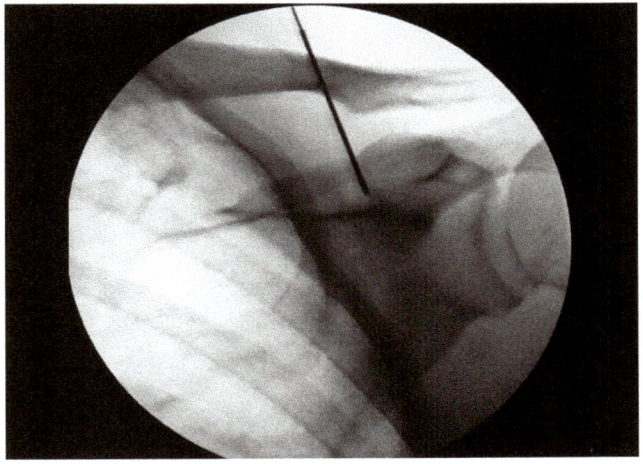

Fig. 13: Radiofrequency cannula in notch anteroposterior view.

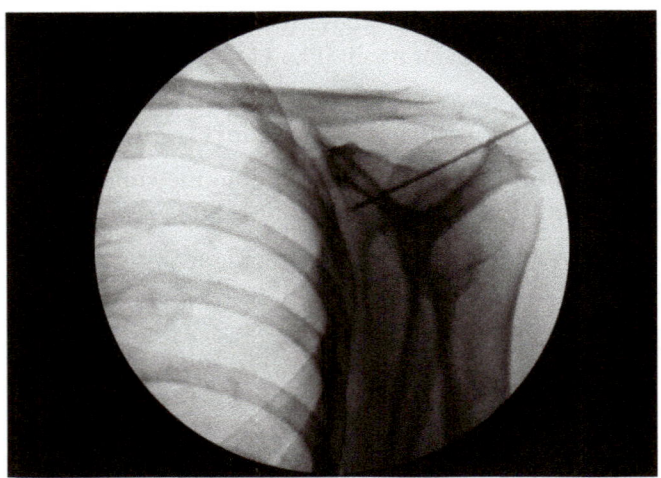

Fig. 14: Radiofrequency cannula in lateral view.

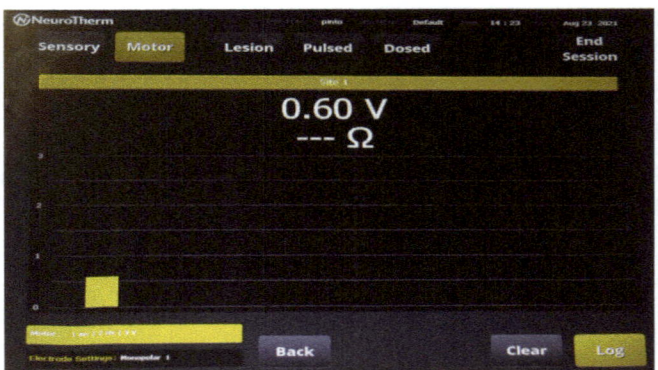

Fig. 15: Motor stimulation.

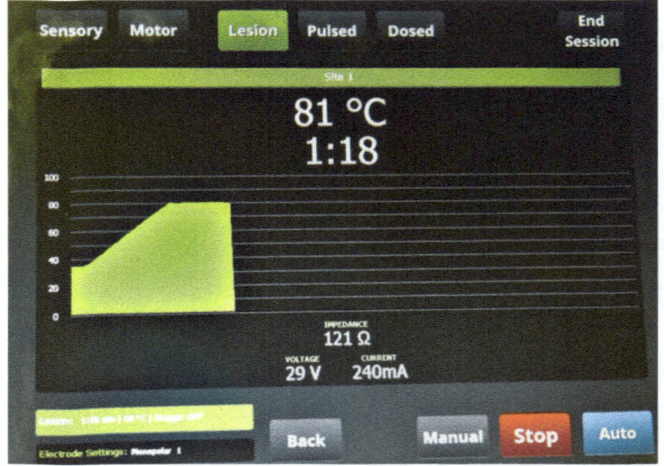

Fig. 16: Lesioning in process.

Step 11: A lateral view of the RF cannula sited in the suprascapular notch, entering from above the scapular spine **(Fig. 14)**.

Step 12: Use motor stimulation (2 Hz) to identify the suprascapular nerve looking for infraspinatus and supraspinatus twitch—aim for stimulation to be present at a voltage <0.5 V (indicates sufficient proximity for successful lesioning) **(Fig. 15)**.

Step 13: Once the RF cannula is at the intended position, inject 2 mL 1% lignocaine. Wait for 2 minutes for it to work.

Step 14: Rotate the C-arm by 90° to obtain a "Y" view of the scapula.

Step 15: Note the RF cannula in the suprascapular notch, entering above the scapular spine, and the tip is clear of the pleural (lung) field.

Step 16: Lesion at 80°C for 90–120 seconds **(Fig. 16)**.

Step 17: Shift the patient to the recovery room for the monitoring of vital signs.

CHAPTER 32

Tennis or Golfer's Elbow

Dwarkadas K Baheti

TENNIS ELBOW

Lateral epicondylitis is a painful condition of elbow, commonly known as "tennis elbow." It involves the tendons that attach to the bone on the outside (lateral) part of the elbow. The tendon involved is extensor carpi radialis brevis which transmits a muscle's force to the bone. The function of this muscle is to help to straighten and stabilize the wrist (**Fig. 1**).

The pathology is degeneration of the tendon's attachment—weakening the anchor site and placing greater stress on the area. The factor is repetitive motions like gripping a racket during a swing which results in excessive strain on the muscles by put too much stress on the tendons.

This occurs with tennis, golf, racquetball, squash, fencing, weightlifting, carpentry, typing, painting, raking, and knitting, which results in occupational hazard.

Tennis elbow, also called golfer's elbow, is another condition which affects the tendon on the inside of the elbow.

Symptoms
- Pain in the arm and tenderness around the elbow
- Pain and tenderness in the bony knob on the outside of elbow
- Swelling in the lateral aspect of elbow
- The pain may also radiate into the upper or lower arm.

Signs
- Tenderness at bony knob—as shown in **Figure 2**.
- Restricted painful movements of elbow
- Tender point—as shown in **Figure 2**, where the injured tendons connect to the bone.

Treatment
Treatment includes the following:
- Modify the activity that induces pain. It is advisable to adopt modification in grips or techniques, such as use of a larger size racket in tennis.
- *Medication:* Analgesics, non-steroidal anti-inflammatory drugs (NSAIDs), analgesic gel or spray. Locally acting patches.
- Local injection mixture of a steroid with local anesthetic helps to reduce pain. At times, adding Inj. Hyaluronidase 1,500 IU will help in faster absorption of the drug.
  - *Platelet-rich plasma (PRP):* Injection into the area of lateral epicondyle will help in some cases.
- *Surgery:* In some cases, surgery may be indicated when the pain is incapacitating.
- Use of brace could reduce the tension and allow to heal.

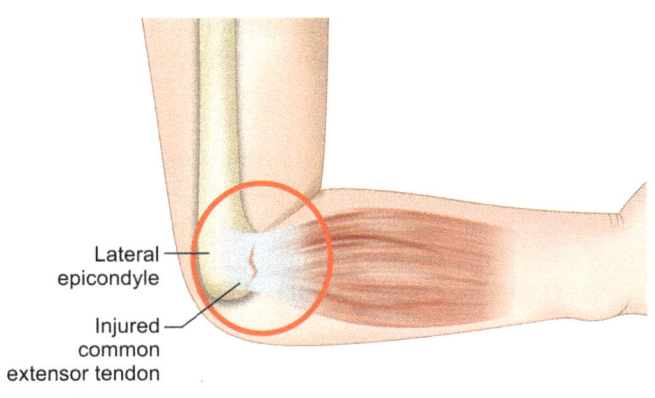

Fig. 1: Injured common tendon.

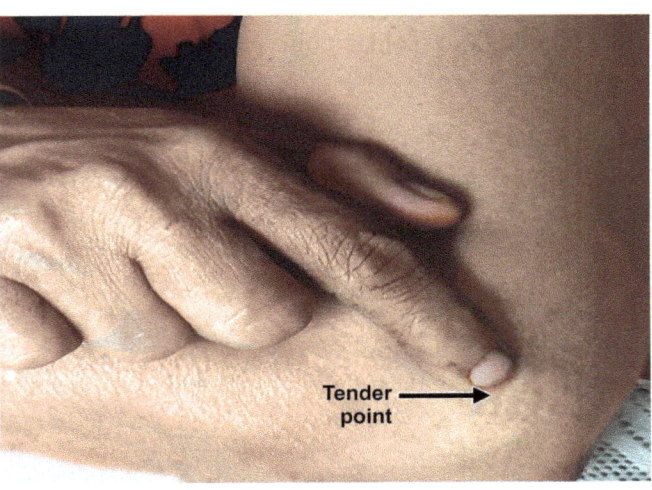

Fig. 2: Tender point for tennis elbow.

- *Physical therapy:* Stretching and/or strengthening exercises, ultrasound, or heat treatments may help in relieving the pain.
  - Exercises such as wrist turn, wrist turn with weight, wrist lift, palm up, elbow bend, and wrist extensor stretch play a vital role in recovery.
- Prevention can be done with reduction in repetitive activities and resting of arm movements. Start exercises as stated above.

Procedure Details

Step 1: Keep the patient's elbow resting on table. Prepare the area with betadine solution.

Step 2: Palpate and pinpoint the needle entry **(Fig. 3)**.

If done under fluoroscopy, the entry point is as shown in **Figure 4**.

Step 3: Injection at tender point can be done with or without fluoroscopy. The needle entry point is reconfirmed with the patient as shown in **Figure 3**. Inject a mixture of local anesthetic, steroid 20 mg, and Inj hyaluronidase 1500 IU at the site of pain.

Step 4: This is an outdoor patient procedure so he/she can leave the hospital.

Step 5: Ask the patient to take hot fomentation at the site three times daily for 2–3 days as it helps in faster absorption and reduction of local edema, if any.

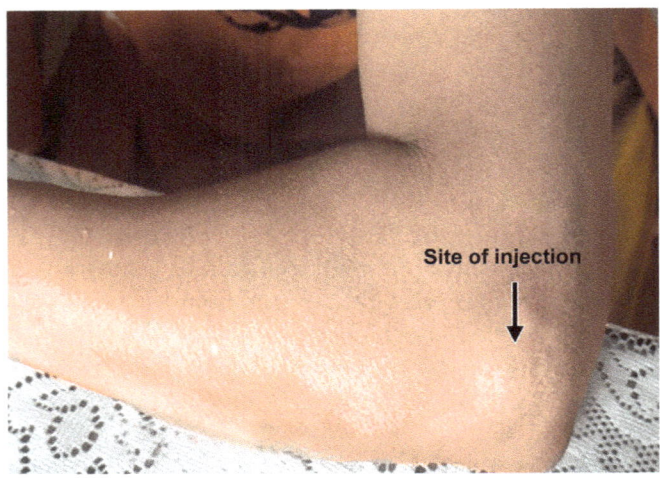

Fig. 3: Site of injection.

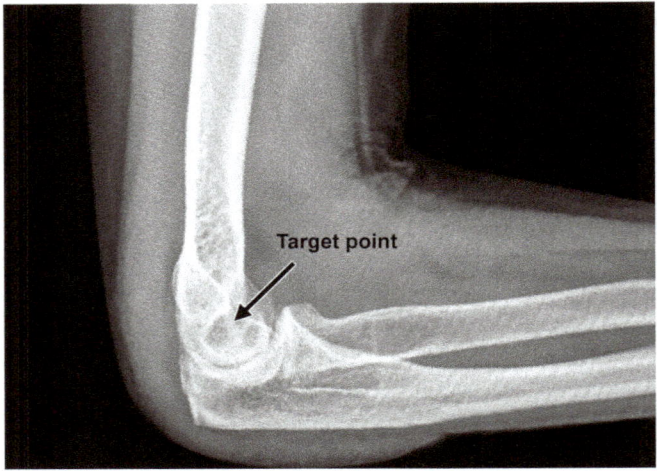

Fig. 4: Target point under fluoroscopy.

GOLFER'S ELBOW

Golfer's elbow is a condition that causes pain where the tendons of your forearm muscles attach to the bony bump on the inside of elbow. The pain might spread into forearm and wrist. Golfer's elbow is like tennis elbow, which occurs on the outside of the elbow; however, it is not limited to golfers.

Pathophysiology

Golfer's elbow, or medial epicondylitis, is tendinosis of the medial epicondyle on the inside of the elbow. The anterior forearm contains several muscles. These are pronator teres, flexor carpi radialis, flexor carpi ulnaris, flexor digitorum superficialis, and palmaris longus.

The function of these muscles is flexion of the digits of the hand and flexion, and pronation of the wrist. The tendons of these muscles come together in a common tendinous sheath, which originates from the medial epicondyle of the humerus at the elbow joint.

The pain is normally caused due to stress on the tendon because of the large amount of grip exerted by the digits and torsion of the wrist which is caused by the use and action of the cluster of muscles on the condyle of the ulna.

Any injury, even a minor one, results in inflammation at the point of insertion and results in pain. The repetitive use of these muscles results in more inflammation and severe pain with restricted painful movements of elbow, arm, and wrist.

Symptoms

Symptoms include pain, inflammation, redness, and restricted painful movements **(Fig. 5)**.

The pain is more on the medial side of elbow.

Investigations such as radiography, ultrasound, and magnetic resonance imaging will be helpful.

Treatment

- Analgesics, NSAIDs, local gel, spray
- Fomentation with heat or ice

CHAPTER 32 | Tennis or Golfer's Elbow

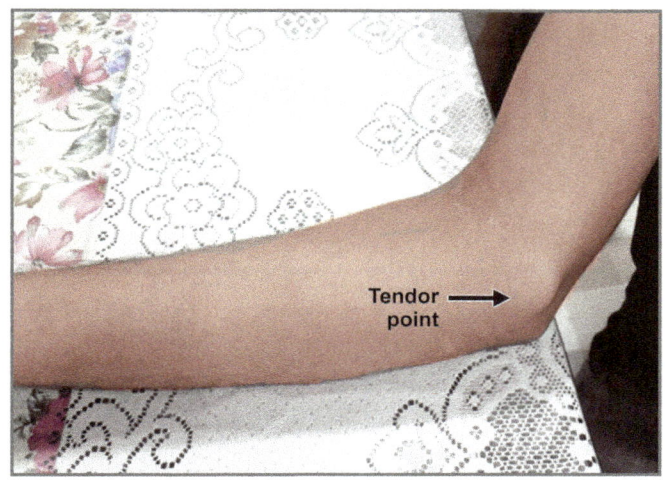

Fig. 5: Golfer's elbow—tender point at medial epicondyle.

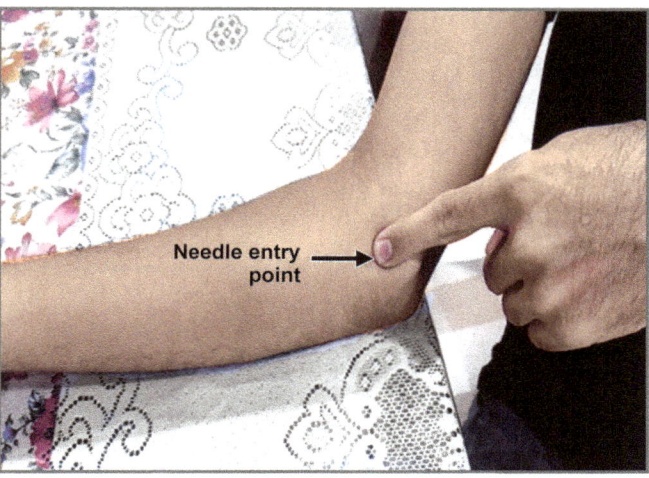

Fig. 6: Golfer's elbow—needle entry point.

- Elbow strap will help to reduce strain and limit the activity. This will reduce further damage. This works on the principle of RICE, i.e., Rest, Ice, Compression, and Elevation.
- In some cases, one may need splint to support elbow and hand.
- Surgery—debridement or cleaning of the area and decompression of the ulnar nerve.

Physical Therapy

Physical therapy includes exercises for reconditioning. It starts with stretching and gradual strengthening of the flexor-pronator muscles.

Procedure Details

Step 1: Keep the patient's elbow resting on table. Prepare the area with betadine solution.

Step 2: Palpate and pinpoint the needle entry.

Injection at the tender point can be done with or without fluoroscopy. The needle entry point is reconfirmed with patient as shown in **Figure 6**.

Step 3: Inject a mixture of local anesthetic, steroid 20 mg, and Inj hyaluronidase 1500 IU at the site of pain, i.e., at the target point as shown with arrow in **Figure 7**.

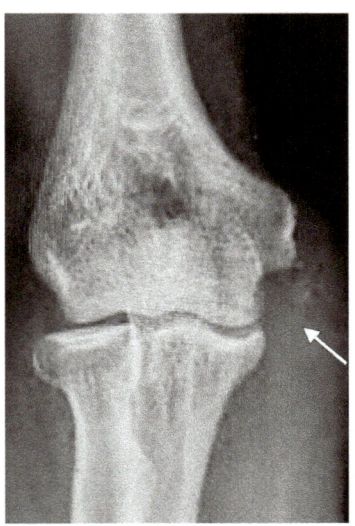

Fig. 7: Arrow at target point.

Step 4: This is an outdoor patient procedure so he can leave the hospital.

Step 5: Ask the patient to take hot fomentation at the site three times daily for 2–3 days as it helps in faster absorption and reduction of local edema, if any.

CHAPTER 33

Hip Joint Injection

Yehia Kamel

INDICATIONS

Intra-articular Pathologies

- Osteoarthritis (OA)
- Rheumatoid arthritis and other causes of arthritis
- Synovitis/capsulitis
- Trauma
- Cartilage degeneration
- Femoro-acetabular impingement

CONTRAINDICATIONS

- Patient refusal
- Systemic or local infection
- Coagulopathy
- Unstable hip joint
- Intra-articular fracture
- True contrast allergy (rare)—could use gadolinium instead when performed using fluoroscopy
- Raised blood sugar/poorly controlled diabetes mellitus (DM) in case of steroids injection

INJECTATE

- *Local anesthetic and steroids:* 5–8 mL of 0.25% bupivacaine/levobupivacaine/lignocaine 1% or 2% + 1 mL/40 mg depo-steroid (triamcinolone or methylprednisolone)
- Hyaluronic acid 5 mL
- Platelet-rich plasma 3–6 mL
- 25% Dextrose + Lignocaine 0.5% 4–8 mL

TECHNIQUE

Fluoroscopy

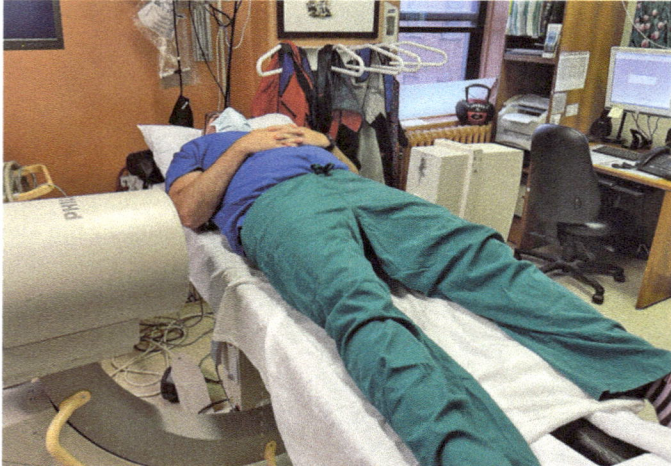

Fig. 1: *Step 1*: Place the patient in the supine position and place the C-arm in a lateral position.

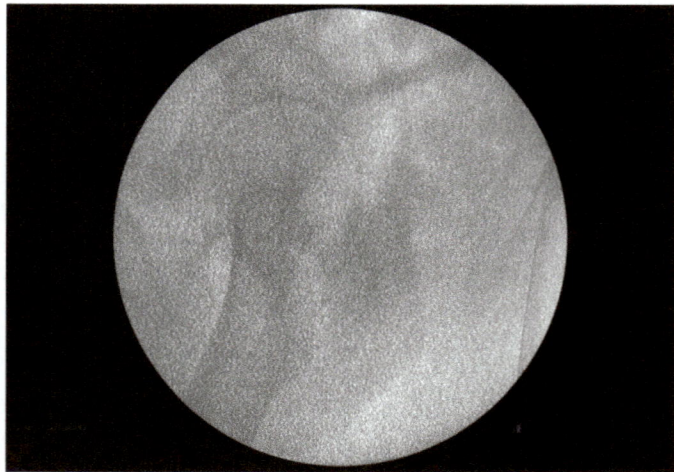

Fig. 2: *Step 2*: Get a lateral image of the hip that shows the greater trochanter, the head of the femur, the neck, and the acetabulum.

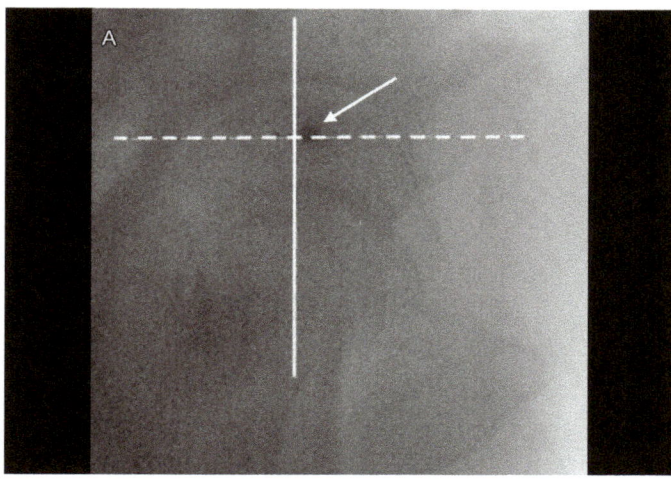

Fig. 3: *Step 3:* Lateral view and needle directed toward head in tunnel vision.

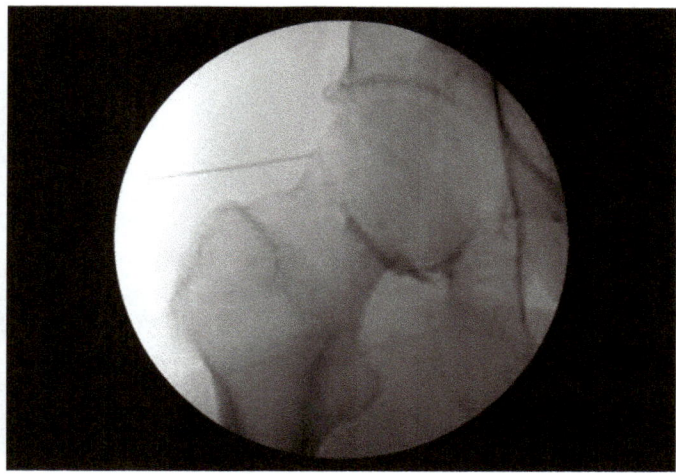

Fig. 4: *Step 4:* Anteroposterior view showing tip of needle at the neck of the femur with contrast around it.

ULTRASOUND

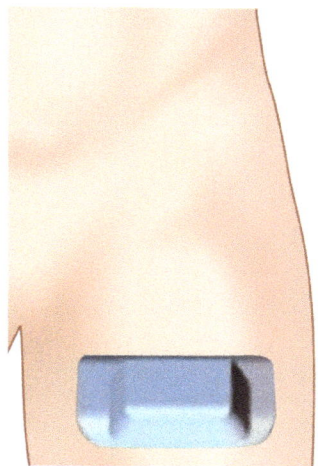

Fig. 5: *Step 1:* Patient supine and use a curvilinear probe 2–6 MHz.

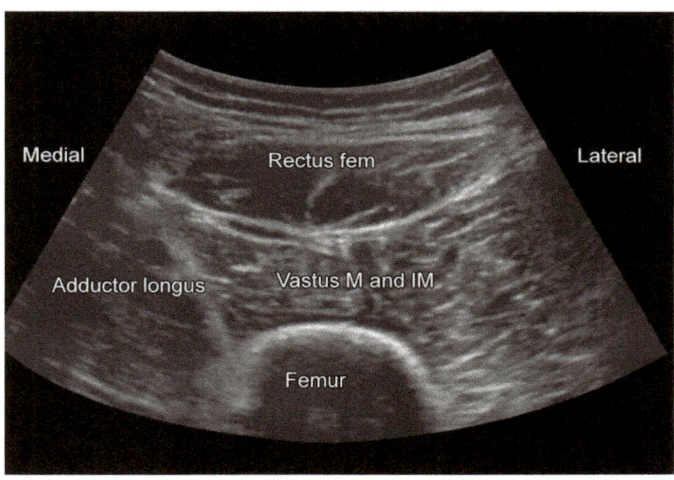

Fig. 6: *Step 2:* Scan of short-axis view of midshaft of the femur up until the convex surface becomes flat denting the greater trochanter.

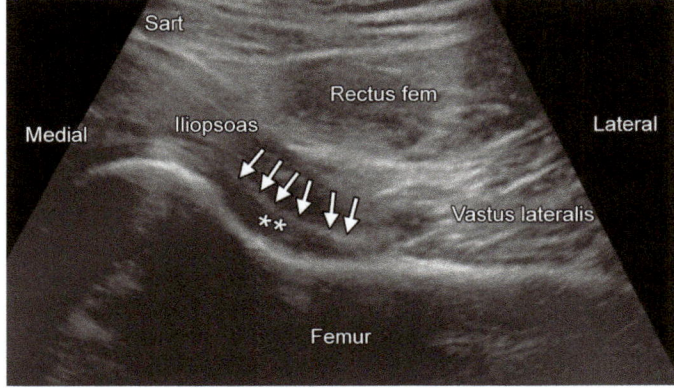

Fig. 7: *Step 3:* Align the probe to get a long-axis view of the acetabulum, head, neck, and shaft of the femur. The capsule and the anterior synovial recess (**) can be seen and accessed.

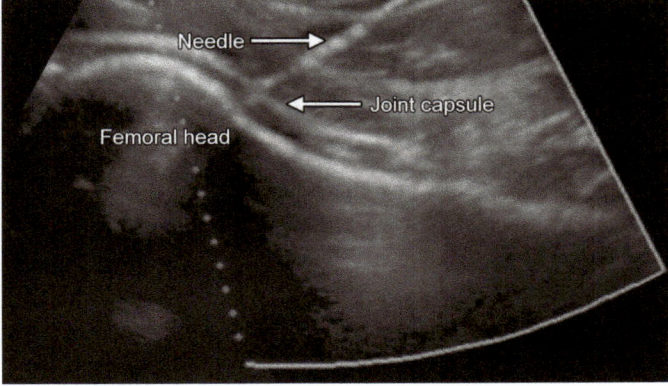

Fig. 8: *Step 4:* Insert the block needle in-plane from inferolateral to superomedial into the anterior synovial recess.

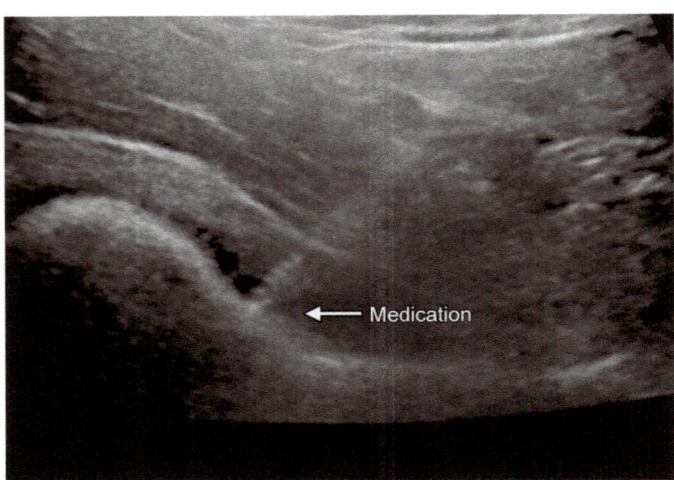

Fig. 9: *Step 5:* Using color Doppler, observe the injectate distending the capsule with cephalad spread.

Chapter 34: Greater Trochanteric Bursa Injection

Yehia Kamel

BASIC INFORMATION

Indications

Greater trochanteric pain syndrome (GTPS): This is a broad term that encompasses various causes of pain on the lateral aspect of the thigh over the greater trochanter. These include:
- Bursae
- Gluteus minimus and/or gluteus medius (most commonly) muscles or tendons
- Piriformis
- Quadrates femoris

Contraindications
- Patient refusal
- Systemic or local infection
- Coagulopathy
- True contrast allergy (in injections under fluoroscopy)
- Raised blood sugar/poorly controlled DM in case of steroids injection

Injectate

LA and steroids: 3-5 mL of 0.25% bupivaicne/levo-bupovacaine/lignocaine 1% or 2% + 1 mL/40 mg depo-steroid (triamcinolone or methylprednisolone)

TECHNIQUE FLUOROSCOPY

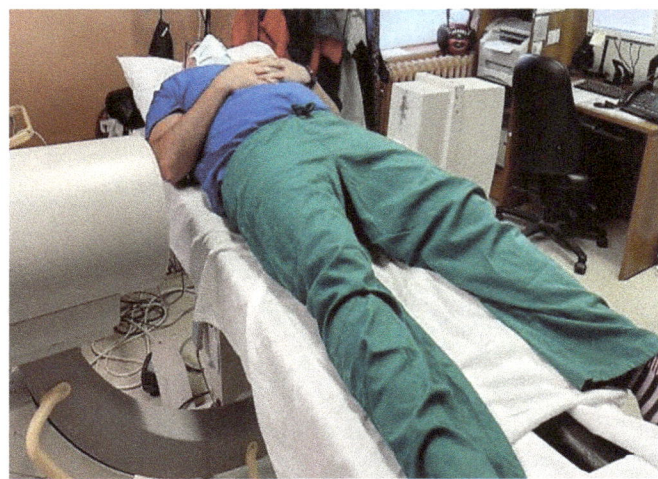

Fig. 1: Patient in supine position and C-arm in lateral position.

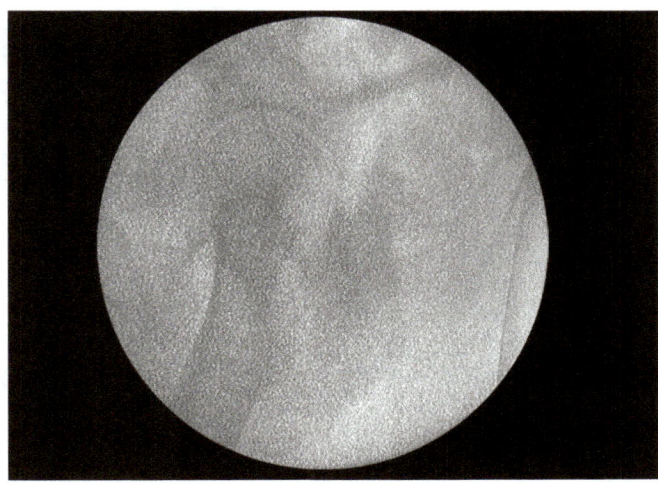

Fig. 2: Greater trochanter and head of femur seen.

Step 1: Place the patient in the supine position and place the C-arm in a lateral position.

Step 2: Get a lateral image of the hip that shows the greater trochanter, the head of the femur, the neck and the acetabulum.

SECTION 7 | Peripheral Blocks

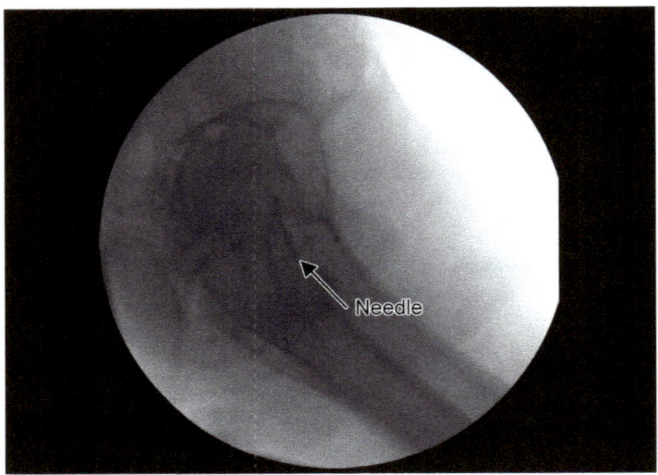

Fig. 3: Needle in tunnel vision aiming at greater trochanter.

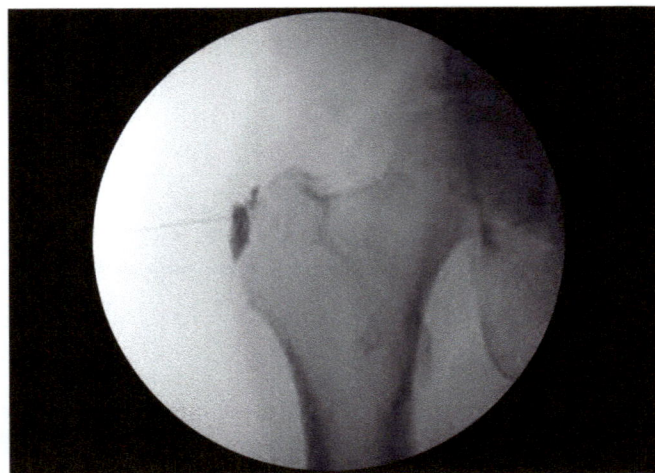

Fig. 4: Contrast spread in AP view.

Step 3: Direct the needle in tunnel vision aiming at the greater trochanter

Step 4: Obtain an AP image and inject contrast. If adequate inject the LA + steroids.

ULTRASOUND

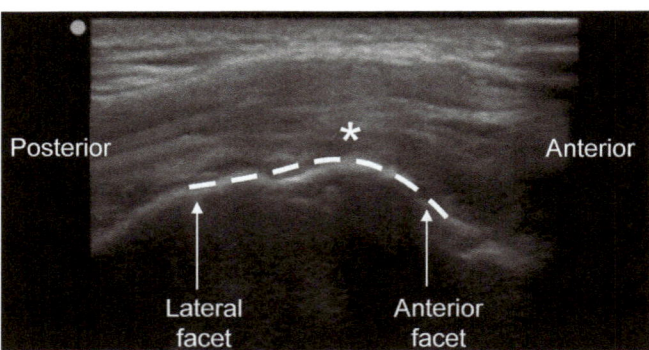

Fig. 5: Scanning of greater trochanter in transverse axis.

Step 1: Palpate the trochanter and scan in a transverse, short axis view until you reach the 'ridge' that separates the trochanter into anterior and lateral facets. Normally use a linear transducer 5–12 MHz unless very obese use a curvilinear probe 2–6 MHz.

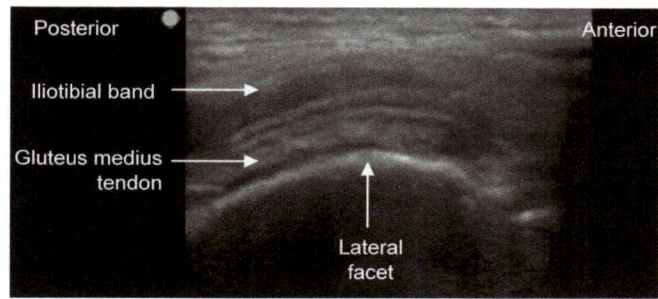

Fig. 6: Attachment of gluteus medius tendon.

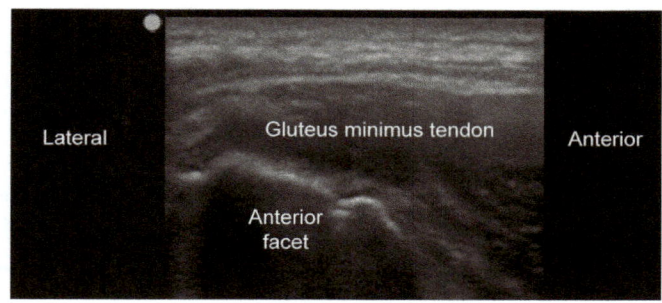

Fig. 7: Attachment of gluteus minimus tendon.

Step 2: Short axis view showing the attachment of the tendon of gluteus medium to the lateral facet of the trochanter.

Step 3: Short axis view showing the attachment of the tendon of gluteus minimum to the anterior facet.

For injection, use an in plane technique above the tendons whether the gluteus medius or minimum.

CHAPTER 35

Popliteal Nerve Block

Yashwant Laxman Nankar, Dwarkadas K Baheti

BASIC INFORMATION

The popliteal block is a proven, safe technique used extensively to provide pain relief for distal lower extremity. In comparison to proximal approaches to the sciatic nerve, the nerve block into the popliteal fossa preserves hamstring function, allowing easier ambulation of the patient.

Indications
- Acute pain management in emergency department
- Postoperative pain therapy at home for an ambulatory surgery setting
- Treatment of patients with complex regional pain syndrome (CRPS) to alleviate pain and allow intense physiotherapy
- Increase blood flow after vascular accidents.
- Trauma patients to be provided analgesia during transport to distal treatment center, especially from battlefield wounds
- Cancer-related pain in lower limbs

Contraindications

Absolute
- Unwilling patient
- Local infection
- Bleeding disorders
- Allergy to local anesthetics

Relative
- Nonavailability of needle insertion site because of a splint/cast/dressing
- Systemic infection

EQUIPMENT
- An insulated stimulating needle (which can be connected to a nerve stimulator)
- Nerve stimulator
- Marker pen, metal marker
- 26-gauge, ½-inch needle for local infiltration
- 18-gauge, 1½-inch needle
- 2-, 5-, and 10-mL syringes

DRUGS
- Inj. lidocaine 2% (maximum dosage 300 mg plain, 500 mg with epinephrine. Duration is 1–1.5 hours plain and 2–3 hours with epinephrine).
- Inj. bupivacaine or ropivacaine, 0.5%, preservative free (maximum dosage 250 mg. Duration is 2–8 hours)
- Inj. normal saline (0.9%)

PREPROCEDURE PREPARATION
- Rule out red flags such as infection, trauma, tumor, and significant neurological deficit.
- Obtain a written informed consent.
- Blood investigations such as bleeding time (BT), clotting time (CT), triple H, and blood sugar
- Secure intravenous line.
- Anesthesiologists standby with monitoring of pulse, blood pressure, oxygen saturation (SaO_2), and electrocardiogram (ECG)
- Antibiotics as per institutional protocol

TIPS
- Studies have shown that inversion of the foot leads to the best sensory and motor block, and dorsiflexion of the foot is second best.
- Occasionally, a local twitch of the biceps femoris muscle is elicited after needle insertion, indicating that needle placement is too lateral and must be redirected slightly medial.
- Conversely, if local twitching of the semitendinosus and semimembranosus muscles occurs, needle placement is too medial and must be redirected slightly more lateral.
- If no motor response is obtained with initial stimulation, then subsequent attempts should be made more lateral (rather than more medial, which causes a risk of inadvertent vascular penetration).
- Vascular puncture and intravascular injection are rare with this block because the nerve is superficial to the popliteal artery and vein at this location.

- Stimulation should be attempted as cephalad as possible in the popliteal fossa, making it less likely that the sciatic nerve has divided at that point, and improving block success.

COMPLICATIONS

- Increased pain in area of injection
- Infection
- Hematoma

PROCEDURE (REFER TO VIDEO NO. 12)

Step 1: After position **(Fig. 1)**, the three landmarks **(Fig. 2)** are identified and marked with pen: (1) Popliteal crease; (2) Tendons of biceps femoris (lateral); and (3) Semitendinosus (medial).

After local anesthesia, a Stimuplex needle is inserted at entry point which is about 7 cm superior to the popliteal crease at the midpoint between each identified tendons, which is approximately 1 cm lateral to the apex of the popliteal triangle **(Fig. 1)**.

Step 2: Needle placement
- Needle is advanced at a 45–60° angle to the skin in a cephalad direction **(Fig. 3)** for about an inch.
- Set the nerve stimulator initially between 1.0 and 1.2 mA.
- Advance anteriorly until the desired nerve is stimulated.

Step 3: Stimulation response (Refer to Video No. 12)
- Inversion of the foot indicates stimulation of the tibial and deep peroneal nerves.
- Eversion of the foot indicates stimulation of the superficial peroneal nerve.
- Plantar flexion indicates stimulation of the posterior tibial nerve.
- Dorsiflexion indicates stimulation of the deep peroneal nerve.

When stimulation response is localized, the output current of the nerve stimulator is then gradually adjusted to the lowest current at which these responses are still obtained (goal is <0.4 mA).

If stimulation is obtained at <0.2 mA, the needle should be slightly withdrawn as stimulation at such a small current intensity may indicate an intraneural placement of the needle.

Step 4: Drug injection

After appropriate stimulation at the desired current level and aspiration of needle to ensure nonintravascular placement, injection of 30–40 cc of local anesthetic may be injected for block.

Drug Injection

After appropriate stimulation at the desired current level and aspiration of needle to ensure nonintravascular placement, injection of 30–40 cc of local anesthetic may be injected for block.

Continuous Technique (Refer to Video No. 12)

With the patient is in the prone position, landmarks are marked. The site of puncture is between the upper muscular borders of the popliteal fossa, in the midline, at least 7 cm above the popliteal skin crease. A Contiplex needle connected to a peripheral nerve stimulator is introduced at an angle of 45° to the skin and advanced in an anterior and cephalad direction. Its position is judged adequate when output <1 mA

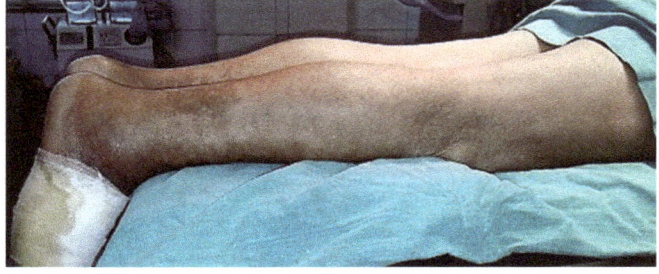

Fig. 1: Position of patient.

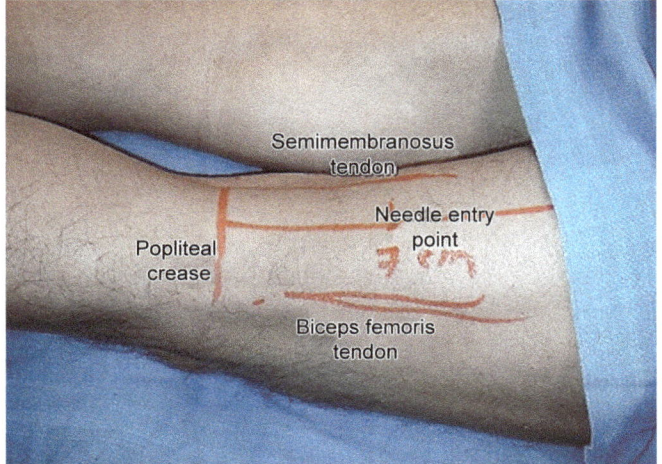

Fig. 2: Surface marking.

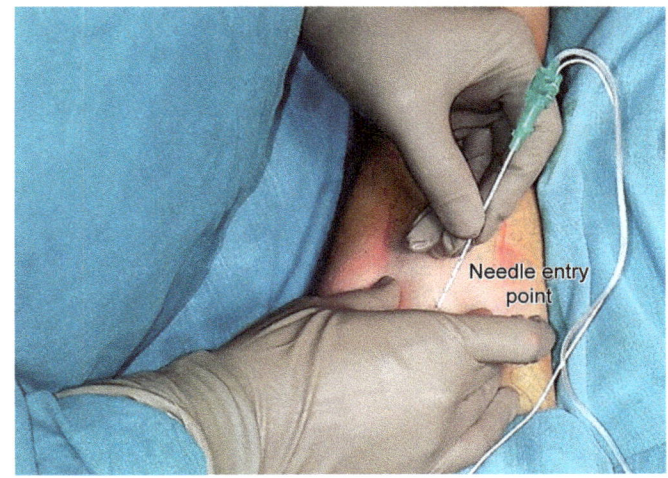

Fig. 3: Needle entry point.

elicits a slight motor response of the foot. The stylet of the needle is then removed, and a catheter is introduced. After an aspiration test, a drug is injected. The needle is removed and dressing applied to fix the catheter. Drug injected intermittently as bolus or continuous infusion with pump.

ULTRASOUND-GUIDED TECHNIQUE POPLITEAL BLOCK

Procedure Details

This procedure can be performed in supine, lateral or prone position. However, lateral position is most preferred one as it is comfortable

Step 1: Position of patient—Lateral **(Fig. 4)**
- Lateral—identify popliteal crease. High-frequency ultrasound (US) probe is used.

Step 2: Identify vessels **(Fig. 5)**
- Begin with the transducer in the transverse position parallel to the popliteal crease; the popliteal artery is identified, aided with the color Doppler ultrasound, when necessary, at a depth of 3–4 cm.
- The popliteal vein accompanies the artery.

Step 3: Identify nerves
- Superficial (i.e., toward the skin surface) and lateral to the artery is the tibial nerve, seen as a hyperechoic, oval, or round structure with a stippled or honeycomb pattern on the interior.
- If difficulty in identifying the nerve is encountered, the patient can be asked to dorsiflex and plantar flex the ankle, which makes the nerve rotate or move in relation to its surroundings.
- Once the tibial nerve is identified, an attempt can be made to visualize the common peroneal nerve, which is located even more superficial and lateral to the tibial nerve.

Step 4: Identify sciatic nerve
- The transducer should be slid proximally until the tibial and peroneal nerves are visualized coming together to form the sciatic nerve before its division **(Figs. 6 and 7)**.

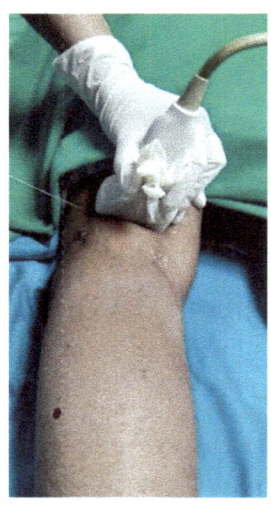

Fig. 4: Position of patient.

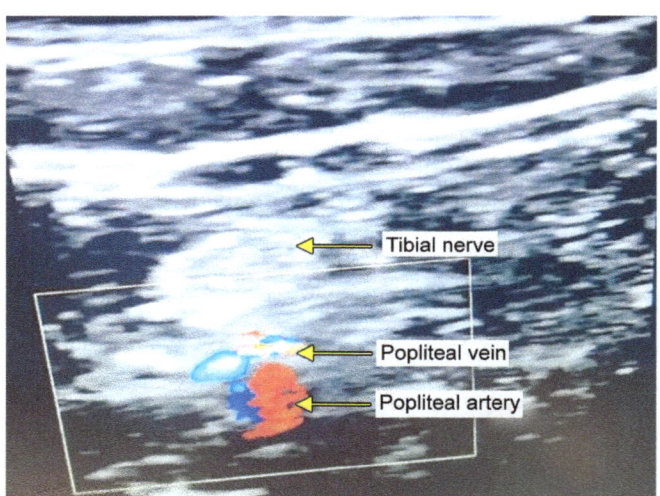

Fig. 5: Identify vessels.

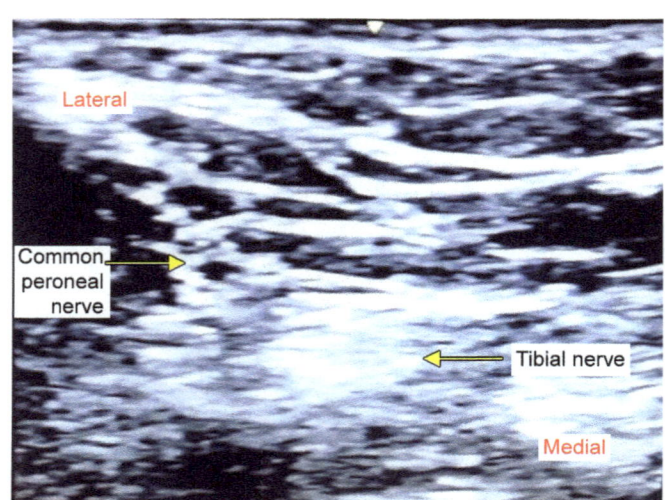

Fig. 6: Identify nerves.

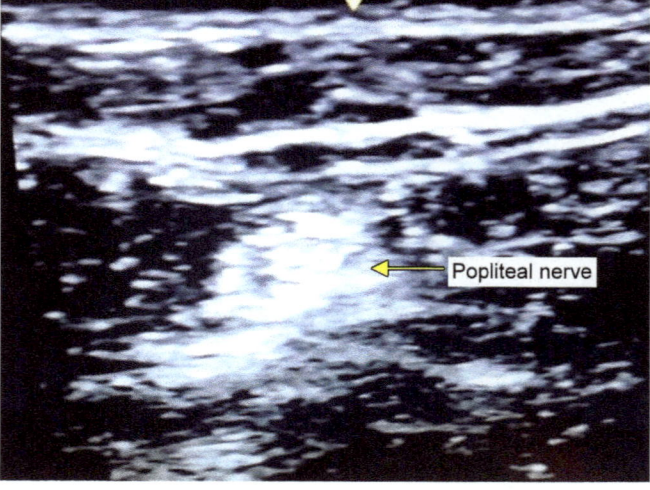

Fig. 7: Identify popliteal nerve.

Step 5:
- Once identified, a skin wheal is made on the lateral aspect of the thigh 2–3 cm above the lateral edge of the transducer.
- Then the needle is inserted in-plane in a horizontal orientation from the lateral aspect of the thigh and advanced toward the sciatic nerve.
- Once the needle tip is witnessed adjacent to the nerve, and after careful aspiration, 1–2 mL of local anesthetic is injected to confirm the proper injection site.
- Such injection should result in distribution of the local anesthetic within the epineural sheath, and often, separation of the tibial nerve (TN) and common peroneal nerve (CPN).

Declaration

Part of the text and some images are taken with permission from M/s Jaypee Brothers Medical Publishers, New Delhi from the chapter "Popliteal Nerve of Sciatic Nerve Block" published in the book, *Interventional Pain Management: Practical Approach* 2009 and 2018 edited by DK Baheti, Sanjay Bakshi, Sanjeeva Gupta, and RP Gehdoo.

CHAPTER 36: Calcaneal Spur Injection

Dwarkadas K Baheti

CALCANEAL SPUR

Basic Information

A calcaneal spur, or commonly known as a heel spur, occurs when a bony outgrowth forms on the heel bone. Calcaneal spurs can be located at the back of the heel (dorsal heel spur) or under the sole (plantar heel spur). The dorsal spurs are often associated with Achilles, while spurs under the sole are associated with plantar fasciitis.

The apex of the spur lies either within the origin of the planter fascia (on the medial tubercle of the calcaneus) or superior to it (in the origin of the flexor digitorum brevis muscle). The relationship between spur formation and the medial tubercle of the calcaneus and intrinsic heel musculature results in a constant pulling effect on the plantar fascia resulting in an inflammatory response.

Causes

Repetitive trauma—result of strained muscles or ligaments in the foot. Athletes, particularly those who run and jump, are at risk of developing this.

- An abnormal gait, or walking pattern, that unevenly distributed weight and pressure on the heel.
- *Running on hard surfaces:* Wearing shoes that do not fit well or that do not provide sufficient support for your arches.
- Being overweight or obese
- Being of an advanced age
- Standing for extended periods of time during the workday
- Diabetes

Symptoms of Heel Spurs

Often, there are no symptoms associated with heel spurs. Pain occurs and is more intense while the patient is walking, running, or jogging. Inflammation can develop which results in pain that many describe as knifing at first and then transitioning into a dull pain.

Treatment Options

The aim is to eliminate inflammation surrounding the spur include painkillers, heel and arch supports, exercises, shock wave therapy, and local steroid injections.

Physiotherapy

- Padding and strapping of the foot
- Therapeutic orthotic insoles for short-term pain relief Achilles and plantar fascia stretching
- Prefabricated OR custom-orthotic device
- Passive and active stretching and strengthening of the muscles of the legs, cold and hot applications (contrast bath)
- Laser treatment

Low-dose radiotherapy (radiation side effects and syndromes): Cryo-ultrasound therapy and cryotherapy are both effective for treating chronic plantar fasciitis with heel spurs.

Thermotherapy: Cold therapy may be used to relieve inflammation and reduce pain. Heat therapy to loosen tense muscles, promote oxygen, and blood flow to the affected area ultrasound.

PROCEDURE

Step 1: After taking detailed history and clinical examination, it is advisable to confirm both ankle joints with X-ray. It could be unilateral or bilateral. The calcaneal spur is shown in **Figure 1**.

Step 2: Once the diagnosis is done, the injection at the site is mainstay in the treatment.

After cleaning and preparing of the respective heel, it is especially important to pinpoint the point of maximum tenderness.

Step 3: Mark the point of entry as shown in **Figure 2**.

Step 4: Do the repeated palpation of the maximum tender point as shown in **Figure 3**.

Step 5: Take a mixture of steroid, local anesthetic, and Inj. hyaluronidase 1,500 IU as shown in **Figure 4**.

Once again palpate the heel gently and mark the tender point as seen in **Figure 3**.

The aim is to inject in-to the target point, i.e., most tender area. The injection should be gentle, slow and in fan shaped fashion to cover wider area (**Fig. 4**).

CHAPTER 36 | Calcaneal Spur Injection

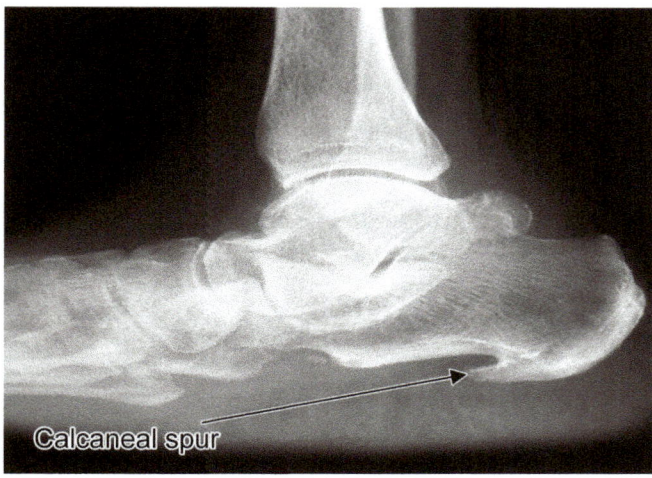

Fig. 1: Calcaneal spur.

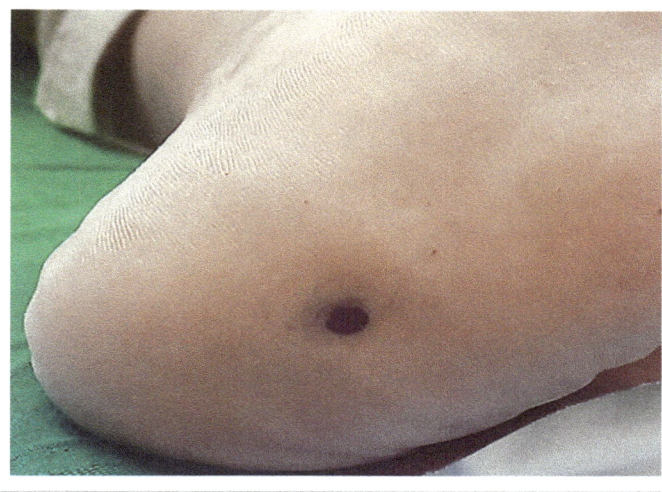

Fig. 2: Point of needle entry.

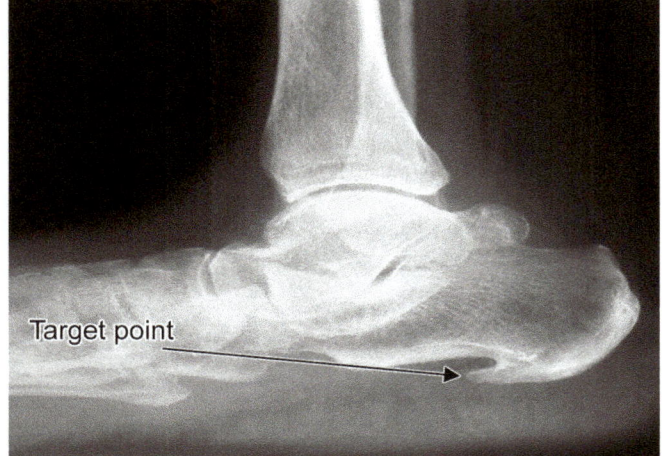

Fig. 3: Target point at spur.

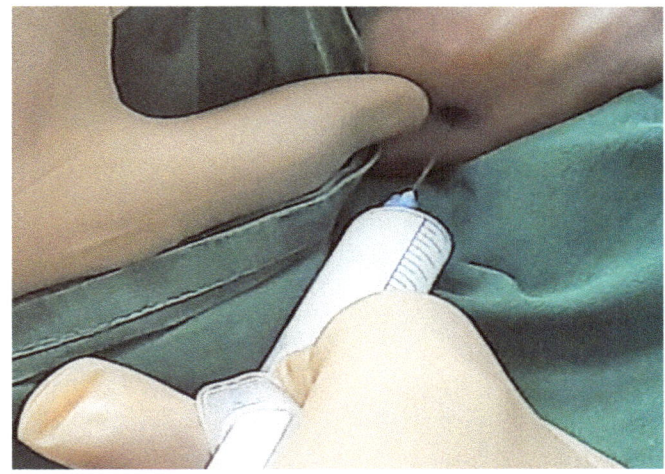

Fig. 4: Injecting the medication.

The total volume about 8–10 to be injected in the target and tender point.

Step 6: Observe and monitor the patient's vitals for 1 hour.

Step 7: Postinjection advice is to do hot fomentation at the heel immediately and at home too. Fomentation will fasten the absorption of the drug.

SECTION 8

Sympathetic Block

- **Stellate Ganglion Block**
  Preeti Doshi

- **Splanchnic Plexus Block: Fluoroscopy Guided**
  Dwarkadas K Baheti

- **CT-guided Splanchinc Plexus Block**
  Dwarkadas K Baheti

- **CT-guided Celiac Plexus Block**
  Dwarkadas K Baheti

- **Celiac Plexus Block: Fluoroscopy Guided**
  Dwarkadas K Baheti

- **Lumbar Sympathetic Plexus Block**
  Dwarkadas K Baheti

- **Superior Hypogastric Plexus Block**
  Dwarkadas K Baheti, Yashwant Laxman Nankar

- **Ganglion of Impar Block**
  Dwarkadas K Baheti

CHAPTER 37

Stellate Ganglion Block

Preeti Doshi

BASIC INFORMATION

Indications
- Pain syndromes of head, face, neck, and upper arm, e.g., complex regional pain syndromes (CRPS) I and II (post-traumatic syndromes), acute herpes zoster and postherpetic neuralgias, phantom limb pain, neoplastic infiltration of brachial plexus, postmastectomy neuropathic pain.
- Orofacial pain syndromes including neuropathic pain following trigeminal ganglion radiofrequency ablation.
- Circulatory insufficiency of the upper extremity, e.g., Raynaud's disease, vasculitis, ischemic pain following accidental intra-arterial injection of drugs such as sodium pentothal.

Contraindications
- Local infection
- Patient refusal
- Patients with coagulopathy or on anticoagulants
- Recent cardiac infarction
- Atrioventricular block
- Glaucoma

APPROACHES

BLIND (not recommended)

Image-guided (CT/Fluoroscopy/Ultrasonography Guided)

Drugs/volumes used: Ropivacaine 0.2% or Lignocaine 1%: 5–10 mL ± Dexamethasone 4 mg

For long-term relief: Radiofrequency ablation/chemical neurolysis (not recommended)

Step 1: Understanding of anatomy

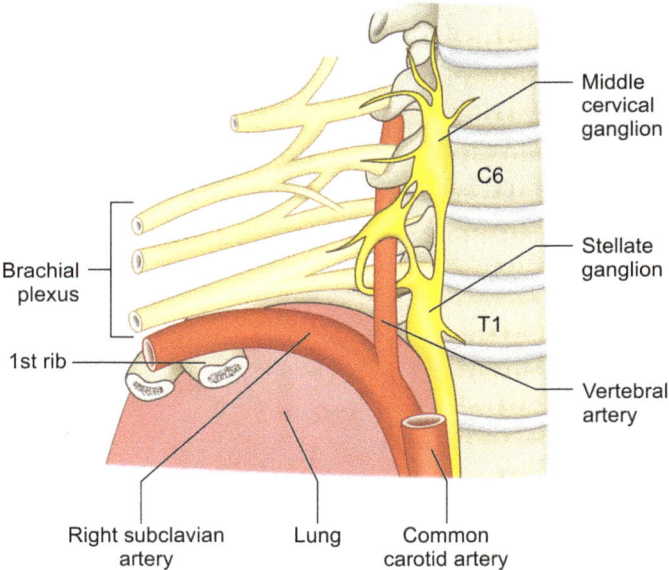

Fig. 1: Diagrammatic depiction of the anatomy of stellate ganglion.

Step 2: Position of patient

Both upper extremities are parallel to the body and anterior neck painted and draped.

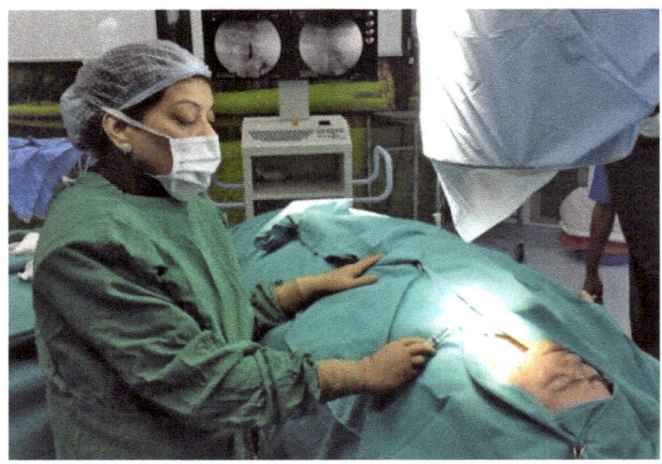

Fig. 2: Patient position—supine with neck extended on a radiolucent table: C-arm positioned for anteroposterior view.

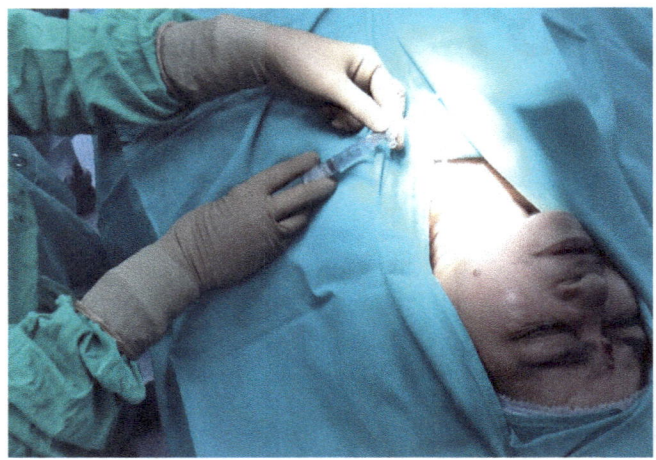

Fig. 3: Patient position—supine with neck extended on radiolucent table—close-up.

FLUOROSCOPIC LANDMARKS AND RELEVANT IMAGES

Step 1: Confirming of marker position

Step 2: Directing the spinal 22G needle at the transverse process of C7 vertebra.

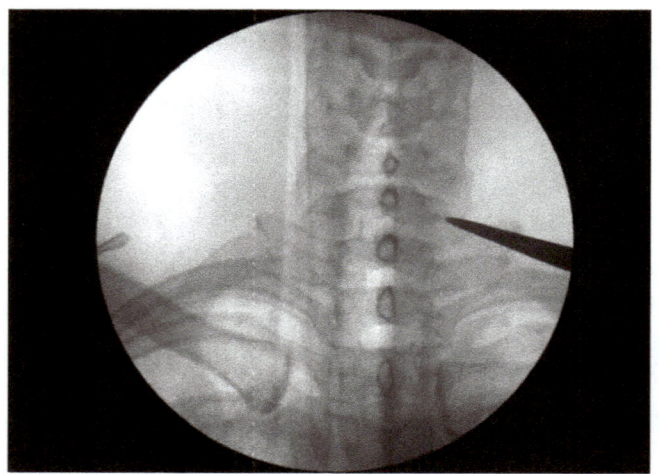

Fig. 4: Radiopaque marker positioned over the transverse process of left C7 vertebra.

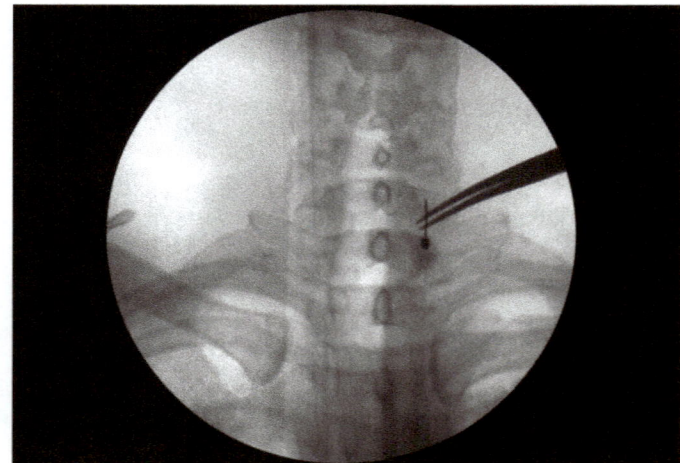

Fig. 5: Spinal needle (22G) positioned and maneuvered with an artery forceps for a tunnel view over the medial aspect of the transverse process of the left C7 vertebra.

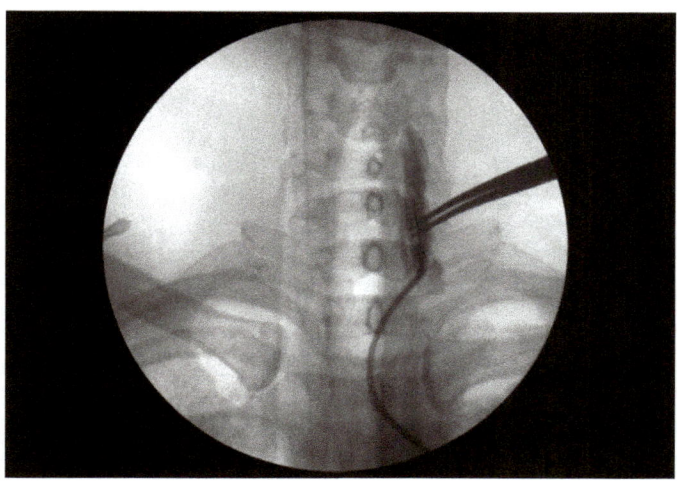

Fig. 6: Vertical spread of nonionic contrast—Iohexol 280 over the longus coli muscle.

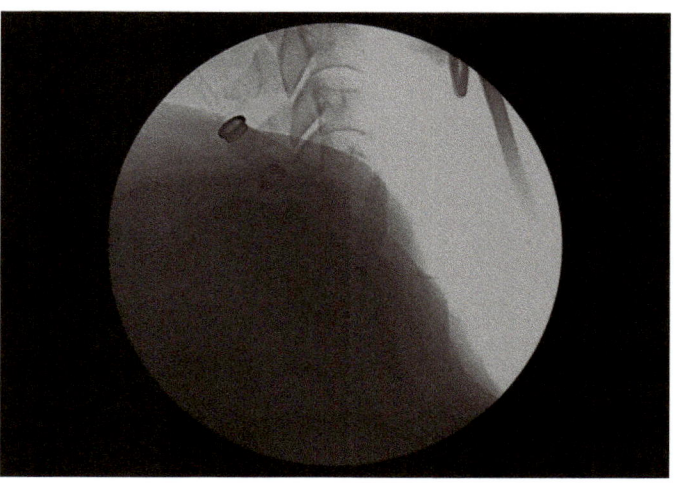

Fig. 7: Lateral view showing contrast spreading up to the anterior aspect of the C5 vertebral body.

POSTPROCEDURE OBSERVATION IN RECOVERY AREA

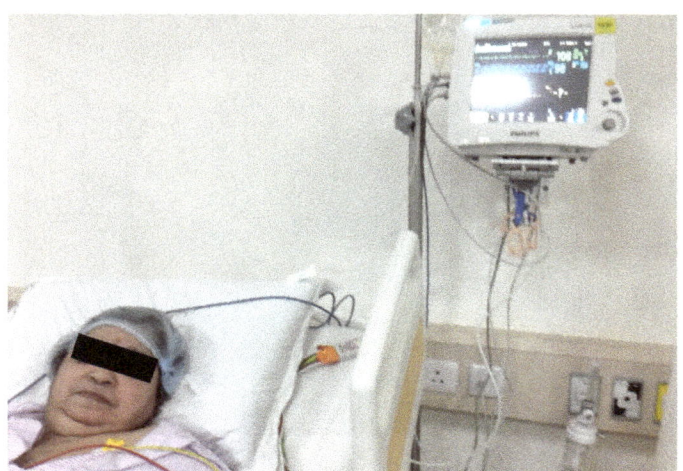

Fig. 8: Patient in the recovery area with vital monitoring attached.

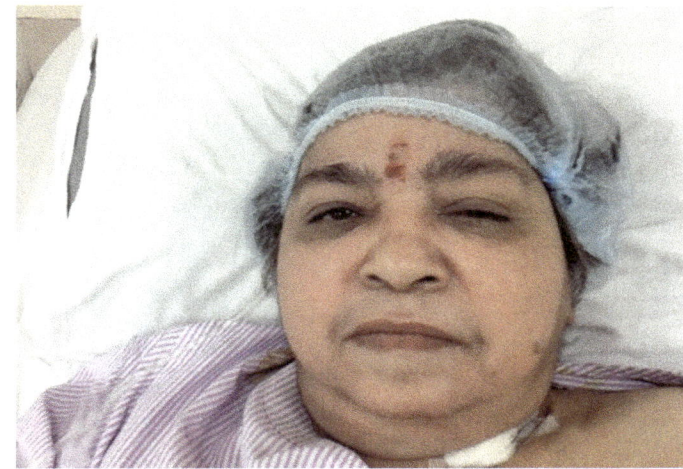

Fig. 9: Patient with features of Horner's syndrome on the left side after stellate ganglion block.

RADIOFREQUENCY ABLATION OF STELLATE GANGLION

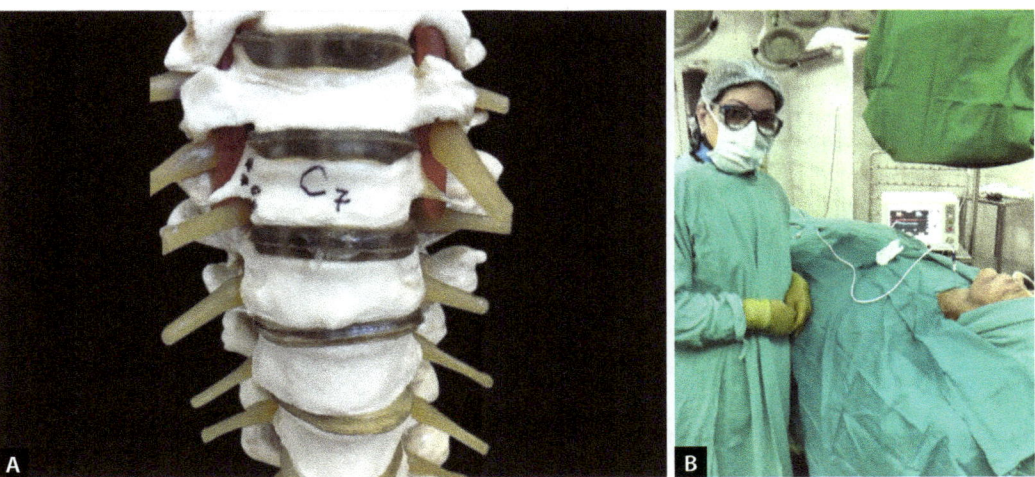

Figs. 10A and B: Three target points and set-up for stellate ganglion radiofrequency ablation.

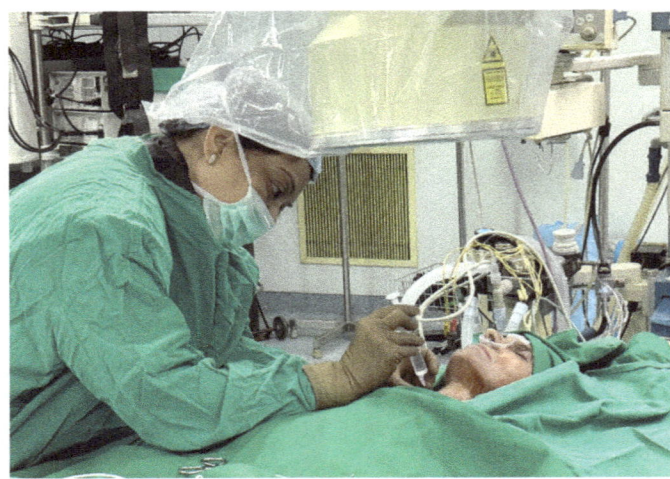

Fig. 11: Supine position of patient for (R) stellate radiofrequency ablation—local anesthesia + monitored care.

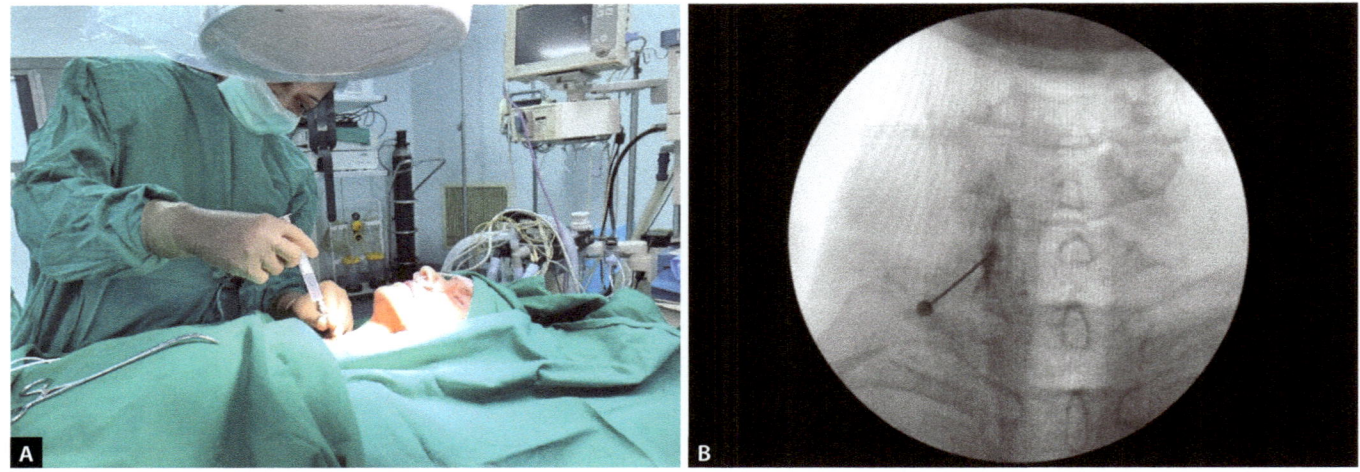

Figs. 12A and B: Injection of contrast medium to confirm radiofrequency needle-tip position over the target point of C7 vertebra.

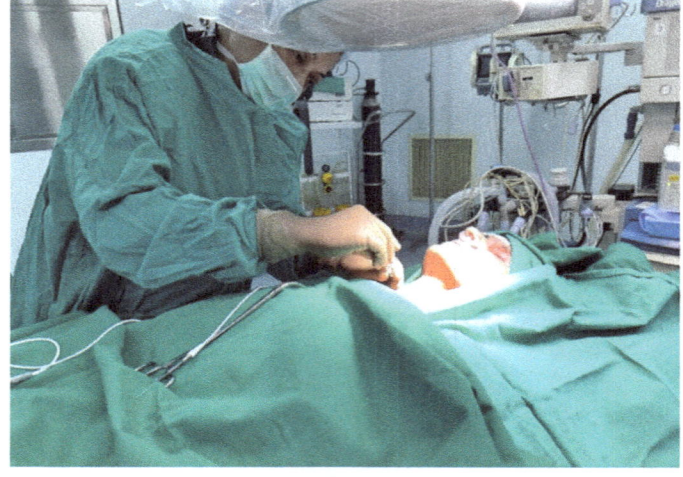

Fig. 13: Thermistor probe assembly ready for introduction through 10-cm 22G, 5-mm tip radiofrequency needle.

ULTRASOUND-GUIDED BLOCK OF STELLATE GANGLION

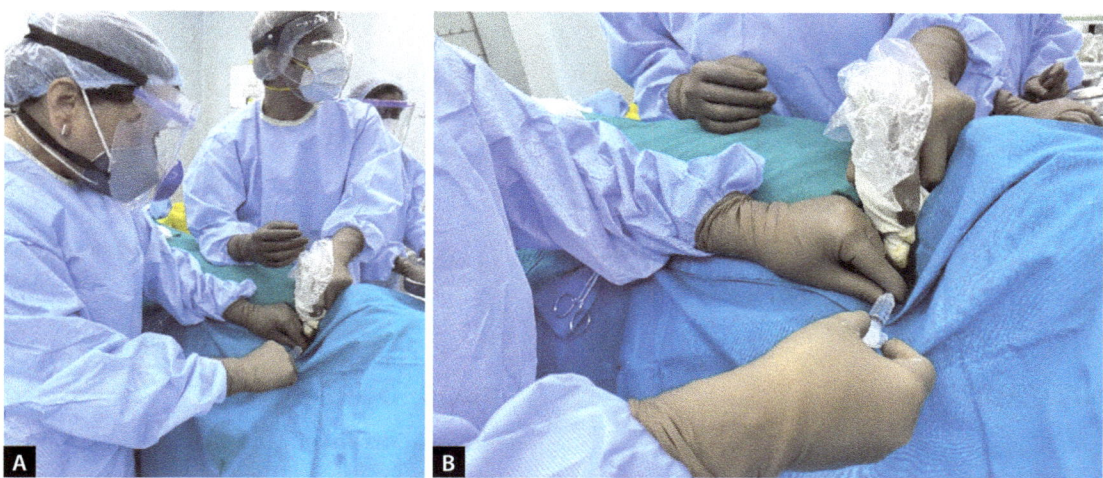

Figs. 14A and B: Left stellate ganglion injection under ultrasound guidance.

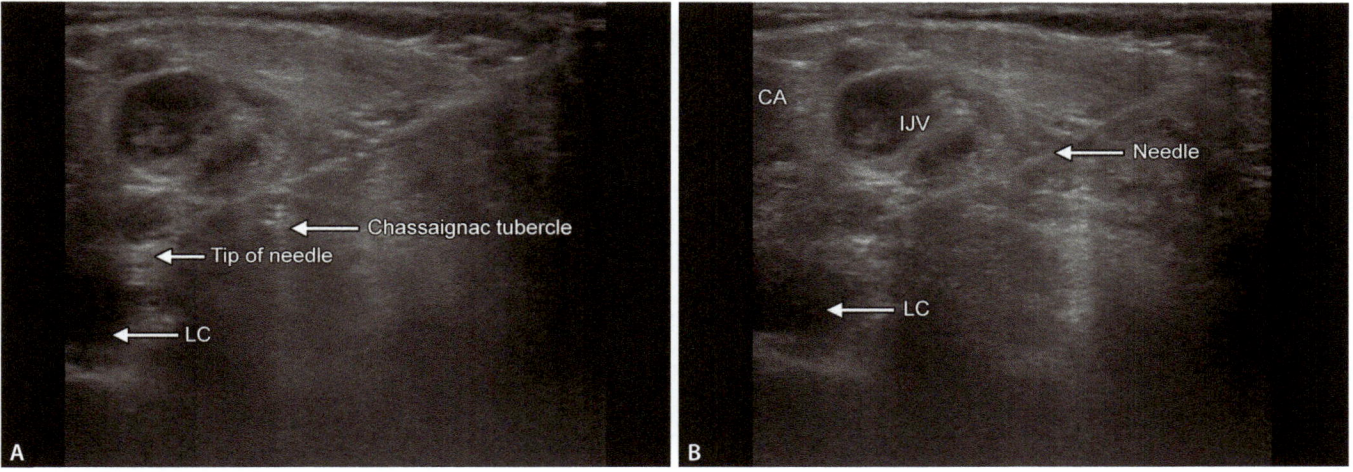

Figs. 15A and B: Sonoanatomy landmarks with needle trajectory for left stellate ganglion injection. (CA: carotid artery; IJV: internal jugular vein; LC: longus coli)

CHAPTER 38

Splanchnic Plexus Block: Fluoroscopy Guided

Dwarkadas K Baheti

BASIC INFORMATION

Indications

- Pain following surgery of stomach, liver, gallbladder, kidney, spleen, pancreas or retroperitoneal structures
- Pain from chronic pancreatitis
- Pain from alcoholic pancreatitis
- Any chronic upper abdominal pain of unknown origin

Contraindications

- On anticoagulant therapy
- Coagulopathies
- Patient with ethanol abuse
- Local skin infection
- Patient on disulfiram therapy for alcohol abuse

DRUGS AND ITS CONCENTRATION

- Inj. lignocaine 2% preservative-free
- Absolute alcohol
- Normal saline
- Inj. bupivacaine 0.5%

Important Tips

- Keep in mind that the procedure is under local anesthesia and sedation.
- Try to be as gentle as possible while redirecting and pushing the needle in deeper plane toward the destination.
- Pushing of the needle in the deeper planes must be slow and gentle and centimeter by centimeter.
- Always confirm the position of needle under fluoroscopy/CT in anteroposterior and lateral positions.
- Repeated negative aspiration at every step.

PROCEDURE DETAILS

Step 1: Position and landmarks

Position: Patient in prone position with pillow under the abdomen (keeps thoracolumbar spine flexed), with head turned to one side and arms as per the patient's comfort (by the side of the patient or hanging freely off the side of the table for the posterior approach).

For a CT-guided block, the anterior approach can also be used making it comfortable for the patient in supine position.

Landmarks: Identify T11 and T12 vertebral bodies with 12th rib in posteroanterior (PA) view. Now with fluoroscopic C-arm rotated 5–10° obliquely toward the ipsilateral side, mark the point below the transverse process, along the pedicle as the entry site of needle. The site of the marker is shown in **Figure 1**.

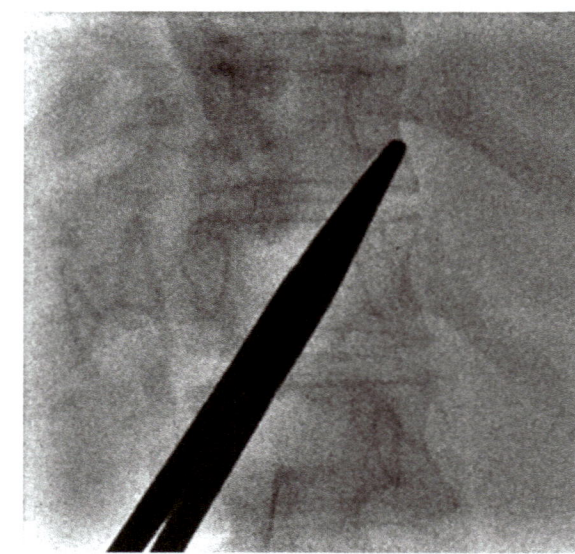

Fig. 1: Position of marker.

Step 2: Needle entry: The entry point is above the twelfth rib 6–8 CM at the edge of the lateral border of the body of the twelfth vertebra, around one third down the vertebral body.

Now, insert 20G, 15-cm styletted (Chiba or long spinal) needle and direct it medially toward the T12 vertebral body by avoiding the injury exiting the nerve root.

Here, the aim is to establish a "tunnel" view of the needle, i.e., the needle should move toward the target as a pinhead **(Fig. 2)**. Now do repeated negative aspiration for blood or cerebrospinal fluid (CSF) to confirm that the needle has not penetrated any vessel or organ.

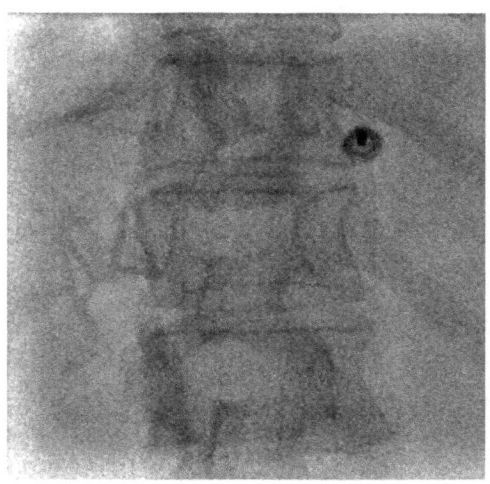

Fig. 2: Tunnel view.

Step 3: Now, push the needle in deeper planes. Here, one may feel the grating sensation as the needle moves along the lateral part of the T12 vertebral body.

Confirm needle placement at the junction of the anterior one-third and posterior two-thirds of the vertebral body in lateral and posteroanterior views **(Figs. 3 and 4)**. Once again, confirm negative aspiration.

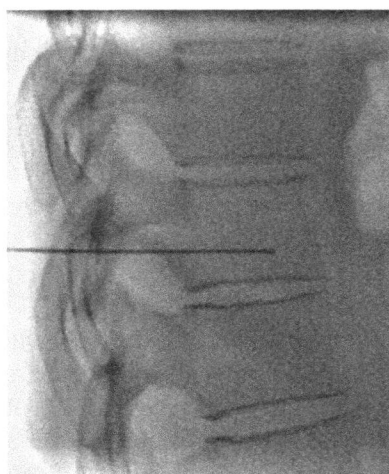

Fig. 3: Needle position in lateral view.

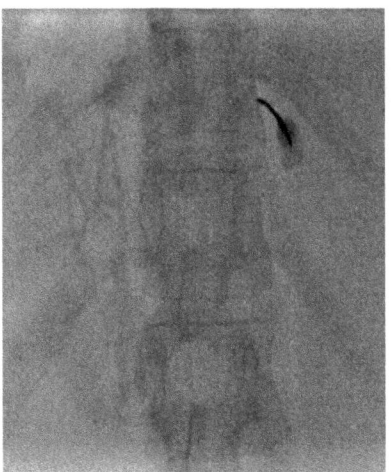

Fig. 4: Needle position in anteroposterior view.

Step 4: After negative aspiration, inject 1–2 mL of Inj. omnipaque (nonionic water-soluble) contrast. Confirm the dye spread in anteroposterior (AP) and lateral views. In AP view, the dye should be along the anterolateral border of T11 and T12 vertebrae in a linear pattern **(Fig. 5)** and in lateral view along the border of vertebra **(Fig. 6)**.

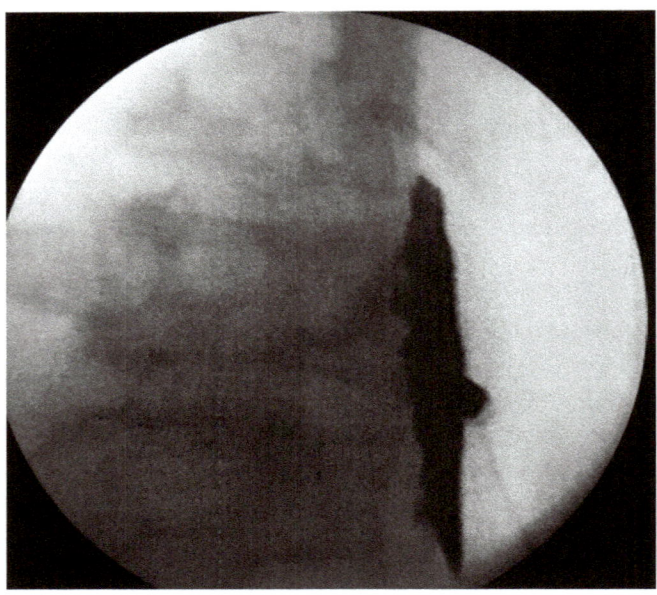

Fig. 5: Dye spread—anteroposterior view.

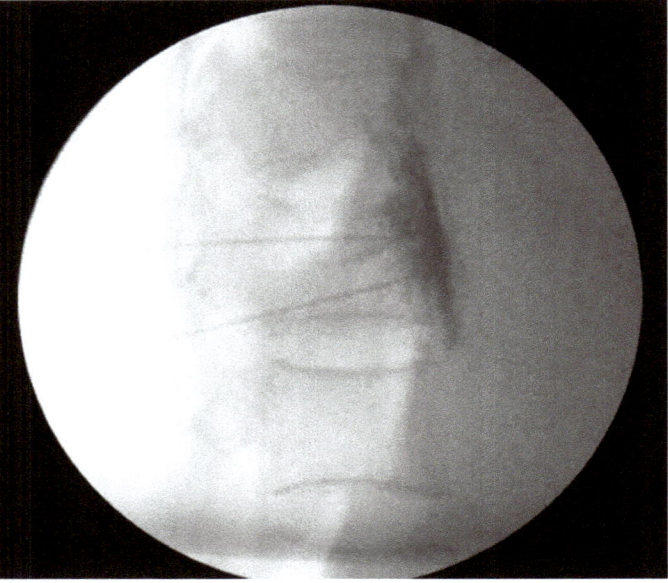

Fig. 6: Dye spread—lateral view.

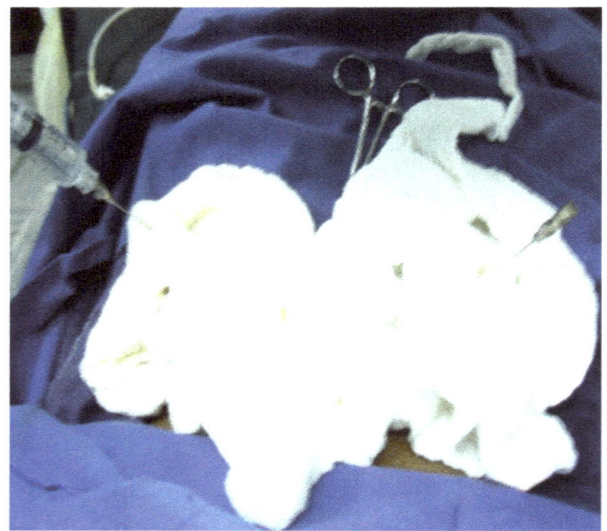

Fig. 7: Sponge around needle.

Step 5: Now, put a sponge around the needle **(Fig. 7)** to avoid spillage of a neurolytic agent on the skin.

After repeated negative aspiration, inject mixture of Inj. alcohol 50% with Inj. bupivacaine 0.25%; 20–25 cc should be injected slowly on both sides with intermittent negative aspiration. Now put the stylet back into the needle to prevent spillage of neurolytic agent on skin.

Last, withdraw needle while injecting local anesthetic into the needle track to decrease postprocedure pain and needle site.

Step 8: Once the vitals of the patient are checked and are within normal limits, then shift him to the recovery room and monitoring of vital signs must be done for at least 2 hours before shifting to the ward.

Declaration

Part of the text and some images are taken with permission from M/s Jaypee Brothers Medical Publishers, New Delhi, from the chapter "Splanchnic Plexus Block" published in the book, *Interventional Pain Management: Practical Approach* 2009 and 2018 edited by DK Baheti, Sanjay Bakshi, Sanjeeva Gupta, and RP Gehdoo.

CHAPTER 39: CT-guided Splanchinc Plexus Block

Dwarkadas K Baheti

BASIC INFORMATION

Indications
- Any pain originating from the upper abdominal viscera such as stomach, liver, gallbladder, kidney, spleen, pancreas, aortic lymphadenopathy, omental mass, and retroperitoneal tumors
- Pain due to chronic pancreatitis and alcoholic pancreatitis
- Any chronic upper abdominal pain of unknown origin

Contraindications
- Anticoagulation therapy or suffer from congenital abnormalities of coagulopathy
- Antiblastic cancer therapy
- Liver abnormalities associated with ethanol abuse
- The local skin infection at needle entry point or intra-abdominal infection and sepsis, intestinal obstruction
- Use of alcohol as a neurolytic agent should be avoided in a patient with disulfiram therapy for alcohol abuse.

Drugs and Concentration
- Inj. lignocaine: 2% (Xylocard—preservative free)
- Absolute alcohol
- Normal saline
- Inj. bupivacaine 0.25%

RECENT ADVANCES AND ITS IMPLICATIONS

The blunt tip needle recently introduced by the author for celiac plexus block and lumbar sympathectomy may further reduce the rate of iatrogenic complications such as injury to vessels and peritoneum and can be reduced.

The blunt tip needle used by the author is a 20G needle (locally made) of stainless steel and can be repeatedly autoclaved.

IMPORTANT TIPS
- Keep in mind that the procedure is under local and sedation.
- Try to be as gentle as possible while redirecting and pushing the needle in deeper plane toward the destination.
- Pushing of the needle in the deeper planes must be slow and gentle and centimeter by centimeter.
- Always confirm the position of the needle under fluoroscopy/CT in anteroposterior and lateral positions.
- Repeated negative aspiration at every step.

PROCEDURE DETAILS

The steps under CT guidance for the block are same as under fluoroscopy. The main difference lies in it being done under CT guidance.

Step 1: Posterior approach using two-needle techniques:
Patient is placed in prone position. Obtain a screening CT scan of T11–L1 area (2-mm slice thickness).

Step 2: Mark the point of insertion of needle with the help of laser on both sides. Estimate the trajectory of needle (**Fig. 1**).

Step 3: Now direct the needles one by one toward the anterior border of T12 vertebra and confirm it under CT (**Fig. 2**).

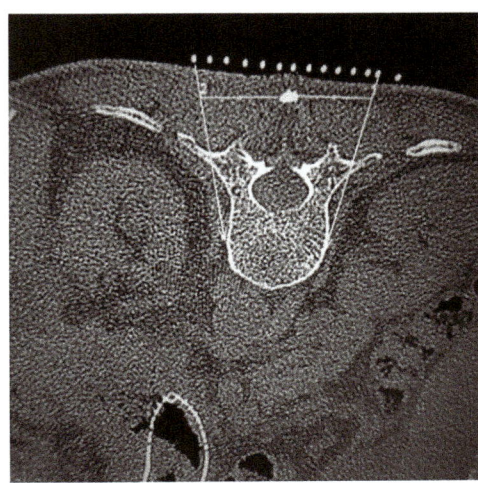

Fig. 1: Distance from skin to body of T12 vertebrae.

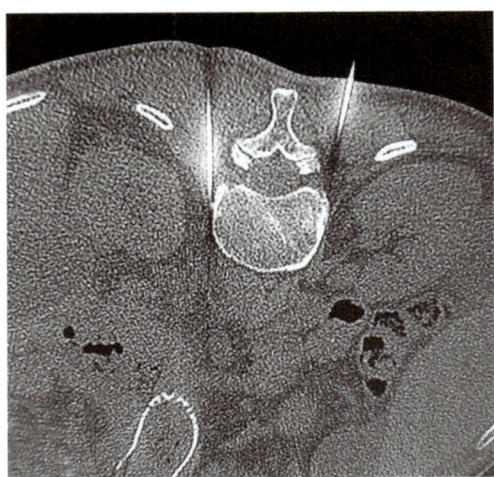 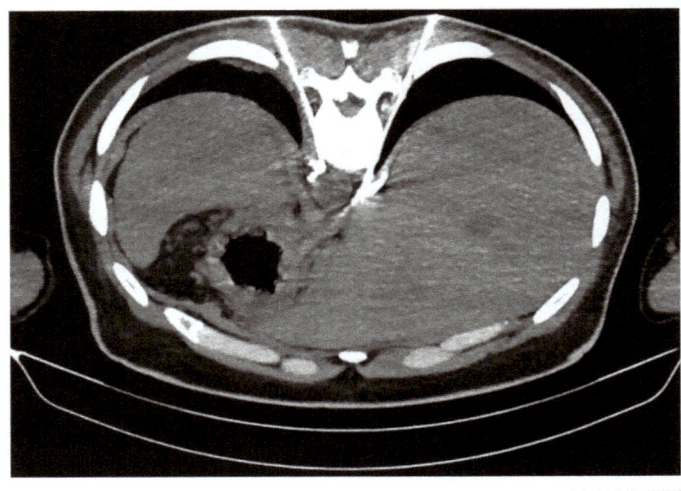

Fig. 2: Lt. needle at T12 vertebrae.

Fig. 3: Dye spread on both sides under CT.

Step 4: Now inject nonionic dye Inj. omnipaque 2–3 cc and confirm the spread of dye **(Fig. 3)**.

Follow the same protocol for injection of neurolytic agent as under fluoroscopy.

If radiofrequency is required, then lesioning is done accordingly.

Observe the patient's vitals for 1 hour and then shift to the ward.

Declaration

Part of the text and some images are taken with permission from M/s Jaypee Brothers Medical Publishers, New Delhi, from the chapter "Splanchnic Plexus Block" published in the book, *Interventional Pain Management: Practical Approach* 2009 and 2018 edited by DK Baheti, Sanjay Bakashi, Sanjeeva Gupta, and RP Gehdoo.

CHAPTER 40

CT-guided Celiac Plexus Block

Dwarkadas K Baheti

BASIC INFORMATION

Indications
- Any pain originating form upper abdominal viscera such as stomach, liver, gallbladder, kidney, spleen, pancreas, aortic lymphadenopathy, omental mass, retroperitoneal tumors, and any chronic upper abdominal pain of unknown origin.
- Pain due to chronic pancreatitis and alcoholic pancreatitis.

Contraindications
- Anticoagulation therapy or suffer from congenital abnormalities of coagulopathy
- Antiblastic cancer therapy
- Liver abnormalities associated with ethanol abuse.
- The local skin infection at needle entry point or intra-abdominal infection and sepsis, intestinal obstruction
- The use of alcohol as neurolytic agent should be avoided in patient with disulfiram therapy for alcohol abuse.

Drugs and Concentration
- Inj. lignocaine—2% (Xylocard—preservative-free)
- Absolute alcohol
- Normal saline
- Inj. bupivacaine 0.25%

Complications
The iatrogenic complications reported during celiac plexus blocks are pneumothorax; partial lower extremity paralysis; temporary paraplegia. Iatrogenic complications such as chylothorax, pleural effusion, renal injury, and injury to veins also have been reported.

IMPORTANT TIPS
- Keep in mind the procedure is under local and sedation try to be as gentle as possible while redirecting and pushing the needle in deeper plane towards the destination.
- Movement of the needle in the deeper planes should be slow and centimeter by centimeter.
- Always confirm position of needle in AP and lateral position
- Repeated negative aspiration at every step.

PROCEDURE DETAILS

Step 1: Position and landmarks: The patient in prone position with a pillow under the abdomen to reverse to thoracolumbar lordosis and to increases the distance between costal margin and iliac crests and transverse processes of adjacent vertebral bodies (**Fig. 1**).

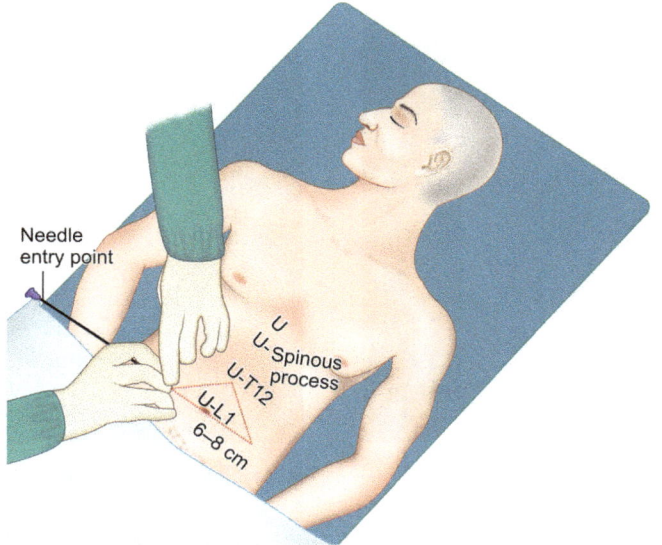

Fig. 1: Surface markings.

Step 2: To start with take initial scan image **(Fig. 2)** to measure the distance from spinous process laterally and depth from entry point to the target, i.e., celiac ganglion or plexus **(Fig. 3)**. Save this image as base line for the procedure.

Now inject preservative-free 1% lidocaine 10 cc deep into the various layers in the direction of the needle as shown in **Figure 3**.

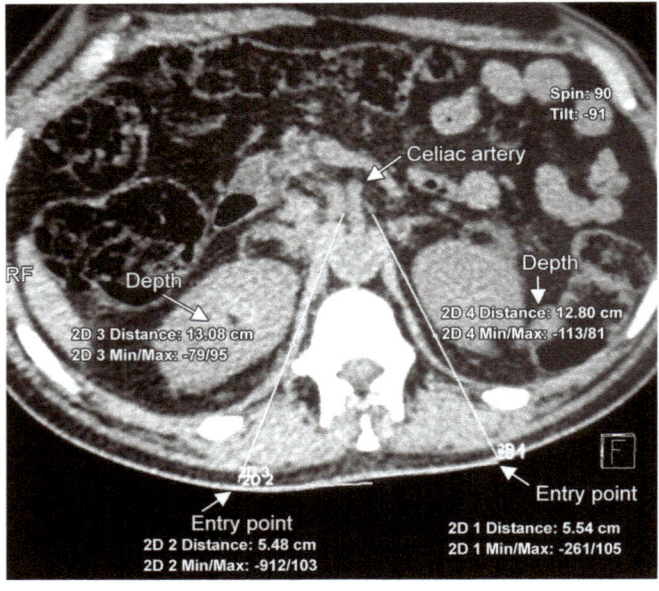

Fig. 2: Basic scan—distance from skin to celiac artery.

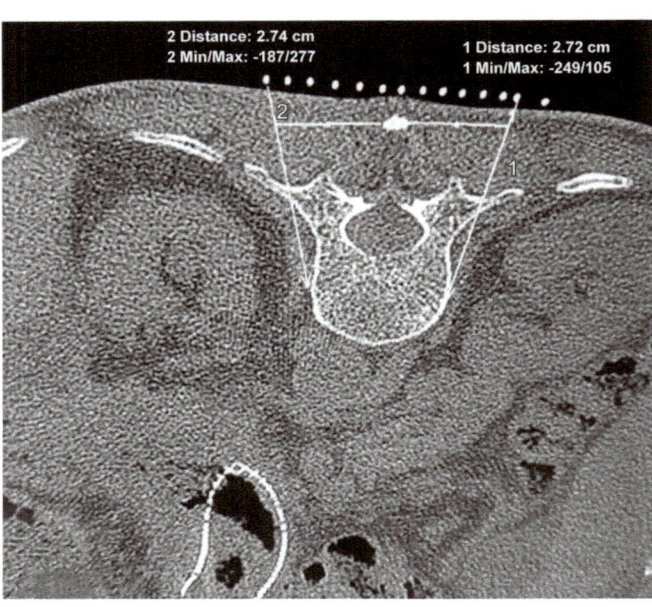

Fig. 3: Measuring distance from skin celiac plexus.

Step 3: A 15-cm long 20-gauge short bevel needle at 45° to the skin, is directed towards midline and cephalad to contact upper part of body of L1 vertebra on one left side and then towards right side.

The position of the needle should be confirmed anteroposterior and lateral views under CT scan. The needle tip should be near aorta and celiac plexus as seen in **Figure 4**.

Step 4: After repeated negative aspiration the 5 cc of 2% lidocaine injected to have immediate pain relief.

Step 5: After repeated negative aspiration 5 cc radiopaque dye iohexol injected on each side and confirmed the spread of the dye on both side of aorta **(Fig. 5)**.

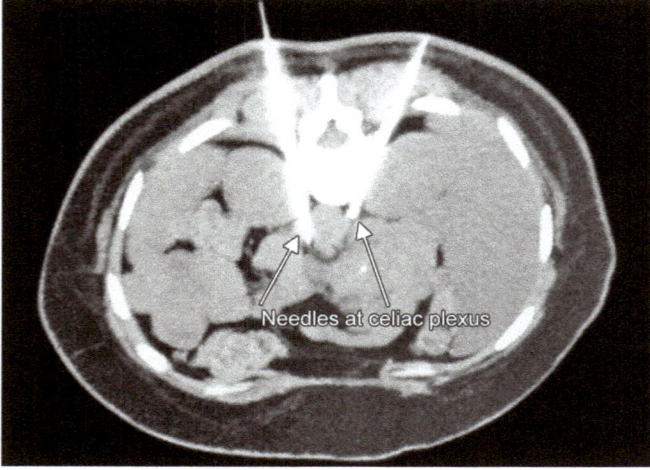

Fig. 4: Needle tips near celiac plexus.

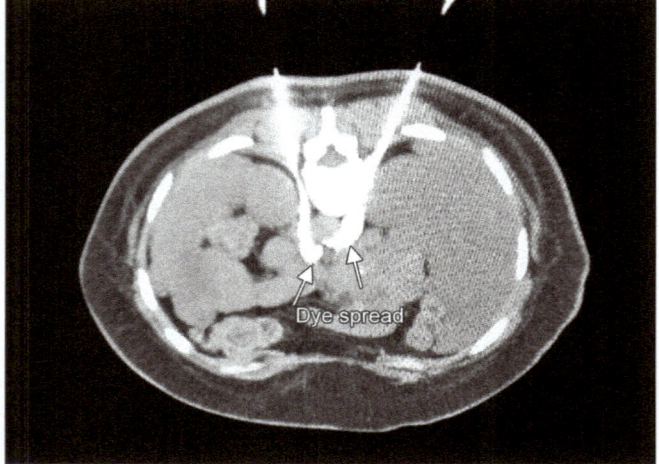

Fig. 5: Bilateral dye spread.

Step 6: Put sponge around needle (**Fig. 6**) to avoid spillage of neurolytic agent on the skin.

Step 7: After repeated negative aspiration, a mixture of injection alcohol 50% with the injection bupivacaine 0.25%, 10 cc should be injected slowly on each side with intermittent negative aspiration. Now put the stylet back into the needle to prevent spillage of neurolytic agent on skin.

Step 8: Lastly withdraw needle while injecting of local anesthetic into the needle track to decrease postprocedure pain and needle site.

Step 9: The patient to be shifted to recovery room and vital signs should be observed for vital signs in the recovery for about 1–2 hours.

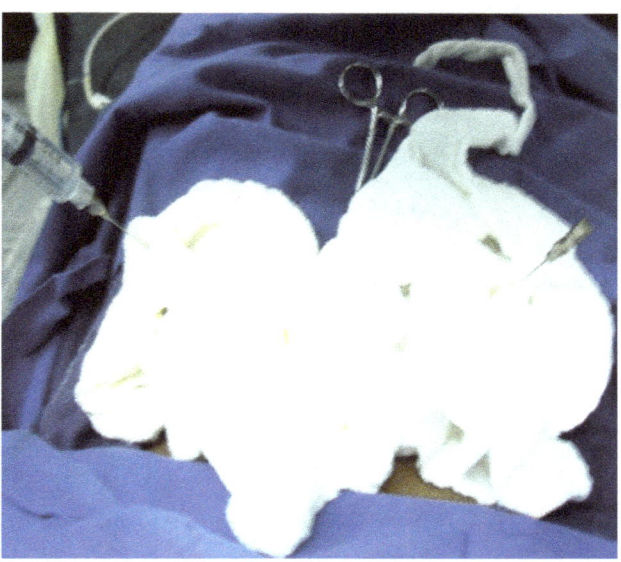

Fig. 6: Sponge around needle.

ADDITIONAL INFORMATION

Advantage of Bending the Needle Tip

In authors experience, the bending of tip of needle to 10°. The bending the tip has following advantages:

- When the needle is deeply placed as seen in **Figure 7** away from target.
- The tip can be turned toward target by holding hub of needle to rotate towards the target as seen in **Figure 8**. The spread of the dye is around aorta as seen in **Figure 9**, when tip is turned inside.

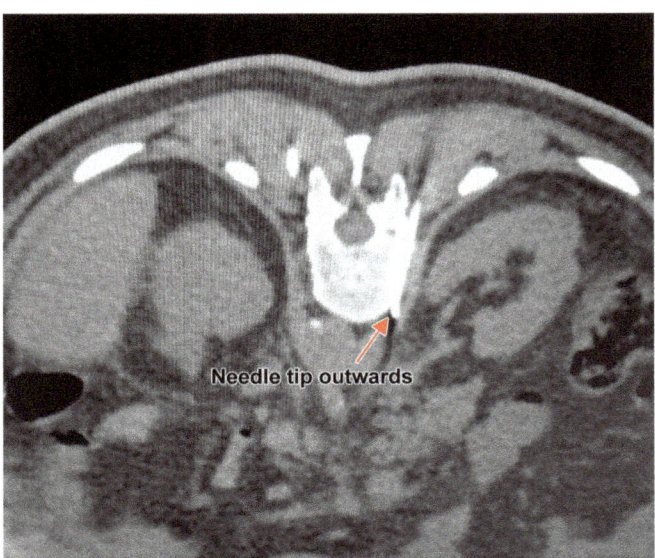

Fig. 7: Needle tip outwards away from target.

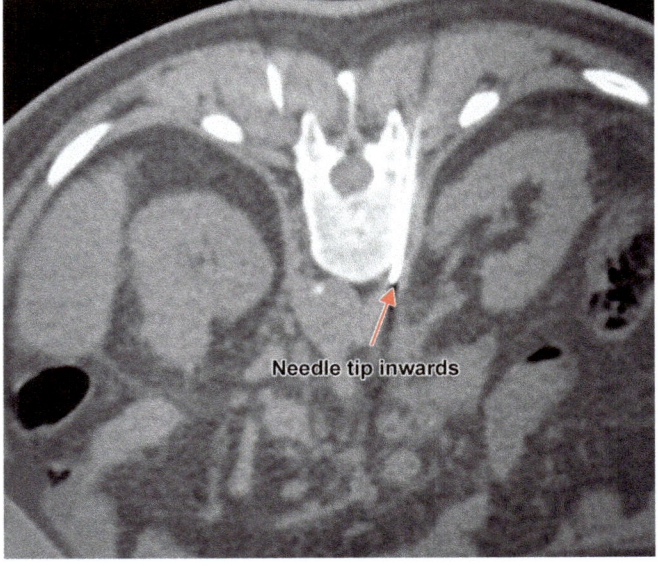

Fig. 8: Needle tip towards target.

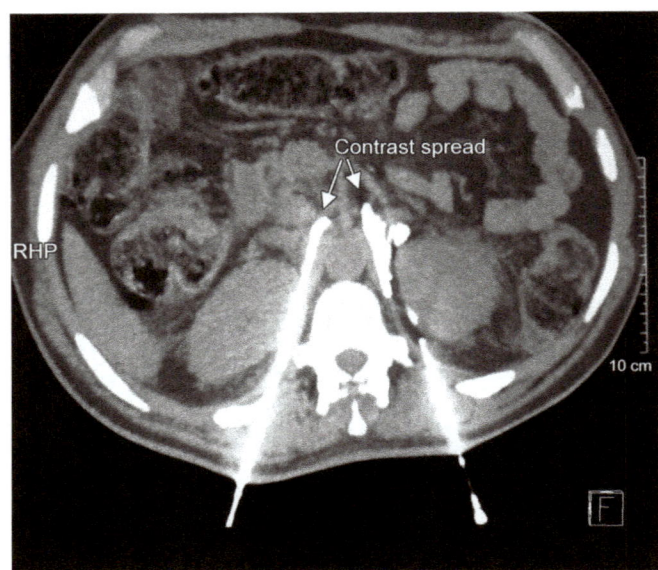

Fig. 9: Dye spread with needle tip turned inside.

Declaration

Part of the text and some images are taken with permission from M/s Jaypee Brothers Medical Publisher, New Delhi, from the chapter "Celiac Plexus Block" published in the book, *Interventional Pain Management: A Practical Approach* 2018 edited by DK Baheti, Sanjay Bakshi, Sanjeeva Gupta, and RP Gehdoo.

CHAPTER 41: Celiac Plexus Block: Fluoroscopy Guided

Dwarkadas K Baheti

BASIC INFORMATION

Indications
- Any pain originating from the upper abdominal viscera such as stomach, liver, gallbladder, kidney, spleen, pancreas, aortic lymphadenopathy, omental mass, retroperitoneal tumors
- Pain due to chronic pancreatitis and alcoholic pancreatitis
- Any chronic upper abdominal pain of unknown origin

Contraindications
- Anticoagulation therapy or suffering from congenital abnormalities of coagulopathy
- Antiblastic cancer therapy
- Liver abnormalities associated with ethanol abuse
- The local skin infection at needle entry point or intra-abdominal infection and sepsis, intestinal obstruction
- The use of alcohol as a neurolytic agent should be avoided in a patient with disulfiram therapy for alcohol abuse.

DRUGS AND CONCENTRATION
- Inj. lignocaine 2% (Xylocard—preservative-free)
- Absolute alcohol
- Normal saline
- Inj. bupivacaine 0.25%

COMPLICATIONS OF NEUROLYTIC CELIAC PLEXUS BLOCK

The iatrogenic complications reported during celiac plexus blocks are pneumothorax, partial lower extremity paralysis, and temporary paraplegia. Iatrogenic complications such as chylothorax, pleural effusion, renal injury, and injury to veins also have been reported.

PROCEDURE DETAILS

Step 1: Position and landmarks
- The patient should lie in prone position with a pillow under the abdomen to reverse to thoracolumbar lordosis and to increase the distance between the costal margin and iliac crests and transverse processes of adjacent vertebral bodies.
- It is advisable to preload the patient with Inj. Ringer's lactate 500–1,000 mL at the start of the procedure.
- The entry points are iliac crests, 12th rib, and spinous processes of T12 and L1 vertebrae. Moore recommended that the intersection of the 12th rib and lateral border of paraspinal muscles on both sides and spine of L1 vertebra which forms an isosceles triangle are shown in **Figure 1**.

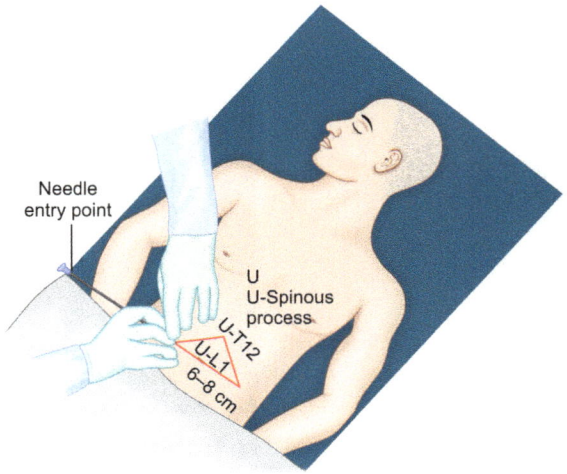

Fig. 1: Prone position and surface marking for celiac plexus block.

Step 2: Needle entry
- The entry point of needle is either four finger-breadths or 6–8 cm from midline. Give Inj. 2% lidocaine about 10 cc intradermally and deep into the various layers in the direction of the needle (**Fig. 1**).

Step 3: Pushing or advancing of needle
- A 15-cm long, 20-gauge, short-bevel needle at 45° to the skin is directed toward the midline and cephalad to contact the upper part of body of L1 vertebra. In the same way, the second needle on the other side is also inserted in the same manner as before. The position of the needle should be confirmed in the anteroposterior and lateral views under fluoroscopy or under CT scan (**Figs. 2 and 3**).

Step 4: In lateral view after repeated negative aspiration, one needle at a time should be redirected toward the anterior border of L1 vertebra. The tip of both the needles should be about 1–2 cm ahead of the anterior border of L1 vertebra (**Figs. 2 and 3**).

It is advised that the tip of the right needle should be little ahead of the left as more fibers of the celiac plexus are on the right side.

Step 5: After repeated negative aspiration, 5 cc of 2% lidocaine is injected to have immediate pain relief. At this stage, there can be sudden fall of blood pressure, which can be treated with either Inj. mephentermine sulfate 3–6 mg or Inj. ringer's lactate 500–1,000 cc.

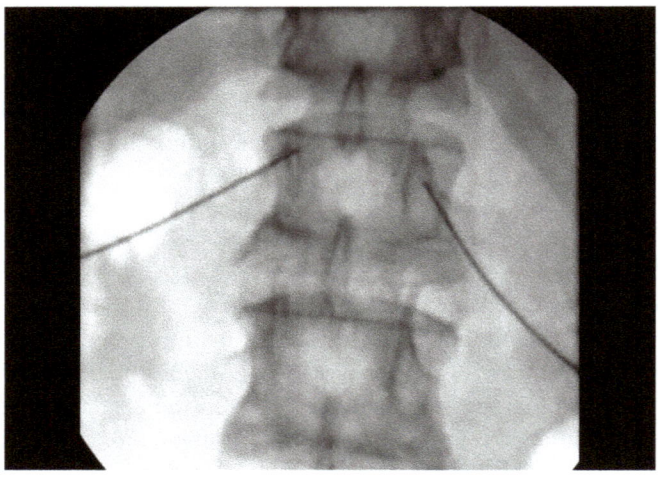

Fig. 2: Needles—anteroposterior view.

Fig. 3: Needles—lateral view.

Step 6: After repeated negative aspiration, 5 cc radiopaque dye Iohexol is injected on each side and spread of the dye is confirmed in anteroposterior and lateral positions (**Figs. 4 and 5**).

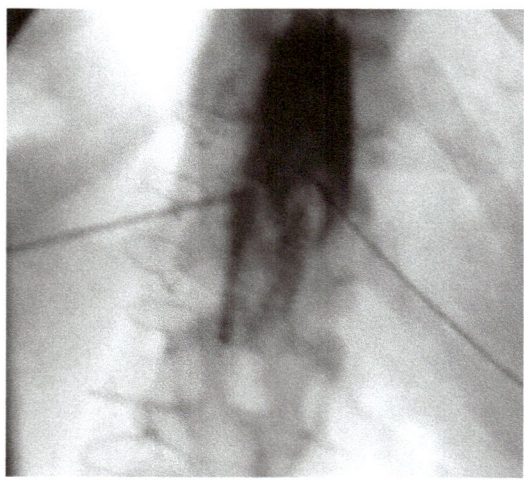

Fig. 4: Dye spread—anteroposterior view.

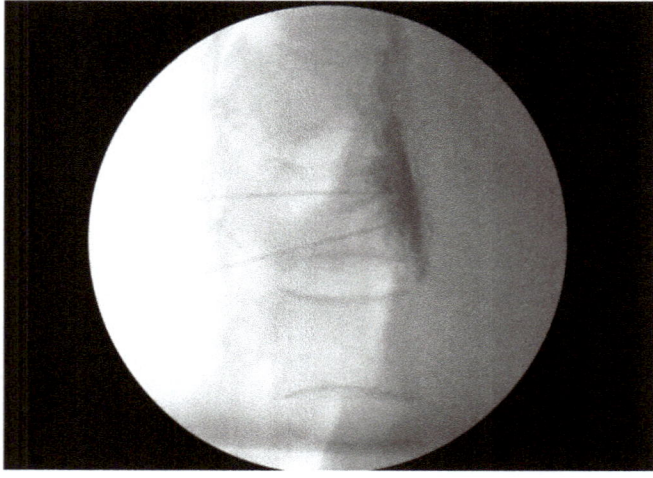

Fig. 5: Dye spread—lateral view.

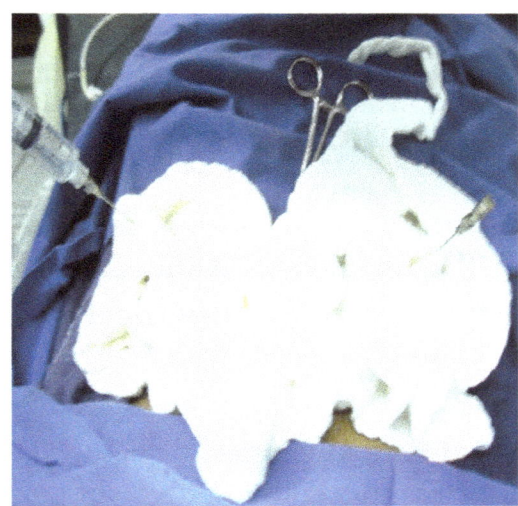

Fig. 6: Sponge around needle.

The spread of the dye should restrict to the body of T12 and L1 vertebrae. Both the pictures should be saved for documentation.

Step 7: Put sponge around needle **(Fig. 6)** to avoid spillage of neurolytic agent on the skin.

After repeated negative aspiration, a mixture of Inj. alcohol 50% and Inj. bupivacaine 0.25%, 20–25 cc should be injected slowly on both sides. Now, put the stylet back into the needle to prevent spillage of the neurolytic agent on skin.

Last, withdraw needle while injecting local anesthetic into the needle track to decrease postprocedure pain and needle site.

Step 8: Lastly shift the patient to the recovery room for monitoring of vital signs and observation for few hours

Declaration

Part of the text and some images are taken with permission from M/s Jaypee Brothers Medical Publishers, New Delhi, from the chapter "Celiac Plexus Block" published in the book, *Interventional Pain Management: A Practical Approach* 2009 and 2018 edited by DK Baheti, Sanjay Bakshi, Sanjeeva Gupta, and RP Gehdoo.

CHAPTER 42

Lumbar Sympathetic Plexus Block

Dwarkadas K Baheti

IMPORTANT TIPS

- Please keep in mind that the procedure is under local anesthesia and sedation. Try to be as gentle as possible while redirecting and pushing the needle in deeper plane toward the destination.
- Movement of the needle in the deeper planes should be slow and centimeter by centimeter.
- Always confirm the position of needle in anteroposterior and lateral positions.
- Repeated negative aspiration at every step.

BASIC INFORMATION

Indications

- *Vascular insufficiency due to*:
  - Peripheral vascular disease
  - Diabetis mallitus
  - Burger's disease
  - Raynaud's disease
- *Miscellaneous*:
  - Complex regional pain syndromes I and II
  - Herpes zoster
  - Stump pain
  - Phantom limb
  - Frostbite
  - Trench foot
  - Renal colic
  - Urogenital pain
  - Hyperhidrosis

Contraindications

- Unwilling or Uncooperative patient
- Allergy to contrast
- Local infection
- Coagulopathy
- Pregnancy

Evidence of Sympatholysis

- Vasodilatation in lower limbs
- Raised temperature in lower limbs
- Decreased edema
- Decreased pain with sympathetic-mediated pain

PROCEDURE

Step 1: Position and landmarks

- Start with obtaining informed consent, patient in prone position with pillow under abdomen reverse to lumbar lordosis, square the endplates ipsilaterally under anteroposterior (AP) fluoroscopy, and identify the levels L2, L3, and L4. The view should obstruct the transverse process of the desired lumbar vertebra.

Step 2: Take AP view of the lumbar spine and see the transverse process as shown in **Figure 1**.

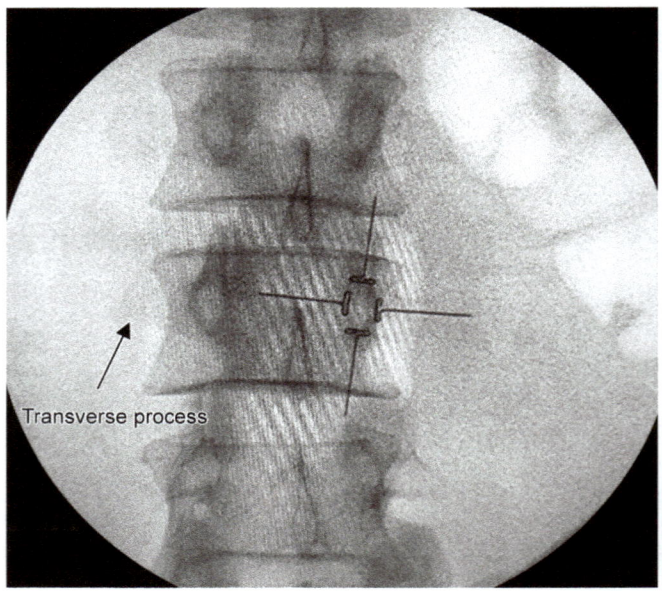

Fig. 1: Lumbar spine AP view.

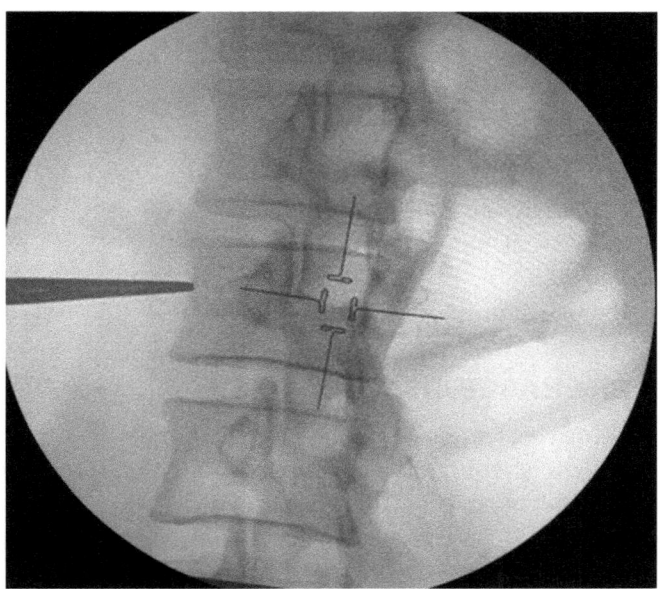

Fig. 2: Marker at entry point—transverse process obliterated.

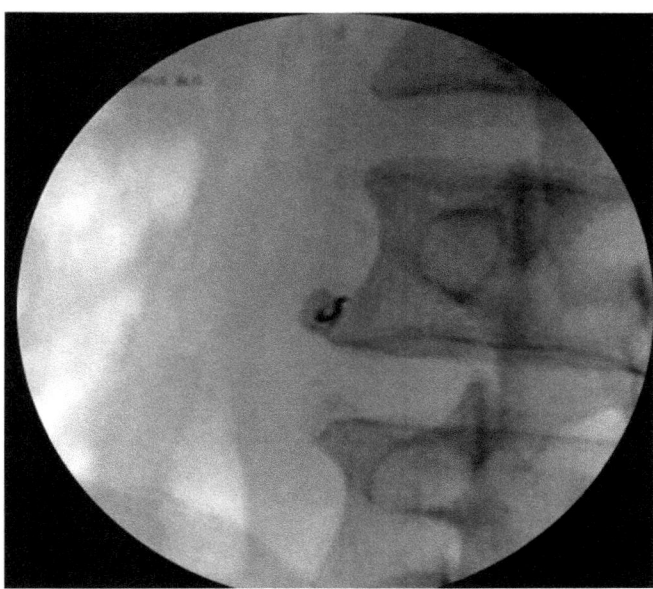

Fig. 3: End on view of needle in AP view.

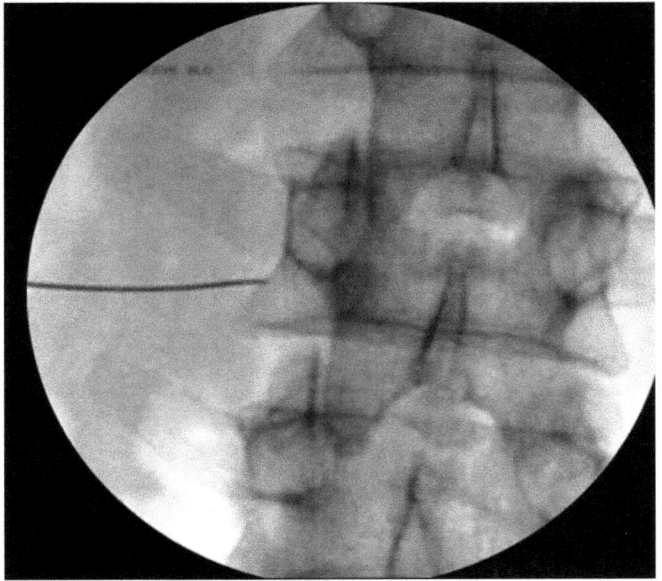

Fig. 4: Needle in anteroposterior view with transverse.

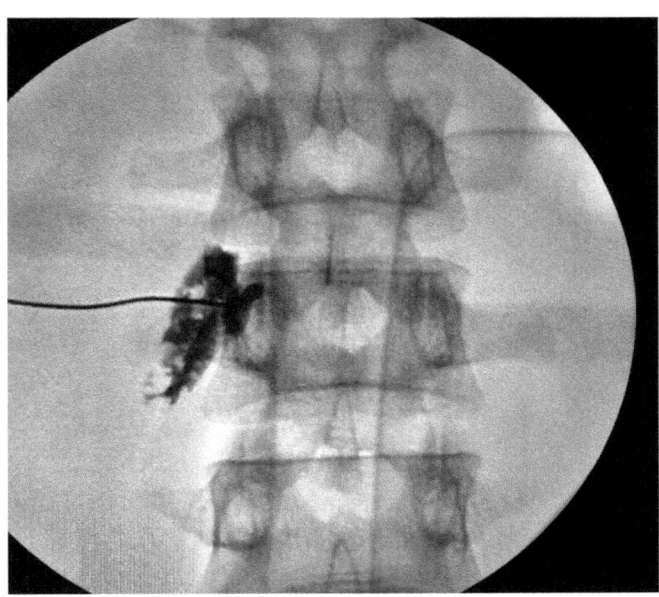

Fig. 5: Dye spread in anteroposterior view.

Then rotate the fluoroscope oblique to obliterate the transverse process, and the midpoint of vertebra is the entry point for the needle (**Fig. 2**). Now, inject Inj. 2% lidocaine about 10 cc intradermally and deep into the various layers in the direction of the needle. The needle is then directed to pass below and slightly medial to the inferior border of the transverse process at an angle of about 10° to the sagittal plane. It is advanced about 2 cm deep to the transverse process, where it should contact the side of the vertebral body. The needle position in end on view after obliteration of transverse process is shown in **Figure 3** and AP view is shown in **Figure 4**.

Step 3: After confirmation of repeated negative aspiration, Inj. omnipaque 4–5 cc is to be injected to confirm the spread of dye. The spread of the dye should be confirmed in both AP and lateral views. In AP view, the dye will hug vertically the spine as shown in **Figure 5**. In lateral view, the dye will spread along the anterior border of the spine as shown in **Figure 6**.

Step 4: Save the images for record purpose.

Step 5: Now depending on the indication, one can inject phenol in glycerin 6–10% about 8–10 cc diluted with Inj. bupivacaine 1% slowly.

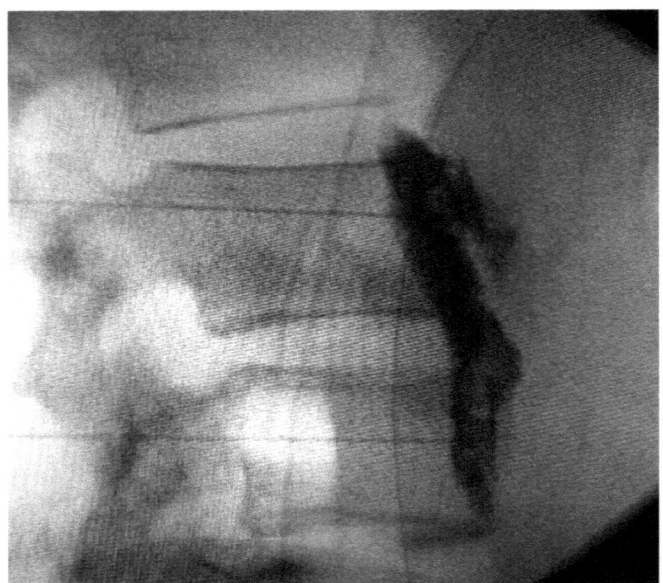

Fig. 6: Dye spread in lateral view.

Step 6: Before withdrawing the needle, put the stylet into it to allow the neurolytic agent to spill the desired area. Inject Inj. xylocaine 2% into the needle track while withdrawing the needle. This will help to reduce the needle pain following the procedure.

Step 7: Lastly shift the patient to the recovery room for monitoring of vital signs and observation for few hours.

Important point: It is advisable to avoid bilateral neurolytic or radiofrequency lumbar sympathectomy in young male patients as it may lead to sexual dysfunction.

PROBLEMS

- Genitofemoral neuralgia up to 15%
- Intravascular injection
- Bleeding
- Hypotension

DISCHARGE INSTRUCTIONS

- No driving for that day.
- Patient should monitor and record the extent and duration of any relief that ensues.
- Contact doctor if headache, fever, chills, increased pain, paralysis, or any other unusual symptoms.
- Resume previous activities over a period of several days.

Declaration

Part of the text and some images are taken with permission from M/s Jaypee Brothers Medical Publishers, New Delhi, from the chapter "Lumbar Sympathetic Block" published in the book, *Interventional Pain Management: Practical Approach* 2009 and 2018 edited by DK Baheti, Sanjay Bakshi, Sanjeeva Gupta, and RP Gehdoo.

CHAPTER 43
Superior Hypogastric Plexus Block

Dwarkadas K Baheti, Yashwant Laxman Nankar

IMPORTANT TIPS

- Keep in mind the procedure is under local and sedation try to be as gentle as possible while redirecting and pushing the needle in deeper plane towards the destination.
- Movement of the needle in the deeper planes should be slow and centimeter by centimeter.
- Always confirm position of needle in anteroposterior (AP) and lateral position.
- Repeated negative aspiration at every step.

BASIC INFORMATION

- The pelvic, rectal, bladder, sigmoid and anal pain are difficult to treat and manage. Overall pharmacological management of patients has become inadequate, and their pain is difficult to manage.
- The superior hypogastric plexus nerve block is a procedure that can provide maximum relief and improve their quality of life. The procedure can be safely performed under fluoroscopy or computed tomography (CT) guidance. Neurolysis is only indicated for tumor pain.

INDICATIONS

- Tumors of uterus/cervix
- Metastatic tumors of colon/rectal malignancy
- Bladder tumor/prostate malignancy
- Chronic pelvic pain
- Testicular tumor/penile cancer

CONTRAINDICATIONS

- Unwilling patient
- Bleeding disorders
- Local skin infection

DRUGS AND CONCENTRATION

- *Injection lignocaine 2%:* (Xylocard-preservative-free)
- Absolute alcohol
- Phenol in glycerin or almond oil 6–10%
- Normal saline
- Inj. bupivacaine 0.25%

Complications

The iatrogenic complication reported during celiac plexus blocks are pneumothorax; partial lower extremity paralysis; temporary paraplegia. Iatrogenic complications such as chylothorax, pleural effusion, renal injury and injury to veins also have been reported.

Procedure

Step 1: First obtain informed consent followed by put patient prone position (**Fig. 1**) with monitors attached.

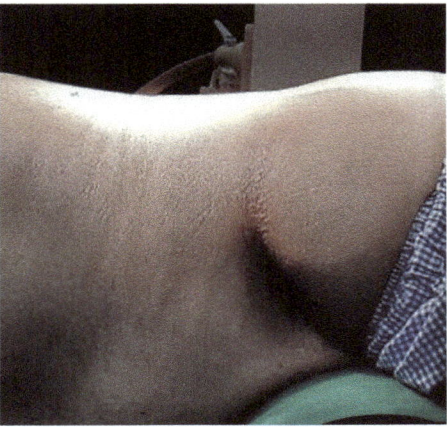

Fig. 1: A pillow is placed under the lower abdomen.

Step 2: Visualize the vertebral bodies of L3–4, L4–5 and L5–S1. A marker is placed at the L4 level of just above the iliac crest 3–5 cm lateral from the midline **(Fig. 2)**.

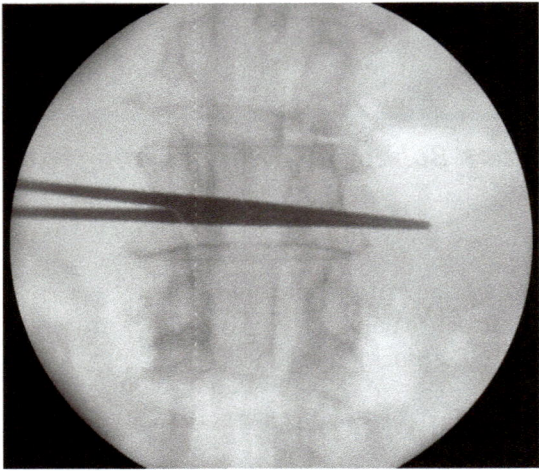

Fig. 2: Marker at L4 vertebra.

Step 3: Put marker at skin entry point about 7 cm away from midline at 4th lumbar interverterbral space as seen in **Figure 3**. Check marker at target point, i.e., at lower border of L5 in oblique view **(Fig. 4)**.

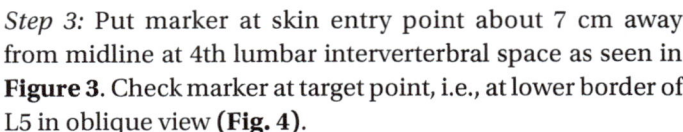
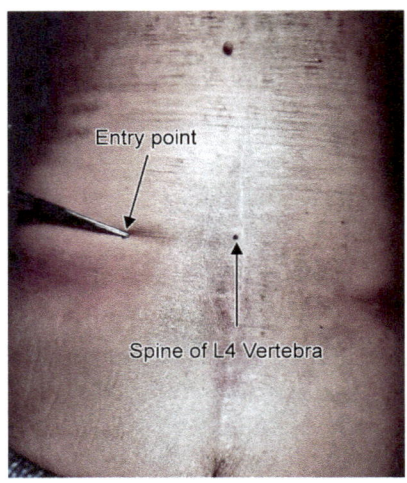

Fig. 3: Marker at skin entry point.

Step 4: After local anesthesia direct a 20-gauge 10-cm needle is pushed in the direction of the sacral promontory.

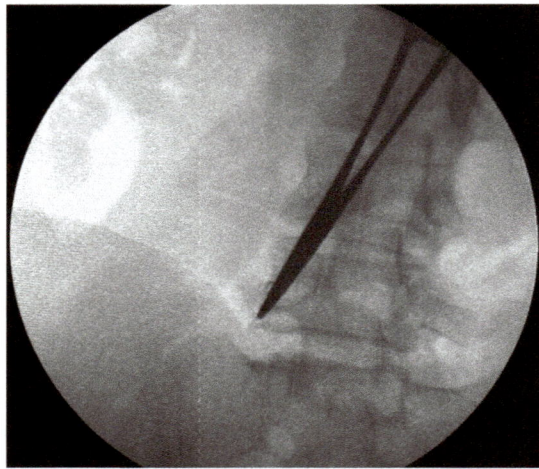

Fig. 4: Marker in oblique view at L5 border.

Step 5: Check in anteroposterior (AP) **(Fig. 5)** and in lateral view **(Fig. 6)**.

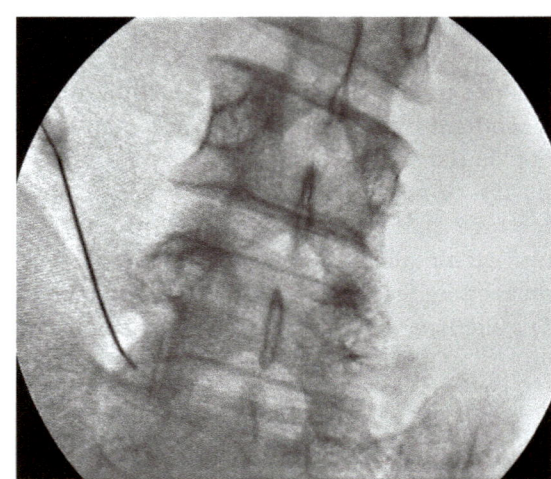

Fig. 5: Needle in AP view.

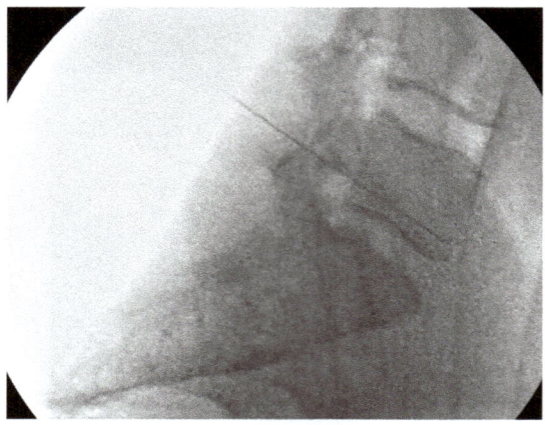

Fig. 6: Needle in lateral view.

CHAPTER 43 | Superior Hypogastric Plexus Block

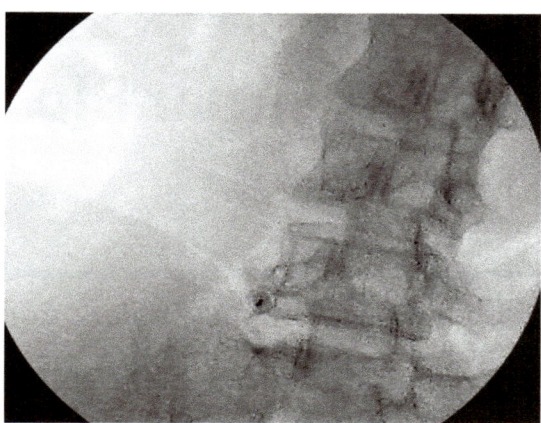

Fig. 7: Tunnel vision oblique view.

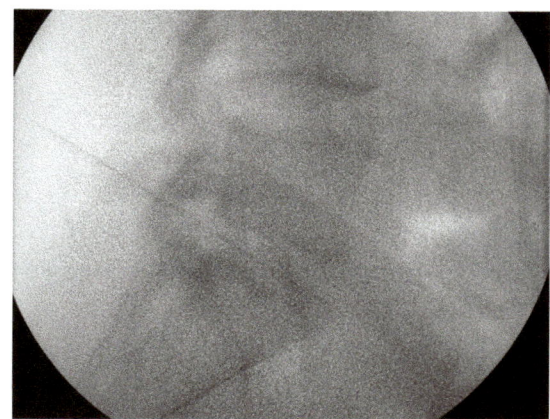

Fig. 8: Needle at sacral promontry lateral view.

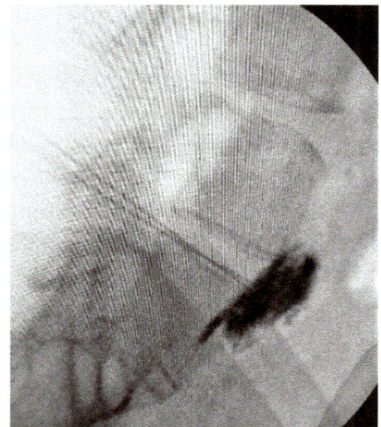

Fig. 9: Dye spread in lateral view.

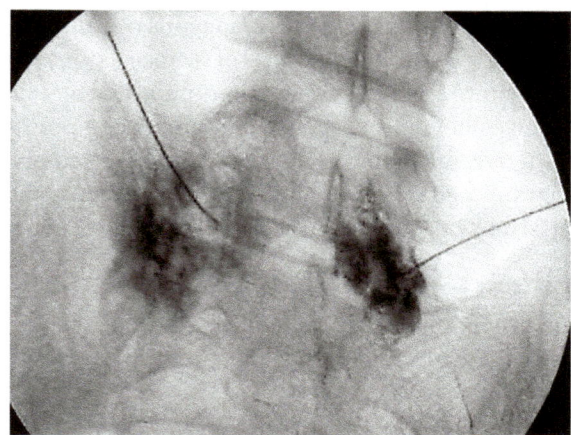

Fig. 10: Dye spread in AP view.

Step 6: Confirm in AP view for tunnel vision as seen in **Figure 7**. Here confirm for negative aspiration for CSF or blood.

Step 7: Now rotate C-arm in lateral view to confirm the tip of needle at the sacral promontory **(Fig. 8)**.

Step 8: Following a negative aspiration, inject 2–3 mL of water-soluble radiopaque contrast and confirmed the spread of dye in lateral **(Fig. 9)** and in AP view **(Fig. 10)**.

Step 9: Now put sponges around the needle to avoid spillage of neurolytic agent on the skin as seen in **Figure 11**.

Step 10: For the diagnostic block 15 mL of 1% lidocaine is injected on both sides. If there is an indication for malignancy, then 10 mL of 50% alcohol or inject Inj. phenol 8–10 cc diluted with local anesthetic slowly with intermittent negative aspiration.

Step 11: The patient to be shifted to recovery room and vital signs should be observed in the recovery for about 1–2 hours.

Declaration

Part of the text and some images are taken with permission from M/s Jaypee Brothers Medical Publishers, New Delhi,

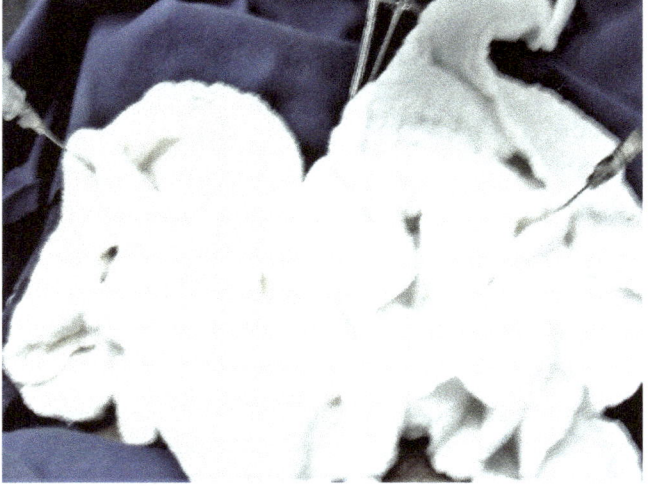

Fig. 11: Sponge around needle.

from the chapter "Superior Hypogastric Plexus Block" published in the book, Interventional *Pain Management: A Practical Approach* 2009 and 2018 edited by DK Baheti, Sanjay Bakshi, Sanjeeva Gupta, and RP Gehdoo.

CHAPTER 44: Ganglion of Impar Block

Dwarkadas K Baheti

BASIC INFORMATION

The ganglion of impar is also known as Ganglion of Walther[1] which is the last ganglion of the sympathetic trunk. It is a single ganglion formed by fusion of two ganglions of both sides and located retroperitoneally at the level of sacrococcygeal junction that marks termination of the paired paravertebral chains. This receives fibers from the lumbar and sacral portions of sympathetic and parasympathetic nervous systems. The pain may be vague, burning, or localized in perineum.

There may be itching and redness around perineum.

Indications

- Pain originating either from pelvic viscera
- Sympathetically maintained pain in the perineum

Contraindications

- Local skin infection
- Intra-abdominal infection and sepsis, and intestinal obstruction
- Anticoagulation therapy or congenital abnormalities of coagulation
- Antiblastic cancer therapy

IMPORTANT TIPS

- Always keep in mind that the procedure is under local anesthesia and sedation. Try to be as gentle as possible while redirecting and pushing the needle in deeper plane toward the destination.
- Movement of the needle in the deeper planes should be slow and centimeter by centimeter.
- Always confirm the position of the needle in antero-posterior (AP) and lateral positions.
- Repeated negative aspiration at every step.

PROCEDURE DETAILS

- Prone position—transcoccygeal or trans-sacrococcygeal approach
- Fluoroscope in AP position

Step 1: Patient should be kept in the procedure room with C-arm fluoroscopy or CT scan along with monitoring and resuscitation facility.

C-arm in AP position and surface marking is done as shown in **Figure 1**.

Now inject Inj. xylocaine 1% at the entry point deep up to the periosteum and around.

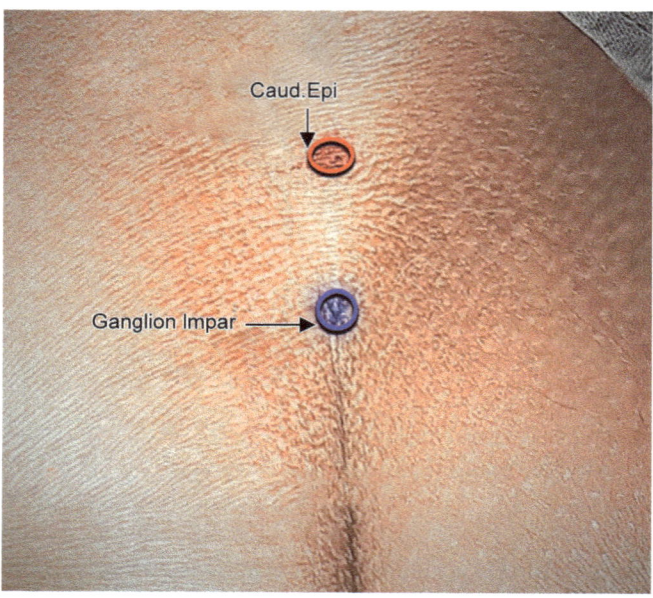

Fig. 1: Surface marking for ganglion of impar.

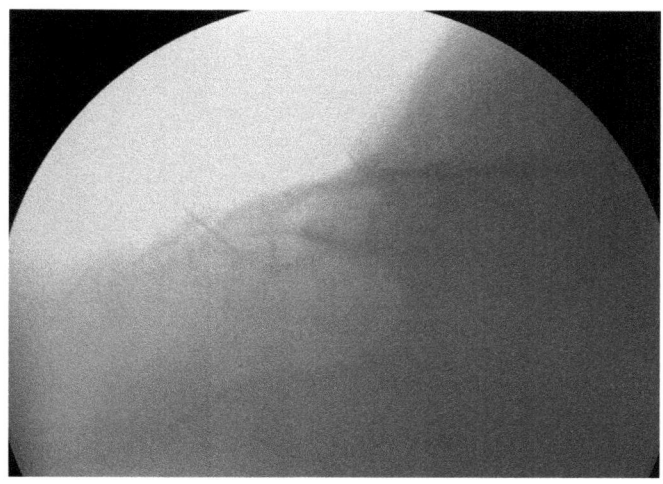
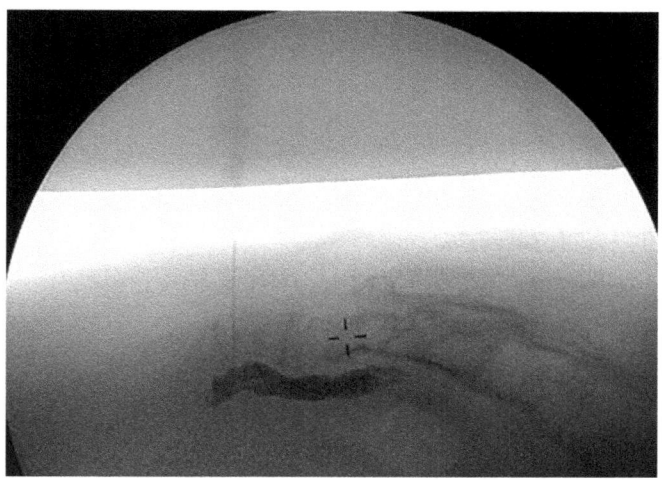

Fig. 2: Needle just crossed the bony margin.

Fig. 3: Dye spread—lateral view.

Step 2: Now under fluoroscopy, direct a 21-gauge spinal needle between coccygeal vertebrae till you feel loss of resistance. Confirm the position of needle under fluoroscopy. The needle should just cross or enter the bony margin as shown in **Figure 2**.

Step 3: After repeated negative aspiration, inject Inj. iohexol 1/2–1 cc and confirm the spread of dye as shown in **Figure 3**.

Step 4: Once again after negative aspiration, inject 2–3 cc of 1% Xylocaine to confirm the pain relief. Injecting of xylocaine before neurolytic decreases the irritation caused after injection of alcohol.

Step 5: Confirm pain relief. Now with the help of insulin syringe inject 1 cc of 100% alcohol slowly with repeated negative aspiration.

Once pain relief is confirmed after repeated negative aspiration with the help of insulin syringe, inject 1 cc of Inj. absolute alcohol 100% very slowly.

Step 6: Now shift the patient to recovery room for observation and monitoring of vital signs.

REFERENCES

1. Warfield CA, Bajwa ZH. Principles and Practice of Pain Medicine, Vol. 1. New Delhi: McGraw-Hill; 2004. p. 366.
2. Lancarte R, Amescua C, Patt R, Allende S. Presacral blockade of ganglion of Walther (ganglion impar). Anesthesiology. 1990;73:A751.

Declaration

Part of the text and some images are taken with permission from M/s Jaypee Brothers Medical Publishers, New Delhi, from the chapter "Ganglion of Impar Block" published in the book, Interventional *Pain Management: A Practical Approach* 2009 and 2018 edited by DK Baheti, Sanjay Bakshi, Sanjeeva Gupta, and RP Gehdoo.

SECTION 9

Ultrasound Guided Block

- **Suprascapular Nerve Block**
  Ritesh Roy, Gaurav Agarwal

- **Brachial Plexus Block (Supraclavicular Approach)**
  Ritesh Roy, Gaurav Agarwal

- **Thoracic Paravertebral Block**
  Archana Areti, Ritesh Roy, Gaurav Agarwal

- **Ultrasound-guided Transversus Abdominis Plane Block**
  Gaurav Agarwal, Ritesh Roy

- **Lumbar Plexus Block**
  Ritesh Roy, Gaurav Agarwal

- **Lateral Femoral Cutaneous Nerve Block**
  Ritesh Roy, Gaurav Agarwal

- **Sacral Plexus Block**
  Ritesh Roy, Gaurav Agarwal

- **Pericapsular Nerve Group Block (For Hip Joint)**
  Ritesh Roy, Gaurav Agarwal

CHAPTER 45

Suprascapular Nerve Block

Ritesh Roy, Gaurav Agarwal

SUPRASCAPULAR NERVE BLOCK

Basic Information

- Suprascapular nerve is formed by the ventral rami of the 5th and 6th cervical nerves. It emerges from the brachial plexus beneath the omohyoid muscle and passes above the suprascapular notch below the superior transverse scapular ligament. It supplies motor branches to the supraspinatus and infraspinatus and sensory branches to the acromioclavicular joint, glenohumeral joint (superior and posterior aspects), coracoclavicular, coracohumeral ligaments, and the subacromial bursa.
- *Indications*: Analgesia for any procedure involving shoulder joint, acute traumatic pain, pain due to adhesive capsulitis, shoulder joint rheumatoid arthritis, cancer pain, or any other chronic shoulder joint pains
- *Contraindications*: Unwilling patient, bleeding disorders, infection at the injection site
- *Medications used*:
  - *Local anesthetic*: 0.1–0.5% Ropivacaine/0.125–0.5% Bupivacaine 15–20 mL with or without adjuvants
  - *Adjuvants that can be used*: Dexmedetomidine 0.5–1 µg/kg, Clonidine 0.5–1 µg/kg, Dexamethasone 0.1–0.2 mg/kg

ANTERIOR SUBOMOHYOID APPROACH

Step 1: Position of patient—supine. Identify clavicle and the tendons of sternocleidomastoid. High-frequency ultrasound (USG) probe placed parallel to clavicle. Scan transverse oblique in a cephalad direction in sweep movement to identify various nerve roots (**Fig. 1**).

Step 2: Scanning cephalad in the transverse oblique direction, identify the 7th cervical nerve root and vertebral artery, at the C7 vertebral level where the anterior tubercle of the C7 transverse process is absent and prominent posterior tubercle is seen (**Fig. 2**).

Fig. 1: Suprascapular nerve block—anterior approach initial probe position.

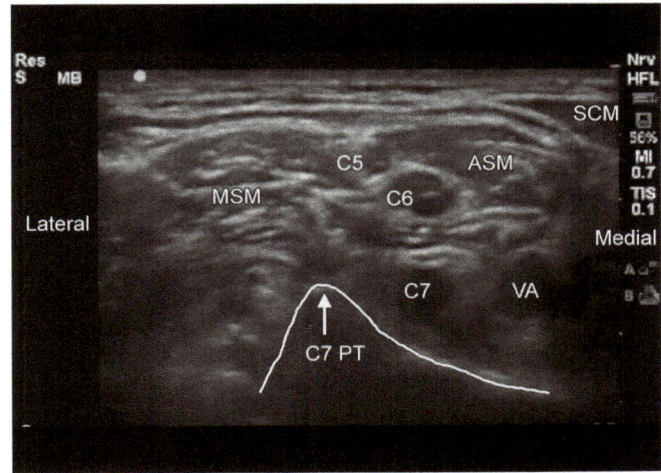

Fig. 2: Image identifying C7. (ASM: anterior scalene muscle; C5: 5th cervical nerve root; C6: 6th cervical nerve root; C7: 7th cervical nerve root; C7 PT: posterior tubercle of the transverse process of the 7th cervical vertebra; MSM: middle scalene muscle; SCM: sternocleidomastoid muscle; VA: vertebral artery)

Step 3: Scanning further cephalad in the transverse oblique direction, identify the 6th cervical nerve root and internal carotid artery, at the C6 vertebral level where the anterior tubercle of the C6 transverse process is the most prominent tubercle in the cervical spine **(Fig. 3)**.

Step 4: Scan further cephalad in the transverse oblique direction. Identify the 5th cervical nerve root and internal carotid artery, at the C5 vertebral level **(Fig. 4)**.

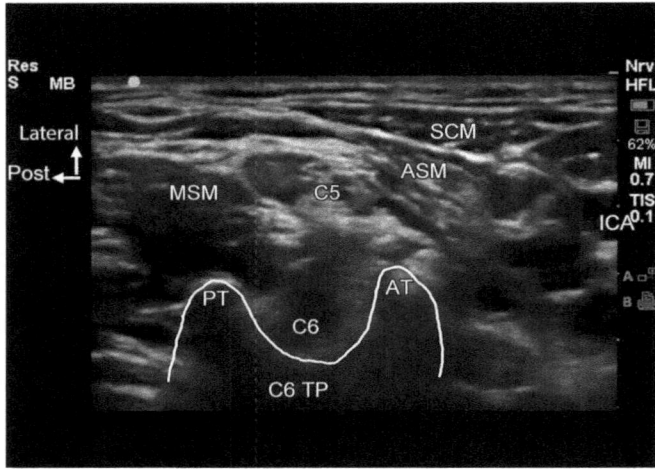

Fig. 3: Image identifying C6. (ASM: anterior scalene muscle; AT: anterior tubercle of the transverse process of the 6th cervical vertebra; C5: 5th cervical nerve root; C6: 6th cervical nerve root; C6 TP: transverse process of the 6th cervical vertebra; ICA: internal carotid artery; MSM: middle scalene muscle; PT: posterior tubercle of the transverse process of the 6th cervical vertebra; SCM: sternocleidomastoid muscle)

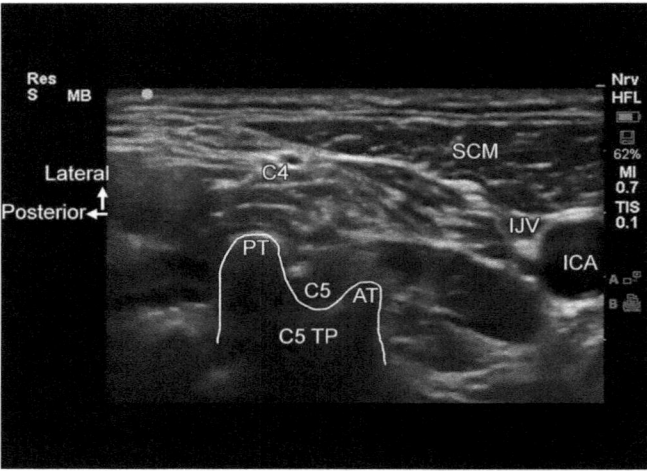

Fig. 4: Image identifying C5. (AT: anterior tubercle of the transverse process of the 5th cervical vertebra; C4: 4th cervical nerve root; C5: 5th cervical nerve root; C5 TP: transverse process of the 5th cervical vertebra; ICA: internal carotid artery; IJV: internal jugular vein; PT: posterior tubercle of the transverse process of the 5th cervical vertebra; SCM: sternocleidomastoid muscle)

Step 5: Scanning back caudad in the transverse oblique direction, identify the 5th and 6th cervical nerve roots, which will form the superior trunk **(Fig. 5)**.

Step 6: Scanning further caudad in the transverse oblique direction, identify the formation of the upper/superior trunk. The dorsal scapular nerve is often seen here crossing the middle scalene muscle **(Fig. 6)**.

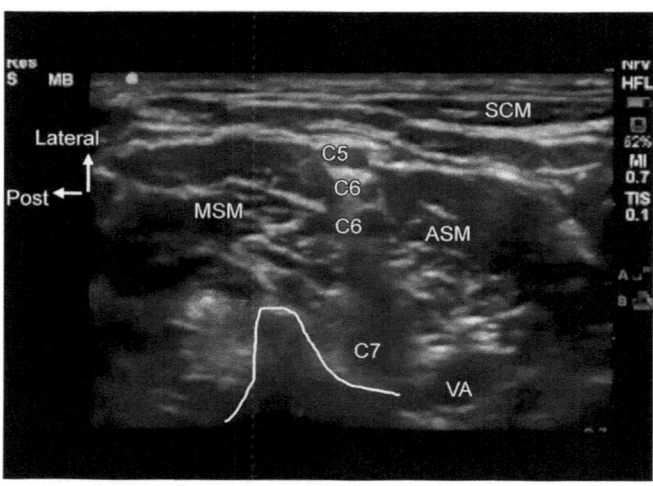

Fig. 5: Image identifying C5 and C6, forming superior trunk of brachial plexus. (ASM: anterior scalene muscle; C5: 5th cervical nerve root; C6: the bifid root of 6th cervical nerve root; MSM: middle scalene muscle; SCM: sternocleidomastoid muscle; VA: vertebral artery)

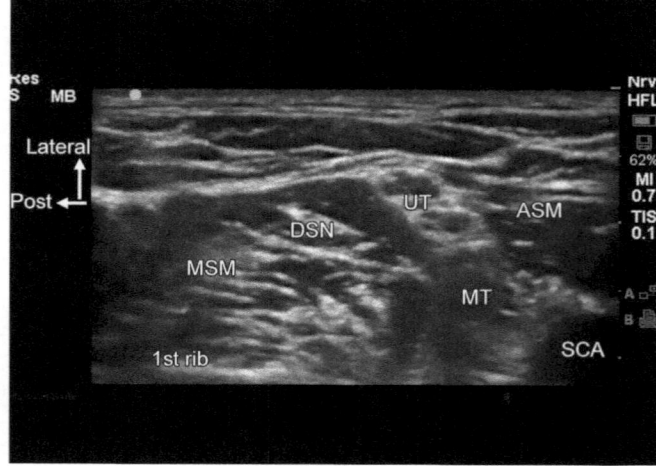

Fig. 6: Image identifying formation of upper trunk. (ASM: anterior scalene muscle; DSN: dorsal scapular nerve; MSM: middle scalene muscle; MT: middle trunk; SCA: subclavian artery; SCM: sternocleidomastoid muscle; UT: upper trunk)

Step 7: Scanning further caudad in the transverse oblique orientation, the divisions of upper trunk can be identified in SPA (Suprascapular nerve, Posterior division, Anterior division) arrangement **(Fig. 7)**.

Step 8: Scanning further caudad in the transverse oblique direction, identify the suprascapular nerve emerging from the upper trunk of the brachial plexus and moving laterally under the belly of omohyoid muscle **(Fig. 8)**.

Step 9: Identifying the suprascapular nerve under the omohyoid muscle as lateral as possible, the needle is advanced in-plane to reach the target and a volume of 4–8 mL of the drug is injected in small aliquots after regular negative aspirations for blood to achieve the block **(Fig. 9)**.

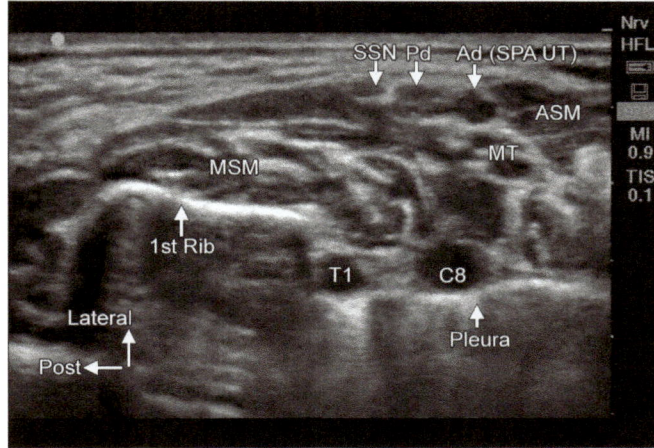

Fig. 7: Scanned image identifying the three divisions of superior trunk (SPA arrangement). (Ad: upper trunk anterior division; ASM: anterior scalene muscle; C8: 8th cervical nerve root; MSM: middle scalene muscle; MT: middle trunk; Pd: upper trunk posterior division; SSN: suprascapular nerve; T1: 1st thoracic nerve root)

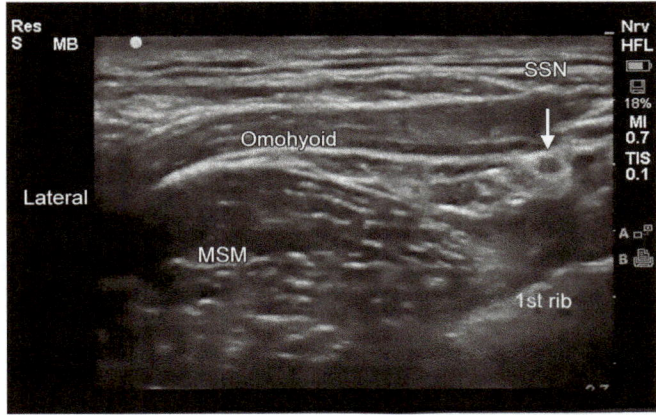

Fig. 8: Image identifying the suprascapular nerve emerging from the upper trunk of brachial plexus. (MSM: middle scalene muscle; SSN: suprascapular nerve)

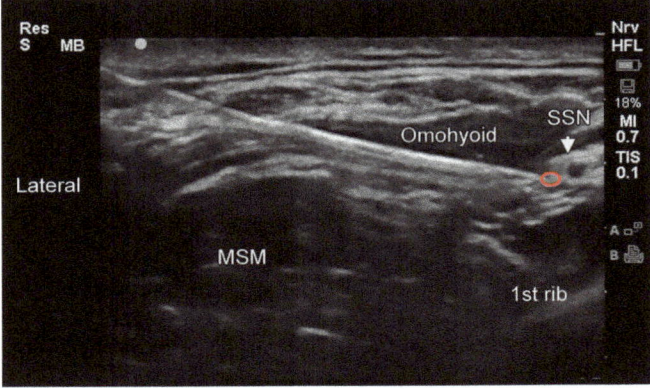

Fig. 9: Injection at the subomohyoid level of the suprascapular nerve. Red circle denotes the needle tip. (MSM: middle scalene muscle; SSN: suprascapular nerve)

POSTERIOR APPROACH

Step 1: Position of patient—sitting. The ipsilateral hand is placed on the contralateral shoulder to make the scapula prominent and lateral. Identify the spine of the scapula and the acromion process of the clavicle **(Fig. 10)**.

Step 2: Place the probe on the spine of scapula and slide anteriorly to identify the suprascapular fossa **(Fig. 11)**.

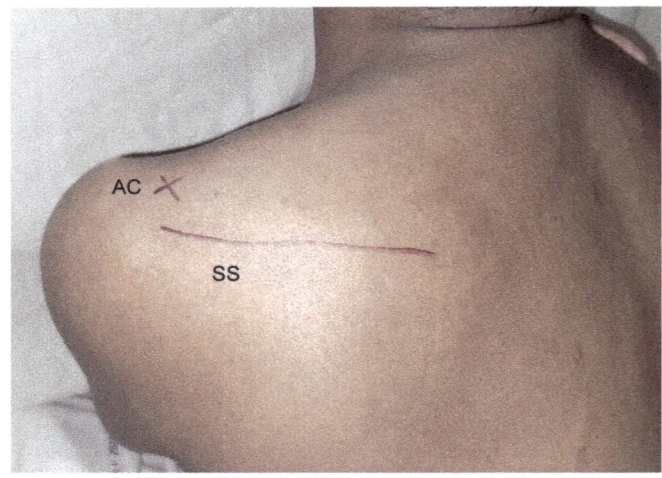

Fig. 10: Suprascapular nerve block posterior approach landmark identification. (AC: acromion of clavicle; SS: spine of scapula)

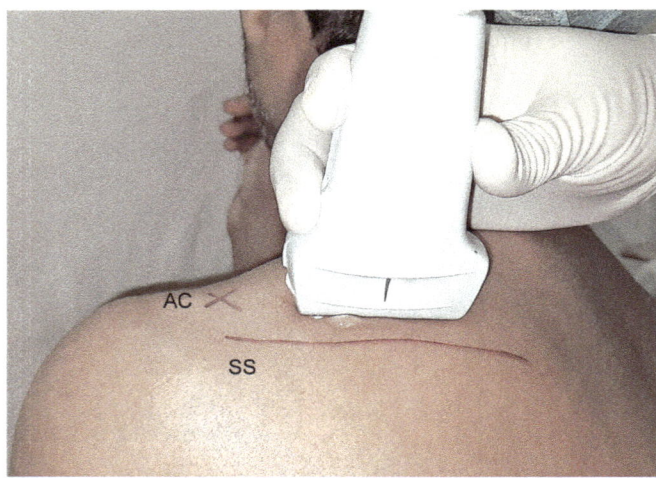

Fig. 11: Suprascapular nerve block posterior approach initial probe position. (AC: acromion of clavicle; SS: spine of scapula)

Step 3: Tilt the probe obliquely to face the cricoid process anteriorly and spine of scapula posteriorly. The suprascapular nerve is perpendicular to this probe position **(Figs. 12 and 13)**.

White arrow denotes the superior transverse scapular ligament (STSL), yellow circle denotes the suprascapular nerve (SSN) below the STSL, and red circle denotes the suprascapular artery (SA) above the STSL.

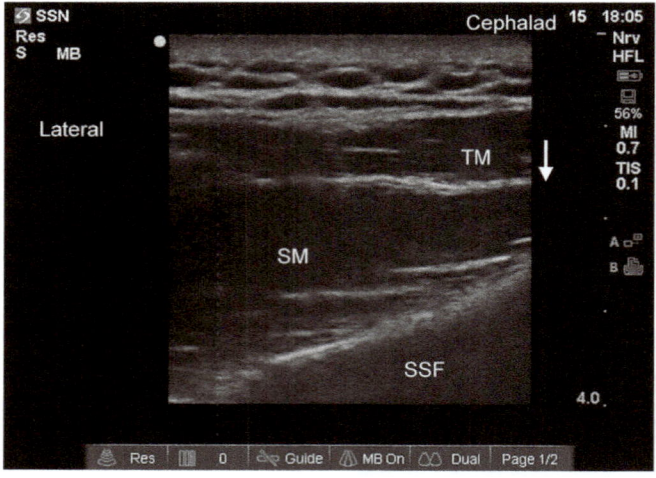

Fig. 12: Sonoanatomy of suprascapular fossa. (SM: supraspinatus muscle; SSF: suprascapular fossa; TM: trapezius muscle)

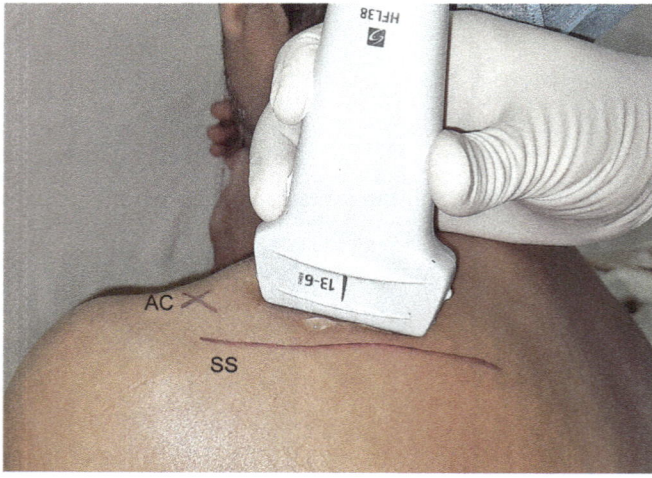

Fig. 13: Probe position to identify the suprascapular notch and the suprascapular nerve. (AC: acromion of clavicle; SS: spine of scapula)

The suprascapular nerve passes below the omohyoid to enter the suprascapular fossa through the suprascapular notch, below the superior transverse scapular ligament. The vessels pass above the superior transvers scapular ligament. The suprascapular nerve and vessels pass together obliquely in the suprascapular fossa below the supraspinatus muscle to enter the supraglenoid fossa **(Fig. 14)**.

Step 4: Scanning further laterally, identify the acromion process of the clavicle in sonoimage and the suprascapular nerve and vessels in the suprascapular fossa **(Fig. 15)**.

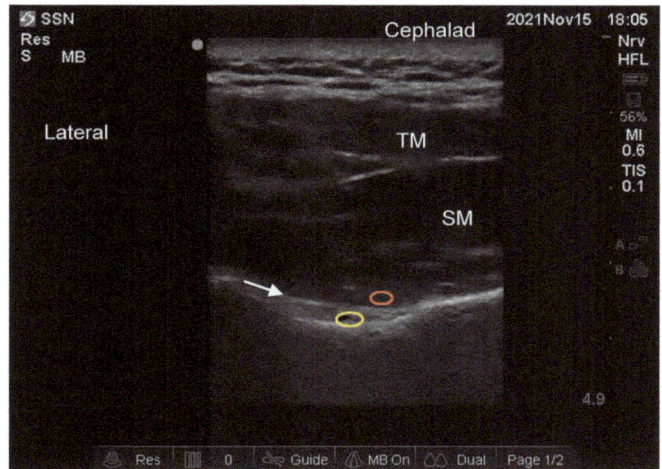

Fig. 14: Sonoanatomy of the suprascapular nerve and the suprascapular fossa.

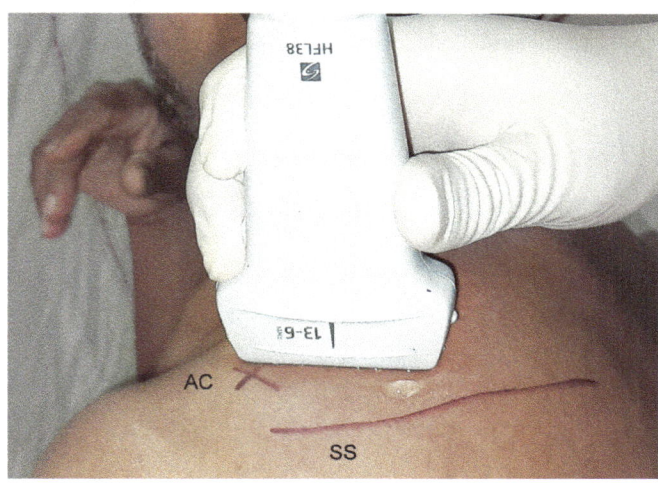

Fig. 15: Probe position to identify the acromion of clavicle. (AC: acromion of clavicle; SS: spine of scapula)

Step 5: Probe in oblique orientation targeting the suprascapular nerve at the mid-point between the suprascapular notch and the supraglenoid notch in the suprascapular fossa. The needle is inserted in-plane from medial to lateral aspect and small aliquots of 4–8 mL of local anesthetic drug are injected **(Figs. 16 and 17)**.

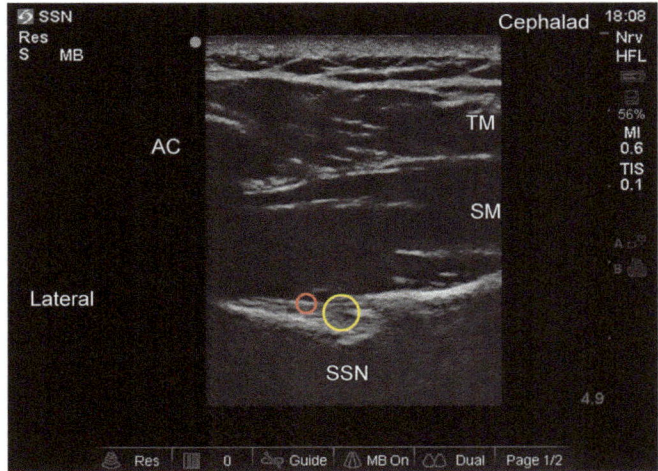

Fig. 16: Sonoanatomy of the suprascapular fossa with the acromion process. Yellow circle denotes the suprascapular nerve (SSN) and red circle denotes the suprascapular artery (SA).(AC: acromion process; SM: supraspinatus muscle; TM: trapezius muscle)

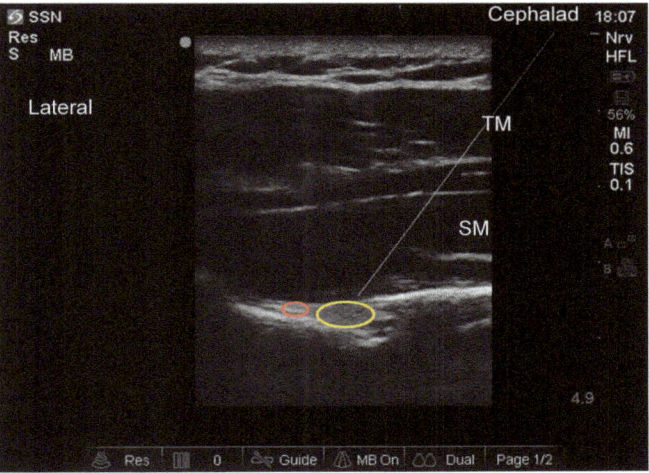

Fig. 17: Injection site of the suprascapular nerve. Yellow circle denotes the suprascapular nerve (SSN), red circle denotes the suprascapular artery (SA), and dashed white line denotes the needle trajectory from medial to lateral. (SM: supraspinatus muscle; TM: trapezius muscle)

FURTHER READING

1. Borglum J, Bartholdy A, Hautopp H, Krogsgaard MR, Jensen K. Ultrasound-guided continuous suprascapular nerve block for adhesive capsulitis: one case and a short topical review. Acta Anesthesiol Scand. 2011;55:242-7.
2. Chan C-W, Peng PWH. Suprascapular nerve block: a narrative review. Reg Anesth Pain Med. 2011;36:358-73.
3. Elsharkawy HA, Abd-Elsayed AA, Cummings KC, Soliman LM. Analgesic efficacy and technique of ultrasound-guided suprascapular nerve catheters after shoulder arthroscopy. Ochsner J. 2014;14:259-63.
4. Ridsall JE, Sharwood-Smith GH. Suprascapular nerve block. New indications and a safer technique. Anesthesia.1992;47:626.
5. Siegenthaler A, Moriggl B, Mlekusch S, Schliessbach J, Haug M, Curatolo M, et al. Ultrasound-guided suprascapular nerve block, description of a novel supraclavicular approach. Reg Anesth Pain Med. 2012;37(3):325-8.
6. Wertheim HM, Rovenstein EA. Suprascapular nerve block. Anesthesiology. 1941;2:541-5.

CHAPTER 46

Brachial Plexus Block (Supraclavicular Approach)

Ritesh Roy, Gaurav Agarwal

BRACHIAL PLEXUS BLOCK

Basic Information

- *Brachial plexus block*: Brachial plexus is formed by the nerve roots from C5 to T1. It blocks the ipsilateral whole of the upper limb.
- *Indications*: Anesthesia and analgesia for any procedure involving upper limb from mid-humerus to the fingertips, cancer pain management involving upper limb, other acute upper limb pains with or without continuous catheters.
- *Contraindications*: Unwilling patient, bleeding disorders, infection at the injection site
- *Medications used*:
  - Local anesthetic: 0.1–0.5% Ropivacaine/0.125–0.5% Bupivacaine 15–20 mL with or without adjuvants
  - Adjuvants that can be used: Dexmedetomidine 0.5–1 μg/kg, Clonidine 0.5–1 μg/kg, Dexamethasone 0.1–0.2 mg/kg

PROCEDURE DETAILS

Step 1: Position of patient: Supine with head turned to the contralateral side. Identify clavicle and the tendons of sternocleidomastoid. High-frequency ultrasonography (USG) probe should be used placed parallel to clavicle. Scan transverse oblique in a cephalad direction in sweep movement to identify different cervical nerve roots **(Fig. 1)**.

Step 2: Identify the brachial plexus bundle posterolateral to the subclavian artery **(Fig. 2)**.

Step 3: Scanning cephalad T1 nerve root can be seen coming out between the pleura and first rib **(Fig. 3)**.

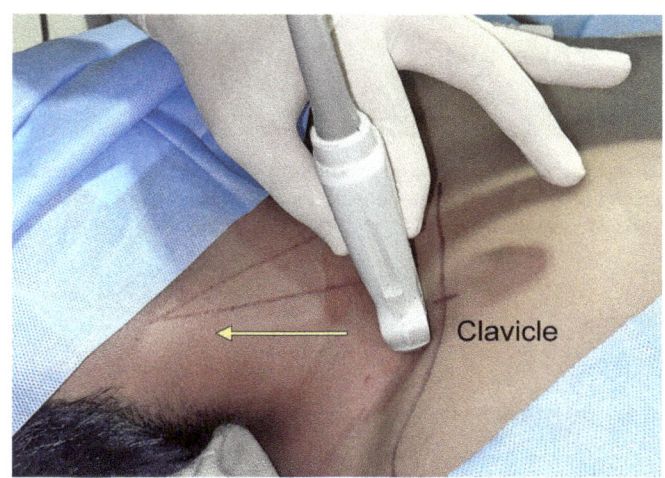

Fig. 1: Brachial plexus block—initial probe position.

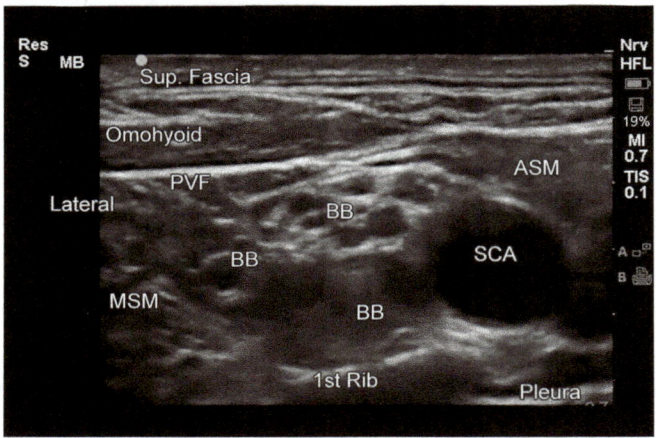

Fig. 2: Sonoanatomy of supraclavicular scanning of brachial plexus. (ASM: anterior scalene muscle; BB: brachial plexus bundles; MSM: middle scalene muscle; PVF: prevertebral fascia; SCA: subclavian artery)

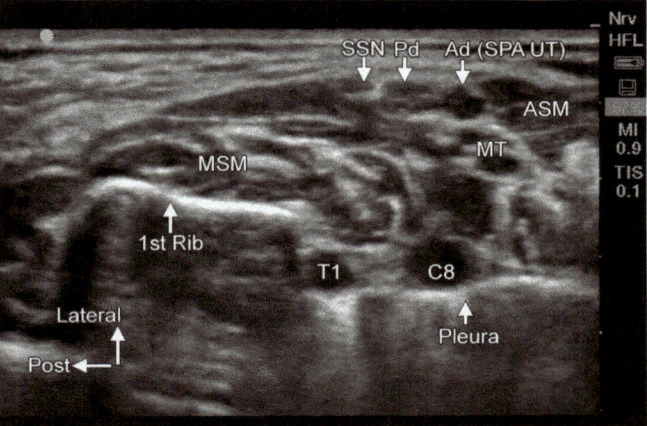

Fig. 3: Scan image identifying T1. (Ad: upper trunk anterior division; Pd: upper trunk posterior division; C8: eighth cervical nerve root; ASM: anterior scalene muscle; MSM: middle scalene muscle; MT: middle trunk; SSN: suprascapular nerve; T1: first thoracic nerve root)

Step 4: Scanning further cephalad in the transverse oblique direction, identify the eighth cervical nerve root (C8) over the first rib **(Fig. 4)**.

Step 5: Scanning further cephalad in the transverse oblique direction, identify the seventh cervical nerve root (C7) and vertebral artery, at the C7 vertebral level where the anterior tubercle of the C7 transverse process is absent and prominent posterior tubercle is seen **(Fig. 5)**.

Step 6: Scanning further cephalad in the transverse oblique direction, identify the sixth cervical nerve root and internal carotid artery, at the C6 vertebral level where the anterior tubercle of the C6 transverse process is the most prominent tubercle in the cervical spine **(Fig. 6)**.

Step 7: Scanning further cephalad in the transverse oblique direction, identify the fifth cervical nerve root (C5) coming out between the two transverse processes of C5 vertebra **(Fig. 7)**.

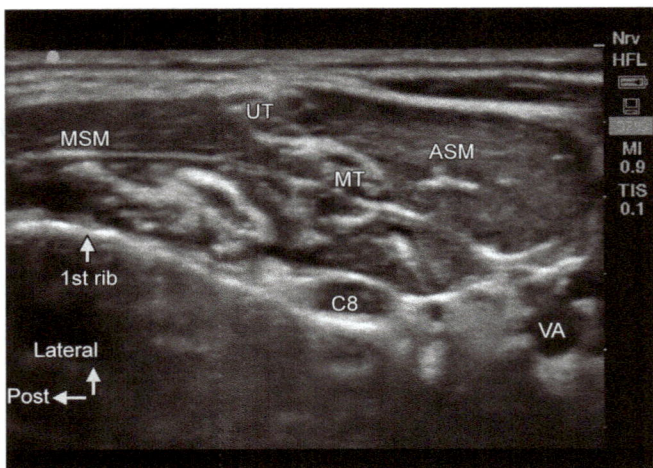

Fig. 4: Brachial plexus image identifying C8. (ASM: anterior scalene muscle; MSM: middle scalene muscle; MT: middle trunk; UT: upper trunk; VA: vertebral artery)

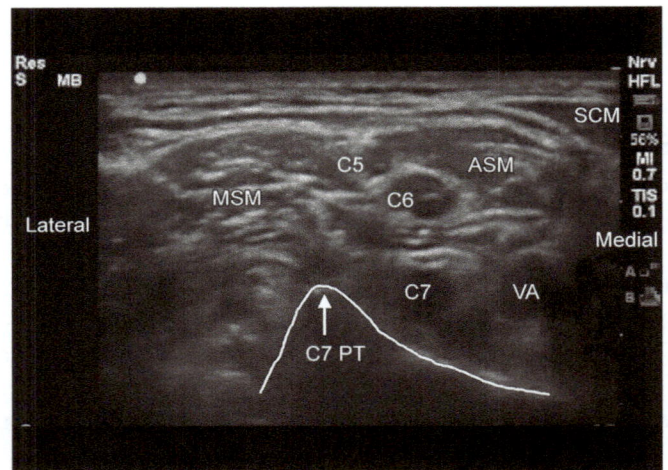

Fig. 5: Brachial plexus image identifying C7. (ASM: anterior scalene muscle; C5: fifth cervical nerve root; C6: sixth cervical nerve root; C7: seventh cervical nerve root; C7 PT: posterior tubercle of the transverse process of the seventh cervical vertebra; MSM: middle scalene muscle; SCM: sternocleidomastoid muscle; VA: vertebral artery)

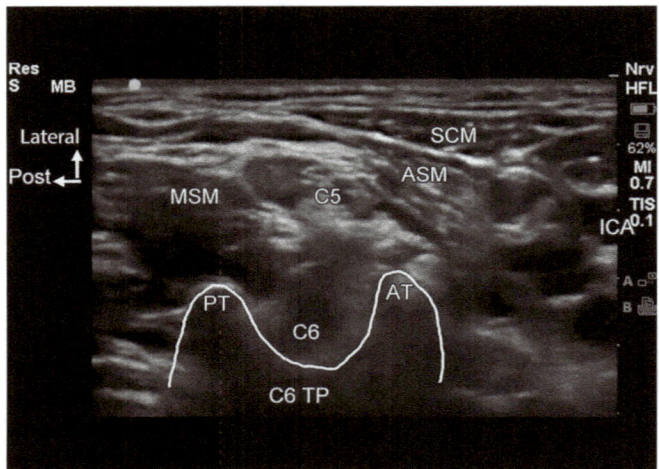

Fig. 6: Brachial plexus image identifying C6. (ASM: anterior scalene muscle; AT: anterior tubercle of the transverse process of the sixth cervical vertebra; C5: fifth cervical nerve root; C6: sixth cervical nerve root; C6 TP: transverse process of the sixth cervical vertebra; ICA: internal carotid artery; MSM: middle scalene muscle; PT: posterior tubercle of the transverse process of the sixth cervical vertebra; SCM: sternocleidomastoid muscle)

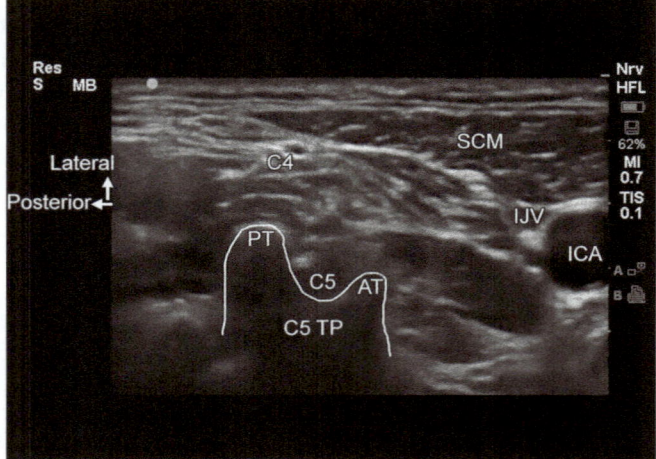

Fig. 7: Brachial plexus image identifying C5. (AT: anterior tubercle of the transverse process of the fifth cervical vertebra; C4: fourth cervical nerve root; C5: fifth cervical nerve root; C5 TP: transverse process of the fifth cervical vertebra; ICA: internal carotid artery; IJV: internal jugular vein; PT: posterior tubercle of the transverse process of the fifth cervical vertebra; SCM: sternocleidomastoid muscle)

Step 8: Scanning back caudad in the transverse oblique direction, identify the fifth and sixth cervical nerve roots, which will form the superior trunk. Earlier, this interscalene traffic light sign was misrepresented as the three cervical nerve roots, which actually is the separation of the nerve root of the sixth cervical nerve root (bifid C6 nerve root) and not seventh cervical nerve root **(Fig. 8)**.

Step 9: Scanning back caudad in the transverse oblique direction, identify the formation of the upper/superior trunk. The dorsal scapular nerve is often seen here crossing the middle scalene muscle **(Fig. 9)**.

Step 10: Scanning back caudad in the transverse oblique direction, identify the formation the middle trunk (continuation of the C7 nerve root) and the starting of division of the upper trunk into SPA (suprascapular nerve, posterior and anterior divisions) is seen **(Fig. 10)**.

Step 11: Scanning back caudad in the transverse oblique direction. The C8 and T1 nerve roots join to form the lower trunk **(Fig. 11)**.

Step 12: Identify all the brachial plexus structures. The needle is guided in-plane to avoid inadvertent arterial or nerve

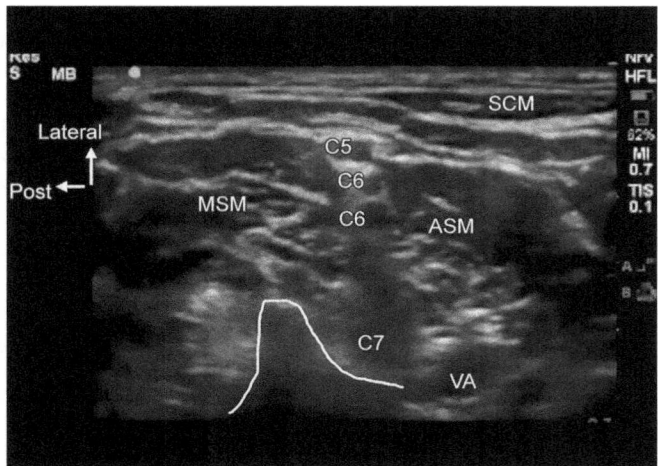

Fig. 8: Brachial plexus image identifying C5 and C6. (ASM: anterior scalene muscle; C5: fifth cervical nerve root; C6: bifid root of the sixth cervical nerve root; MSM: middle scalene muscle; SCM: sternocleidomastoid muscle; VA: vertebral artery)

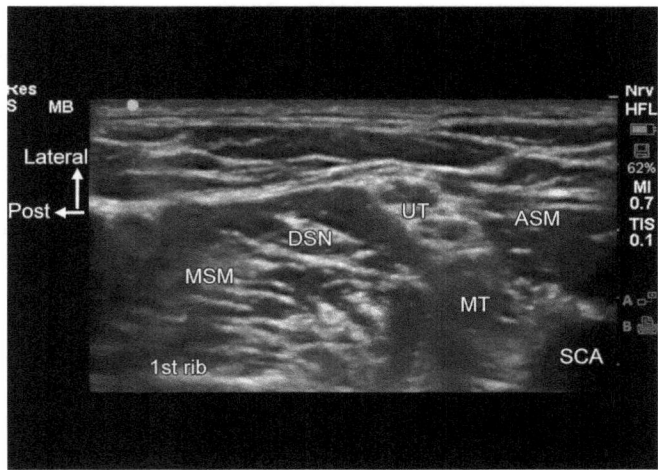

Fig. 9: Brachial plexus image identifying formation of upper trunk. (ASM: anterior scalene muscle; DSN: dorsal scapular nerve; MSM: middle scalene muscle; MT: middle trunk; SCA: subclavian artery; SCM: sternocleidomastoid muscle; UT: upper trunk)

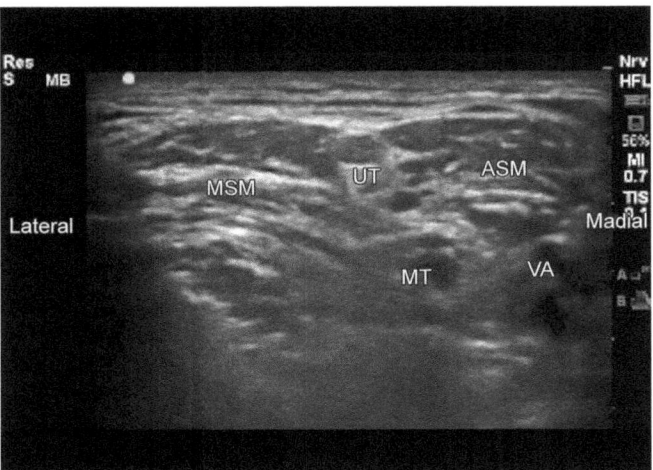

Fig. 10: Brachial plexus image identifying formation of middle trunk. (ASM: anterior scalene muscle; MSM: middle scalene muscle; MT: middle trunk; SCM: sternocleidomastoid muscle; UT: upper trunk; VA: vertebral artery)

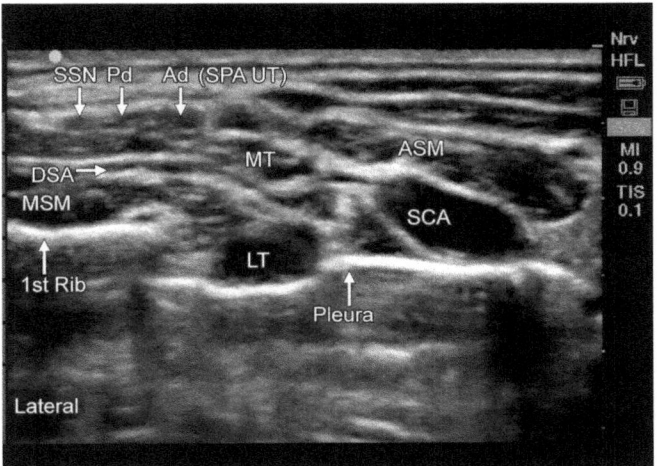

Fig. 11: Brachial plexus image. Identify C8 and T1. Join to form the lower trunk. [ASM: anterior scalene muscle; DSA: dorsal scapular artery; LT: lower trunk; MSM: middle scalene muscle; MT: middle trunk; SCA: subclavian artery; UT: upper trunk—the three divisions (SSN: suprascapular nerve; Pd: posterior division; Ad: anterior division)]

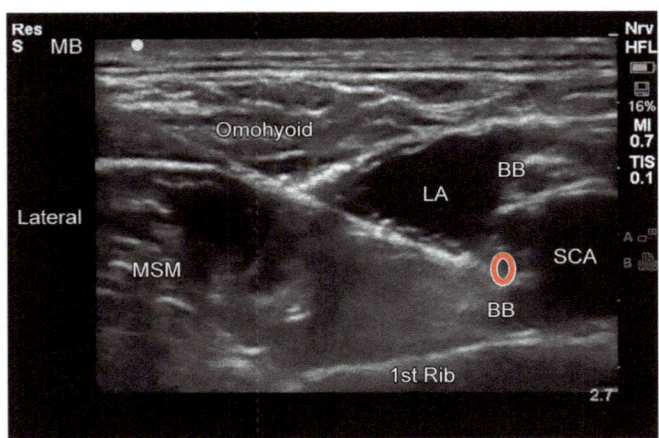

Fig. 12: Brachial plexus image injection at the supraclavicular fossa. Red circle denotes the needle tip. (ASM: anterior scalene muscle; BB: brachial plexus bundles; LA: local anesthesia; MSM: middle scalene muscle; SCA: subclavian artery)

puncture, first to the corner pocket formed by the subclavian artery and the first rib to avoid ulnar nerve sparing and then redirected. A total volume of 15–20 mL of the drug is injected in small aliquots after regular negative aspirations for blood to achieve the block **(Fig. 12)**.

FURTHER READING

1. Collins AB, Gray AT, Kessler J. Ultrasound-guided supraclavicular brachial plexus nerve block: a modified Plumb-Bob technique. Reg Anesth Pain Med. 2006;31:591-2.
2. Cornish P. Supraclavicular nerve block: new perspectives. Reg Anesth Pain Med. 2009;34:607-8.
3. Hanumanthaiah D, Vaidiyanathan S, Garstka M, Szucs S, Iohom G. Ultrasound-guided supraclavicular nerve block. Med Ultrason. 2013;15:224-9.
4. Heil JW, Ilfeld BM, Loland VJ, Mariano ER. Preliminary experience with a novel ultrasound-guided supraclavicular perineural catheter insertion technique for perioperative analgesia of the upper extremity. J Ultrasound Med. 2010;29:1481-5.
5. Karmakar MK, Pakpirom J, Songthamwat B, Areeruk P. High definition ultrasound imaging of the individual elements of the brachial plexus above the clavicle. Reg Anesth Pain Med. 2020;45(5):344-50.
6. Zinboonyahgoon N, Vlassakov K, Abrecht CR, Srinivasan S, Narang S. Brachial plexus block for cancer-related pain: a case series. Pain Physician. 2015;18(5):E917-24.

47. Thoracic Paravertebral Block

Archana Areti, Ritesh Roy, Gaurav Agarwal

THORACIC PARAVERTEBRAL BLOCK

Basic Information

- The thoracic paravertebral space begins at T1 and extends caudally to terminate at T12.
- The thoracic paravertebral space is wedge shaped. The vertebral body, intervertebral discs, and intervertebral foramina form the medial wall. Anterolaterally, it is bounded by the parietal pleura. Posteriorly, it is bounded by the transverse process of the thoracic vertebrae, the heads of the ribs, and the superior costotransverse ligament.
- The TPVB is the deposition of local anesthetic in the thoracic paravertebral space close to the intervertebral foramen where the spinal nerves emerge.
- It produces ipsilateral, segmental, somatic, and sympathetic nerve blockade in contiguous thoracic dermatomes.
- It is used for acute and chronic pain management of unilateral origin from the thorax and abdomen.
- *Indications*:
  - Anesthesia for unilateral surgery:
    – Breast surgery
    – Thoracic surgery
    – Cholecystectomy
    – Renal surgery
  - Analgesia for rib fractures
  - *Chronic pain management*:
    – Neuropathic chest or abdominal pain (postsurgical or postherpetic)
    – Complex regional pain syndrome
    – Relief of cancer pain
  - *Relative contraindications*:
    – Patient refusal
    – Local sepsis
    – Tumors in the paravertebral space at the level of injection
    – Severe coagulopathy
    – Allergy to local anesthetic drugs
    – Severe respiratory distress
    – Severe spinal deformity
    – Pleurodesis
- *Complications*:
  - Pleural puncture
  - Pneumothorax
  - Vascular puncture
  - Hypotension
  - Ipsilateral Horner's syndrome

TRANSVERSE OR AXIAL SCAN TECHNIQUE

Position of Patient

Sitting/prone/lateral decubitus

Step 1: Patient is placed in lateral/sitting/prone position.

A low-frequency curvilinear or high-frequency linear transducer is placed in transverse orientation as shown in **Figures 1 to 3**.

Note: Probe selection is dependent on the body habitus of the patient. If the intended target is within 4 cm, then a high-frequency linear probe can be used; otherwise, a curvilinear probe is selected.

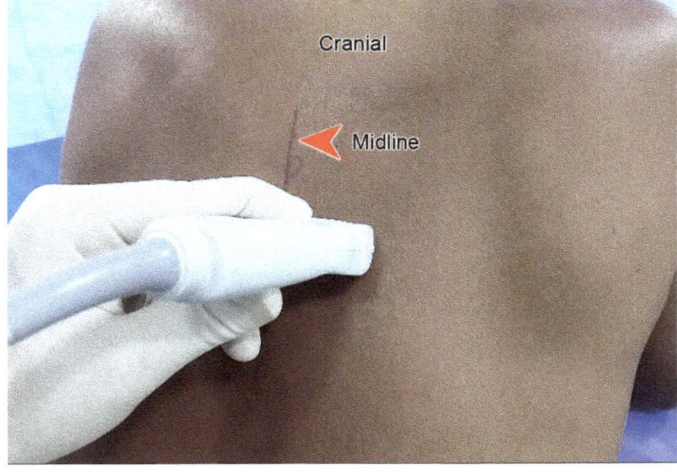

Fig. 1: Transverse ultrasound scan of the mid-thoracic paravertebral region with the patient in sitting position using a linear high-frequency transducer. Note the position of probe relative to midline.

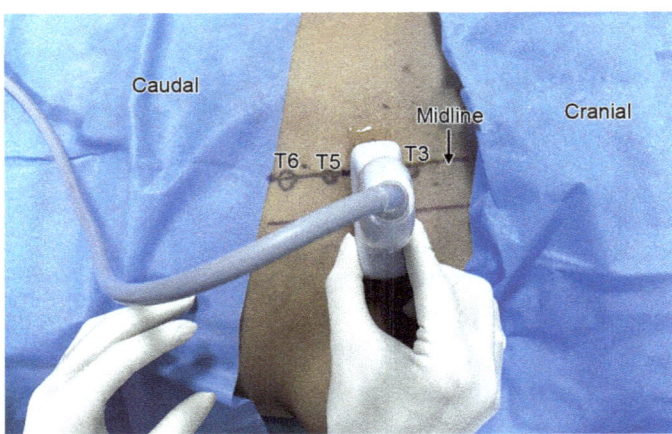

Fig. 2: Transverse ultrasound scan of the mid-thoracic paravertebral region with the patient in right lateral position using a curvilinear low-frequency transducer. Note the position of probe relative to midline.

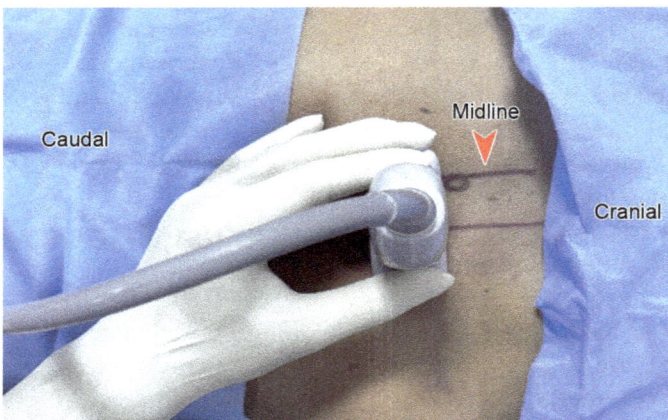

Fig. 3: Transverse ultrasound scan of the mid-thoracic paravertebral region with the patient in prone position using a curvilinear low-frequency transducer. Note the position of probe relative to midline.

Scanning Sequence with Sonoanatomy

Step 2: A stepwise scanning is started from position 1 to position 4 of the transducer **(Fig. 4)**.

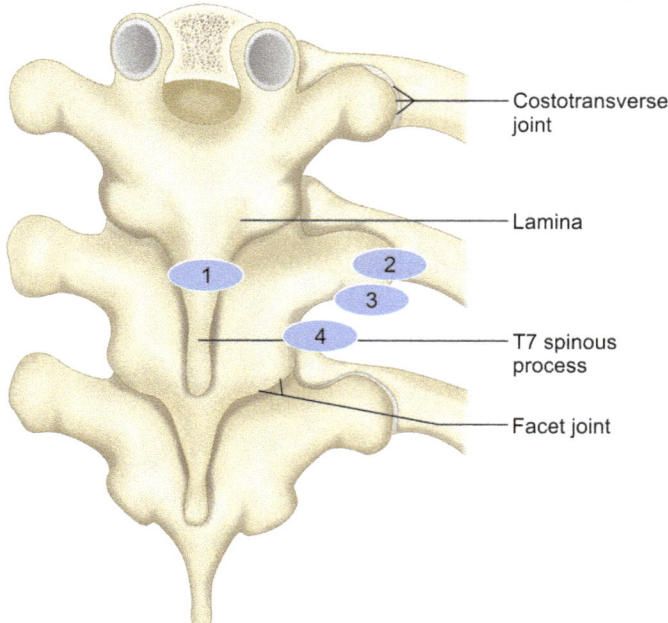

Fig. 4: Image showing mid-thoracic region of the spine with a stepwise approach (1 to 4) for transverse scan of the thoracic paravertebral region. Blue ovals represent the transducer.

Position 1: Transducer in midline over the thoracic spinous process **(Figs. 5 and 6)**.

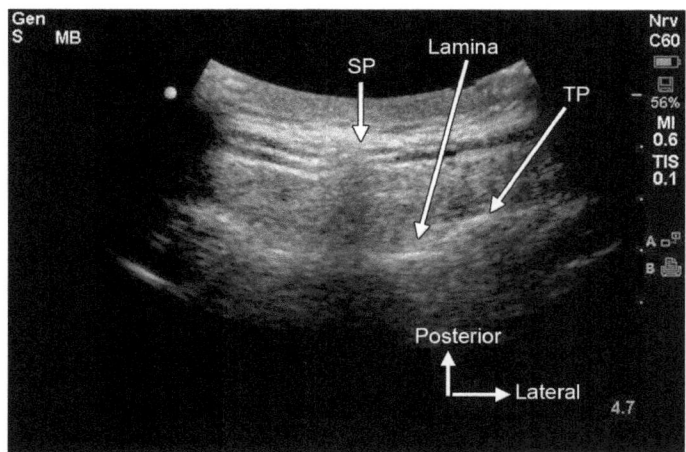 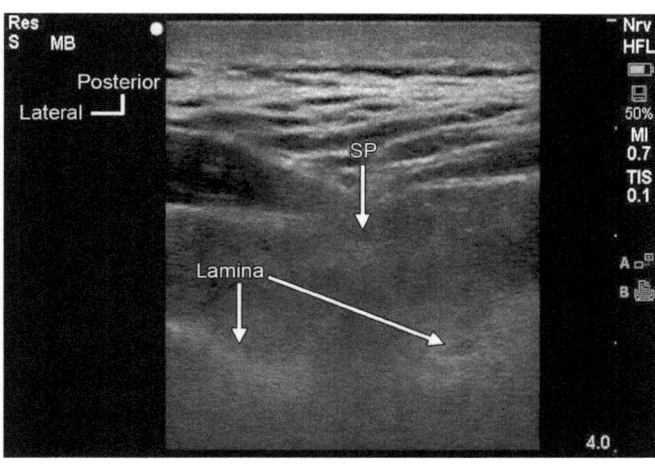

Fig. 5: Transverse midline scan of the mid-thoracic spine using a curvilinear low-frequency transducer with ultrasound rays over the spinous process (Position 1 in **Figure 4**). Note the formation of a "flying swan" sonographic pattern produced by the acoustic shadow of spinous process (SP), transverse process (TP), and lamina.

Fig. 6: Transverse midline scan of the mid-thoracic spine using a linear high-frequency transducer with ultrasound rays over the spinous process (Position 1 in **Figure 4**). (SP: spinous process)

Position 2: Transducer at the level of the transverse process (TP) and rib **(Figs. 7 to 9)**.

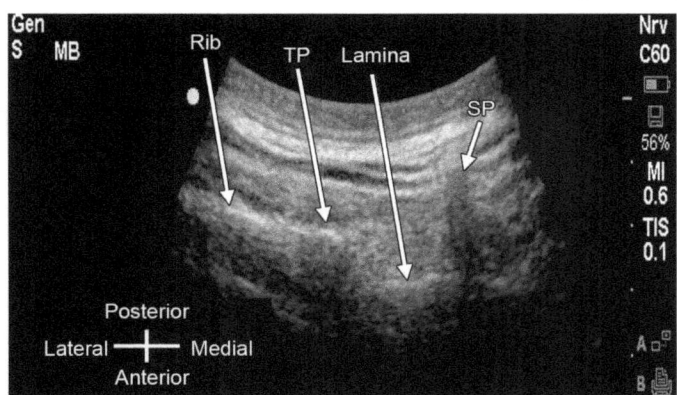 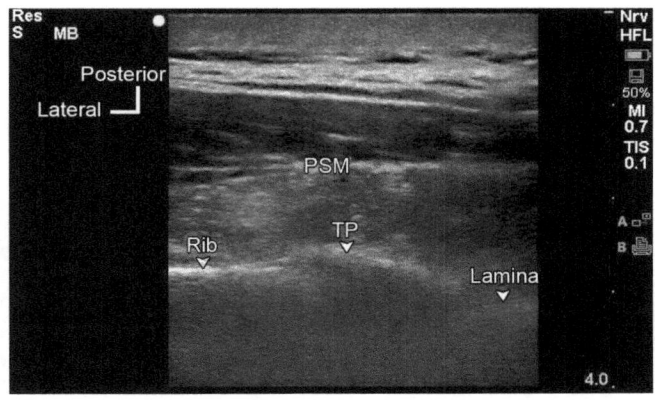

Fig. 7: Paramedian transverse scan of mid-thoracic spine using a curvilinear low-frequency transducer with ultrasound rays over the spinous process (SP), lamina, transverse process (TP), and ribs (Position 2 in **Figure 4**).

Fig. 8: Paramedian transverse scan of the mid-thoracic spine using a linear high-frequency transducer with ultrasound rays over the lamina, transverse process (TP), and ribs (Position 2 in **Figure 4**). (PSM: paraspinal muscle)

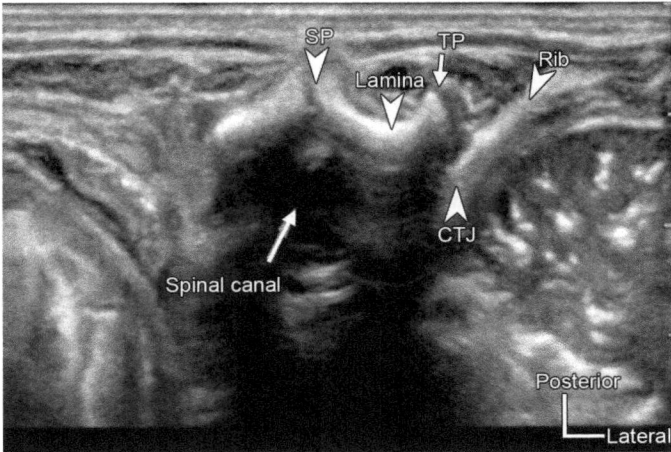

Fig. 9: Paramedian transverse scan of the mid-thoracic spine in a neonate using a linear high-frequency transducer with ultrasound rays over the spinous process (SP), lamina, transverse process (TP), ribs, and costotransverse joint (CTJ) (Position 2 in **Figure 4**).

Position 3: Transducer at the level of the TP (**Figs. 10 and 11**).

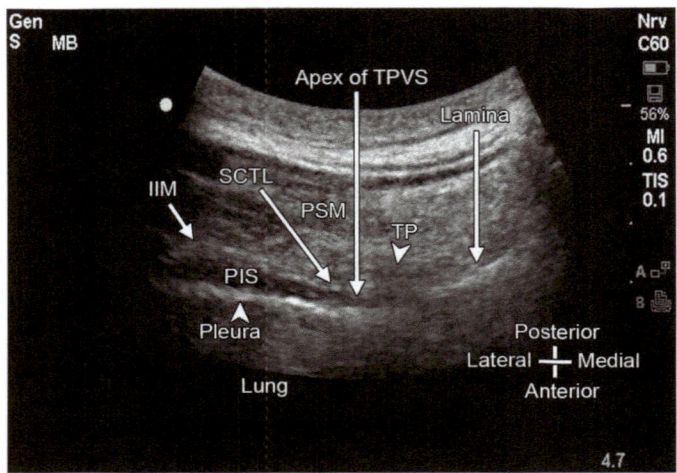 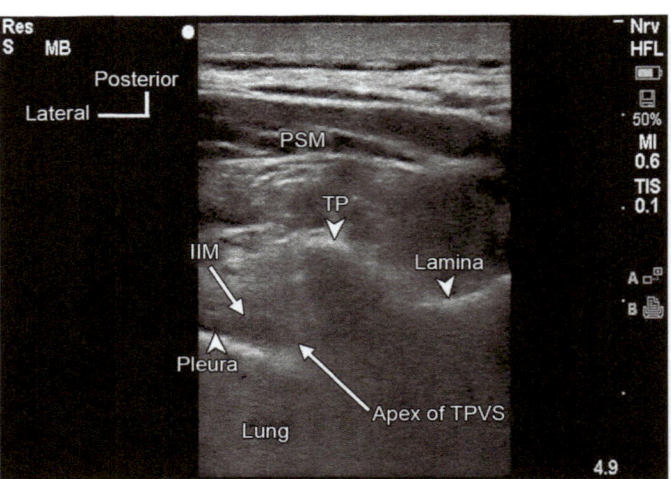

Fig. 10: Paramedian transverse scan of the mid-thoracic paravertebral region using a curvilinear low-frequency transducer with ultrasound rays over the transverse process (TP) (Position 3 in **Figure 4**). Note the hyperechoic TP with its acoustic shadow. The apex of the thoracic paravertebral space (TPVS), superior costotransverse ligament (SCTL), and pleura are seen lateral to the TP. (IIM: internal intercostal membrane; PIS: posterior intercostal space; PSM: paraspinal muscle)

Fig. 11: Paramedian transverse scan of the mid-thoracic paravertebral region using a linear high-frequency transducer with ultrasound rays over the transverse process (TP) (Position 3 in **Figure 4**). Note the hyperechoic TP with its acoustic shadow. The apex of the thoracic paravertebral space (TPVS) and pleura are seen lateral to the TP. (IIM: internal intercostal membrane; PSM: paraspinal muscle)

Position 4: Transducer at the level of the articular process [position at which a thoracic paravertebral block (TPVB) is given] (**Figs. 12 to 14**).

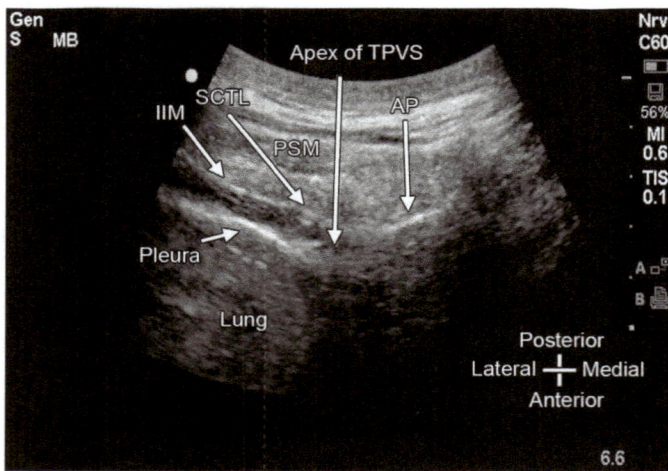 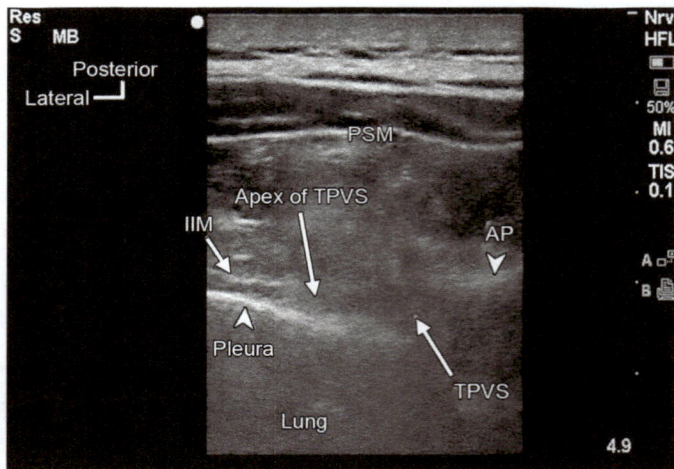

Fig. 12: Paramedian transverse scan of the mid-thoracic paravertebral region using a curvilinear low-frequency transducer with ultrasound rays through the intertransverse space (Position 4 in **Figure 4**). Note the hyperechoic articular process (AP) with its acoustic shadow. The apex of the thoracic paravertebral space (TPVS), superior costotransverse ligament (SCTL), and pleura are seen laterally. (IIM: internal intercostal membrane; PSM: paraspinal muscle)

Fig. 13: Paramedian transverse scan of the mid-thoracic paravertebral region using a transverse high-frequency transducer with ultrasound rays through the intertransverse space (Position 4 in **Figure 4**). Note the hyperechoic articular process (AP) with its acoustic shadow. The thoracic paravertebral space (TPVS), apex of the (TPVS, and pleura are seen laterally. (IIM: internal intercostal membrane; PSM: paraspinal muscle)

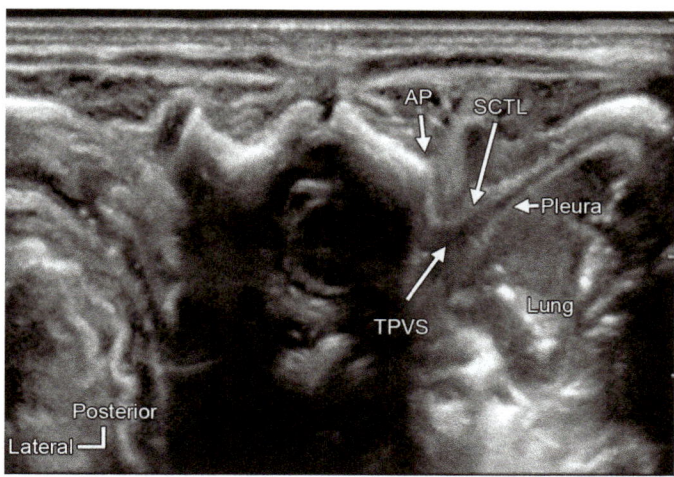

Fig. 14: Paramedian transverse scan of the mid-thoracic paravertebral region in a neonate using a transverse high-frequency transducer with ultrasound rays through the intertransverse space (Position 4 in **Figure 4**). Note the hyperechoic articular process (AP) with its acoustic shadow. The thoracic paravertebral space (TPVS), superior costotransverse ligament (SCTL), and pleura are seen laterally.

Needling and Drug Deposition

Step 3: In-plane needling from lateral to medial with the probe at position 4 (**Figs. 4 and 11**) and 5–7 mL of local anesthetic to be deposited at each level (**Fig. 15**).

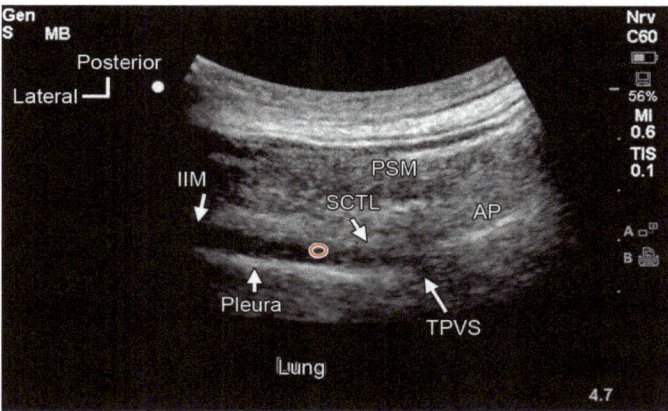

Fig. 15: Paramedian transverse scan of the mid-thoracic paravertebral region using a curvilinear low-frequency transducer with ultrasound rays through the intertransverse space (Position 4 in **Figure 4**) with in-plane needling from lateral to medial. Red dot denotes the needle tip. Note the hyperechoic articular process (AP) with its acoustic shadow. The apex of the thoracic paravertebral space (TPVS), superior costotransverse ligament (SCTL), and pleura are seen laterally. (IIM: internal intercostal membrane; PSM: paraspinal muscle)

FURTHER READING

1. Abdallah FW, Brull R. Off side! A simple modification to the parasagittal in-plane approach for paravertebral block. Reg Anesth Pain Med. 2014;39:240-2.
2. Ardon AE, Lee J, Franco CD, Riutort KT, Greengrass RA. Paravertebral block: anatomy and relevant safety issues. Korean J Anesthesiol. 2020;73(5):394-400.
3. Cowie B, McGlade D, Ivanusic J, Barrington MJ. Ultrasound-guided thoracic paravertebral blockade: a cadaveric study. Anesth Analg. 2010;110:1735-9.
4. Karmakar MK. Thoracic paravertebral block (review article). Anesthesiology. 2001;95:771-80.
5. Karmakar MK. Ultrasound-guided thoracic paravertebral block. In Narouze S (Ed). Atlas of Ultrasound-guided Procedures in Interventional Pain Management, 1st edition. New York: Springer; 2010. pp. 134-47.
6. Krediet AC, Moayeri N, van Geffen GJ, Bruhn J, Renes S, Bigeleisen PE, et al. Different approaches to ultrasound-guided thoracic paravertebral block: an illustrated review. Anesthesiology. 2015;123(2):459-74.
7. Marhofer P, Kettner SC, Hajbok L, Dubsky P, Fleischmann E. Lateral ultrasound-guided paravertebral blockade: an anatomical-based description of a new technique. Br J Anaesth. 2010;105:526-32.
8. O Riain SC, Donnell BO, Cuffe T, Harmon DC, Fraher JP, Shorten G. Thoracic paravertebral block using real-time ultrasound guidance. Anesth Analg. 2010;110:248-51.
9. Paraskeuopoulos T, Saranteas T, Kouladouros K, Krepi H, Nakou M, Kostopanagiotou G, et al. Thoracic paravertebral spread using two different ultrasound-guided intercostal injection techniques in human cadavers. Clin Anat. 2010;23: 840-7.
10. Purcell-Jones G, Pither CE, Justins DM. Paravertebral somatic nerve block: a clinical, radiographic, and computed tomographic study in chronic pain patients. Anesth Analg. 1989;68:32-9.

CHAPTER 48: Ultrasound-guided Transversus Abdominis Plane Block

Gaurav Agarwal, Ritesh Roy

TRANSVERSUS ABDOMINIS PLANE BLOCK

Basic Information

- TAP block—blocks the anterior cutaneous branches of the thoracic nerves which lie in the plane between the internal oblique muscles and the transversus abdominis muscle. Posterior TAP block is a more lateral approach to blocking the anterior and lateral cutaneous branches of the T10–L1 nerves.
- *Indications*: Part of multimodal analgesia for various abdominal surgeries, hernia repairs, procedure involving anterior abdominal wall, cesarean section, appendicectomy, laparoscopic surgery, pain from the anterior abdominal wall.
- *Contraindications*: Unwilling patient, bleeding disorders, infection at the injection site.
- *Types of TAP block*:
  - *Subcostal TAP block*: Blocks the anterior cutaneous branches of T6–T9 nerves.
  - *Classical TAP block*: Blocks the anterior cutaneous branches of T10–T12 nerves.
  - *Posterior TAP block*: Blocks the anterior and lateral cutaneous branches of T10–L1 nerves.
- *Medications used*:
  - *Local anesthetic*: 0.1–0.2% ropivacaine, 0.125–0.25% bupivacaine 15–20 mL with or without adjuvants.
  - *Adjuvants that can be used*: Dexmedetomidine 0.5–1 µg/kg, clonidine 0.5–1 µg/kg, dexamethasone 0.1–0.2 mg/kg.

SUBCOSTAL TRANSVERSUS ABDOMINIS PLANE BLOCK

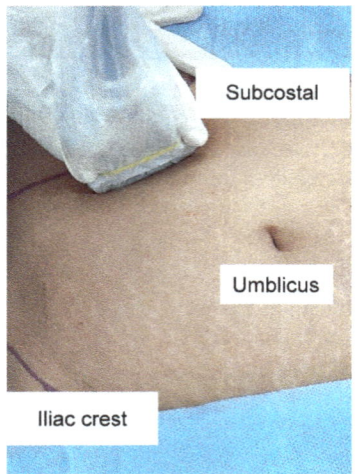

Fig. 1: Probe position of subcostal transversus abdominis plane block.

Step 1: Position of patient—supine. Identify subcostal line. A high-frequency ultrasonography (USG) probe is placed parallel to the subcostal line **(Fig. 1)**.

Step 2: Identify the layers of the abdominal wall—EO (external oblique), IO (internal oblique), TA (transversus abdominis), RA (rectus abdominis), ARS (anterior rectus sheath), LS (linea semilunaris) **(Figs. 2 and 3)**.

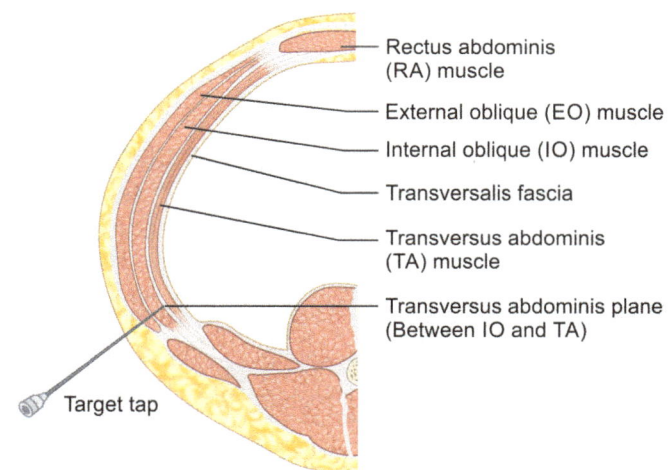

Fig. 2: Target transversus abdominis plane. (IO: internal oblique; TA: transversus abdominis)

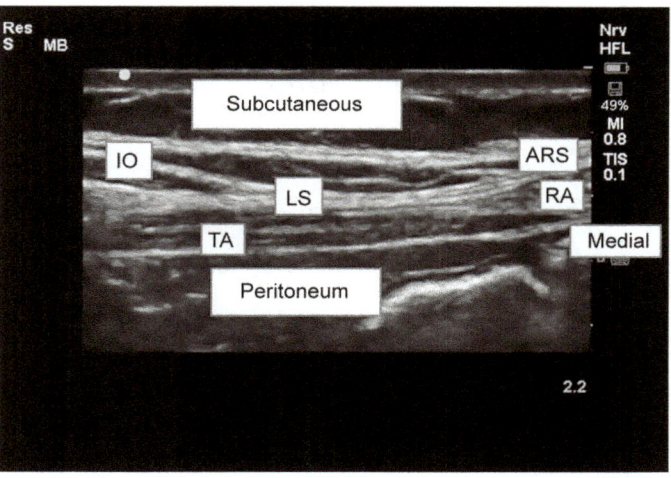

Fig. 3: Sonoanatomy of subcostal transversus abdominis plane. Target is between RA and TA at the linea semilunaris level. (ARS: anterior rectus sheath; EO: external oblique; IO: internal oblique; LS: linea semilunaris; RA: rectus abdominis; TA: transversus abdominis)

Step 3: After skin local anesthesia (LA) infiltration, insert the needle in-plane (under vision) to reach the target between rectus abdominis and transversus abdominis muscles **(Fig. 4)**.

Step 4: After confirming the needle tip in the target plane and negative aspiration of blood, inject the desired LA in small aliquots with a total of 15–20 mL, on each side for the block **(Fig. 5)**.

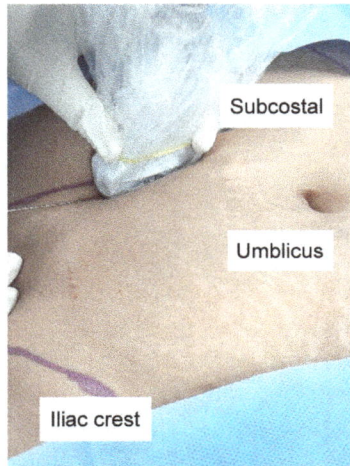

Fig. 4: Needle insertion in plane.

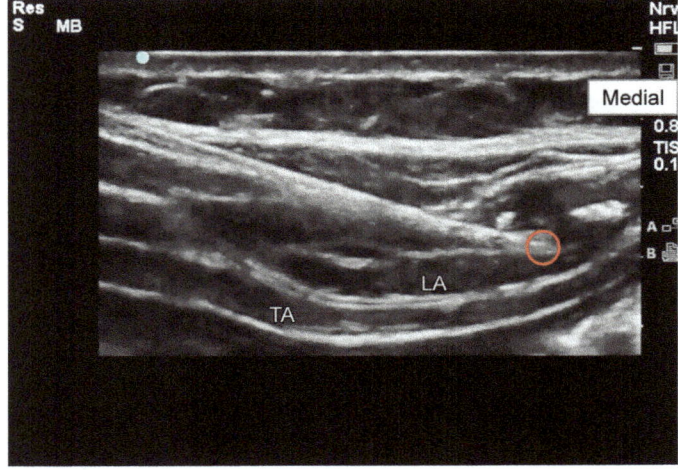

Fig. 5: LA injection at the target site. Red circle denotes the needle tip. (LA: local anesthetic; TA: transversus abdominis)

CLASSICAL TRANSVERSUS ABDOMINIS PLANE BLOCK

Step 1: Position of the patient—supine. Anterior superior iliac spine—iliac crest and subcostal line identified. High-frequency USG probe is placed at the mid-axillary line between the two landmarks **(Fig. 6)**.

Step 2: Identify the layers of the abdominal wall—EO (external oblique), IO (internal oblique), and TA (transversus abdominis) **(Fig. 7)**.

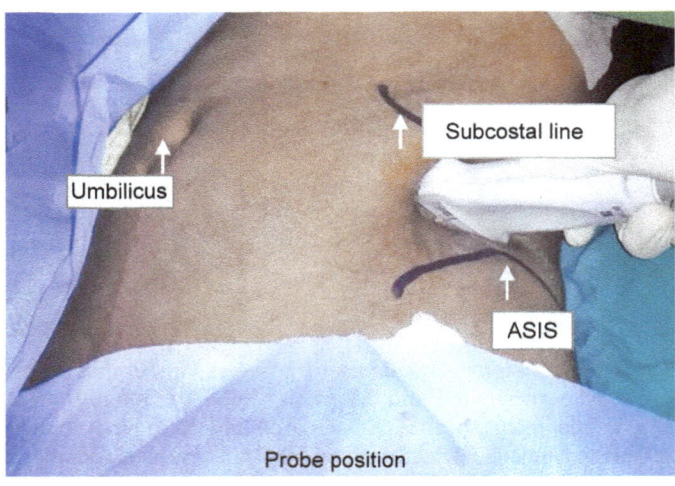

Fig. 6: Classical transversus abdominis plane probe position.

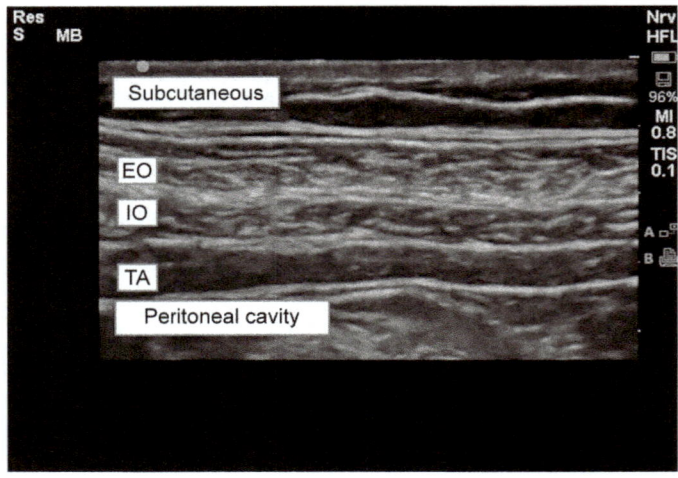

Fig. 7: Sonoanatomy of the classical transversus abdominis plane. Target is between the internal oblique and transversus abdominis.

Step 3: After skin LA infiltration, insert the needle in-plane (under vision) to reach the target between internal oblique and transversus abdominis **(Fig. 8)**.

Step 4: After confirming the needle tip in the target plane and negative aspiration of blood, inject the desired LA in small aliquots with a total of 15–20 mL, on each side for the block **(Fig. 9)**.

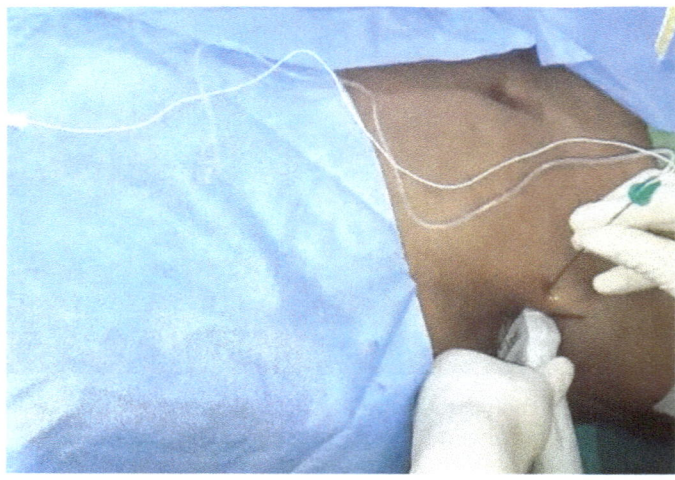

Fig. 8: Needle insertion in plane.

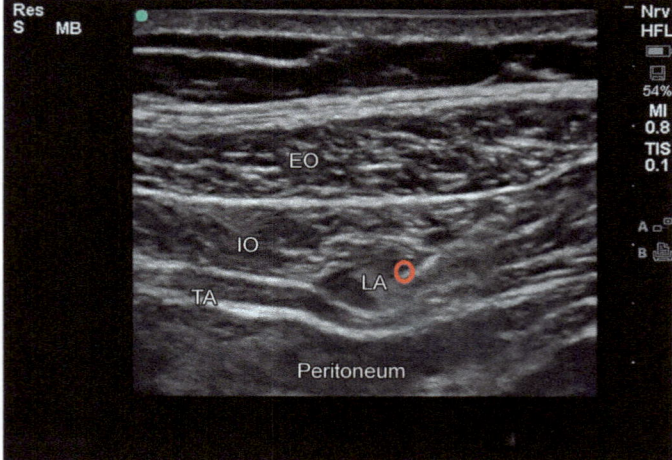

Fig. 9: LA injection at the target site. Red circle denotes the needle tip. (EO: external oblique; IO: internal oblique; TA: transversus abdominis; LA: local anesthetic).

POSTERIOR TRANSVERSUS ABDOMINIS PLANE BLOCK

Step 1: Position of patient—supine. Anterior superior iliac spine (ASIS)—iliac crest and subcostal line identified. High-frequency USG probe is placed at the posterior-axillary line between the two landmarks, to identify the abdominal layers and the fascia transversalis **(Fig. 10)**.

Step 2: Identify the layers of the abdominal wall—EO (external oblique), IO (internal oblique), TA (transversus abdominis), and TA aponeurosis (transversus abdominis aponeurosis) **(Fig. 11)**.

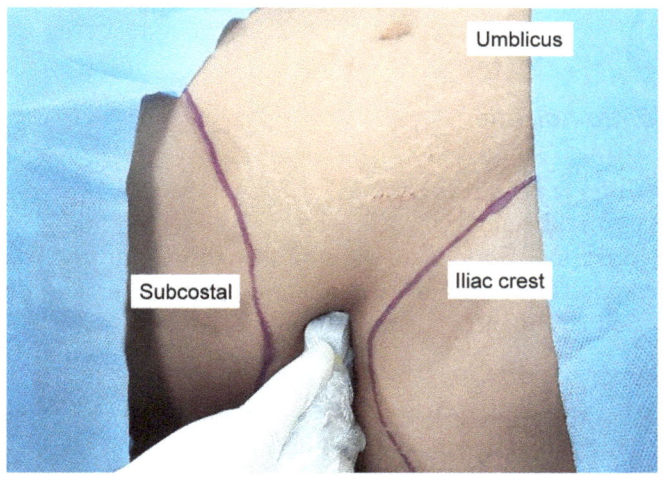

Fig. 10: Posterior transversus abdominis plane probe position. (IC: iliac crest)

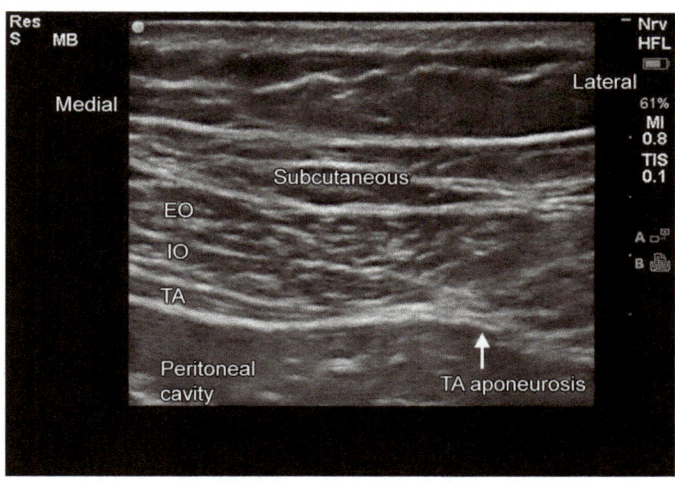

Fig. 11: Sonoanatomy of the posterior transversus abdominis plane. Target is between the internal oblique and transversus abdominis aponeurosis.

Step 3: After skin local anesthesia infiltration, insert the needle in-plane (under vision) to reach the target between IO and TA **(Fig. 12)**.

Step 4: After confirming the needle tip in the target plane and negative aspiration of blood, inject the desired LA in small aliquots with a total of 15–20 mL, on each side for the block **(Fig. 13)**.

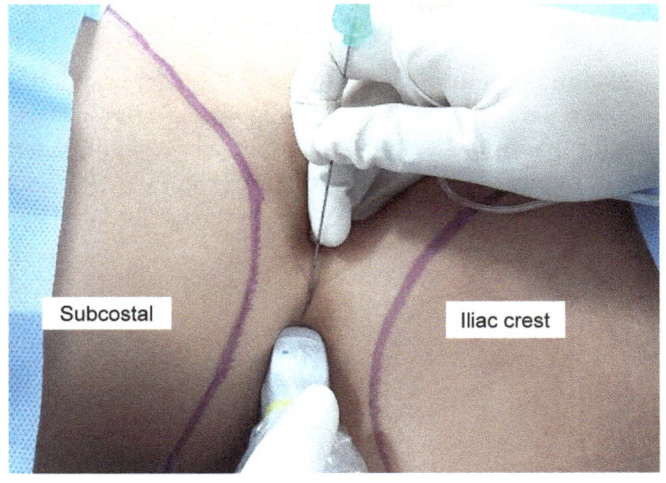

Fig. 12: Needle insertion in-plane for posterior transversus plane block.

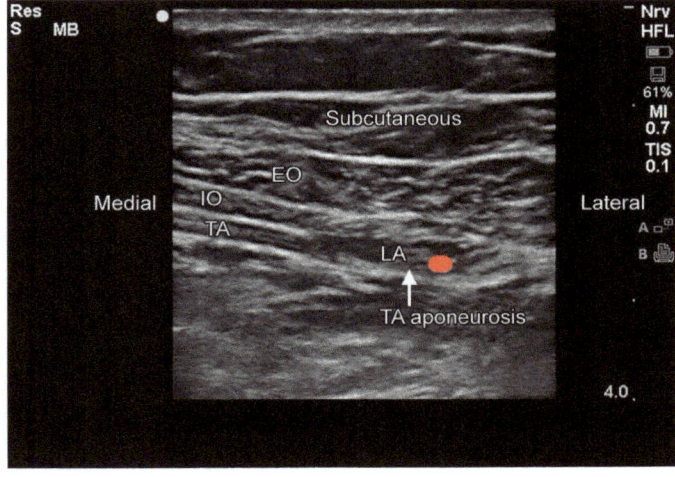

Fig. 13: LA injection at the target site. (EO: external oblique; IO: internal oblique; LA: local anesthesia; TA: transversus abdominis)

Lumbar Plexus Block

Ritesh Roy, Gaurav Agarwal

BASIC INFORMATION

- The lumbar plexus is formed of ventral primary rami of the L1, L2, L3, and L4 spinal nerves.
- The lumbar plexus is located in an intramuscular fascial compartment, also called psoas compartment, between the anterior two-thirds and posterior one-third of the psoas muscle.
- Lateral femoral cutaneous nerve (LFCN), femoral nerve (FN), and obturator nerve (ON) originate from the lumbar plexus.
- The lumbar plexus block (LPB) is an injection of local anesthetic in a fascial plane within the posterior part of psoas muscle to produce complete blockade of the major component of the ipsilateral lumbar plexus, namely lateral femoral cutaneous nerve (LFCN), femoral nerve (FN), and obturator nerve (ON).

Indications

- Surgical anesthesia for lower limb surgery along with sacral plexus block.
- Analgesia following hip or thigh surgery or injury (e.g., acetabular fractures, femoral neck or mid-shaft fractures, hip replacement, hip arthroscopy, knee replacement).
- Chronic pain conditions such as herpes zoster.
- Diagnostic and therapeutic tool for chronic hip pain disorders.

Contraindications

- Patient refusal
- Allergy to local anesthetics
- Local infection
- Systemic anticoagulation [international normalized ratio (INR) >1.5 or inadequate time since cessation of anticoagulant]

Complications

- Local anesthetic spread to the epidural space
- Intrathecal injection and spinal anesthesia
- Renal injury
- Local anesthetic systemic toxicity (LAST)
- Retroperitoneal or psoas hematoma or other vascular injuries.

PARAMEDIAN TRANSVERSE OBLIQUE APPROACH

Position of Patient

Step 1: The patient is positioned in lateral position with hips and knees flexed and the side to be blocked placed up.

The following anatomical landmarks are identified and marked:

A—interspinous line (midline), B—intercristal line, C—a line parallel to midline passing through the posterior superior iliac spine (PSIS), which intersects the intercristal line (B) roughly 4 cm lateral to midline (**Fig. 1**).

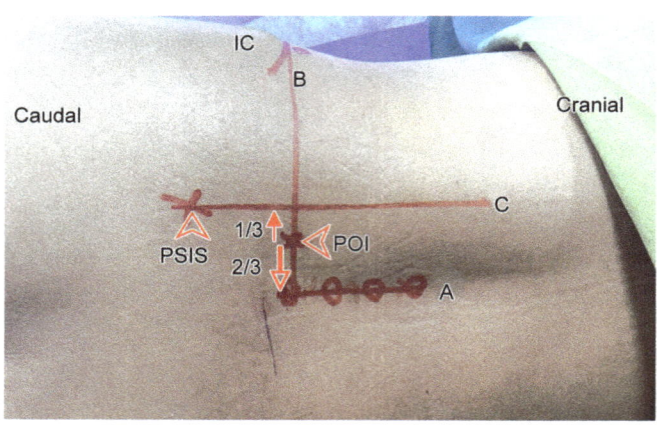

Fig. 1: Position of the patient with anatomical landmark marking. (IC: iliac crest; POI: point-of-needle insertion; PSIS: posterior superior iliac spine)

Scan Technique

Step 2: A curvilinear probe is placed in a paramedian transverse oblique orientation to identify the target structures (**Figs. 2 and 3**).

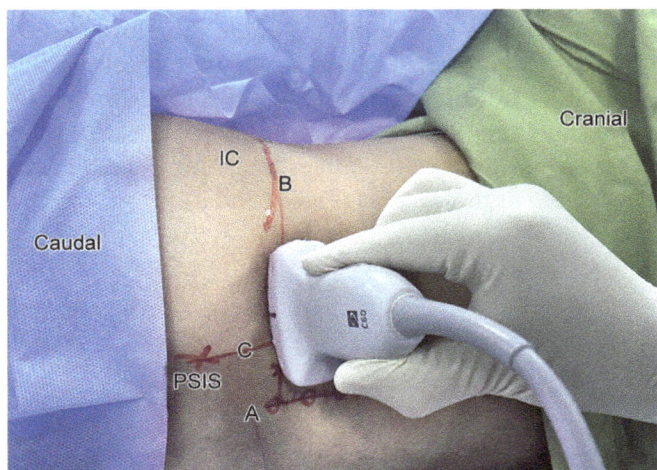

Fig. 2: Probe placement. (IC: iliac crest; PSIS: posterior superior iliac spine)

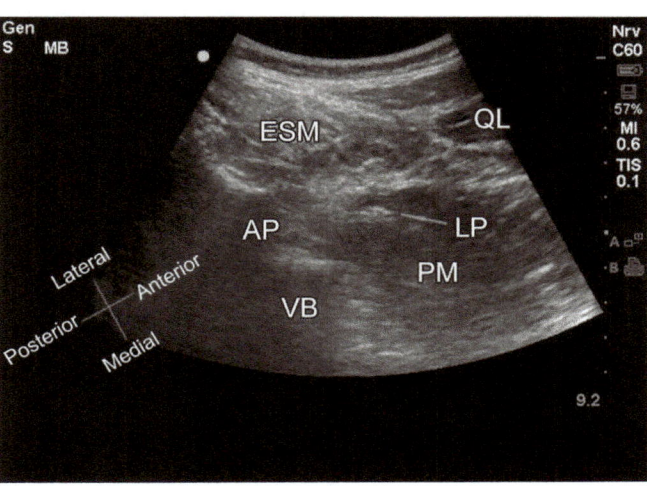

Fig. 3: Sonoanatomy of paramedian transverse oblique scan view. (AP: articular process; ESM: erector spinae muscle; LP: lumbar plexus; PM: psoas major; QL: quadratus lumborum; VB: vertebral body)

Needling and Drug Deposition

Step 3: Needling is done using dual modality of ultrasound-guided in-plane needling and peripheral nerve stimulation. The initial stimulation current is set at 1.5 mA; once the desired stimulation of quadriceps muscle contraction is achieved, current is reduced to 0.5 mA. [*Note*: The quadriceps contraction should be abolished <0.5 mA; needle hub/drug injection port should not be attached to syringe and kept open to air to check for cerebrospinal fluid (CSF)/blood]. 15–20 mL of local anesthesia is injected in small aliquots after repeated negative aspiration. Drug deposition can be visualized real time under ultrasound (**Figs. 4 and 5**).

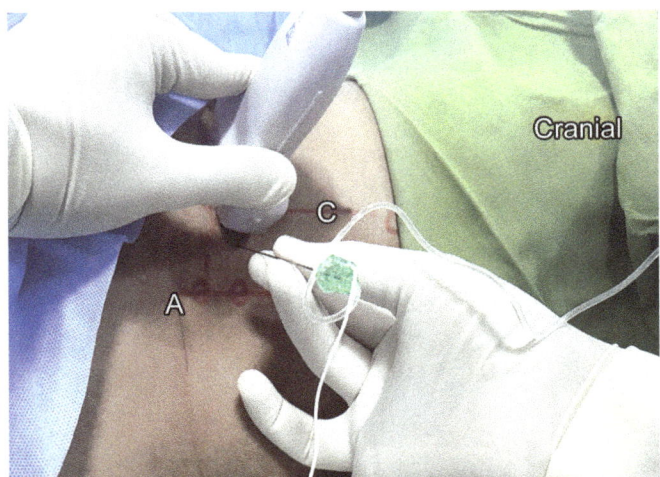

Fig. 4: In-plane needling for a paramedian transverse oblique approach.

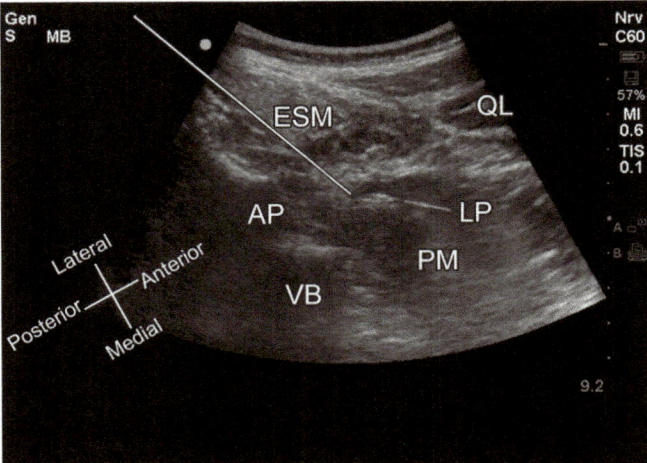

Fig. 5: Sonoimage of in-plane needling. White line denotes the needle trajectory. (AP: articular process; ESM: erector spinae muscle; LP: lumbar plexus; PM: psoas major muscle; QL: quadratus lumborum; VB: vertebral body)

SHAMROCK'S APPROACH

Position of Patient

Step 1: The patient is positioned in lateral position with hips and knees flexed and the side to be blocked placed up.

The following anatomical landmarks are identified and marked:

A—interspinous line (midline), B—intercristal line; C—a line parallel to midline passing through posterior superior iliac spine which intersects the intercristal line (B) roughly 4 cm lateral to midline **(Fig. 6)**.

Scan Technique

Step 2: A curvilinear probe is placed in transverse orientation above the iliac crest to identify the target structures.

The sonoanatomy arrangement of the three muscles [psoas muscle (anterior), quadratus lumborum muscle (lying at apex) and erector spinae muscle (posterior)] around the transverse process resembles a Shamrock with muscle representing its three leaves **(Figs. 7 and 8)**.

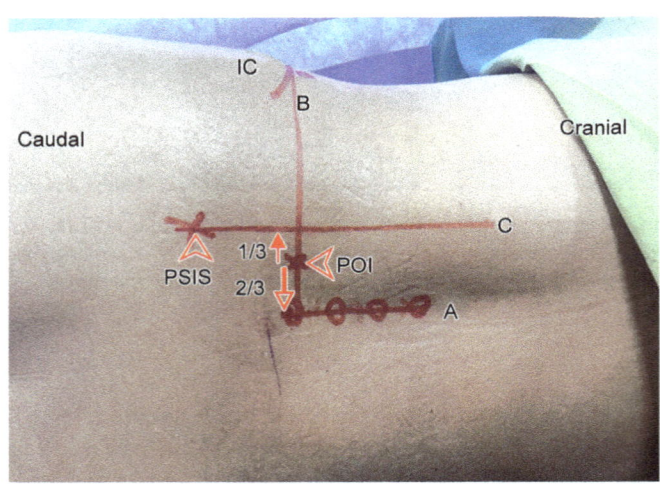

Fig. 6: Position of patient with anatomical landmark marking. (IC: iliac crest; POI: point-of-needle insertion; PSIS: posterior superior iliac spine)

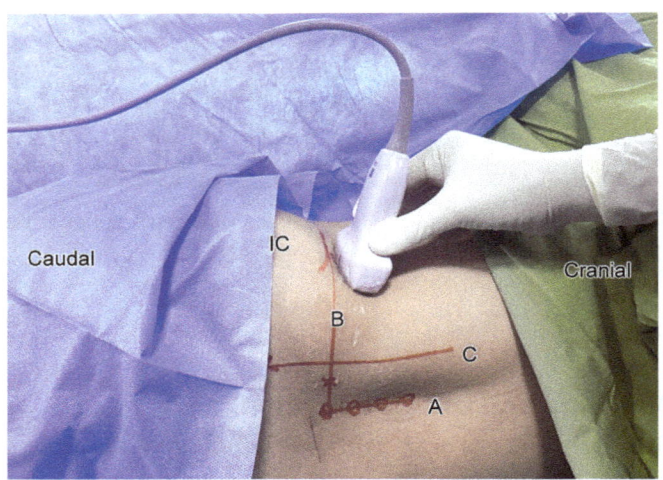

Fig. 7: Probe placement. (IC: iliac crest)

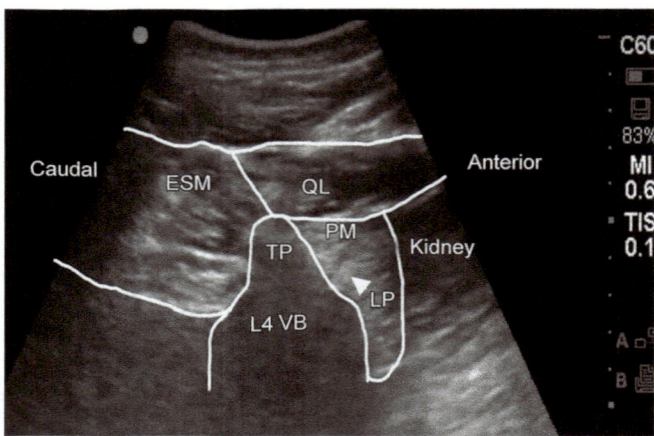

Fig. 8: Sonoanatomy of Shamrock's approach. (ESM: erector spinae muscle; QL: quadratus lumborum; LP: lumbar plexus; PM: psoas major; TP: transverse process; VB: vertebral body)

Needling and Drug Deposition

Step 3: Needling is done using dual modality of ultrasound-guided in-plane needling and peripheral nerve stimulation. The initial stimulation current is set at 1.5 mA; once the desired stimulation of quadriceps muscle contraction is achieved, current is reduced to 0.5 mA (*Note*: The quadriceps contraction should be abolished <0.5 mA; needle hub/drug injection port should not be attached to the syringe and kept open to air to check for CSF/blood). 15–20 mL of local anesthesia is injected in small aliquots after repeated negative aspiration. Drug deposition can be visualized real time under ultrasound **(Figs. 9 to 11)**.

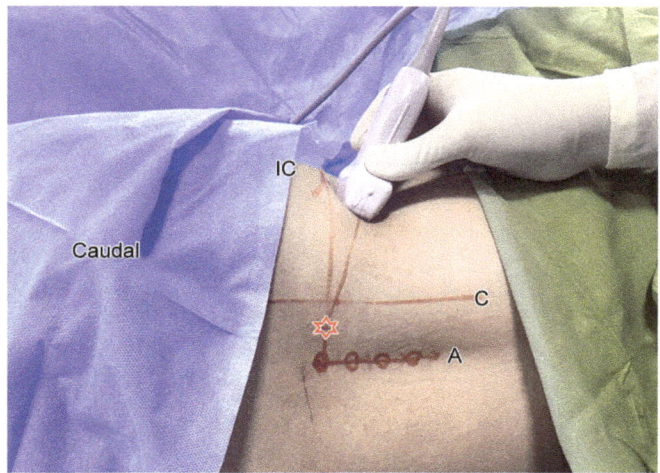

Fig. 9: In-plane needling point for Shamrock's approach. A straight line is drawn from the midpoint of the probe to intersect the intercristal line which is the point of needle insertion. Red star denotes the point of needle insertion.

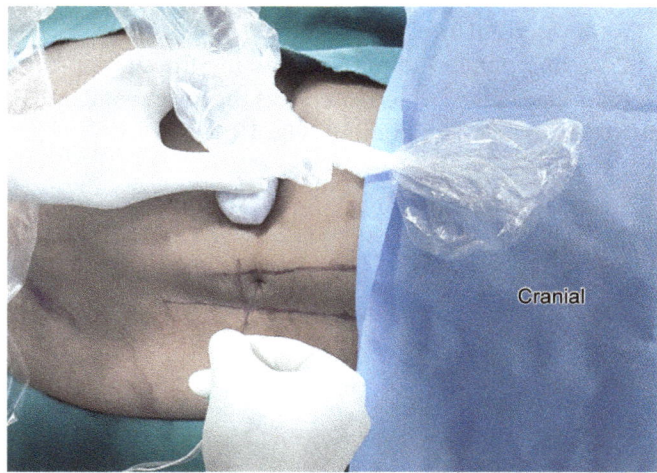

Fig 10: In-plane needling point for Shamrock's approach.

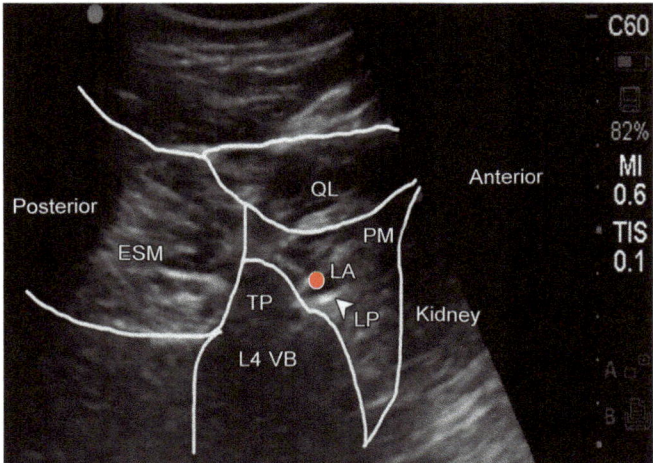

Fig. 11: Sonoimage of in-plane needling in Shamrock's approach. Red dot indicates the needle tip. (ESM: erector spinae muscle LA: local anesthesia; LP: lumbar plexus; PM: psoas major; QL: quadratus lumborum muscle; VB: vertebral body; TP: transverse process)

PARAMEDIAN SAGITTAL TRIDENT VIEW APPROACH

Position of Patient

Step 1: The patient is positioned in lateral position with hips and knees flexed and the side to be blocked placed up.

The following anatomical landmarks are identified and marked:
- A—interspinous line (midline)
- B—intercristal line
- C—a line parallel to midline passing through posterior superior iliac spine) which intersects the intercristal line (B) roughly 4 cm lateral to midline **(Fig. 12)**.

Scan Technique

Step 2: A curvilinear probe is placed in a paramedian sagittal orientation to identify the target structures.

The hyperechoic reflection of transverse processes of L3, L4, and L5 along with the acoustic shadow in the paramedian sagittal scan resembles a trident of Poseidon (the Greek god of sea) or the Trishul of the Hindu God Shiva **(Figs. 13 and 14)**.

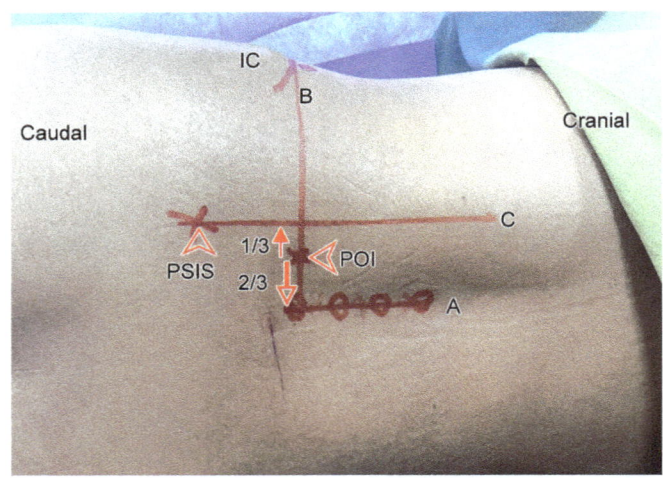

Fig. 12: Position of a patient with anatomical landmark marking. (IC: iliac crest; POI: point of needle insertion; PSIS: posterior superior iliac spine)

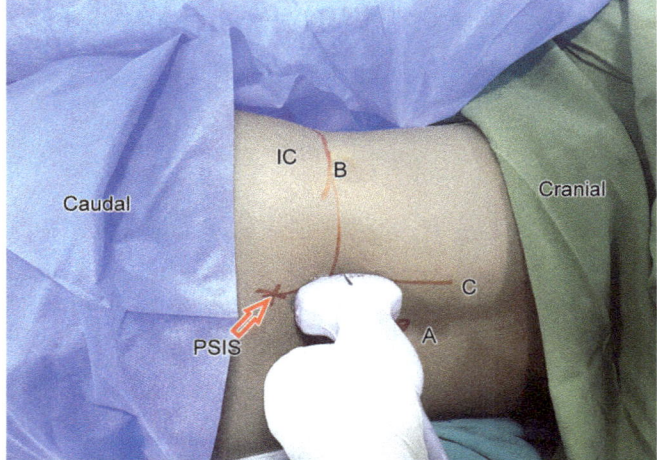

Fig. 13: Probe placement. (IC: iliac crest; PSIS: posterior superior iliac spine)

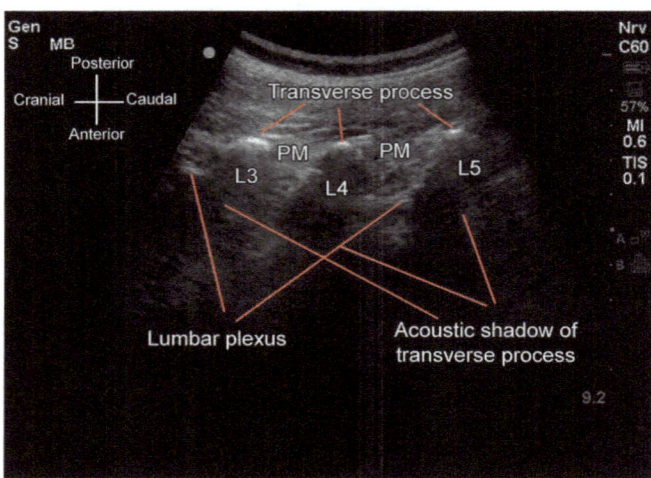

Fig. 14: Sonoanatomy of paramedian sagittal scan view (Trident sign). (PM: psoas major)

Needling and Drug Deposition

Step 3: Needling is done using the dual modality of ultrasound-guided in-plane needling and peripheral nerve stimulation. The initial stimulation current is set at 1.5 mA; once the desired stimulation of quadriceps muscle contraction is achieved, the current is reduced to 0.5 mA (*Note*: The quadriceps contraction should be abolished <0.5 mA; needle hub/drug injection port should not be attached to syringe and kept open to air to check for CSF/blood). 15–20 mL of local anesthesia is injected in small aliquots after repeated negative aspiration. Drug deposition can be visualized real time under ultrasound **(Fig. 15)**.

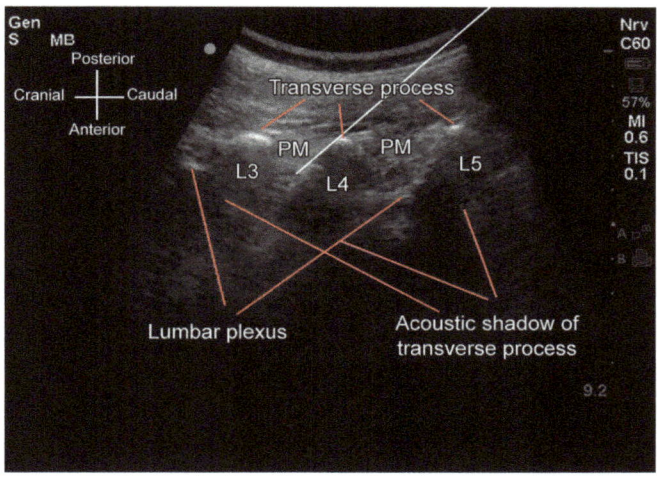

Fig. 15: In-plane needling from caudad to cephalad in the paramedian sagittal approach. White line denotes the needle trajectory. (PM: psoas major)

FURTHER READING

1. Bendtsen TF, Pedersen EM, Haroutounian S, Søballe K, Moriggl B, Nikolajsen L, et al. The suprasacral parallel shift vs lumbar plexus blockade with ultrasound guidance in healthy volunteers: a randomised controlled trial. Anesthesia. 2014;69:1227-40.
2. Capdevila X, Coimbra C, Choquet O. Approaches to the lumbar plexus: success, risks, and outcome. Reg Anesth Pain Med. 2005;30:150-62.
3. Doi K, Sakura S, Hara K. A modified posterior approach to lumbar plexus block using a transverse ultrasound image and an approach from the lateral border of the transducer. Anaesth Intensive Care. 2010;38:213-4.
4. Karmakar MK, Ho AM, Li X, Kwok WH, Tsang K, Kee WD. Ultrasound-guided lumbar plexus block through the acoustic window of the lumbar ultrasound trident. Br J Anaesth. 2008;100:533-7.
5. Kirchmair L, Entner T, Kapral S, Mitterschiffthaler G. Ultrasound guidance for the psoas compartment block: an imaging study. Anesth Analg. 2002;94:706-10.
6. Kirchmair L, Entner T, Wissel J, Moriggl B, Kapral S, Mitterschiffthaler G. A study of the paravertebral anatomy for ultrasound-guided posterior lumbar plexus block. Anesth Analg. 2001;93:477-81.
7. Sauter AR, Ullensvang K, Bendtsen TF, Boerglum J. The "Shamrock Method"—a new and promising technique for ultrasound-guided lumbar plexus blocks [letter]. Br J Anaesth. [online] Available from: http://bja.oxfordjournals.org/forum/topic/brjana_el%3B9814 [Last accessed March, 2022].

CHAPTER 50

Lateral Femoral Cutaneous Nerve Block

Ritesh Roy, Gaurav Agarwal

BASIC INFORMATION

- *LFCN block:* It blocks the lateral femoral cutaneous nerve which innervates the anterolateral aspect of the thigh.
- *Indications:* Analgesia for any procedure involving lateral and anterior portion of the thigh; postoperative analgesia for hip surgery, hip arthroscopy and hip arthroplasty; and meralgia paresthetica.
- *Contraindications:* Unwilling patient, bleeding disorders, infection at the injection site.
- *Medications used:*
  - *Local anesthetic:* 0.1–0.2% Ropivacaine/0.125–0.25% Bupivacaine 7–10 mL with or without adjuvants.
  - *Adjuvants that can be used:* Dexmedetomidine 0.5–1 µg/kg, clonidine 0.5–1 µg/kg, dexamethasone 0.1–0.2 mg/kg.

Step 1: Position of patient—supine. Identify femoral crease. High-frequency USG probe is placed parallel to femoral crease. Scan laterally toward anterior superior iliac spine (ASIS) to identify the lateral margin of Sartorius.

LFCN lies in a fat-filled space between the tensor fascia lata (TFL) muscle and sartorius muscle below the fascia lata **(Figs. 1 to 3)**.

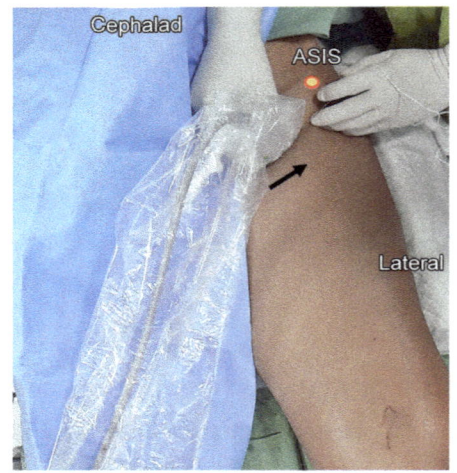

Fig. 1: Lateral femoral cutaneous nerve (LFCN) block.

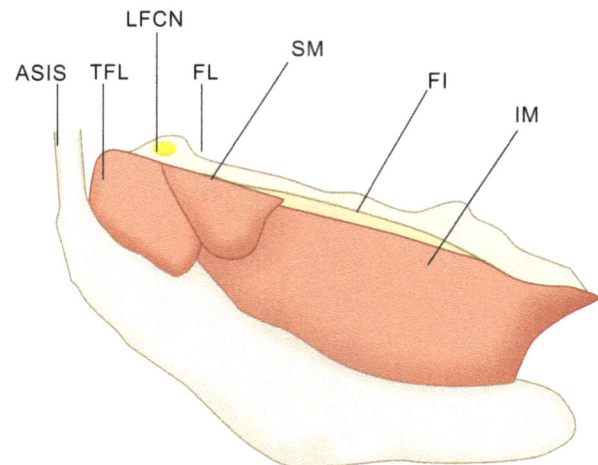

Fig. 2: Image illustrating the plane of LFCN. (ASIS: anterior superior iliac spine; FI: fascia iliaca; FL: fascia lata; IM: iliacus muscle; LFCN: lateral femoral cutaneous nerve; SM: sartorius muscle; TFL: tensor fascia lata)

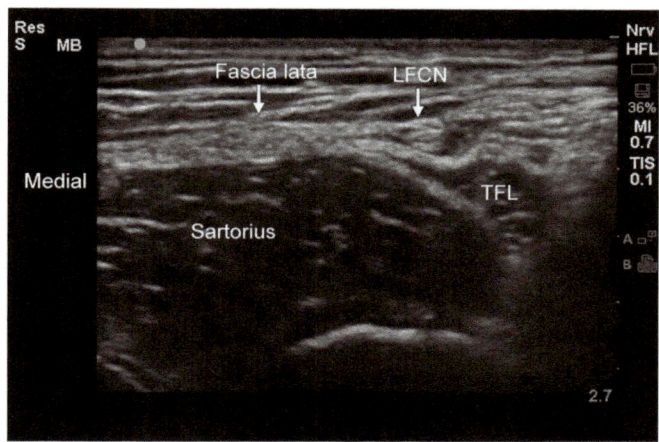

Fig. 3: Sonoanatomy of lateral femoral cutaneous nerve (LFCN). Target is in the pocket between fascia lata, lateral margin of Sartorius, and medial margin of tensor fascia lata (TFL).

Step 2: After skin local anesthesia infiltration, insert the needle in-plane (under vision) to reach the target between TFL (tensor fascia lata), Sartorius and facia lata **(Fig. 4)**.

Step 3: After confirming the needle tip in the target plane, confirm negative aspiration of blood and inject the desired local anesthetic (LA) in small aliquots with a total of 7–10 mL for the block **(Fig. 5)**.

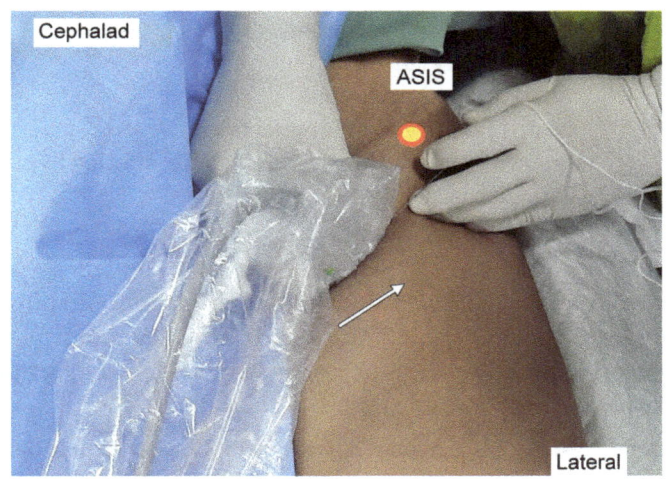

Fig. 4: Needle insertion in plane. (ASIS: anterior superior iliac spine)

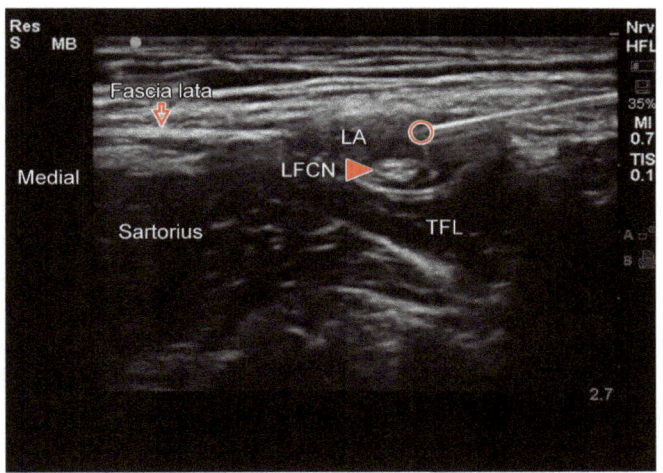

Fig. 5: LA injection at the target site. Red circle denotes the needle tip. (LA: local anesthetic; LFCN: lateral femoral cutaneous nerve; TFL: tensor fascia lata)

FURTHER READING

1. Bodner G, Bernathova M, Galiano K, Putz D, Martinoli C, Felfernig M. Ultrasound of the lateral femoral cutaneous nerve: normal findings in a cadaver and in volunteers. Reg Anesth Pain Med. 2009;34:265-8.
2. Corujo A, Franco CD, Williams JM. The sensory territory of the lateral cutaneous nerve of the thigh as determined by anatomic dissections and ultrasound-guided blocks. Reg Anesth Pain Med. 2012;37:561-4.
3. Hara K, Sakura S, Shido A. Ultrasound-guided lateral femoral cutaneous nerve block: comparison of two techniques. Anaesth Intensive Care. 2011;39:69-72.
4. Moritz T, Prosch H, Berzaczy D, Happak W, Lieba-Samal D, Bernathova M, et al. Common anatomical variation in patients with idiopathic meralgia paresthetica: a high resolution ultrasound case-control study. Pain Physician. 2013;16:E287-93.
5. Ng I, Vaghadia H, Choi PT, Helmy N. Ultrasound imaging accurately identifies the lateral femoral cutaneous nerve. Anesth Analg. 2008;107:1070-4.
6. Shteynberg A, Riina LH, Glickman LT, Meringolo JN, Simpson RL. Ultrasound-guided lateral femoral cutaneous nerve (LFCN) block: safe and simple anesthesia for harvesting skin grafts. Burns. 2013;39:146-9.
7. Zhu J, Zhao Y, Liu F, Huang Y, Shao J, Hu B. Ultrasound of the lateral femoral cutaneous nerve in asymptomatic adults. BMC Musculoskelet Disord. 2012;13:227.

CHAPTER 51: Sacral Plexus Block

Ritesh Roy, Gaurav Agarwal

SACRAL PLEXUS BLOCK OR PARASACRAL SCIATIC NERVE BLOCK

INTRODUCTION

Sacral plexus block or parasacral sciatic nerve block is the injection of local anesthesia in a plane around the nerves of sacral plexus (in the greater sciatic foramen) before the formation of sciatic nerve.

BASIC INFORMATION

- Sacral plexus block or parasacral sciatic nerve block is the injection of local anesthesia in a plane around the nerves of sacral plexus (in the greater sciatic foramen) before the formation of the sciatic nerve.
- The advantage is the ability to achieve anesthesia of sciatic nerve, posterior cutaneous nerve of thigh, superior gluteal nerve, inferior gluteal nerve, and nerve to quadratus femoris by single injection.
- *Indications*:
  - Surgical anesthesia for lower limb surgery along with lumbar plexus block.
  - Postoperative pain management after knee, leg, and foot surgery.
  - Catheters can be inserted for continuous infusion.
- *Contraindications*:
  - Infection at puncture site
  - Coagulation disorders
  - Sacral decubitus
  - Lack of patient cooperation
  - Inability of achieve lateral or semiprone position
- *Complications*:
  - Pelvic hematoma formation
  - Visceral injury (ureter or colon)
  - Transient sciatic neuralgia
  - Inadvertent intravascular injection
  - Urinary retention due to blockade of inferior hypogastric plexus.

ANATOMY

Sacral plexus is derived from the anterior rami of spinal nerves L4, L5, S1, S2, S3, and S4. It provides motor and sensory nerves to part of pelvis, posterior thigh, leg except the medial portion, and entire foot **(Figs. 1 and 2)**.

Sacral plexus or parasacral sciatic nerve block scan techniques:
- Parasacral parallel shift (PSPS)
- Taha's technique

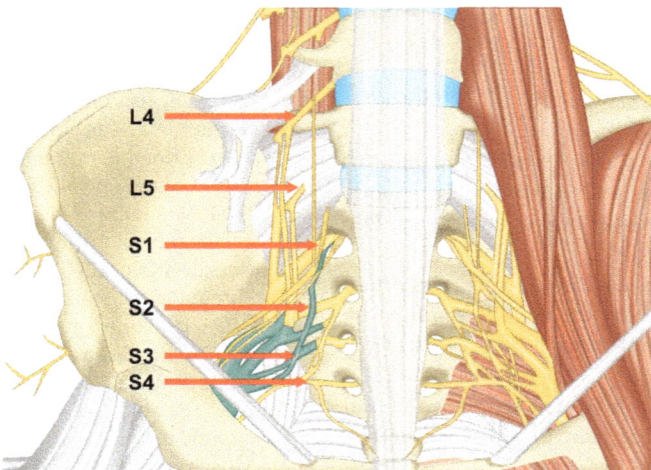

Fig. 1: Formation of sacral plexus.

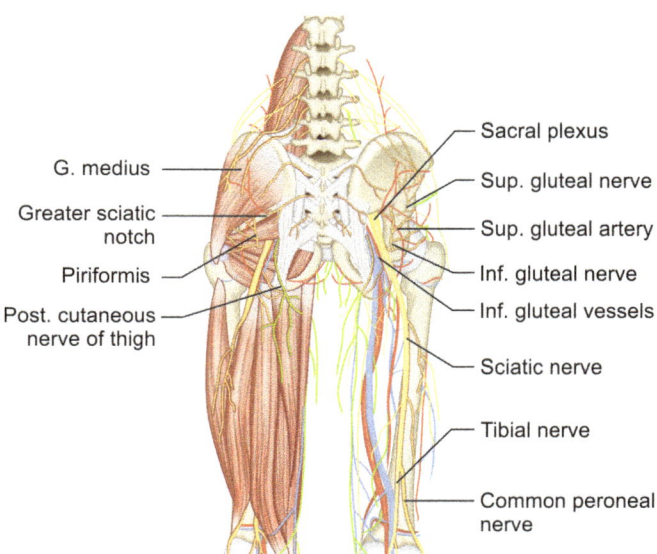

Fig. 2: Anatomical illustration showing the exit of sacral plexus from the pelvis through the greater sciatic notch or foramen. The following structures also exit through the greater sciatic notch: (1) piriformis muscle, (2) superior gluteal vessels and nerve above the piriformis muscle, (3) inferior gluteal vessels and nerve, sciatic nerve, posterior cutaneous nerve of thigh, pudendal nerve and vessels, nerve to obturator internus and nerve to quadratus femoris below the piriformis muscle.

Parasacral Parallel Shift

Step 1: Position of the patient—semiprone (Sims') position with the side to be blocked and upper hip flexed to around 90°. Palpate and mark GT (greater trochanter of femur) and PSIS (posterior superior iliac spine). Draw a line connecting GT and PSIS and divide the line into two equal halves **(Figs. 3 and 4)**.

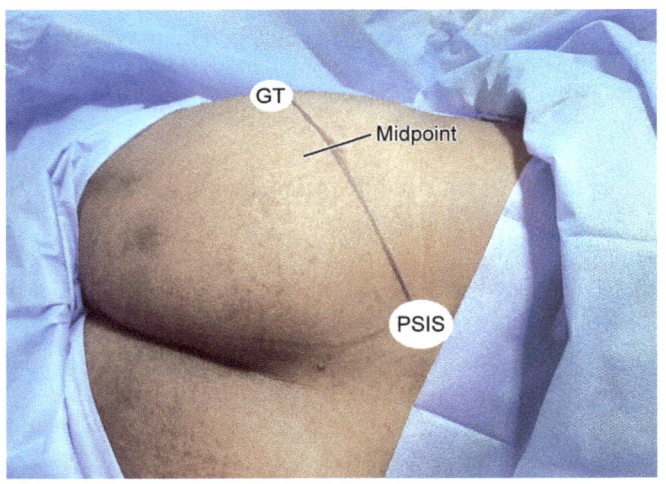

Fig. 3: Position of patient.

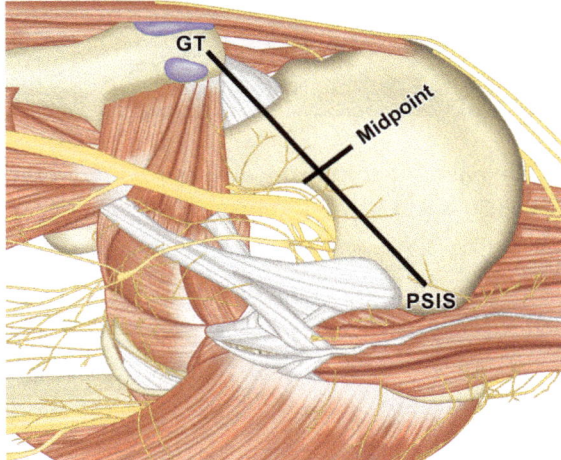

Fig. 4: Image showing the semiprone (Sims') position of patient with side to be blocked up and marking of GT (greater trochanter) and PSIS (posterior superior iliac spine).

Step 2: The curvilinear transducer is aligned between the posterior superior iliac spine (PSIS) and the midpoint of the line connecting the PSIS and the greater trochanter (GT) (**Figs. 5 to 7**).

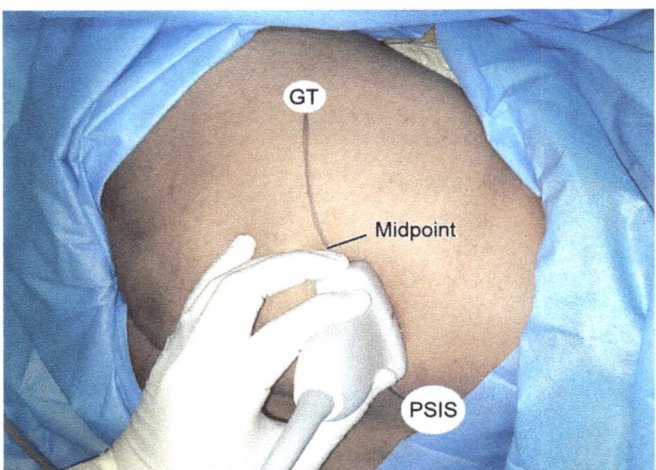

Fig. 5: Starting position of scanning.

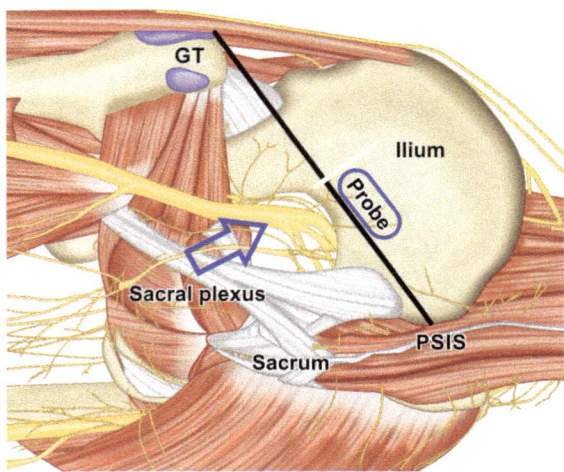

Fig. 6: Image showing the starting position of scanning. (GT: greater trochanter; PSIS: posterior superior iliac spine)

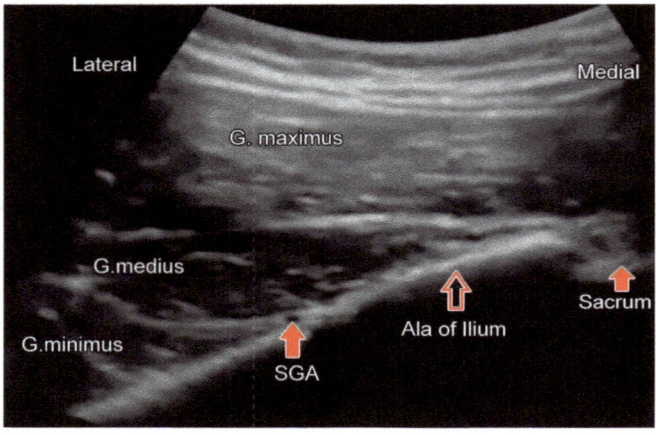

Fig. 7: Sonoanatomy at the start of scanning. Note the continuity of the iliac bone (ala of ilium). (G. maximus: gluteus maximus; G. medius: gluteus medius; G. minimus: gluteus minimus; SGA: superior gluteal artery)

Step 3: The curvilinear transducer is moved inferomedially with PSPS (**Figs. 8 to 10**). The transducer beam arrives at the greater sciatic notch, and the ultrasonographic continuity of the iliac bone line is interrupted. The sacral plexus exits the

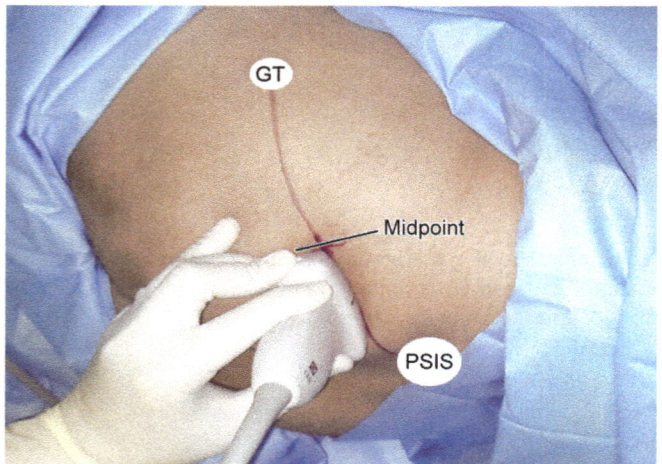

Fig. 8: Parasacral parallel shift of the transducer.

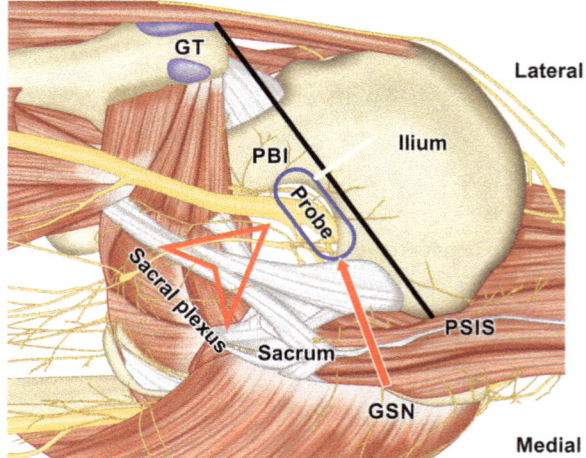

Fig. 9: Image showing the parasacral parallel shift of transducer. *Note*: The break in continuity of the iliac bone and appearance of greater sciatic notch as the probe is moved inferomedially. (GSN: greater sciatic notch; GT: greater trochanter; PBI: posterior border of ischium; PSIS: posterior superior iliac spine)

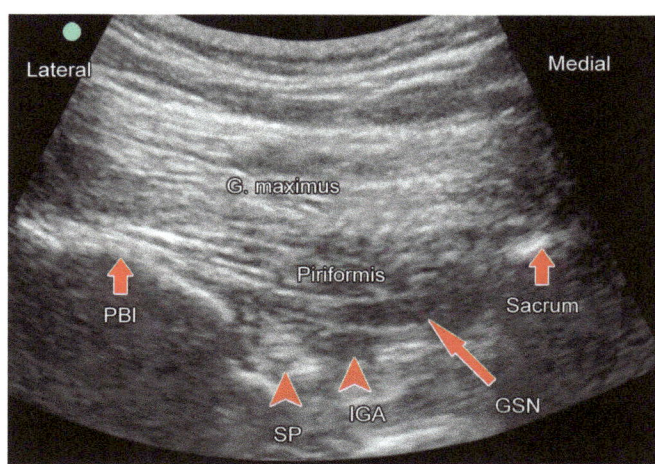

Fig. 10: Sonoanatomy with parasacral parallel shift of the transducer. Note the sacral plexus (SP) coming out of the greater sciatic notch (GSN) below the piriformis muscle between the sacrum and the posterior border of ischium (PBI). The sacral plexus lies just medial to PBI. The inferior gluteal artery (IGA) lies just medial to SP.

pelvis through the greater sciatic notch. A slight caudal tilt of the transducer helps in visualization of the sacral plexus between the sacrum and the posterior border of ischium beneath the dark triangular piriformis muscle.

Step 4: The needle is advanced in-plane from the lateral to the medial till the needle tip (red dot) reaches the sacral plexus **(Figs. 11 and 12)**. The confirmation of the sacral plexus is done by dual guidance by nerve stimulation with a sciatic

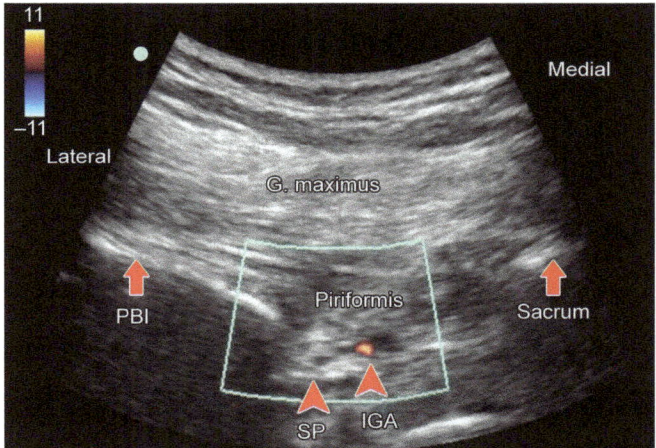

Fig. 11: Sonoanatomy showing inferior gluteal artery (IGA) medial to sacral plexus (SP) in color Doppler mode.

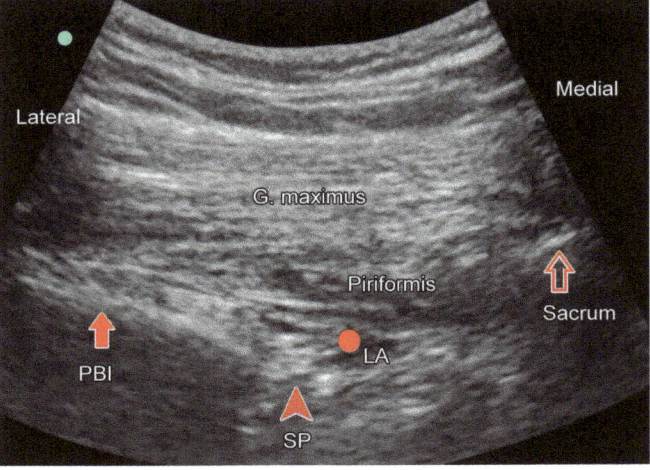

Fig. 12: Sonoanatomy showing needling and local anesthesia (LA) deposition around sacral plexus (SP).

motor response in the range of 0.3–0.5 mA. 20–25 mL of ropivacaine 0.5% is injected with sonographic observation of perineural spread as the endpoint with reposition of the needle tip if necessary using solely ultrasonographic guidance.

Taha's Technique

Step 1: Position of the patient—semiprone (Sims') position with the side to be blocked up and upper hip flexed to around 90°. Mark the highest point of natal or gluteal cleft. Mark a point 8 cm lateral from the highest point of natal cleft (**Figs. 13 and 14**).

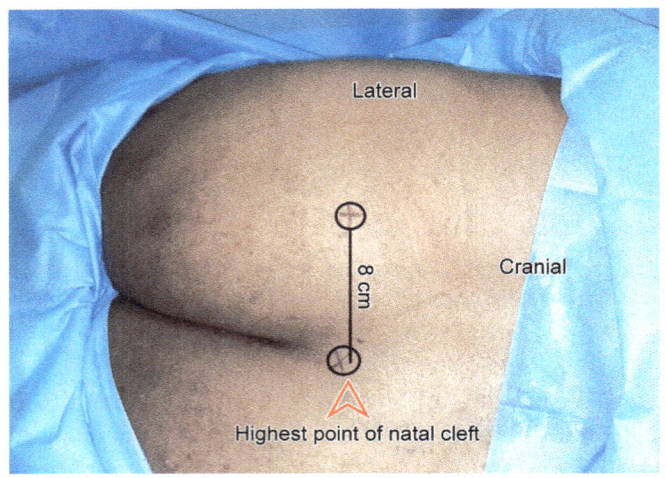

Fig. 13: Position of patient.

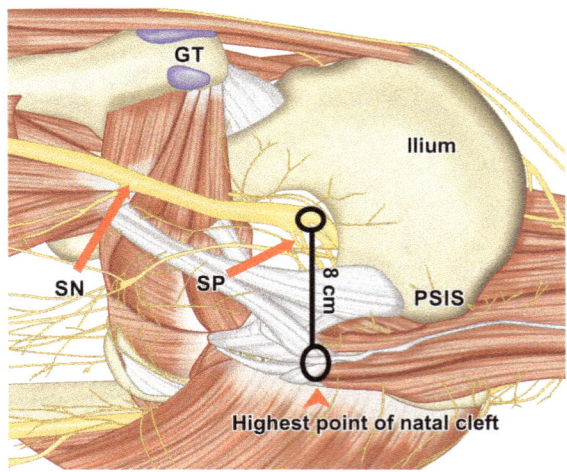

Fig. 14: Image showing patient position and markings. (GT: greater trochanter; PSIS: posterior superior iliac spine; SP: sacral plexus; SN: sciatic nerve)

Step 2: The curvilinear probe is placed on an axial plane 8 cm lateral to the uppermost point of the natal or gluteal cleft. The transducer beam arrives at the greater sciatic notch. The sacral plexus exits the pelvis through the greater sciatic notch. A slight caudal tilt of the transducer helps in visualization of the sacral plexus between the sacrum and the posterior border of ischium beneath the dark triangular piriformis muscle (**Figs. 15 and 16**).

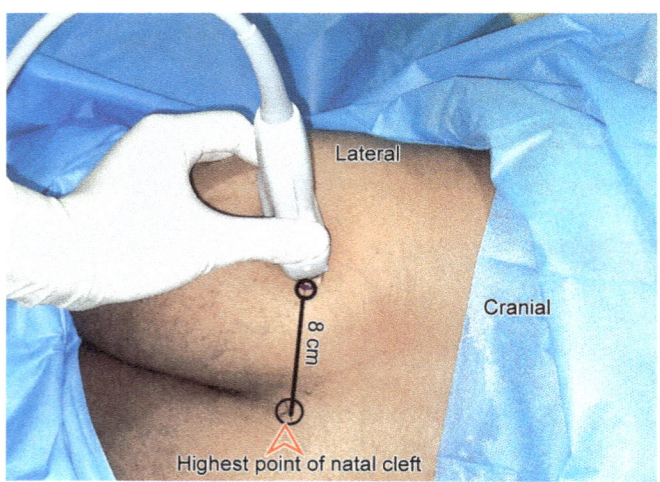

Fig. 15: Probe position.

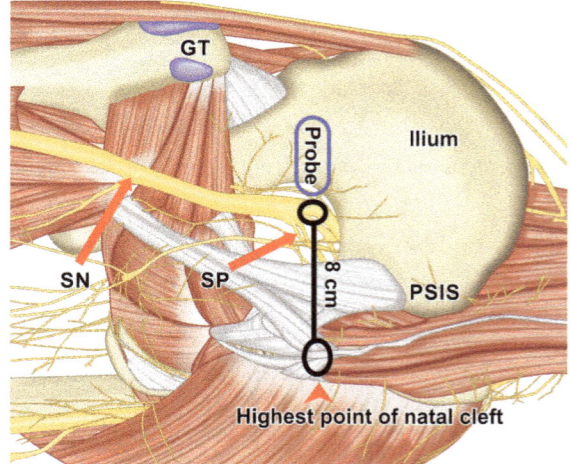

Fig. 16: Image showing the placement of probe. (GT: greater trochanter; PSIS: posterior superior iliac spine; SP: sacral plexus; SN: sciatic nerve). Blue circle denotes the probe.

Step 3 (optional): If in the initial probe placement **(Fig. 7)** sonoanatomy is visualized, slide the probe downward maintaining the same orientation of probe and with a slight caudal tilt **(Fig. 17)** sonoanatomy will be visualized.

Step 4: The needle is advanced in plane from the lateral to the medial till the needle tip (red dot) reaches the sacral plexus **(Fig. 12)**. The confirmation of the sacral plexus is done by dual guidance by nerve stimulation with a sciatic motor response in the range of 0.3–0.5 mA. 20–25 mL of ropivacaine 0.5% is injected with sonographic observation of perineural spread as the endpoint with reposition of the needle tip if necessary using solely ultrasonographic guidance.

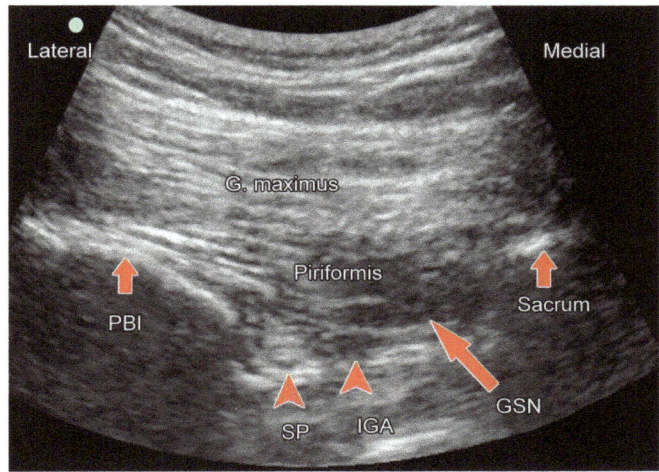

Fig. 17: Sonoanatomy with probe placed on an axial plane 8 cm lateral to the uppermost point of the natal or gluteal cleft. Note the sacral plexus (SP) coming out of the greater sciatic notch (GSN) below the piriformis muscle between the sacrum and the posterior border of ischium (PBI). The sacral plexus lies just medial to the posterior border of ischium (PBI). The inferior gluteal artery (IGA) lies just medial to SP.

FURTHER READING

1. Ben-Ari AY, Joshi R, Uskova A, Chelly JE. Ultrasound localization of the sacral plexus using a parasacral approach. Anesth Analg. 2009;108:1977-80.
2. Bendtsen TF, Lonnqvist PA, Jepsen KV, Petersen M, Knudsen L, Borgium J. Preliminary results of a new ultrasound-guided approach to block the sacral plexus: the parasacral parallel shift. Br J Anaesth. 2011;107:278-80.
3. Gaertner E, Lascurain P, Venet C, Maschino X, Zamfir A, Lupescu R, et al. Continuous parasacral sciatic block: a radiographic study. Anesth Analg. 2004;98:831-4.
4. Helayel PE, Ceccon MS, Knaesel JA, Conceicao DB, de Oliveira Filho GR. Urinary incontinence after bilateral parasacral sciatic nerve block: report of two cases. Reg Anesth Pain Med. 2006;31:368-71.
5. O'Connor M, Coleman M, Wallis F, Harmon D. An anatomical study of the parasacral block using magnetic resonance imaging of healthy volunteers. Anesth Analg. 2009;108:1708-12.
6. Taha. A simple and successful sonographic technique to identify the sciatic nerve in the parasacral area. Can J Anesth. 2012;59:263-7.
7. Walker PL. Greater sciatic notch morphology: sex, age, and population differences. Am J Phys Anthropol. 2005;127:385-91.

CHAPTER 52
Pericapsular Nerve Group Block (For Hip Joint)

Ritesh Roy, Gaurav Agarwal

PERICAPSULAR NERVE GROUP BLOCK

Basic Information

- *PENG (pericapsular nerve group) block:* Blocks the articular branches of the hip joint capsule from the femoral, obturator and accessory obturator nerves which lie in the plane between the psoas tendon and the superior pubic ramus at the IPE (ilio-pubic eminence).
- *Indications:* Analgesia for acute pain for hip fractures; along with LFCN (lateral femoral cutaneous nerve) block postoperative analgesia for hip replacement, proximal femur and head of femur surgery, and hip arthroscopy; vaso-oclusive sickle crisis hip pain and other persistent hip pain. PENG radiofrequency ablation for persistent hip pain has also been reported.
- *Contraindications:* Unwilling patient, bleeding disorders, Infection at the injection site
- *Medications used:*
  - *Local anesthetic:* 0.1–0.2% ropivacaine/0.125%–0.25% bupivacaine 15–20 mL with or without adjuvants
  - *Adjuvants that can be used:* Dexmedetomidine 0.5–1 µg/kg, clonidine 0.5–1 µg/kg, dexamethasone 0.1–0.2 mg/kg

PERICAPSULAR NERVE GROUP BLOCK—SLIDING APPROACH

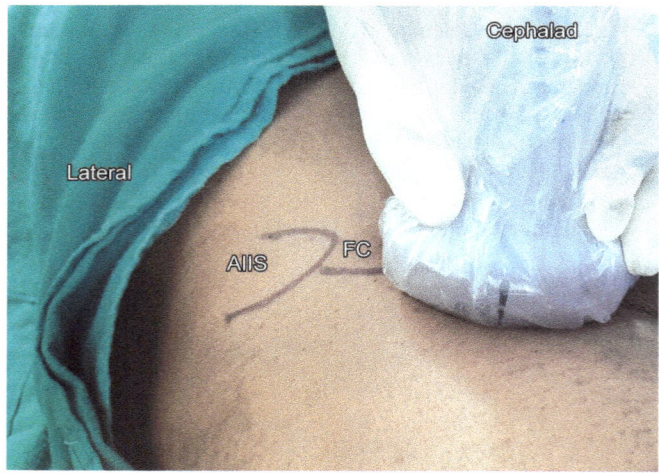

Fig. 1: Pericapsular nerve group block—sliding approach—probe position. (AIIS: anterior inferior iliac spine; FC: femoral crease)

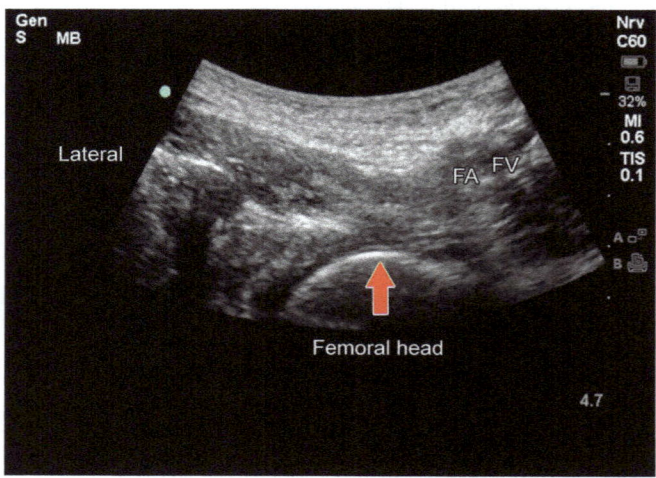

Fig. 2: Sonoanatomy of the starting position—sliding approach. (FA: femoral artery; FV: femoral vein)

Step 1: Position of patient—supine. Identify anterior inferior iliac spine (AIIS) and the femoral crease (FC). Low-frequency USG probe is placed on a line 1–1.5 cm below and parallel to FC **(Fig. 1)**.

Step 2: Identify the femoral head and the femoral vessels **(Fig. 2)**.

Step 3: The probe is slid proximally (cephalad) closer to the femoral crease to identify the superior pubic ramus and Iliopubic eminence.

Step 4: Sliding the probe cephalad; identify the IPE (Iliopubic eminence) on the ilio-pubic ramus from AIIS (anterior inferior iliac spine), PT (Psoas tendon), Iliacus muscle, FN (femoral nerve), FA (femoral artery), FV (femoral vein). The target lies in between the PT and superior pubic ramus at IPE **(Fig. 4)**.

Step 5: Needle is inserted from lateral to medial to reach the target between the psoas tendon (PT) and the superior pubic ramus at IPE, 12–20 mL of local anesthetic (LA) is injected after negative aspiration in small aliquots after repeated negative aspirations for blood **(Fig. 5)**.

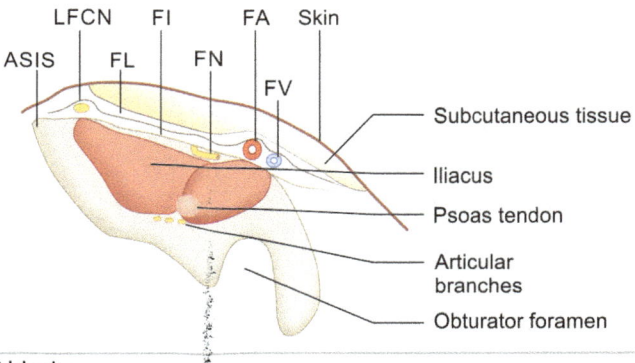

Fig. 3: Anatomical illustration of PENG block.
(ASIS: anterior superior iliac spine; LFCN: lateral femoral cutaneous nerve; FL: fascia lata; FI: fascia Iliaca; FN: femoral nerve; FV: femoral vein; FA: femoral artery)

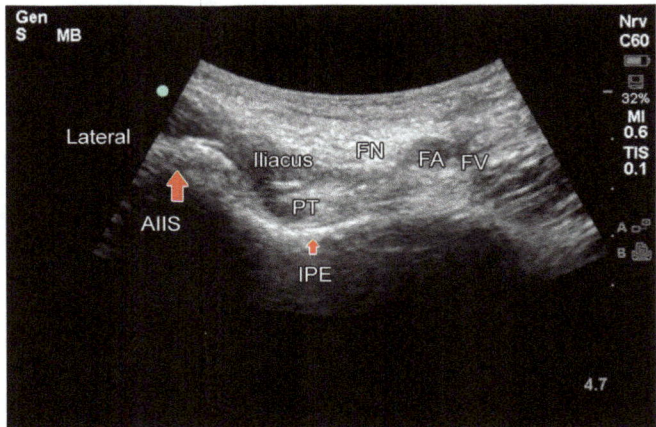

Fig. 4: Sonoanatomy of PENG.

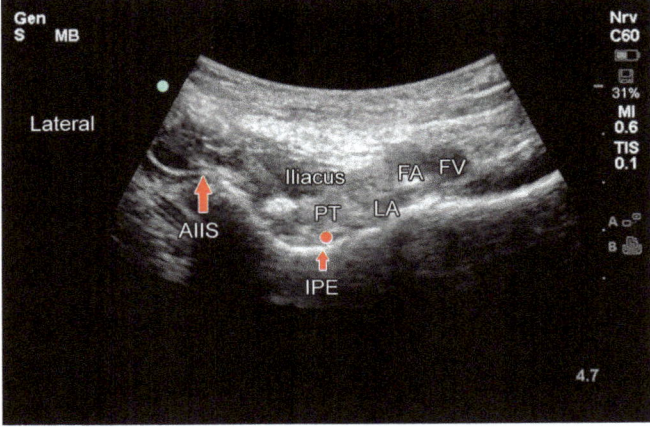

Fig. 5: Injection of drug in PENG; Red circle – Needle tip.

PENG BLOCK—CLASSICAL APPROACH

Step 1: Position of patient—supine. Identify ASIS (anterior superior iliac spine and AIIS (Anterior inferior iliac spine); low frequency USG probe placed on a transverse line on AIIS **(Fig. 6)**.

Step 2: Identify the AIIS **(Fig. 7)**.

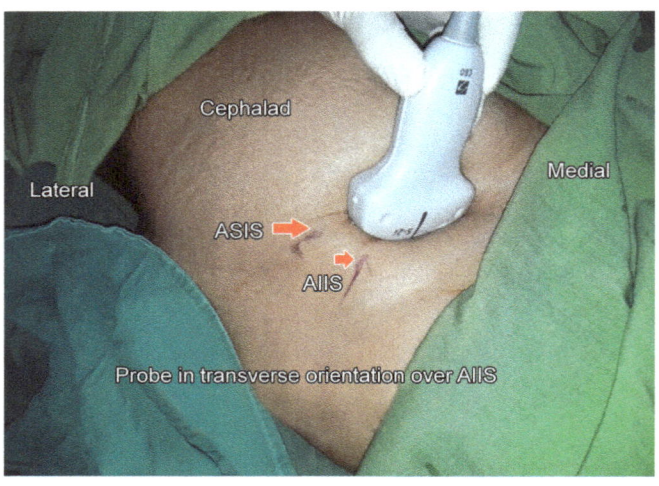

Fig. 6: PENG Block—Classical approach: Probe position.

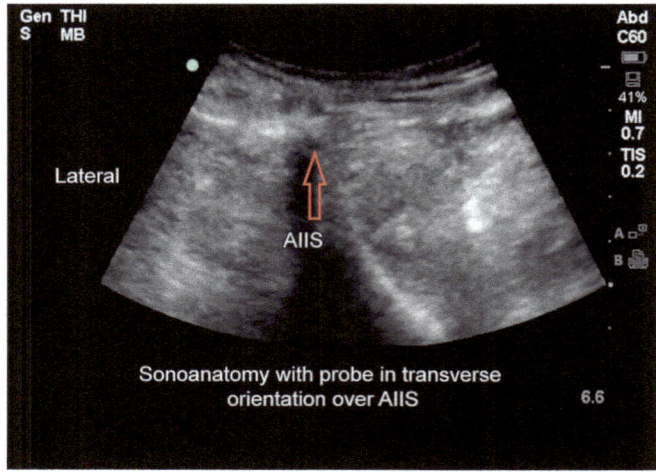

Fig. 7: Sonoanatomy of starting position—Classical approach.

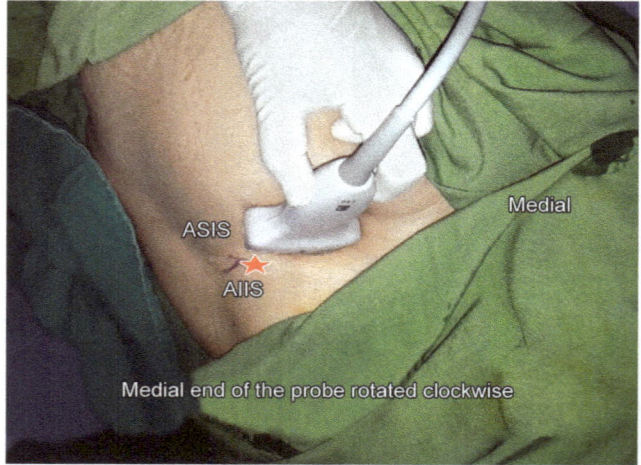

Fig. 8: Probe rotation to target location.

Fig. 9: Sonoanatomy of PENG.

Step 3: The medial end of the probe is rotated clockwise for right-sided block and anticlockwise for left-sided block to achieve the target location **(Fig. 8)**.

Step 4: Rotating the medial end of the probe; identify the IPE (Iliopubic eminence) on the ilio-pubic ramus from AIIS (anterior inferior iliac spine), PT (psoas tendon), iliacus muscle, FN (femoral nerve), FA (femoral artery), FV (femoral vein). The target lies in between the PT and superior pubic ramus at IPE **(Fig. 9)**.

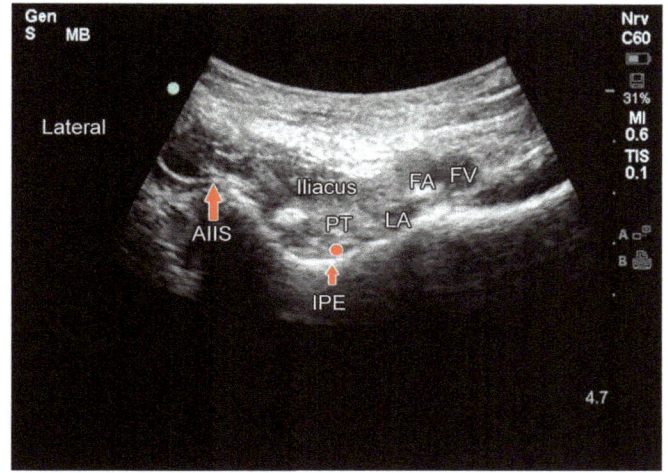

Fig. 10: Injection of drug in PENG; Red circle – Needle tip.

Step 5: Needle is inserted from lateral to medial to reach the target between the psoas tendon (PT) and the superior pubic ramus at IPE (iliopubic emienence), 12–20 mL of local anesthetic (LA) is injected after negative aspiration in small aliquots after repeated negative aspirations for blood **(Fig. 10)**.

FURTHER READING

1. Del Buono R, Padua E, Pascarella G, Costa F, Tognù A, Terranova G, et al. Pericapsular nerve group block: an overview. Minerva Anestesiol. 2021;87:458-66.
2. Girón-Arango L, Peng PW, Chin KJ, Brull R, Perlas A. Pericapsular nerve group (PENG) block for hip fracture. Reg Anesth Pain Med. 2018;43:859-63.
3. Jaramillo S, Muñoz D, Orozco S, Herrera AM. Percutaneous bipolar radiofrequency of the pericapsular nerve group (PENG) for chronic pain relief in hip osteoarthrosis. J Clin Anesth. 2020;64:109830.
4. Mysore K, Sancheti SA, Howells SR, Ballah EE, Sutton JL, Uppal V. Postoperative analgesia with pericapsular nerve group (PENG) block for primary total hip arthroplasty: a retrospective study. Can J Anaesth. 2020;67:1673-4.
5. Pagano T, Scarpato F, Chicone G, Carbone D, Bussemi CB, Albano F, et al. Analgesic evaluation of ultrasound-guided pericapsular nerve group (PENG) block for emergency hip surgery in fragile patients: a case series. Arthroplasty. 2019;1:18.
6. Roy R, Agarwal G, Pradhan C, Kuanar D. Total postoperative analgesia for hip surgeries, PENG block with LFCN block. Reg Anesth Pain Med. 2019;44:684.
7. Wyatt KE, Pranav H, Henry T, Liu CJ. Pericapsular nerve group blockade for sickle cell disease vaso-occlusive crisis. J Clin Anesth. 2020;66:109932.

SECTION 10

Ultrasound-guided Dry Needling

- **Ultrasound-guided Dry Needling**
  Lakshmi Vas

CHAPTER 53

Ultrasound-guided Dry Needling

Lakshmi Vas

BASIC INFORMATION

- *Indications*: Every chronic pain. Myofascial pain syndrome (MPS) affects up to 95% of people with chronic pain disorders and is a common finding in specialty pain management centers. As such, ultrasound-guided dry needling (USGDN) has the potential to revolutionize the outcomes in chronic pain if it were to be universally utilized.
- It may be used as a sole treatment or as an adjunct to spine injections, nerve block, and radiofrequency (RF) procedures, particularly pulsed RF and regenerative therapies. The prerequisites to the use of USGDN are thorough knowledge of muscle anatomy, sonoanatomy, and the ability to visualize and steer the fine 32-gauge needles with ultrasound visualization. Most importantly though, it is the readiness to acknowledge the importance of neuromyopathy in neuropathic pains and the clinical acumen to diagnose the prevalence of myofascial pains in all chronic pains that lead to success **(Fig. 1)**.
- *Contraindications*: Unwilling patient. Patients with fear of needles can be usually managed with prior application of prilocaine lignocaine mixture (Prilox® cream).
- *Type of USGDN*: Depends on the pain location. The muscles underlying the painful area are treated. When the nerve is involved, all the muscles supplied by it are addressed. For example, in L4–5 radiculopathy, not only the back but also the limb musculature along the line of pain is treated with USGDN. **Figures 2 to 5** demonstrate USGDN of back buttock, thighs, and leg for radicular pain with backpain. **Figure 6** shows USGDN of thorax, **Figure 7** shows USGDN of abdomen, **Figure 8** shows USGDN of groin, and **Figure 9** shows USGDN of masticatory muscles to relieve pain in trigeminal neuralgia. There are two clinical videos of the technique of USGDN and the ultrasound videos of actual needling of back, buttock, and thigh muscles as well as USGDN of thorax which are available.
- *Medications used*: There is no injection in USGDN but based on the findings of USGDN, ultrasound-guided Botox injection may be used with great benefit to the patient. Small dose of steroid may also be used for ultrasound-guided trigger point injections.

PROCEDURE DETAILS

Step 1: Choose the type and length of needle.

Solid filiform 30–32-gauge needles used for USGDN. Needles are inserted under ultrasound guidance into muscles to relieve myofascial pains. — 1.3 cm, 2.5 cm

Karel Lewit (Pain 1979) called the immediate analgesia produced by needle insertion distinct and independent of any injections, "the needle effect". — 4 cm, 5 cm

He further proposed that there are very many MTrPs in the body that could cause myriad pains. — 6 cm

— 7.5 cm

— 10 cm

Fig. 1: Needles used for USGDN.
(MTrPs: myofascial trigger points)

Step 2: Decide the site and position of probe to understand sonoanatomy.

Ultrasound demonstrates individual muscles and the depth to which needles have to be inserted to address each **Figure 2A** shows the probe position for USGDN of paravertebral muscles. **Figure 2B** shows the three parts of erector spinae: spinalis (SP), longissimus (L), iliocostalis (IC), and quadratus lumborum (QL) outlined for understanding.

USGDN operates on the principle that the whole of the muscle with the taut bands harboring myofascial trigger points (MTrPs) has to be addressed. This is unlike ordinary blindly performed DN which targets only few most painful points where MTrPs are demonstrable during DN. Hence, **Figure 2C** shows about 40 needles of which 20 needles are inserted into just medial paravertebral muscles (spinalis multifidus and medial longissimus).

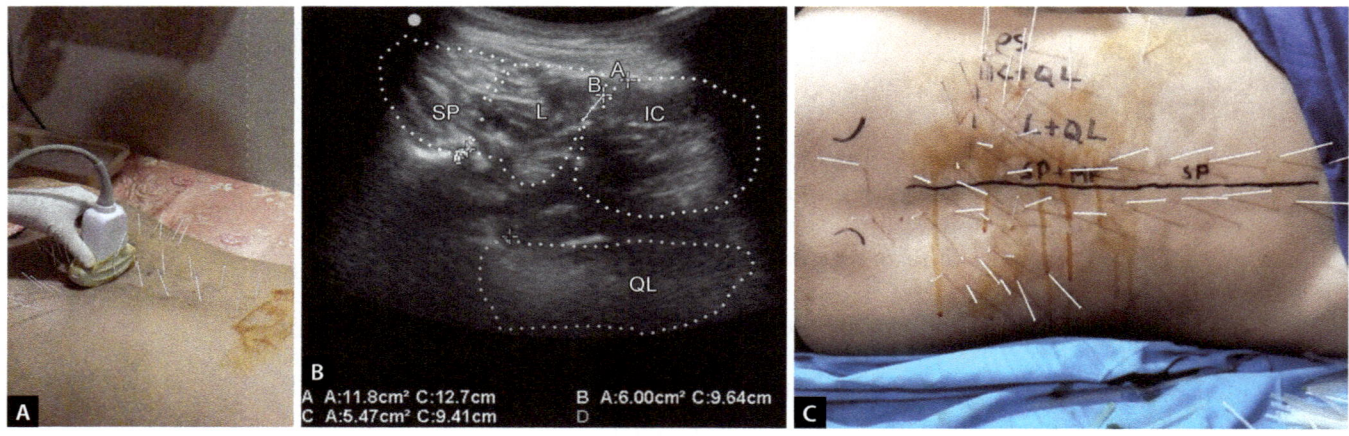

Figs. 2A to C: Probe position for (A) back USGDN; (B) Sonoanatomy muscles; (C) Needles in situ.

Step 3: The patient shown in **Figure 3** had pyriformis syndrome but two CT-guided and one USG-guided pyriformis trigger injections had failed to relieve his pain due to which he continued to be bedridden. He improved with USGDN of the gemelli and obturator internus indicating that his sciatic nerve was being scissored between the gemelli and the piriformis rather than piriformis acting as a knife on the nerve. **Figure 3A** shows gluteus maximus (GM) over lying piriformis (PYR). **Figure 3B** with the probe a little lower shows gluteus maximus (G Max) and the superior gemellus and inferior gemellus (G) above and below obturator internus (OI). **Figure 3C** shows how the muscles scissor the sciatic nerve.

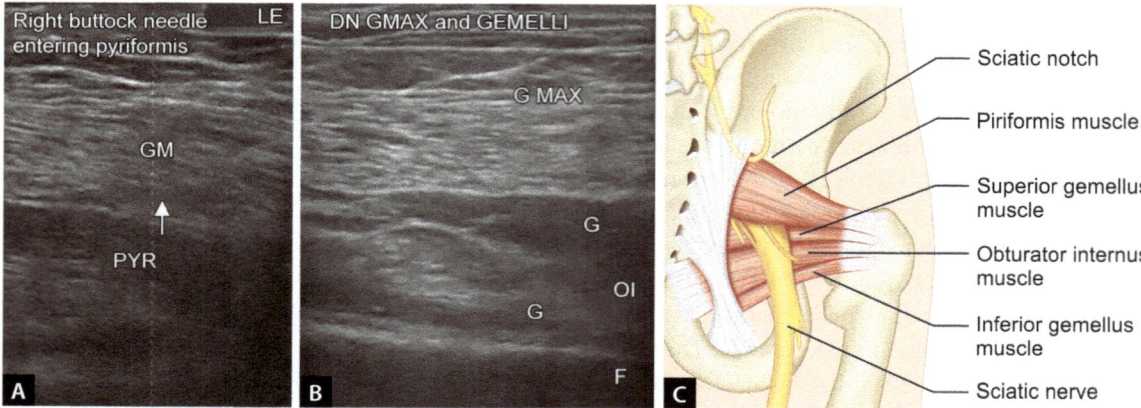

Figs. 3A to C: USGDN of buttock muscles.

Figure 4A shows the semimembranosus and semitendinosis (SMST). **Figure 4B** shows a 100-mm long, 30G needle (arrow) visualized in the biceps femoris (BF) superficial to the sciatic nerve (SN). USGDN resolved the pain and mechanical effects from the taut bands in the muscle to relieve the pulling pain from radiculopathy in this patient with persistent pain after transforaminal epidural steroid injection at L4–5.

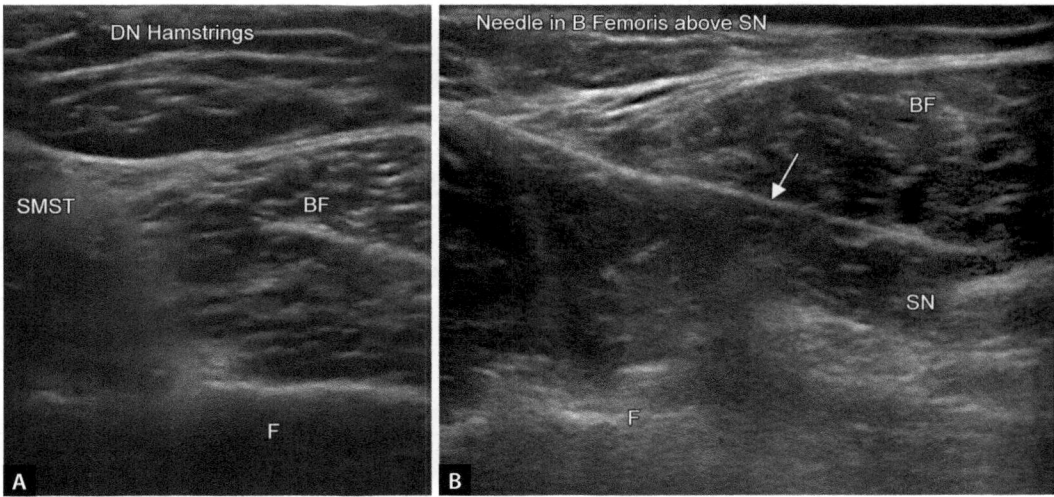

Figs. 4A and B: USGDN of hamstring muscles.

Figure 5A shows the needle passing through tibialis anterior (TA) and the extensor digitorum (EXT). The arrow in **Figure 5B** shows the needle passing through gastrocnemius (Gastroc) overlying the soleus (SOL) muscle.

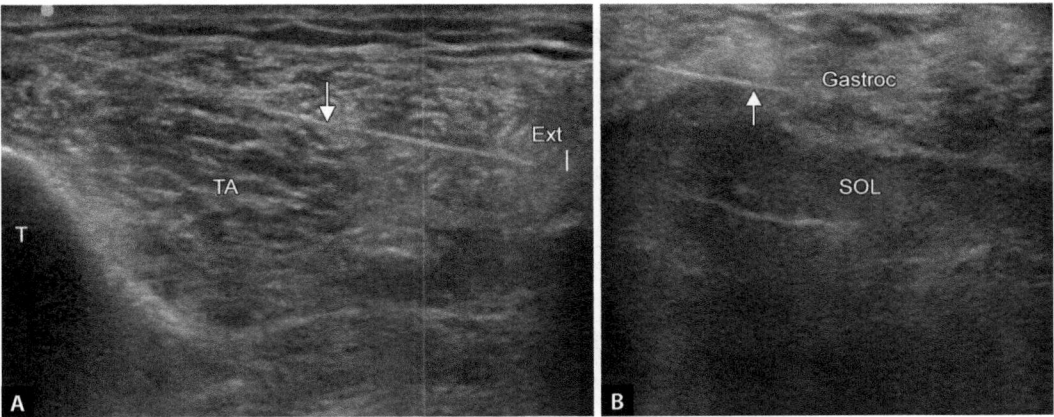

Figs. 5A and B: USGDN of calf and shin muscles involved in radicular pain.

Figures 6A to D show USGDN of intercostal muscles overlying the pericardium and pleura to treat severe chest wall pain in a post-mastectomy pain syndrome (PMPS) patient. She had persistent pain in spite of radiofrequency ablation of stellate ganglion + oral morphine + neuromodulators + transdermal fentanyl. Combination of ultrasound-guided Botox injection and USGDN kept her PMPS under control (at 2–3 VRS) for 6 months till her peaceful demise. **Figure 6A** shows the needle entering the intercostal muscle (ICM) over the pericardium. **Figure 6B** shows USGDN of lateral chest wall muscles—latissimus dorsi (LD), serratus anterior (SA), and intercostal muscle (ICM) next to the rib (R) responsible for her lateral chest wall pain in the same patient. **Figure 6C** shows USGDN of the interscapular area with the needle passing through rhomboids (RH) to enter the intercostal muscle (ICM) between 2 ribs (R) with the pleura (PL) in between. **Figure 6D** shows USGDN of trapezius (TR), levator scapulae (LS), rhomboids (RH), intercostal muscles (ICM), and pleura (PL) in a younger patient with simple myofascial pain syndrome.

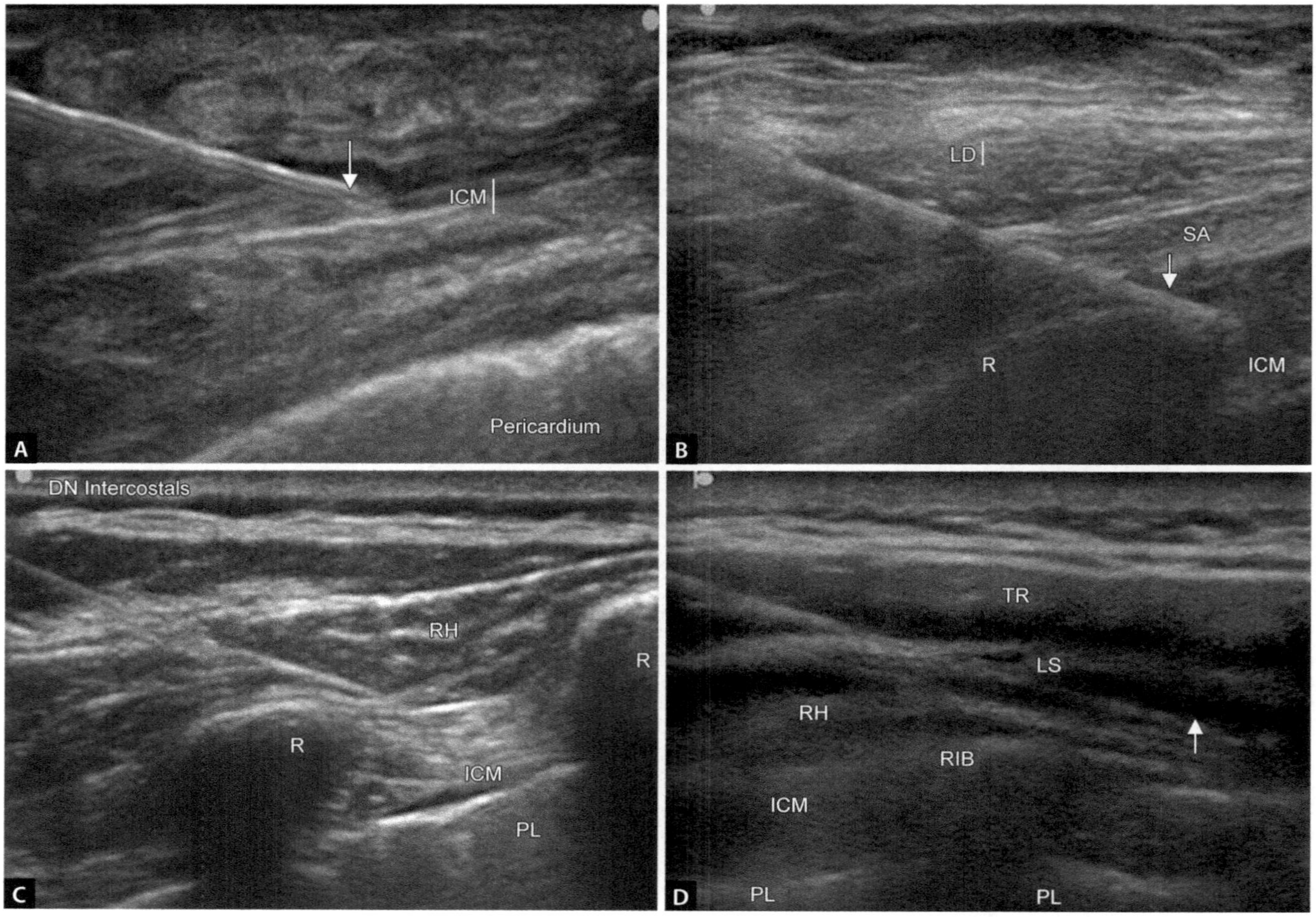

Figs. 6A to D: Ultrasound safeguards injury to pleura and pericardium during USGDN for relieving chest wall pains in postmastectomy pain syndrome (PMPS).

Figures 7A and B show USGDN of rectus abdominis (R abdominis) and the oblique muscles; external oblique (EO), internal oblique (IO) and transversus abdominis (TA) in an 18-year-old patient with chronic pancreatitis who had failed to respond to two celiac plexus blocks—one with fluoroscopy guidance and another through the endoscope. His pain was completely relieved after five USGDN sessions with weight gain and return to normal life.

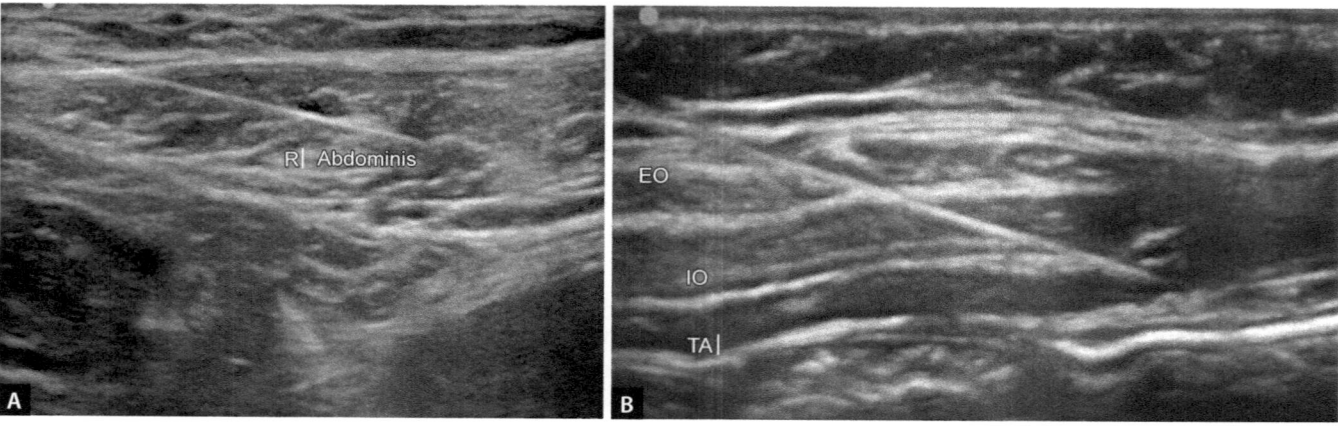

Figs. 7A and B: USGDN of abdominal muscles.

Figure 8 shows needle (arrow) passing through pectineus (P), adductor longus (AL), brevis (AB), and adductor magnus (AM) in a patient with groin pain. Medial edge of femoral vein (FV) is seen in the upper left corner.

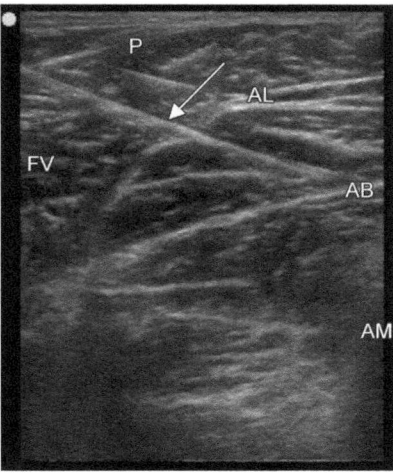

Fig. 8: USGDN for groin pain.

Figures 9A and B show USGDN of masticatory muscles relieved trigeminal neuralgia persisting at numerical rating scale 8–9 pain in spite of radiofrequency ablation of trigeminal ganglion 18 months prior. Systematic USGDN of all masticatory muscles relieved her pains as well as reduced her medications. Pulsed radiofrequency of mandibular nerve was performed to reduce the intense masticatory muscle spasm at presentation. Combination of neural treatments with USGDN achieves the optimal results. **Figure 9A** shows needles in masseter (Mass) overlying the mandible (Man) and **Figure 9B** shows needling around mental foremen to relieve local pain. This is to be followed by USGDN of masticatory muscles.

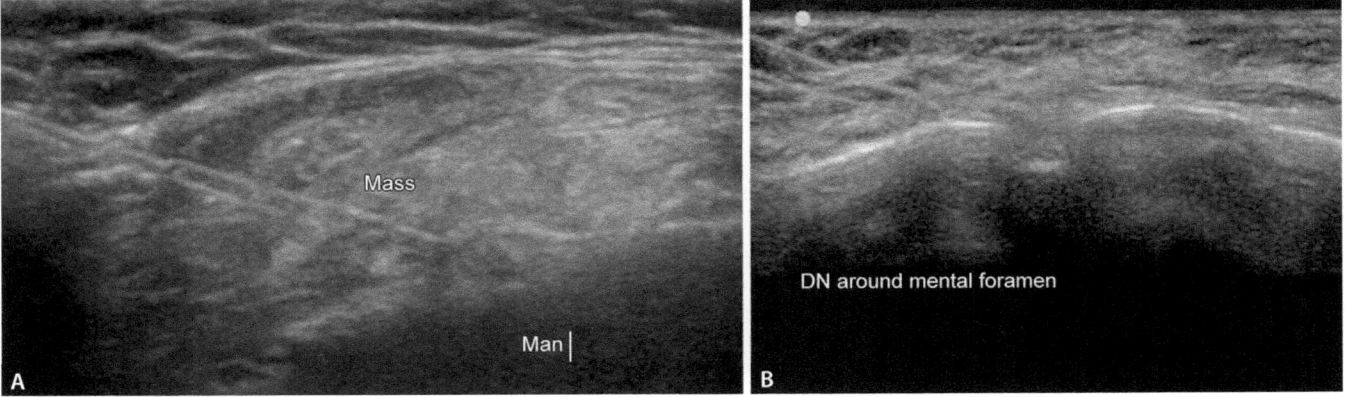

Figs. 9A and B: USGDN masticatory muscles.

SECTION 11

Advanced Pain Management

- **Spinal Cord Stimulation**
  Timothy Ray Deer

- **Intrathecal Drug Delivery System**
  Samir Ranjit Jani, Dwarkadas K Baheti

- **Transforaminal Endoscopic Discectomy**
  Kailash M Kothari, Manish Raj, Shiraz Ahmed Munshi

- **Kyphoplasty**
  Samir Ranjit Jani

CHAPTER 54

Spinal Cord Stimulation

Timothy Ray Deer

SPINAL CORD STIMULATION

Basic Information

- *Common indications*: Lumbar radiculopathy, post-laminectomy syndrome, neuropathic pain of the trunk or limbs, complex regional pain syndrome, cervical radiculopathy, post-herpetic neuralgia
- *Relative contraindications*: Bleeding disorders, local infection at the implant site, systemic infection, poorly controlled diabetes, improper spinal anatomy
- *Regions of potential treatment*:
  - Cervical
  - Thoracic
  - Lumbar
  - Sacral
- *Equipment used*:
  - 14-gauge needle (curved or straight)
  - Spinal cord stimulation (SCS) lead(s)
  - Trialing system with cable
  - Materials to secure the trial system

Permanent: Same as trial and in addition:
- Generator
- Tunneling rod
- Closure materials and proper suture, skin adhesive, or staples
- Neuromonitoring equipment, if needed.

Step 1: Pad, position, and properly drape the patient.

Step 2: Assure a widespread prep and drape to secure a sterile area.

Step 3: Take initial scout films and use local anesthesia for planned needle entry.

Step 4: Make a small stab wound at the planned needle entry.

Step 5: Needle placement is paramedian at an angle of 30–45°.

Step 6: Loss of resistance is used to confirm the epidural space.

Confirm in anteroposterior and lateral views fluoroscopically **(Figs. 1 and 2)**.

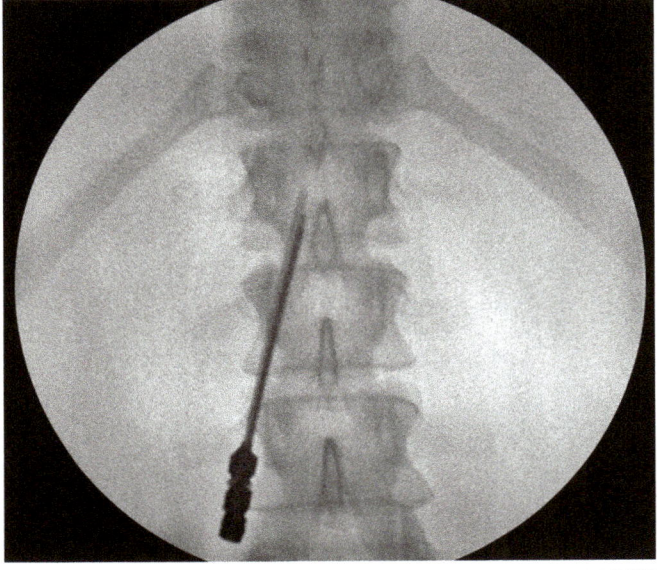

Fig. 1: Needles in epidural space in anteroposterior view.

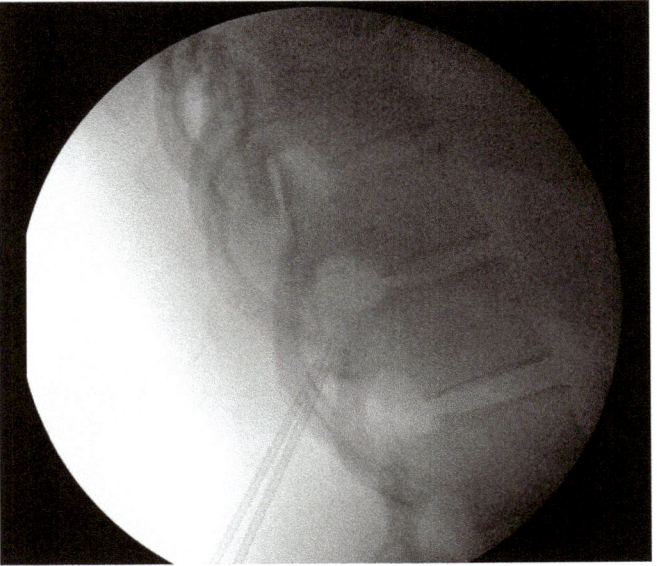

Fig. 2: Needles in epidural space in lateral view.

Step 7: Low exposure live fluoroscopy is used to position the lead.

Confirm both leads in epidural space in anteroposterior and lateral views fluoroscopically **(Figs. 3 and 4)**.

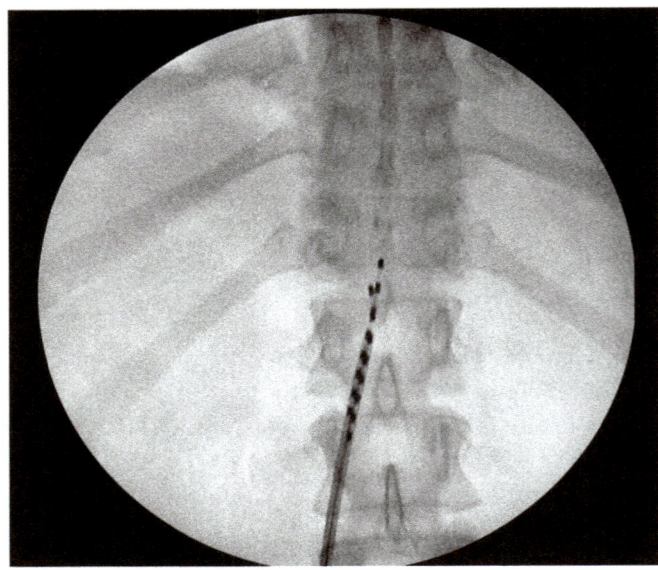

Fig. 3: Lead in epidural space in anteroposterior view.

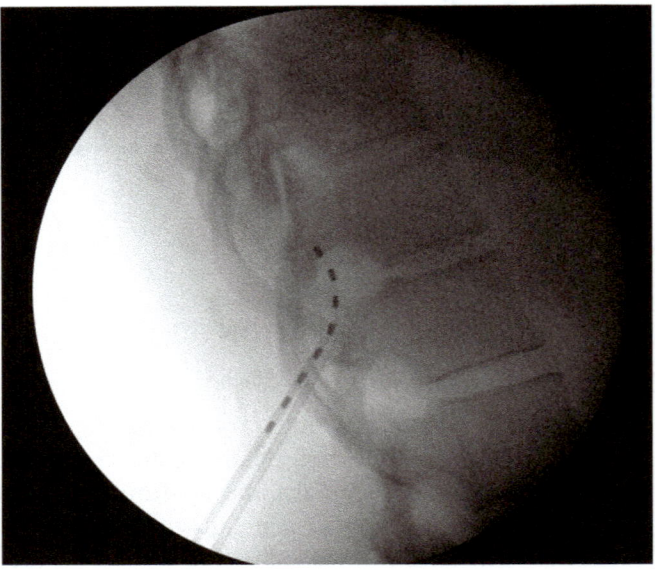

Fig. 4: Lead in epidural space in lateral view.

Step 8: Once the position of leads reaches the desired dermatome or level, which needs to be confirmed with the patient.

Step 9: Now fix the lead and tunnel it under skin near the proposed site of hardware **(Figs. 5 and 6)**.

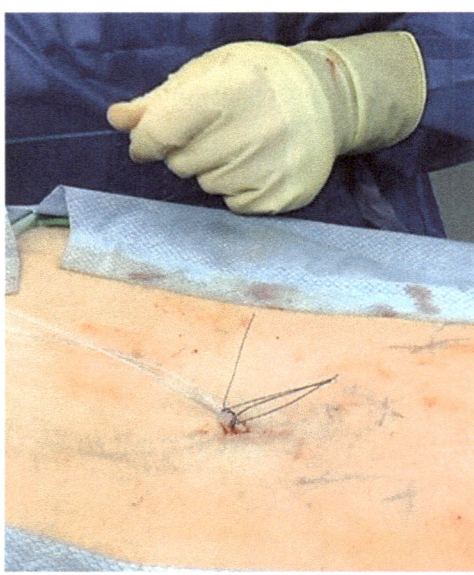

Fig. 5: Fixation of leads.

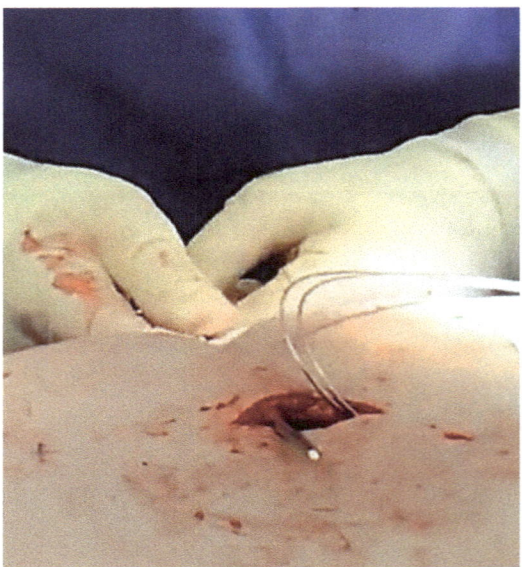

Fig. 6: Tunneling of leads.

Step 10: Make a pocket for hardware and insert the hardware into the pocket **(Figs. 7 and 8)**.

Step 11: Once hardware is inserted into the pocket, take a final picture of hardware with leads attached fluoroscopically and program with the programmer **(Figs. 9 and 10)**.

Step 12: After lead placement is radiologically confirmed, prepare to test the leads.

Step 13: Connect to a trialing system of your choice.

Step 14: Once the leads are trialed, remove the needles if it is a trial system and secure the leads.

Permanent: The permanent procedure requires additional steps:

Step 15: Plan the pocket position and anchor the leads.

Step 16: Anchor and tunnel the leads.

Step 17: Connect the leads to the generator and test impedances and mapping if needed.

Step 18: Complete pocketing and wound closure.

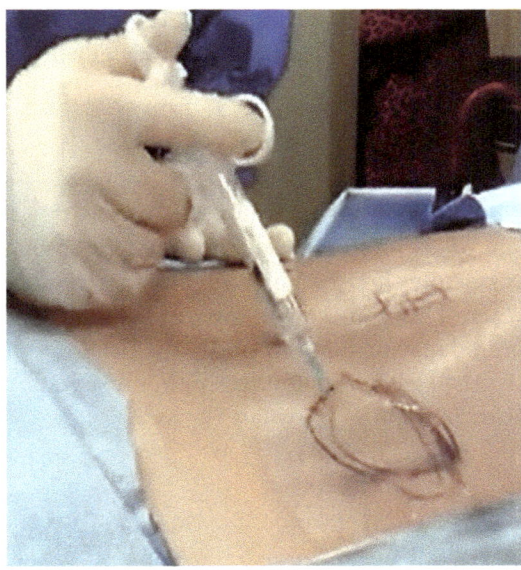

Fig. 7: Making pocket for hardware.

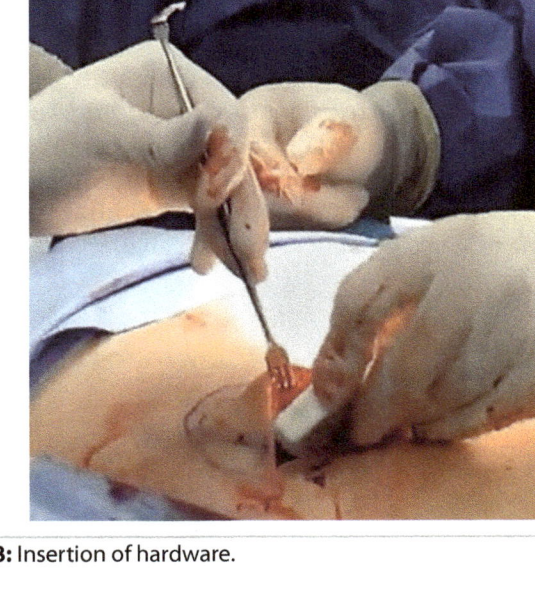

Fig. 8: Insertion of hardware.

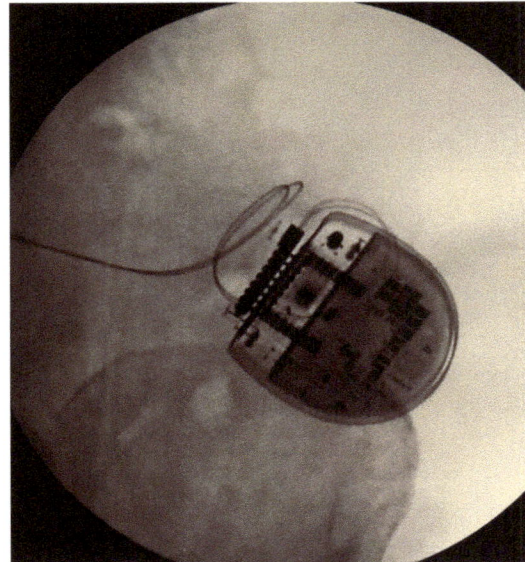

Fig. 9: Hardware with leads in situ.

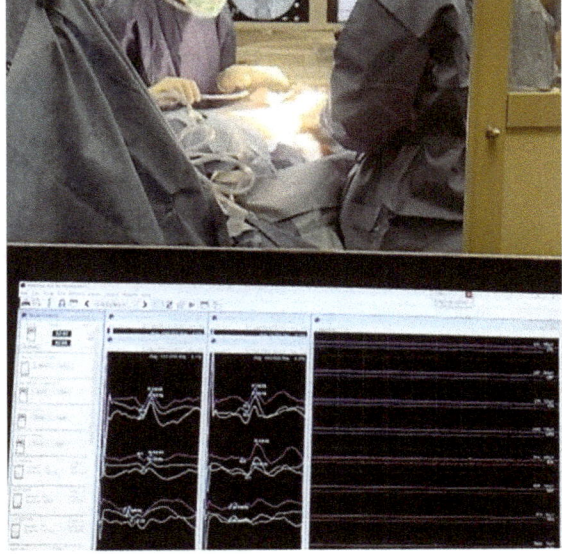

Fig. 10: Intraoperative monitoring.

CHAPTER 55

Intrathecal Drug Delivery System

Samir Ranjit Jani, Dwarkadas K Baheti

BASIC INFORMATION

Indications
- Intractable chronic pain
- Cancer pain with life expectancy >6 months
- Significant adverse reactions to systemic opioid use
- Poor response to more conservative management (nonopioid medications, injections, neurostimulation)
- Successful intrathecal pump trial (epidural trial preferable to single shot but both acceptable)

Contraindications
- Patient refusal
- Active infection (cellulitis, sepsis)
- Anticoagulation that cannot be held or bleeding diathesis
- Severe depression (psychological evaluation beneficial)
- Unreliable patient (IT opioid withdrawal can be severe and life-threatening)

PROCEDURE

Step 1: Position the patient in the prone position for placement of IT pump into back (well tolerated by patient, easier surgically, less catheter means less risk of kinks/damage, etc.). Eliminate lumbar lordosis and optimize alignment by placing a pillow under the pelvis as shown in **Figure 1**. Also, have a diagrammatic representation of the final picture in mind as shown in **Figure 2**.

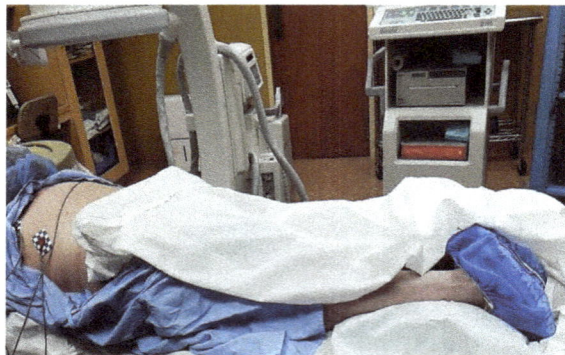

Fig. 1: Patient position.

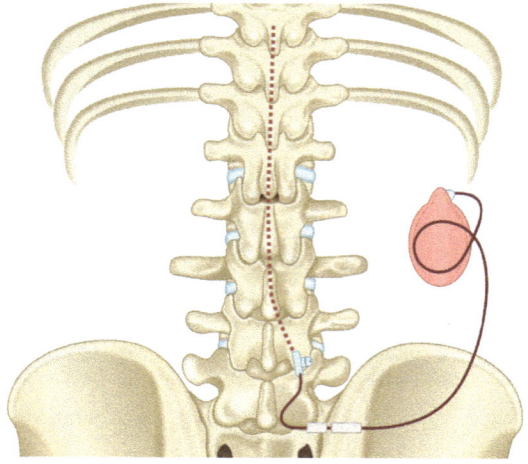

Fig. 2: Diagrammatic representation of intrathecal drug delivery system.

Step 2: After anesthesia, prepare and drape the patient. Obtain anteroposterior fluoroscopy and tilt C-arm cephalad or caudad to optimize view and square off the superior endplate **(Figs. 3 and 4)**.

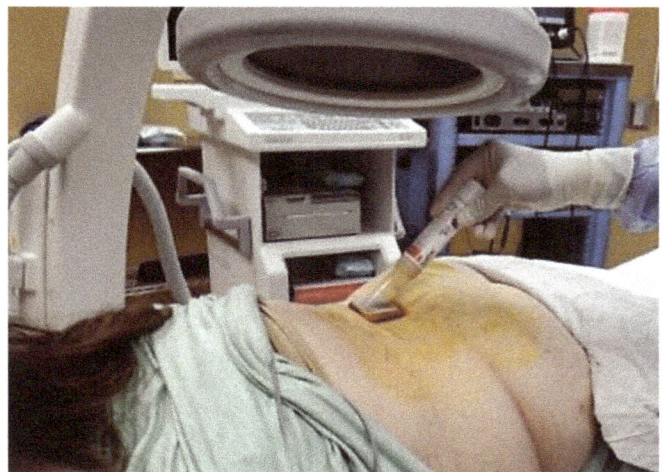

Fig. 3: C-arm anteroposterior view.

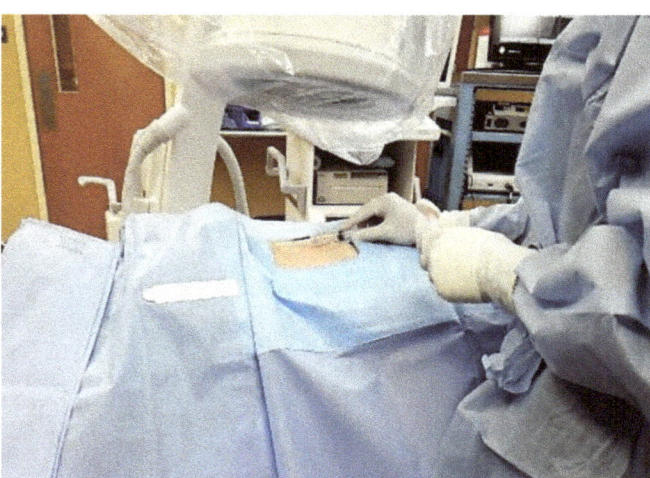

Fig. 4: C-arm tilt to optimize view.

Step 3: First decide the site of needle entry point **(Fig. 5)** (approximately 1 vertebral body lower on the medial pedicle border; see the figure). Now inject Inj. lidocaine 1% 2 mL into soft tissue.

Step 4: Using a paramedian approach, enter the epidural space with a similar angle to that for spinal cord stimulation (SCS) lead insertion **(Fig. 6)**.

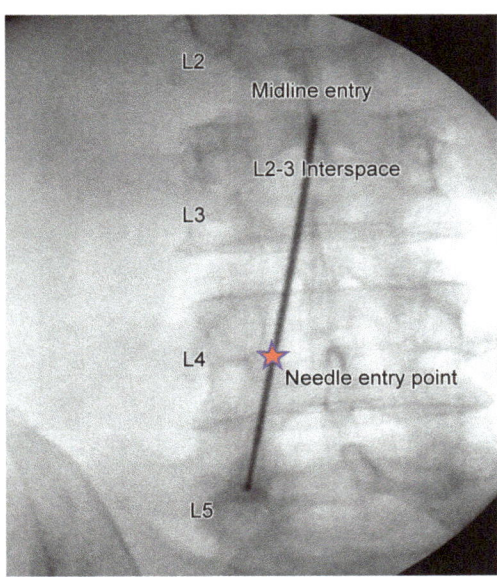

Fig. 5: Needle entry point.

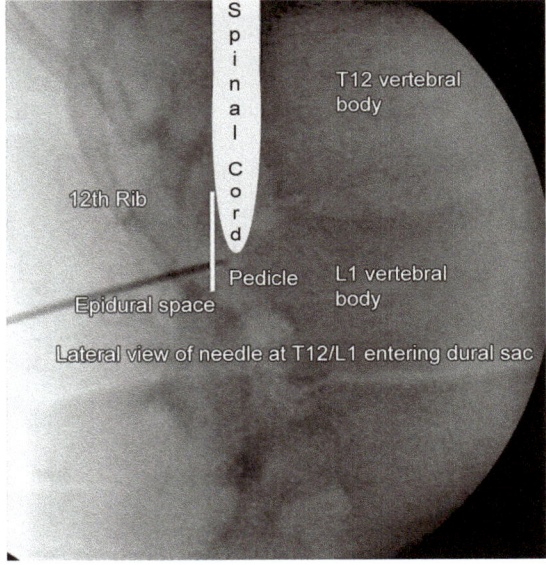

Fig. 6: Needle in epidural space.

Step 5: Ideally, aim for L1/2 or L2/3 (as seen above). Enter below conus for safety and obtain lateral view to confirm needle location. Cerebrospinal fluid (CSF) should be free flowing and robust **(Fig. 7)**.

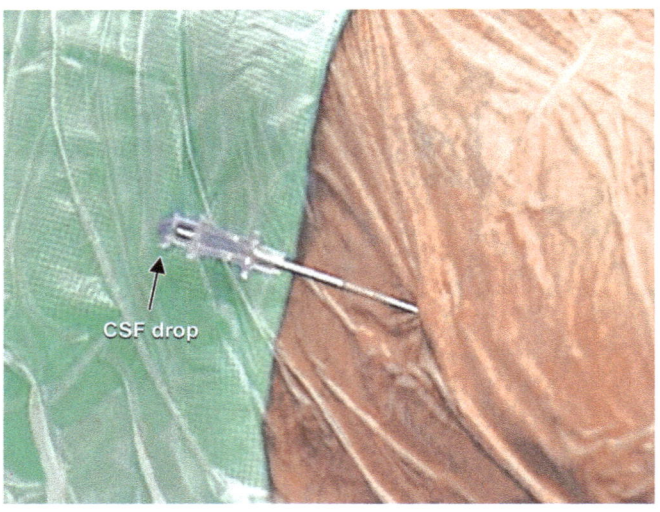

Fig. 7: Free flow of cerebrospinal fluid (CSF).

Step 6: Advance catheter toward the desired thoracic level **(Fig. 8)** staying dorsal as best as possible. The catheter tip should be ideally situated posterior and midline **(Figs. 9 and 10)**.

The dermatomes are brachial plexus C3–C5; arm C3–C5; breast T1–T2; upper chest wall T3–T4; visceral abdomen T5–T6; lower chest wall T6–T7; abdominal wall T6–T7; pelvis T9–T12; back/leg T10 and sacrum—conus.

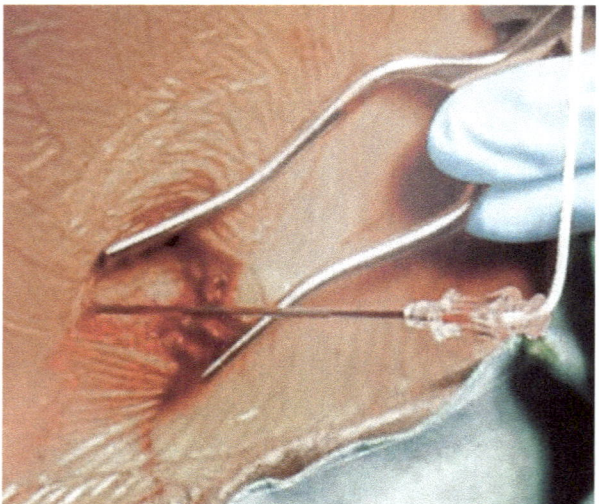

Fig. 8: Insertion and advancing of catheter.

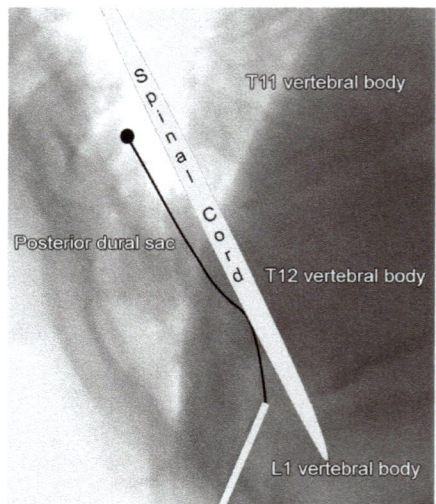

Fig. 9: Intrathecal catheter in anteroposterior view.

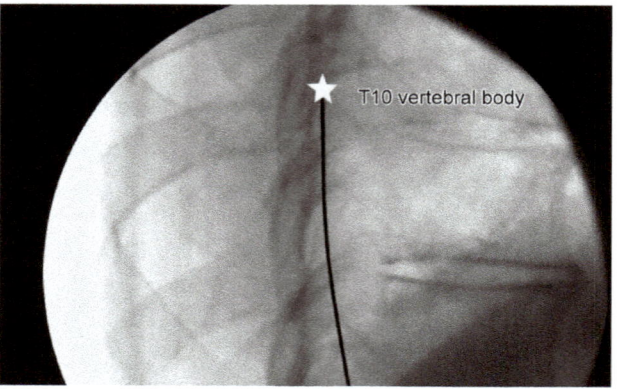

Fig. 10: Intrathecal catheter in lateral view.

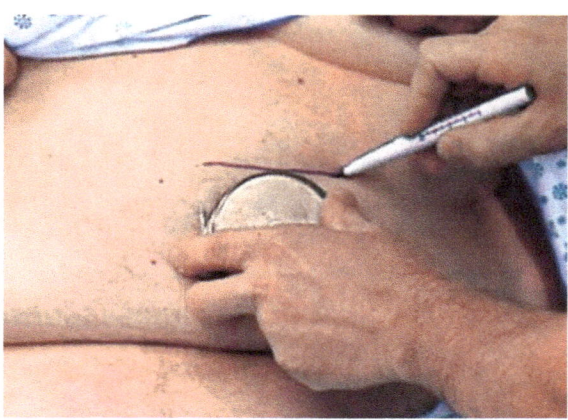

Fig. 11: Making pocket for pump.

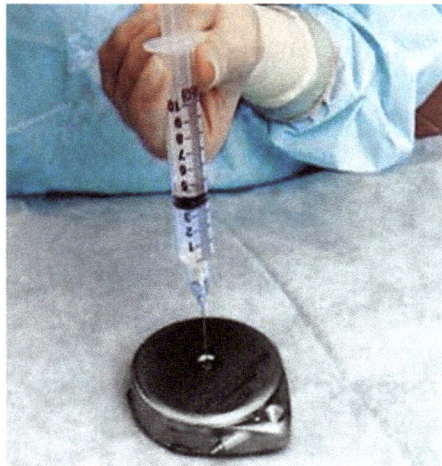

Fig. 12: Filling of pump with medication.

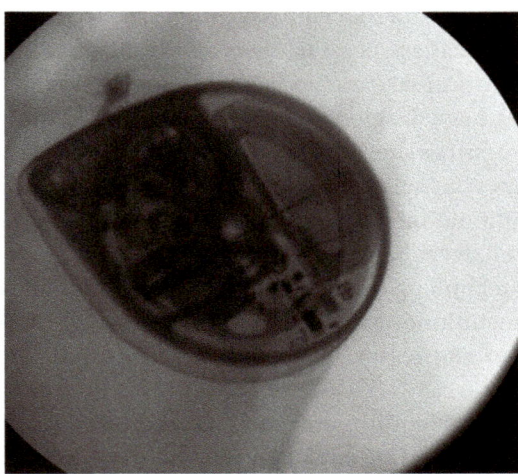

Fig. 13: Pump in situ.

Step 7: Confirm adequate CSF flow from the distal end of the catheter; if no flow, manipulate catheter or retry placement.

Step 8: Confirm the position of the intrathecal catheter in the anteroposterior view fluoroscopically.

Step 9: Create adequate pocket for pump **(Fig. 11)**. One must make sure of bleeding points in the pocket as little blood collection can be the source of infection.

Step 10: Now create a midline pocket for anchoring catheter. Inject 1% lidocaine 5 mL and make a 2–3-cm vertical midline incision over the needle. Here too, cauterize any bleeding points. Also, one can use blunt (finger) and sharp scissor or electrocautery to create adequate pocket to accommodate anchor.

Step 11: Now gently remove Touhy needle without removing the catheter and using prepackaged anchor tool, place the anchor over the catheter and deploy the anchor catheter to thoracolumbar fascia using 2-0 silk suture. Now cut excess catheter length and note removed length for pump setup.

Step 12: Tunnel catheter from the midline pocket to the pump site using supplied tunneling tool or Touhy needle and connect the pump segment catheter to the intrathecal catheter.

Step 13: Aspirate from the side port to ensure adequate CSF return. To prevent any collection or dead tissue due to cautery, irrigate both wounds with antibiotic wash.

Step 14: Make sure that there is no collection of blood. Then close both incisions and apply firm and proper bandage at the pocket and needle site.

Step 15: Filling of intrathecal pump to be done by pain physician or assistant side-by-side and keep it ready as shown in **Figure 12**.

Step 16: Take X-ray of pump in situ **(Fig. 13)**.

Refills will need to be done periodically every 1–4 months as needed.

Step 17: Shift the patient to recovery room for monitoring and observation.

Declaration

Part of the text and some images are taken with permission from M/s Jaypee Brothers Medical Publishers, New Delhi, from the chapter "Intrathecal Pump" published in the book, *Interventional Pain Management: Practical Approach* 2009 and 2018 edited by DK Baheti, Sanjay Bakshi, Sanjeeva Gupta and RP Gehdoo.

CHAPTER 56

Transforaminal Endoscopic Discectomy

Kailash M Kothari, Manish Raj, Shiraz Ahmed Munshi

INTRODUCTION

Pain medicine as a specialty has progressed immensely over the last 5 decades. As researchers agreed that it is important to preserve normal structures while doing surgery, all surgical branches have developed various techniques of minimally invasive surgeries. Interventional pain management techniques have also developed during this period and many interventional minimally invasive techniques to treat disc have been developed by various researchers.

The technological advances have helped to make these newer techniques simple and effective. Few examples are IDET, DeKompressor, Nucleotome, DiscFx, Epiduroscopy, etc.

Advanced equipment such as radiofrequency (RF), lasers, optics, and radioimaging helped in making minimally invasive pain management procedures a more acceptable and effective treatment option compared to open surgeries.

Transforaminal lumbar endoscopic decompression is one such technique which is being practiced by pain physicians across the globe. The endoscopic treatment of lumbar spine is now advancing to various other approaches, e.g., interlaminar decompression, interlaminar stenotic decompression, unilateral biportal decompression surgery (UBS).

HISTORY

1934: Mixter and Barr treated herniated lumbar/thoracic and cervical disc prolapse causing radicular pain with laminectomy.

1964: Chemonucleolysis using a needle inserted percutaneously in the disc (first minimally invasive technique described for disc), though as patients developed transverse myelitis as the side effect, this technique was abandoned.

1973: Kambin used Craig cannula to perform nucleotomy to decompress the disc through the posterolateral approach.

1983: Forst and Hausmann used a modified arthroscope in the disc.

1985: Onik et al. introduced a motorized aspiration shaver for nucleotomy, called automated percutaneous nucleotomy.

1988: For the first time in history, Kambin published a discoscopic view of nucleus pulposus.

1989: Schreiber et al. for the first time used indigo carmine dye to stain abnormal nucleus and annular fissures.

1990: Kambin introduced the triangular working zone called Kambin's triangle. The borders of Kambin's triangle are—anteriorly the exiting roots, posteriorly superior articular process of inferior vertebra, and inferiorly superior endplate of lower vertebra and medially traversing nerve root.

1993: Mayer and Brock used an angled lens scope to focus on the annular tear.

1999: Foley presented treatment of far lateral disc using an endoscope.

1996: Mathew used a foraminal approach to endoscopic discectomy successfully.

1996: Kambin and Zhou used 300Scopes, forceps, and trephines for decompression of annulus and osteophytes.

1997: Tsou and Yeung introduced a rigid endoscope with lens and multiple channels.

2007: Knight et al. used a laser [holmium:yttrium-aluminum-garnet (Ho: YAG)].

2002:
- Intradiscal Electrothermal Therapy (IDET) was introduced for low back pain due to disc.
- Yeung and Tsou presented their work on transforaminal endoscopic discectomy and concluded that results are comparable to open surgery.

2003: Yeung Endoscopic Spine System (YESS) was introduced.

2005: Schubert and Hoogland used reamers to perform foraminoplasty and get access to sequestrated disc.

BASIC INFORMATION

Indications

- Lumbar disc herniation/prolapse not responding to conservative treatment

Drugs

- Local anesthetic
- IV sedation if planned
- Indigo carmine contrast
- Steroid—dexamethasone or triamcinolone (Kenalog)
- Antibiotics—cefuroxime 1.5 g preoperative within 30 minutes of the start of the procedure
- Preservative-free saline 3 L for irrigation

Contraindications

- Unwilling patient
- Untreated infection
- Pregnancy
- Bleeding problems or blood thinners
- Allergy to medications
- Presence of red flags

Complications

- Incomplete removal
- Hematoma
- Infection
- Nerve root injury
- Paralysis/paraplegia
- Recurrent disc herniation

ADDITIONAL TIPS

- Review the latest MRI scan images and any fluoroscopic images of any procedure.
- Obtain informed written consent.

ANATOMY

- Lumbar intervertebral disc (Fig. 1)

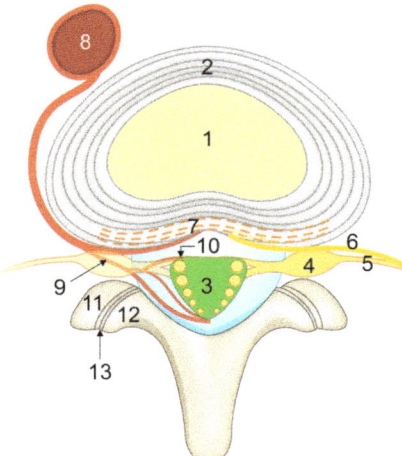

Lumbar Intervertebral Disc
1. Nucleus pulposus
2. Annulus
3. Thecal sac with nerve roots arranged in the spinal canal
4. Dorsal root ganglion (DRG)
5. Exiting nerve root
6. Sinu-vertebral nerve
7. Unmyelinated free nerve endings supplying outer third of the annulus
8. Aorta
9. Radicular artery
10. Anterior spinal artery
11. Superior articular facet
12. Inferior articular facet
13. Facet joint

Fig. 1: *Image Courtesy:* Sakshi Kothari

- Lumbar motion segment with Kambin's triangle (Fig. 2A)

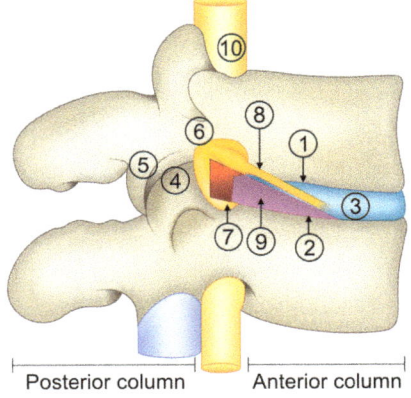

Lumbar Motion Segment with Kambin's Triangle
1. Inferior endplate of upper vertebra
2. Superior endplate of lower vertebra
3. Intervertebral disc
4. Superior facet
5. Inferior facet
6. Pedicle
7. Intervertebral foramen
8. Exiting root with DRG
9. Kambin's triangle
10. Traversing nerve root

Fig. 2A: *Image Courtesy:* Sakshi Kothari

Lumbar motion segment consisting of three joints—one facet joint on each side and a joint between the upper and the lower vertebral body with intervertebral disc in between.

Kambin's triangle: The hypotenuse is the exiting nerve root, the base (width) is the superior border of the caudal vertebra, and the height is the dura/traversing nerve root.

Kambin's triangle provides access to the "hidden zone" of Macnab by foraminoplasty (by cutting the tip of the superior articulate process and the ventral aspect of the superior articular facet). The foramen and lateral recess access is achieved by foraminoplasty so we can reach to the axilla between the traversing and the exiting nerve.

- Intervertebral foraminal ligamentum (**Fig. 2B**)

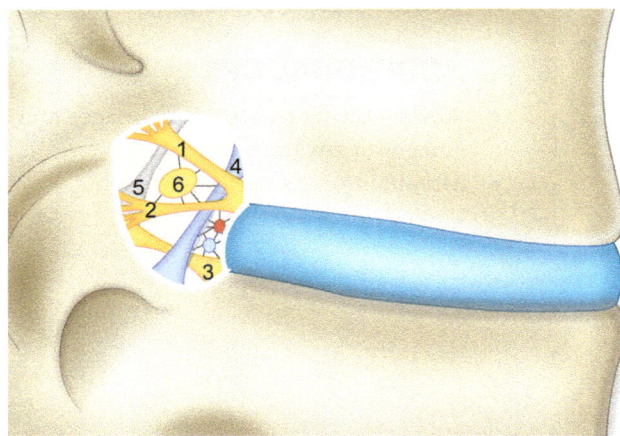

Lumbar Foraminal Ligaments
1. Superior transforaminal ligament
2. Mid-transforaminal ligament
3. Inferior transforaminal ligament
4. Superior corporo-pedicular ligament
5. Inferior corporo-pedicular ligament
6. Nerve roots
7. Vessels

Fig. 2B: *Image Courtesy:* Sakshi Kothari

OPERATING ROOM SET-UP (FIG. 3)

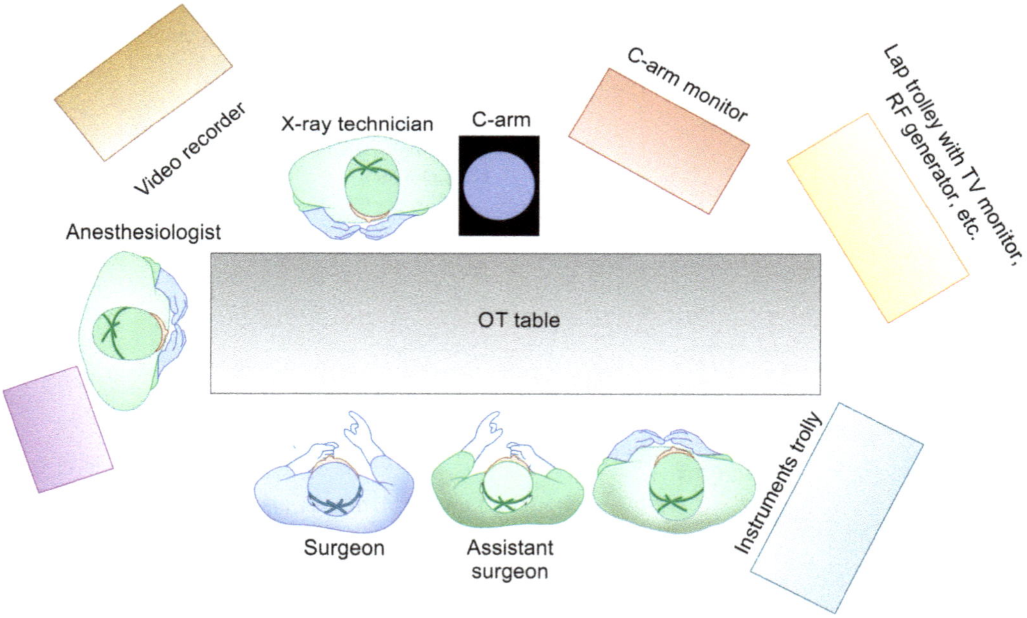

Fig. 3: *Image Courtesy:* Sakshi Kothari

Skin Markings

Markings: Mark the lines using the marker to measure and identify the correct entry point at the skin level.

Under Fluoroscopic Guidance (in Anteroposterior View)

- Vertical line **(Figs. 4A and B)**, joining lumbar spinous processes

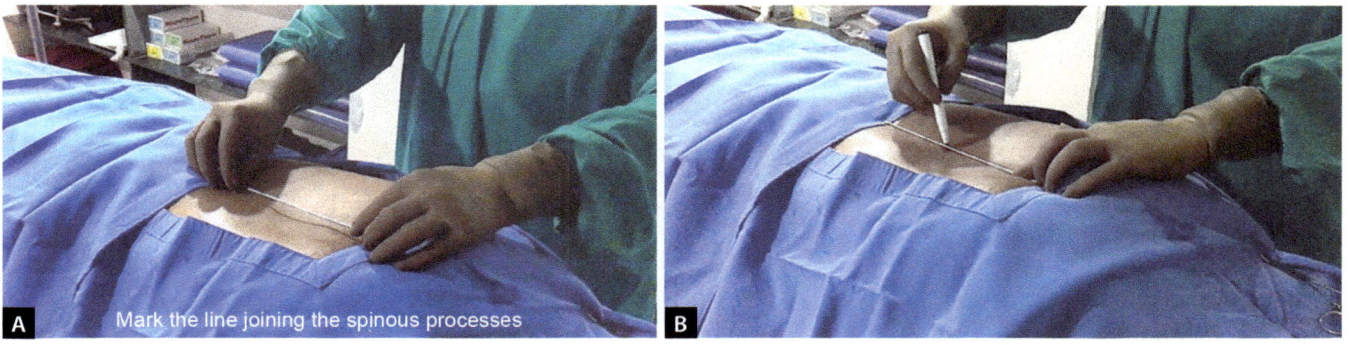

Figs. 4A and B: *Image Courtesy:* Pain Clinic of India

- Horizontal line **(Figs. 5A and B)**, from the center of the disc to be operated

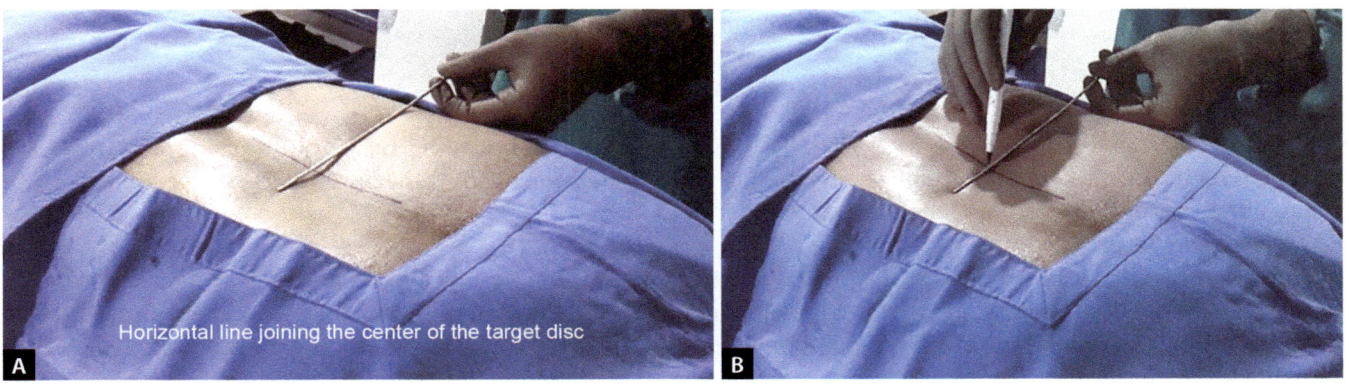

Figs. 5A and B: *Image Courtesy:* Pain Clinic of India

- For L5–S1 disc—draw an oblique line from the center of the disc and draw above the iliac crest **(Figs. 6A and B)**.

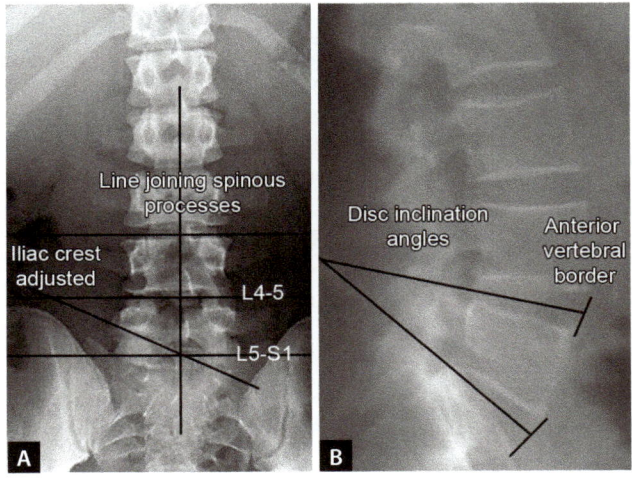

Figs. 6A and B: *Image Courtesy:* Pain Clinic of India

Lateral View

Disc inclination line **(Figs. 7A and B):** Draw a line from along and from the anterior border of the center of the disc and take it all the way to the posterior back where it crosses the horizontal line (vertical line point A).

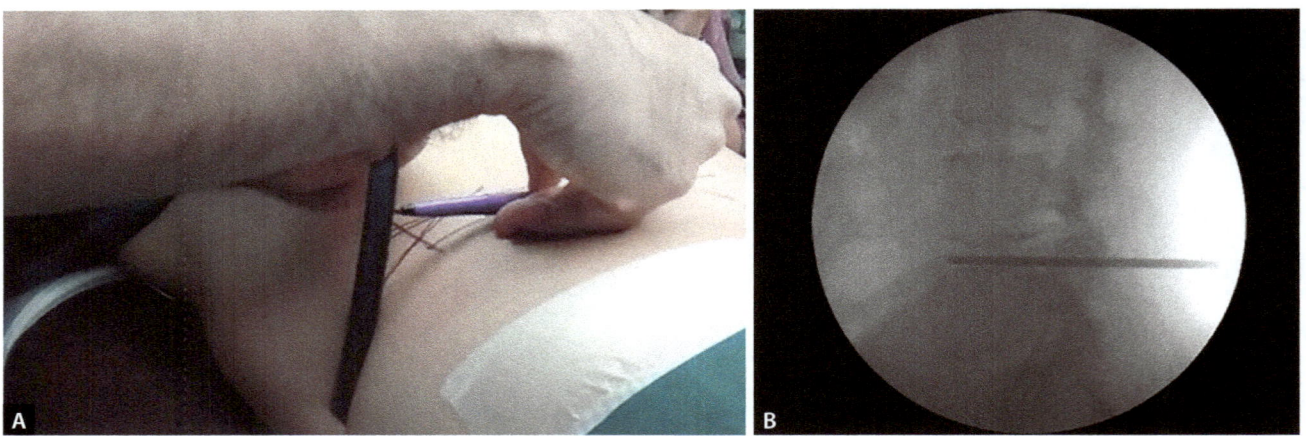

Figs. 7A and B: (A) Drawing of line; (B) Marker crossing the vertical line.
Image Courtesy: Pain Clinic of India

Patient Position and Preoperative Counseling

- The patient is lying prone, comfortable enough so that he does not move for the duration of the procedure.
- Awake during the procedure.
- With the bolsters at the chest and abdomen with abdomen being free of any pressure, so that good kyphosis is achieved at the site of procedure (lumbar)
- He should be counseled and educated about the procedure.
- He should be informed about the feeling of injection and instruments entering the back.
- Alert the operator if he feels any tingling or sharp shooting pain going down the leg during the procedure,

Anesthesia

- Proper cleaning and draping
- Sedation can be given as per the patient's anxiety level.
- The most common point of skin entry is between 10 and 12 cm from the midline.
- Xylocaine 2% infiltration is done—skin wheel, deep in the muscles up to facet joint using spinal needle **(Fig. 8)**.

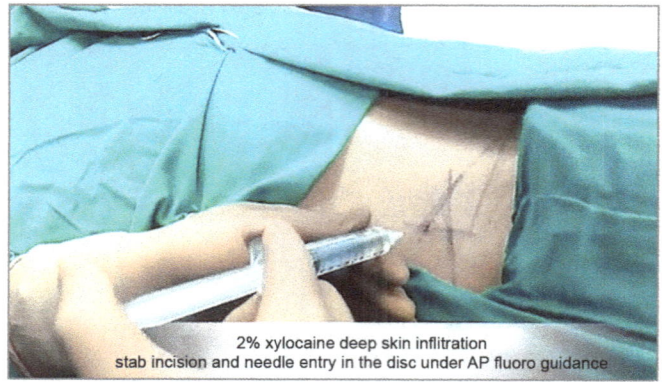

Fig. 8: Injecting local anesthetic.
Image Courtesy: Pain Clinic of India

Procedure: Step-wise Description

- *Stab incision and needle entry (Figs. 9A and B):* By using an 11-sizes stab knife, a stab incision is taken (approximately 1.5–2 cm long). This will avoid direct contact of the instruments with skin and in turn reduce the chances of bacteria (the most being *Staphylococcus aureus*) entering the disc.

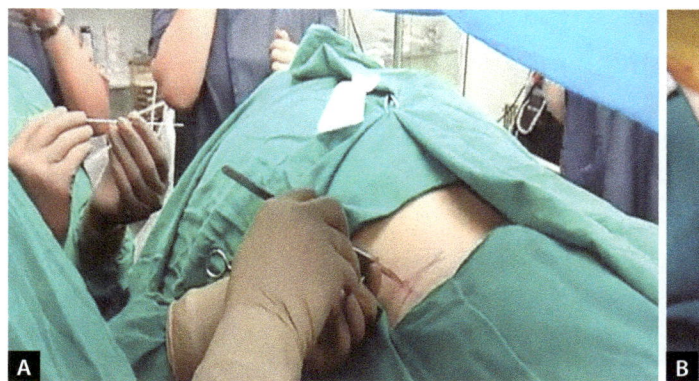
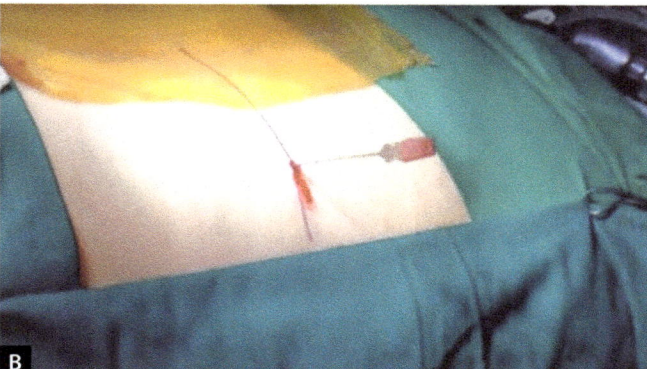

Figs. 9A and B: (A) Skin incision; (B) Skin entry point.
Image Courtesy: Pain Clinic of India

- The needle is slowly inserted toward the facet in the AP view of fluoroscopy and confirmed in lateral view, till the needle hits the facet joint. 1% xylocaine can be injected over this point to provide pain relief during manipulation of needle **(Figs. 10A to H)**.
- Needle tip is then manipulated in such a way that it walks off the facet and enters the disc.

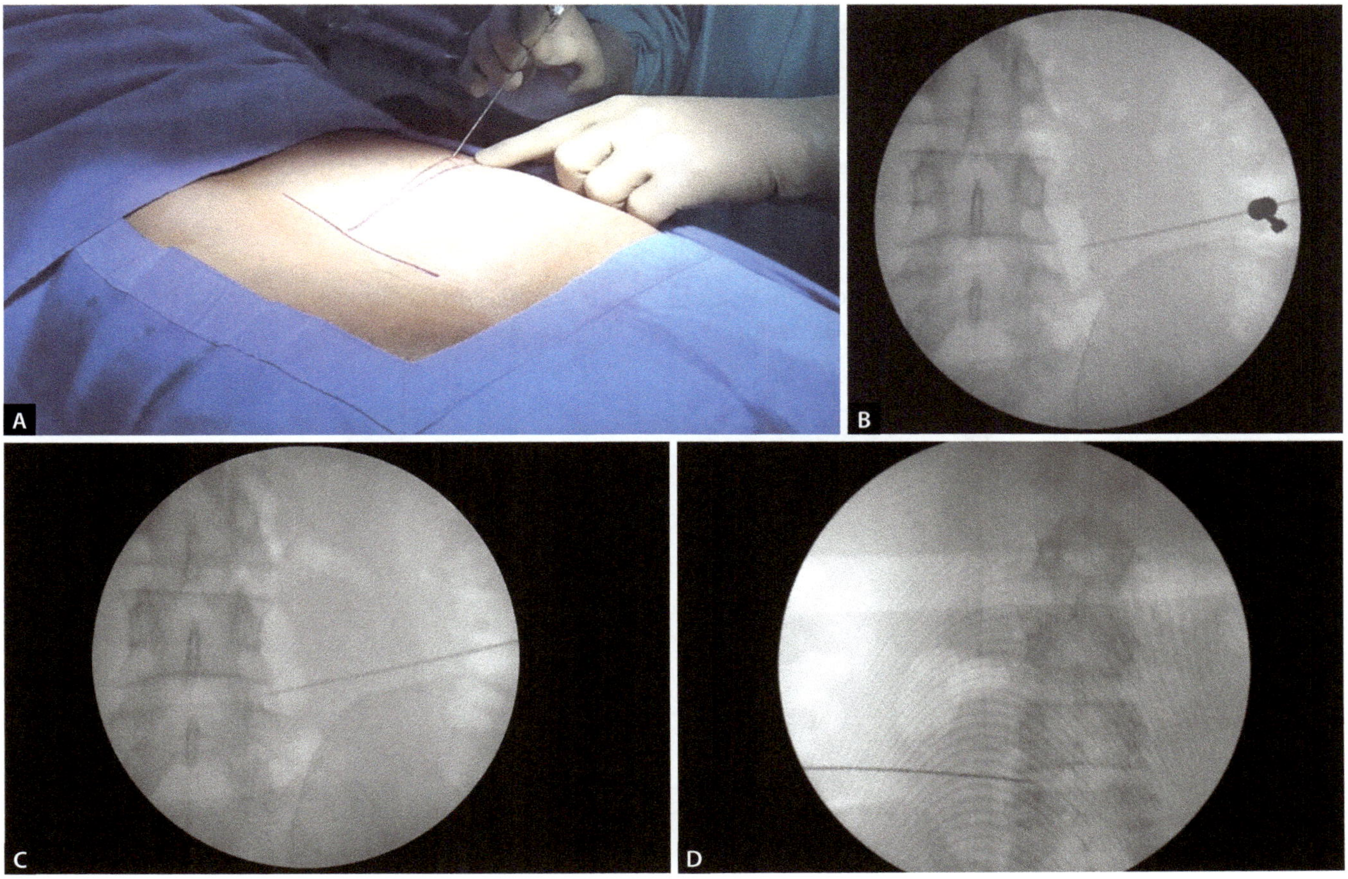

Figs. 10A to D: (A and B) Needle insertion; (C and D) Manipulation of the needle tip.
Image Courtesy: Pain Clinic of India

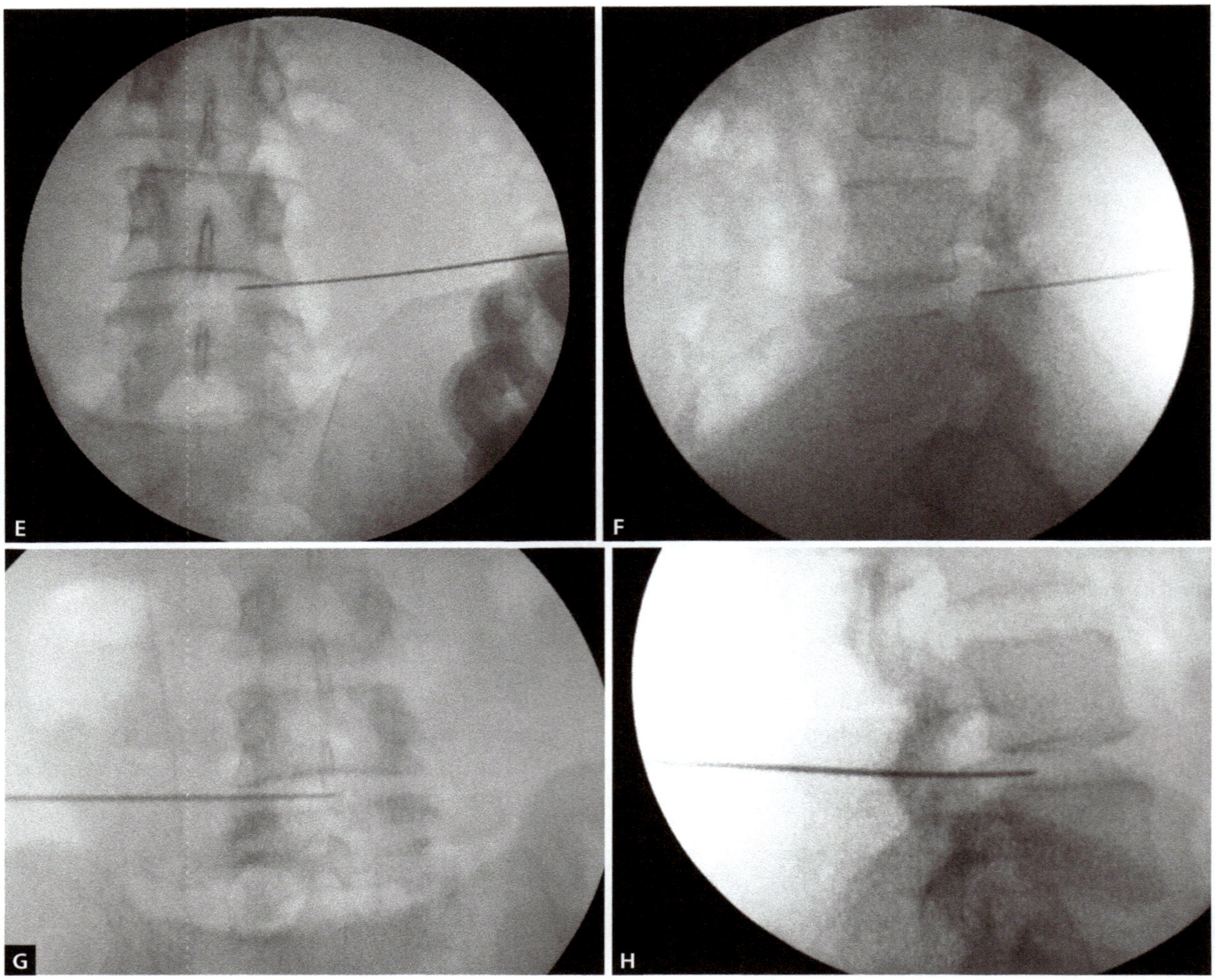

Figs. 10E to H: (E and F) Needle tip about to reach centre the disc AP and lateral views; (G) Needle tip at the center of the disc in anteroposterior view; (H) Needle tip in lateral view.
Image Courtesy: Pain Clinic of India

- Once the needle tip is in the center of the disc in AP and in posterior third of the disc, discography is performed using a dye called indigo carmine which stains the acidic abnormal damaged nucleus. There is no staining of the normal nucleus **(Fig. 10I)**.

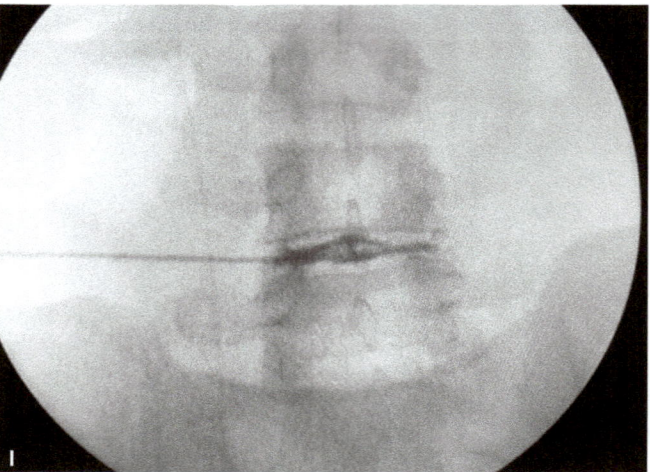

Fig. 10I: Discogram.
Image Courtesy: Pain Clinic of India

- Guidewire is being inserted through the needle in to the disc **(Fig. 11)**.

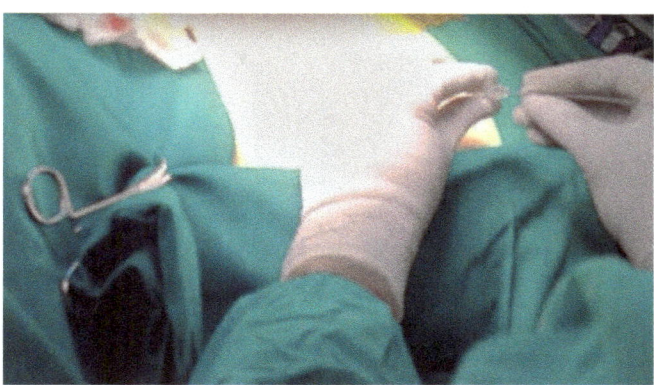

Fig. 11: Insertion of guidewire.
Image Courtesy: Pain Clinic of India

- Needle is removed leaving the guidewire in the disc.
- In patients with foraminal stenosis or facet hypertrophy, reaming or drilling the undersurface (anterior surface) of the superior facet is required. Manual bone drilling or reaming is performed by inserting reamers of various sizes (smaller to larger) over guidewire under fluoroscopic guidance up to the medial border of the facet **(Fig. 12)**. This helps in creating enough space for other instruments to enter the disc.

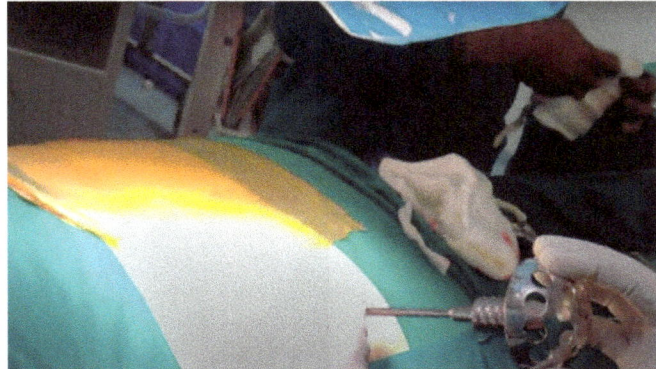

Fig. 12: Needle removed. Foraminotomy—various sizes of bone reamers inserted till the facet medial border to drill the undersurface of the facet. *Note*: This is a fluoroscopic-guided drilling and needs very careful execution with constant feedback from patient.
Image Courtesy: Pain Clinic of India

- The dilator is then inserted over the guidewire **(Figs. 13A and B)**.

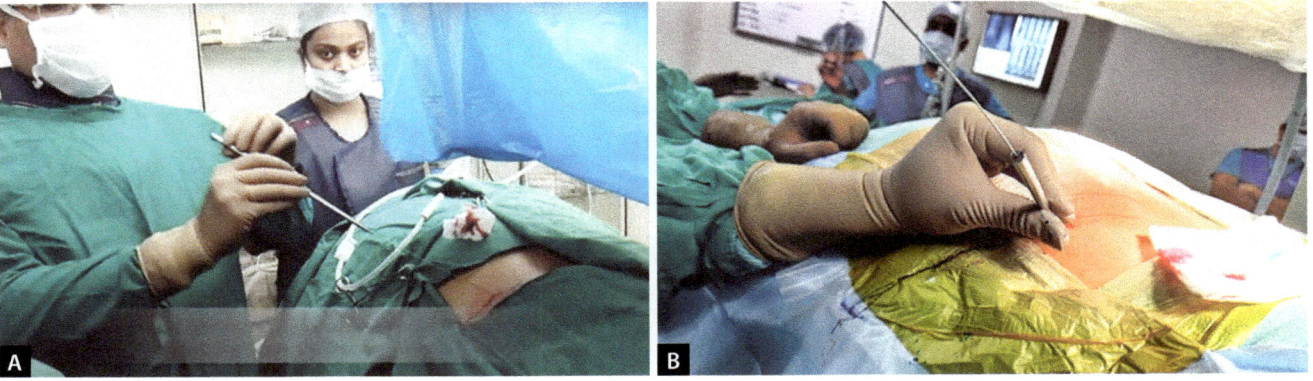

Figs. 13A to B: (A) Insertion of dilator over guidewire; (B) Insertion of guidewire in process.
Image Courtesy: Pain Clinic of India

- When the dilator reaches up to the disc, as the annulus is very sensitive, the annulus is anesthetized using a long needle inserted through the second channel present in the dilator **(Figs. 13C and D)**.

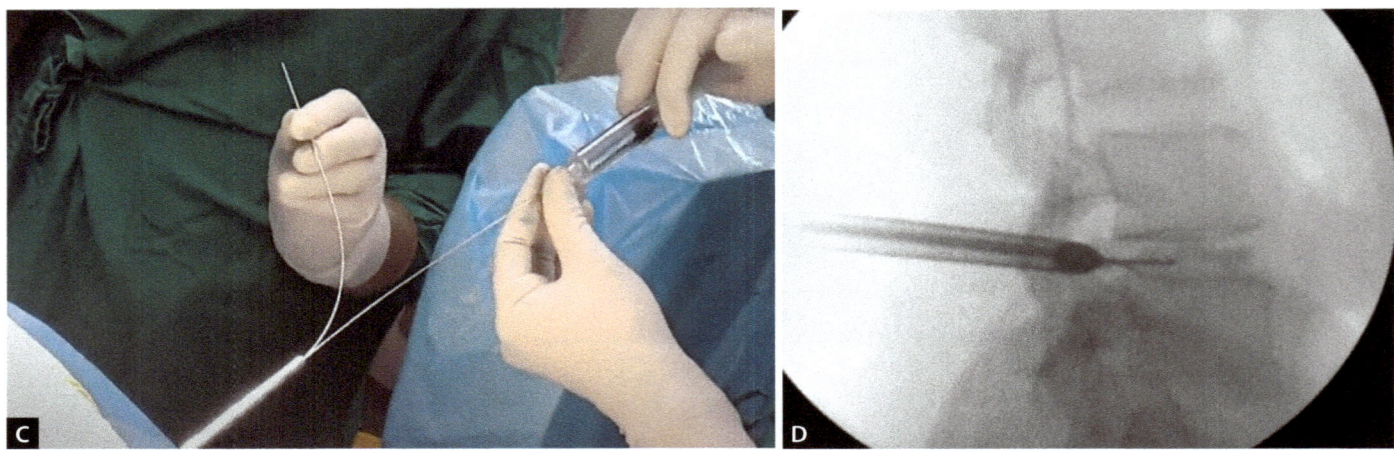

Figs. 13C to D: (C) Injection of local anesthetic; (D) Guidewire in disc.
Image Courtesy: Pain Clinic of India

- Once the annulus is anesthetized, it is pain free to insert dilator in the disc **(Figs. 13E and F)**.

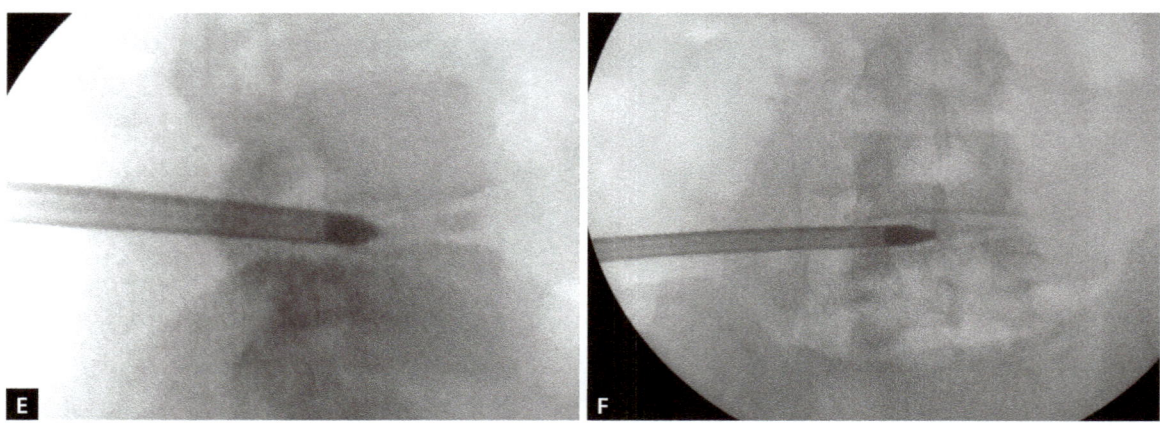

Figs. 13E to F: (E) Dilator into the posterior one-third of the disc; (F) Dilator into the center of the disc.
Image Courtesy: Pain Clinic of India

- Passing the sleeve over the dilator **(Figs. 14A to E)**.

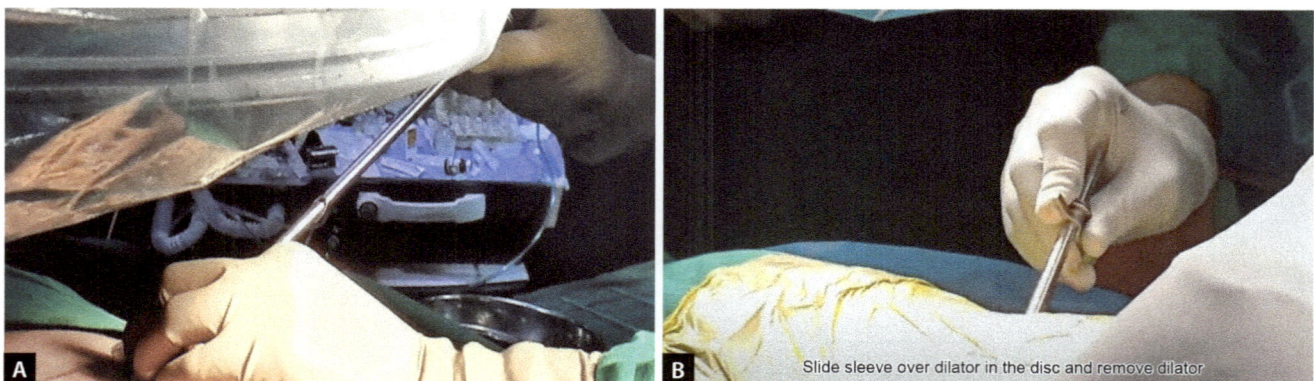

Figs. 14A and B: (A) Passing of sleeve over dilator; (B) Passing of sleeve.
Image Courtesy: Pain Clinic of India

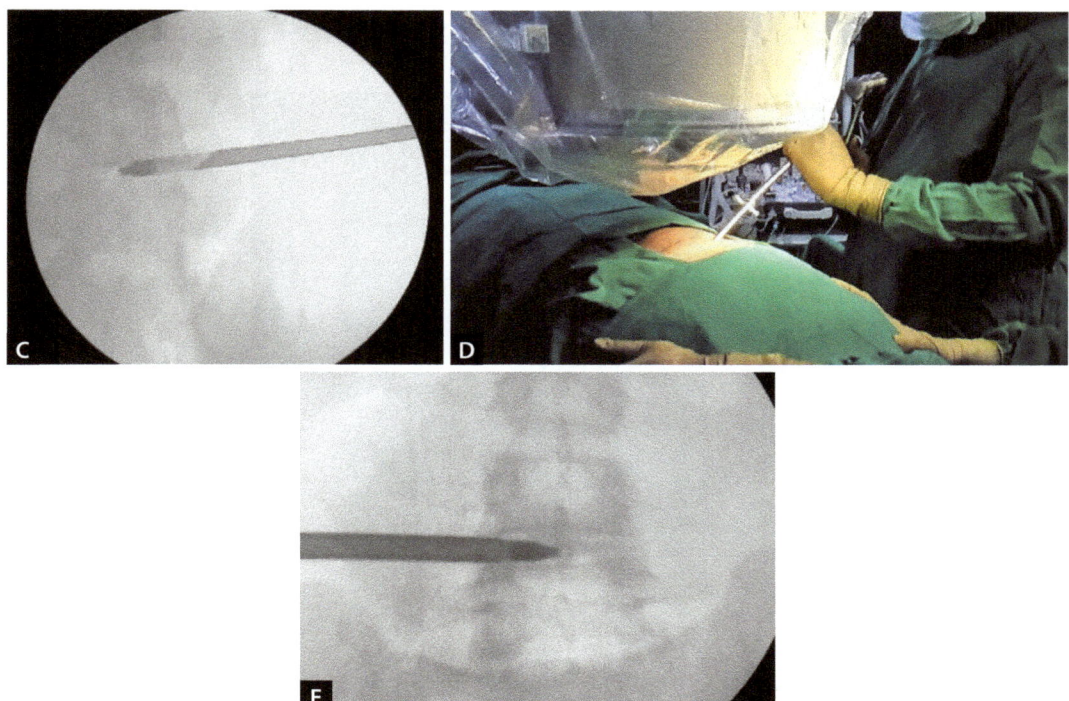

Figs. 14C to E: (C) Sleeve over dilator lateral view; (D) Guidewire in the disc; (E) Sleeve over dilator in the disc.
Image Courtesy: Pain Clinic of India

- Remove the dilator and insert the endoscope **(Fig. 15A)**.

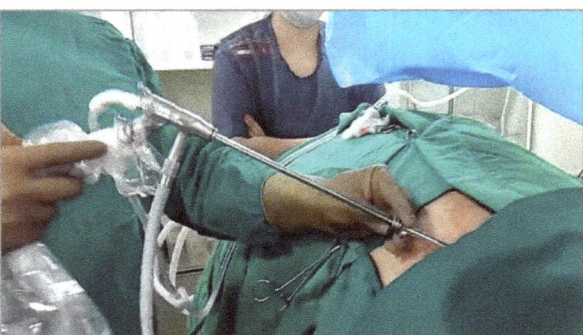

Fig. 15A: Insertion of an endoscope.
Image Courtesy: Pain Clinic of India

- The endoscope design contains optics in the bottom center. On both sides of the optics, there is an irrigation channel and above that the largest channel is the working channel **(Fig. 15B)**.

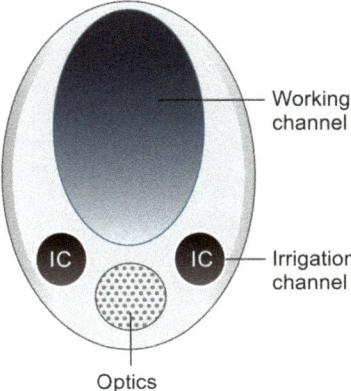

Fig. 15B: Lumbar endoscope.
Image Courtesy: Sakshi Kothari

- *Half-in-half-out technique*: The bevel is partially inside the disc. The disc and some portion of the epidural space containing traversing root and epidural fat are visualized **(Fig. 15C)**.

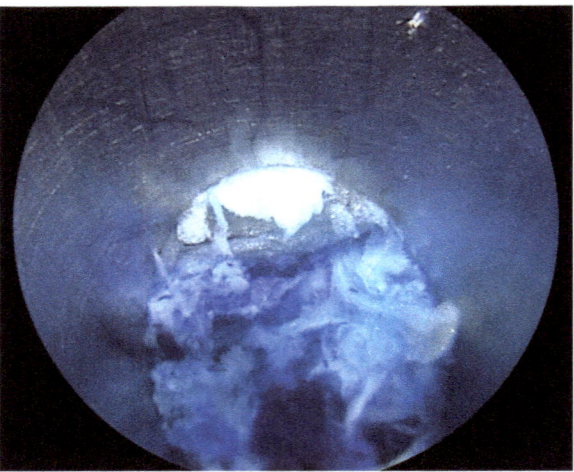

Fig. 15C: Visualization of epidural fat.
Image Courtesy: Pain Clinic of India

- *Inside-out technique:* The whole sleeve bevel is inside the disc. Only the disc is visualized and no epidural space.
- Insert disc removal forceps and remove stained abnormal nucleus **(Fig. 16A)**.

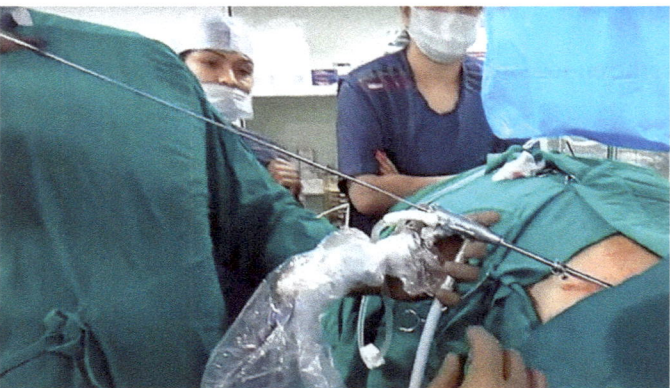

Fig. 16A: Insertion of disc forceps.
Image Courtesy: Pain Clinic of India

- Always close the mouth of the instruments when inserting and removing through the scope. This is very important to avoid direct damage to the optics of the scope **(Fig. 16B)**.

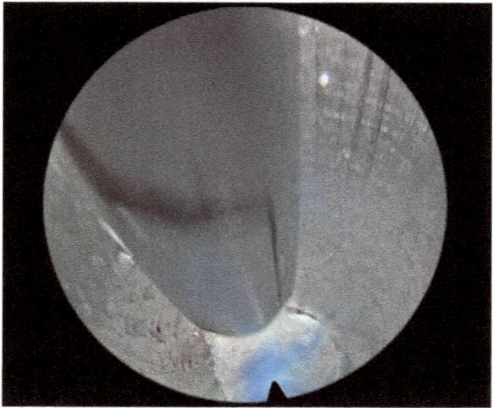

Fig. 16B: Instruments in scope.
Image Courtesy: Pain Clinic of India

- When your placement of the sleeve is over the herniated disc, many times the herniated disc can come as a single long piece, which will give immediate feeling of relief for the patient. As they are awake, they will inform the operator about the relaxing feeling over the back and leg **(Figs. 17A and B)**.

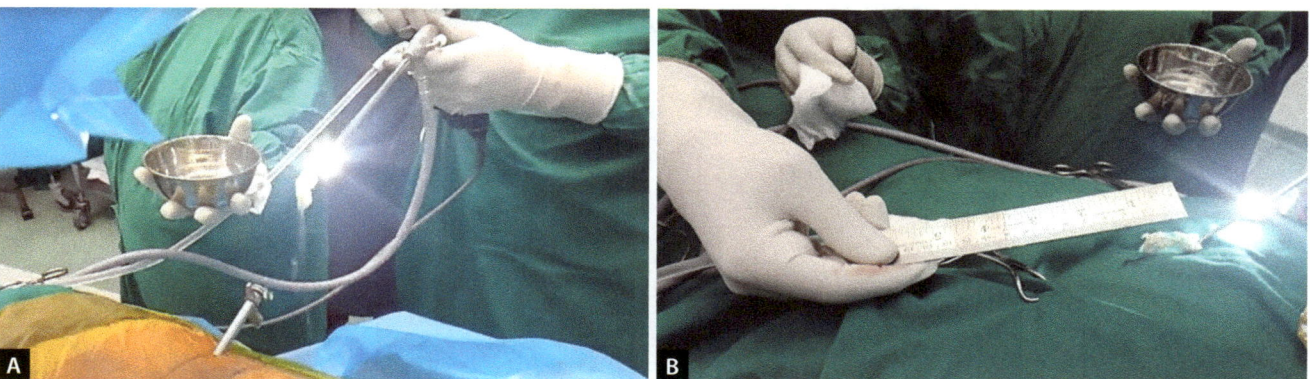

Figs. 17A and B: (A) Removal of piece of disc; (B) Disc nucleus removed.
Image Courtesy: Pain Clinic of India

- Always check the position of the instruments under intermittent fluoroscopy—center, paracentral, foramen, axilla, shoulder, or epidural space **(Figs. 18A to C)**.

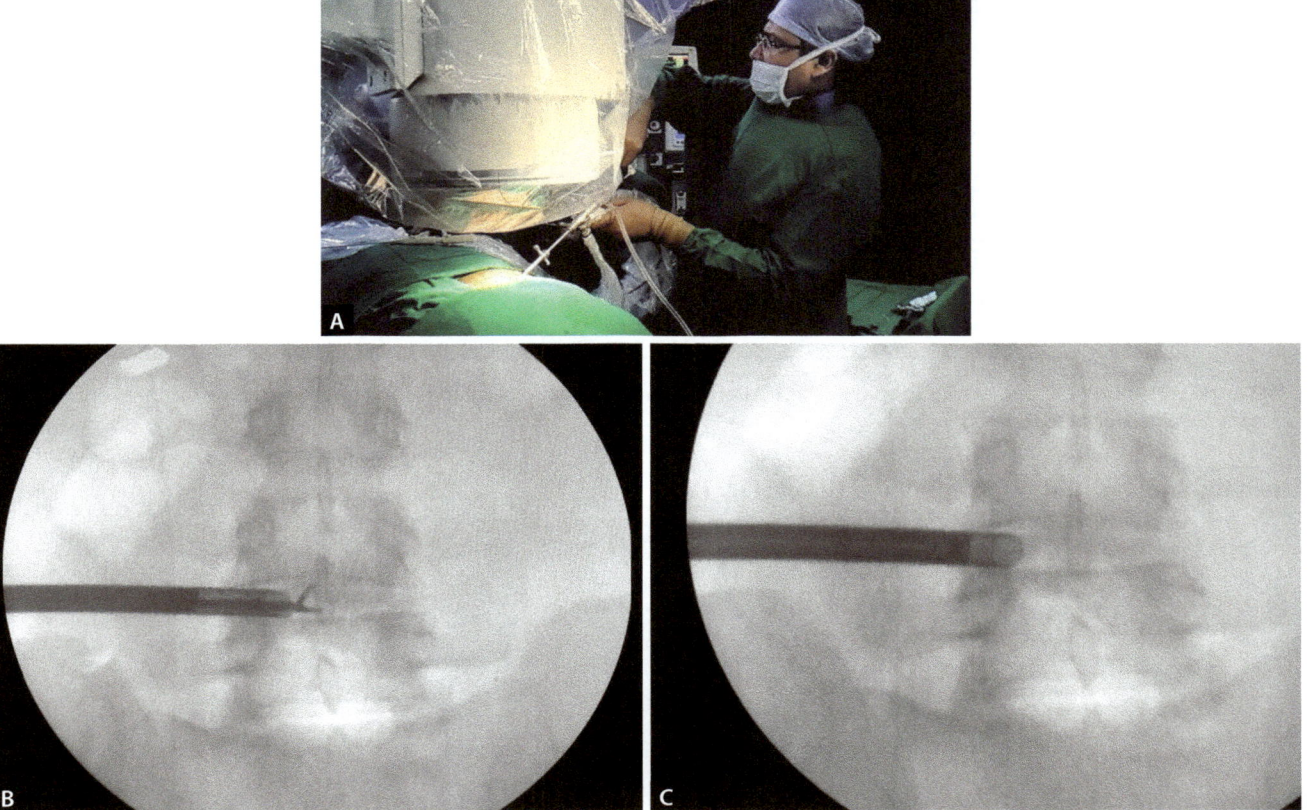

Figs. 18A to C: (A) Use of disc removal forceps; (B) Annular fibers in the epidural area; (C) Sleeve in foramen.
Image Courtesy: Pain Clinic of India

- Once the adequate nucleus is removed and the floor of the working area is cleared, the roof, i.e., annulus, will fall down along with epidural contents.
- *Cutting the annulus (annulectomy)*: Bring the annulus to be cut in the center of the endoscopic view **(Fig. 19A)**.

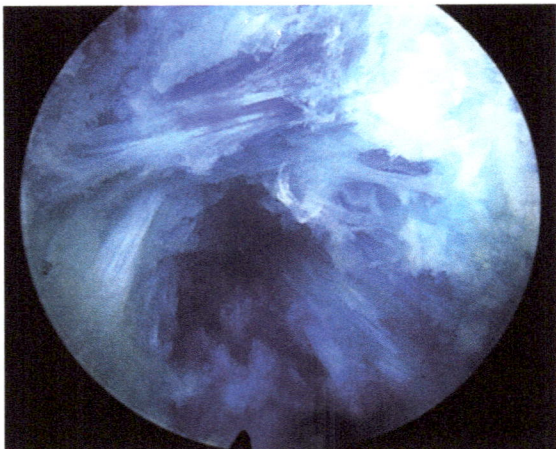

Fig. 19A: Annulus visualized.
Image Courtesy: Pain Clinic of India

- Camera to move near the annulus to be cut with epidural space visualized clearly **(Figs. 19B and C)**.

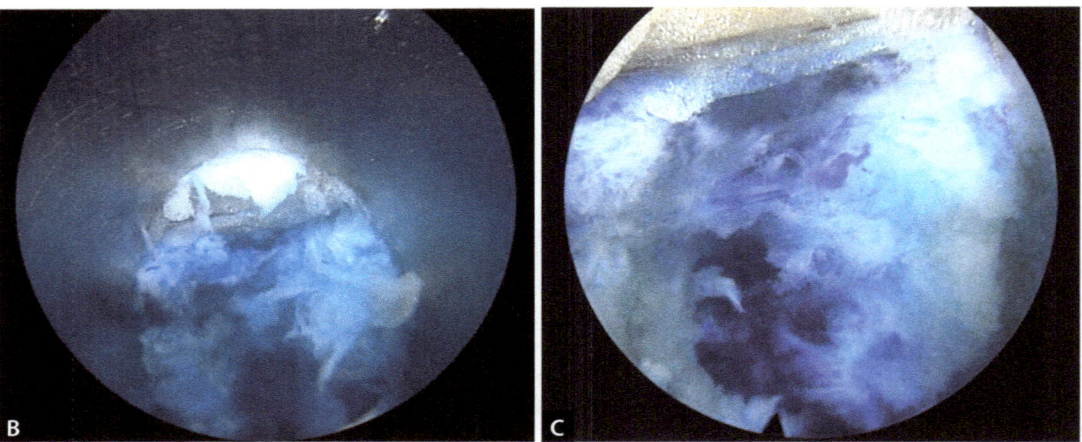

Figs. 19B and C: (B) Annulus fibers anterior to epidural fat; (C) Before annulectomy, epidural space and traversing nerve root are kept in the vision.
Image Courtesy: Pain Clinic of India

- Open the annular cutting forceps under vision **(Fig. 19D)**

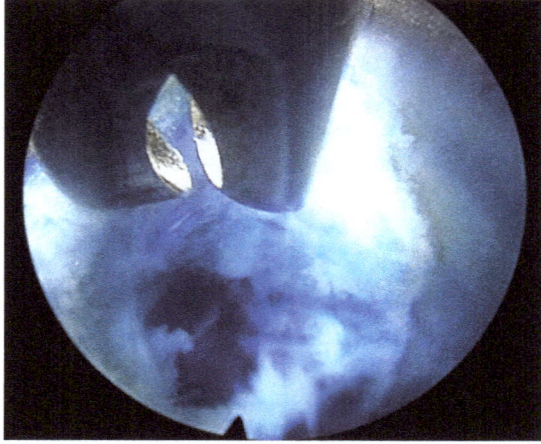

Fig. 19D: Annular cutter is inserted and the mouth is opened under direct vision.
Image Courtesy: Pain Clinic of India

- Slowly insert upper lip of the annular cutter between the annulus and the traversing nerve root, hold the annulus and compress it, ask patient if he feels any sharp shooting pain (nerve) going down in the dermatomal fashion, if the response is negative, cut the annulus **(Figs. 19E to G)**.

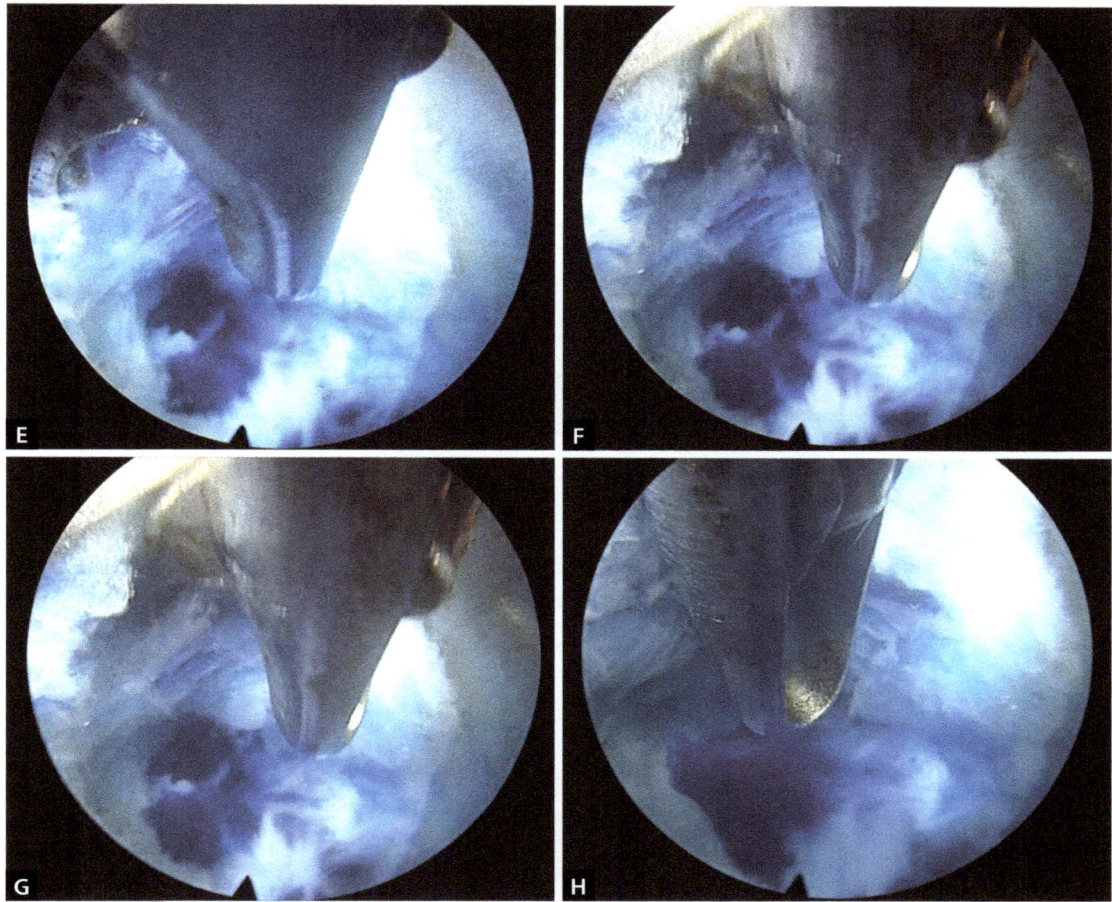

Figs. 19E to H: (E) Carefully and gentle insertion of the upper lip of the annular cutter in between the annulus; (F) Pushing of annular cutter's upper lip between the annulus and the epidural space; (G) Keep the entire field under vision while cutting the annulus. Never go blindly to avoid direct nerve injury; (H) Compress the annulus and ask the patient if he feels any sharp pain going in the leg; if not, we are safe to cut the annulus. Cut it and a nice click is heard.
Image Courtesy: Pain Clinic of India

- A click will be felt while cutting the annulus. Free annular fibers are seen after cutting, which can be shrunken using the RF probe to make the operative area clear **(Fig. 19H)**.

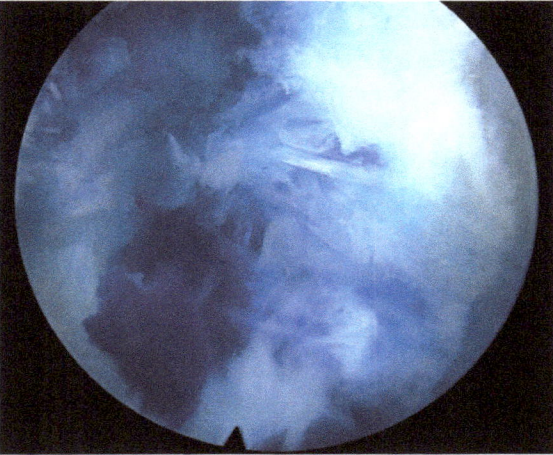

Fig. 19I: Post-annulus dissection.
Image Courtesy: Pain Clinic of India

- After good nucleotomy and annulectomy, the camera is rotated superiorly and slightly pulled in the foramen to see the free pulsating exiting nerve root **(Fig. 20)**.

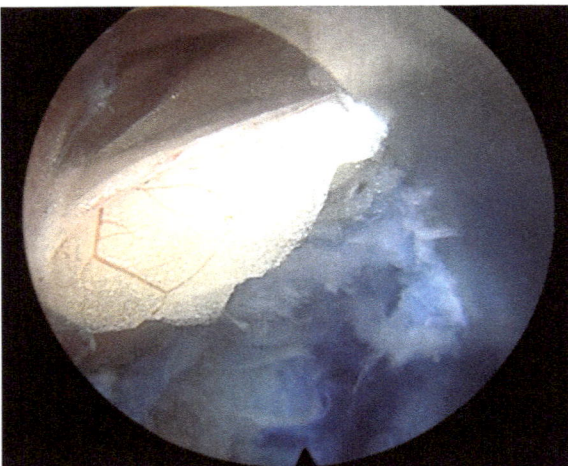

Fig. 20: Free pulsating exiting nerve root with overlying fat visualized with the bevel of the sleeve rotated superiorly.
Image Courtesy: Pain Clinic of India

- Sometimes, the herniated disc can be seen stuck in annulus (herniated portion). The straight instruments may not reach there. We use angular forceps and other angular instruments to remove such disc and tissues **(Figs. 21A and B)**.

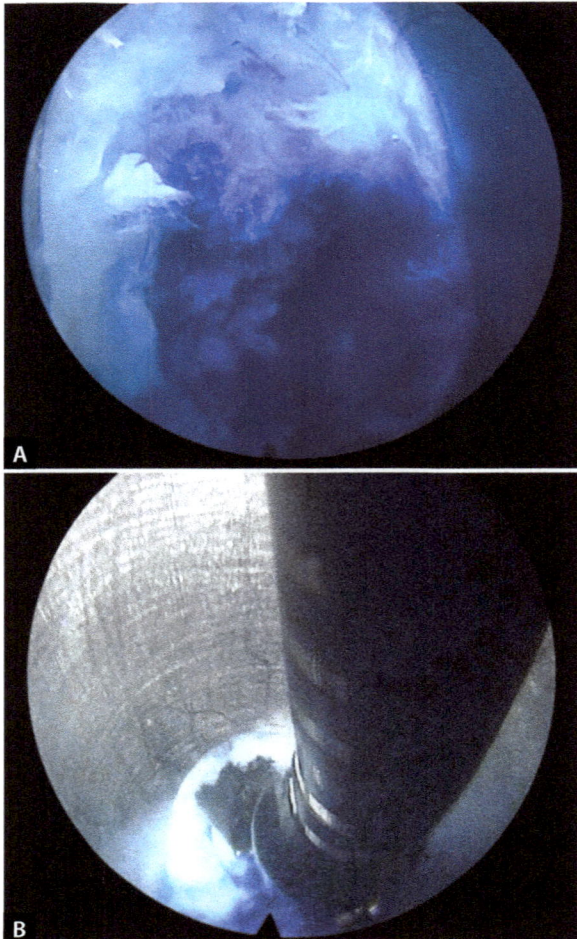

Figs. 21A and B: (A) Many times, disc material is noted at a difficult angle which is difficult to remove with straight forceps; (B) Use of flexible curved disc forceps to remove disc at a difficult angle.
Image Courtesy: Pain Clinic of India

- A high-frequency 4.1-MHz RF probe is used to coagulate the bleeders and shrink the tissues which are floating free, to clear the operative field **(Figs. 22A to E)**.

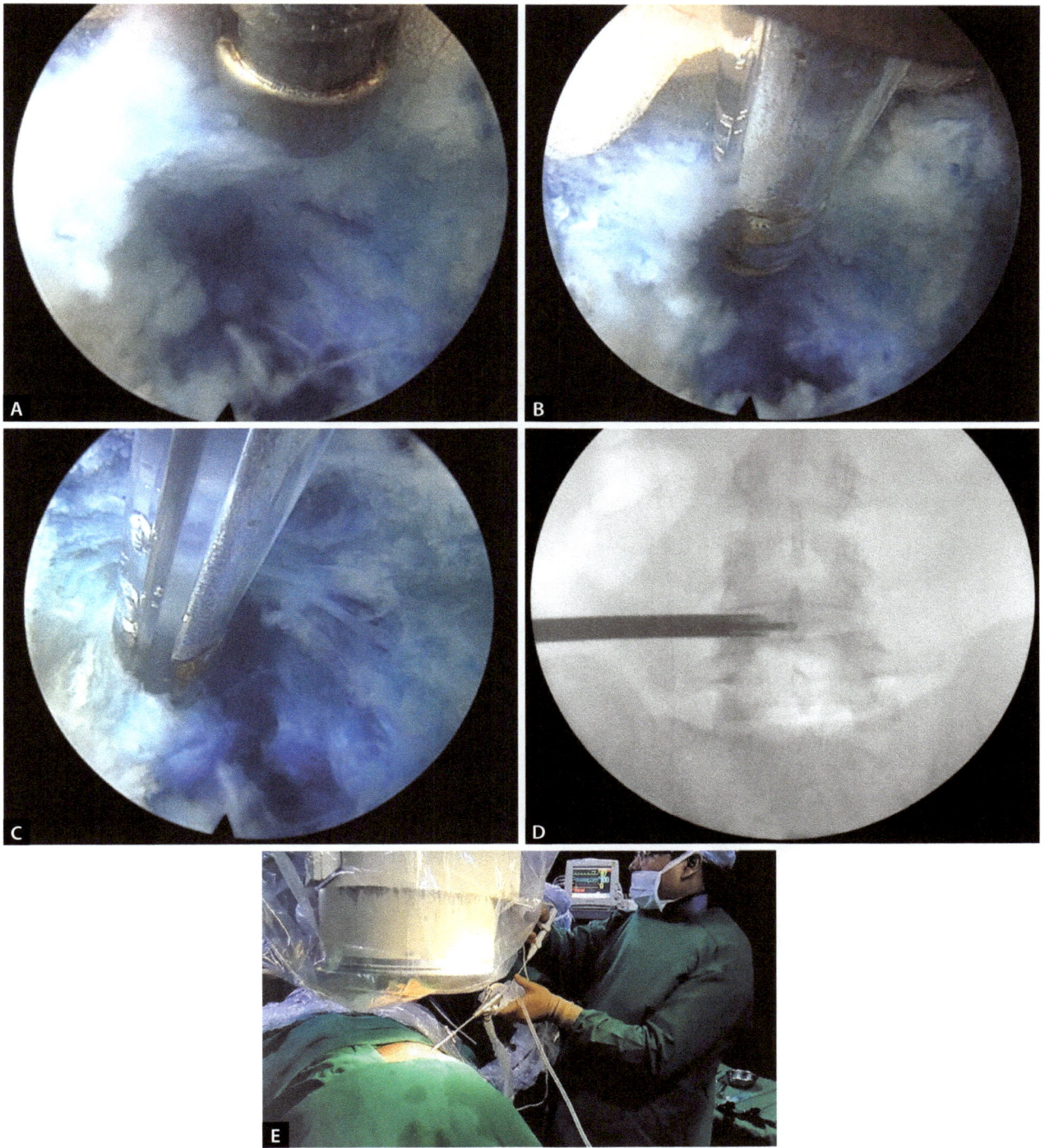

Figs. 22A to E: (A to C) Use of high-frequency RF probe to coagulate the bleeders and shrinking the loose tissues; (D) RF probe should be used with the live fluoroscopic image in anteroposterior view to know the exact location of the probe in the epidural space or disc; (E) Use of RF probe. (RF: radiofrequency)
Image Courtesy: Pain Clinic of India

- Side-firing laser is another good option to achieve this much faster.
- Once the freely pulsating traversing and exiting nerve roots are visualized, the scope is slowly withdrawn and any bleeder if present is coagulated using RF.
- The irrigation is stopped and the instruments are removed.
- The water in the tract is removed with gentle pressure from medial to lateral side.
- Usually, the incision does not require any stitches. A simple dressing is enough **(Fig. 23)**.

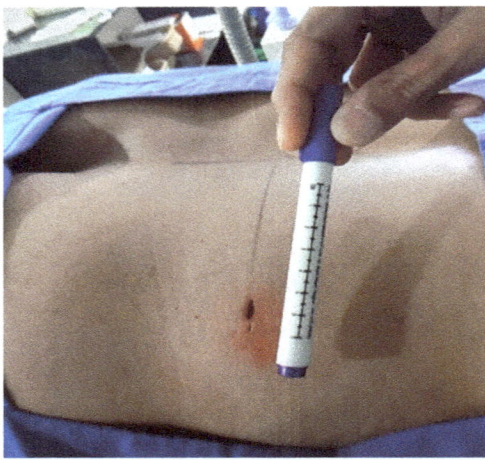

Fig. 23: Small incision at the end of procedure.
Image Courtesy: Pain Clinic of India

- MRI pictures pre- and post-endoscopic discectomy **(Figs. 24 to 28)**.

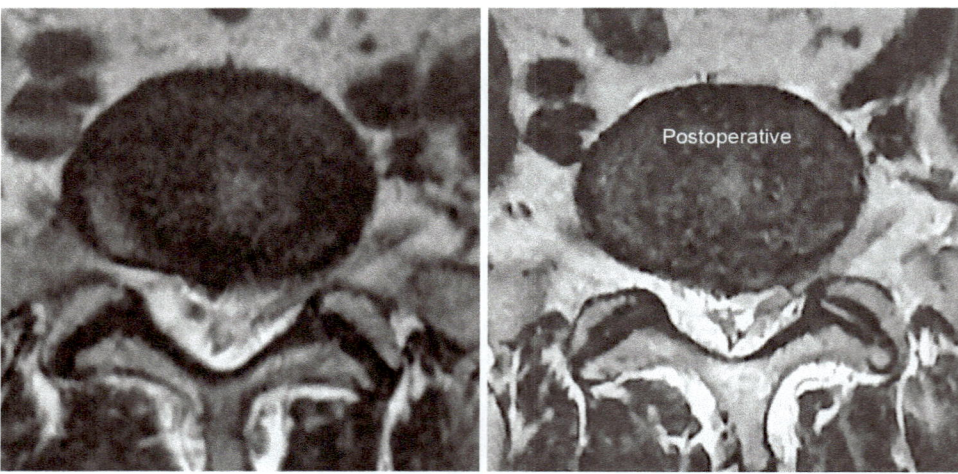

Fig. 24: *Image Courtesy:* Dr Manish Raj

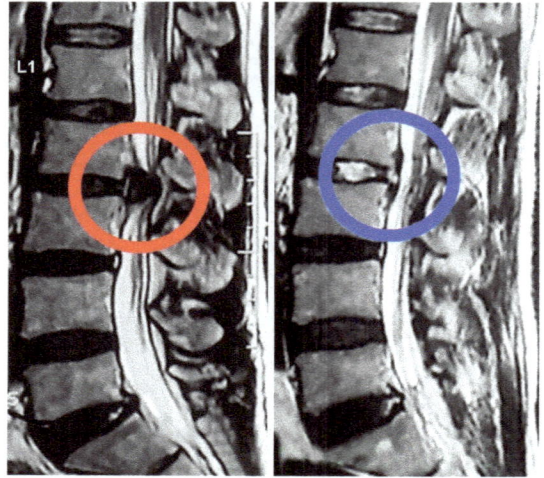

Fig. 25: *Image Courtesy:* Dr Manish Raj

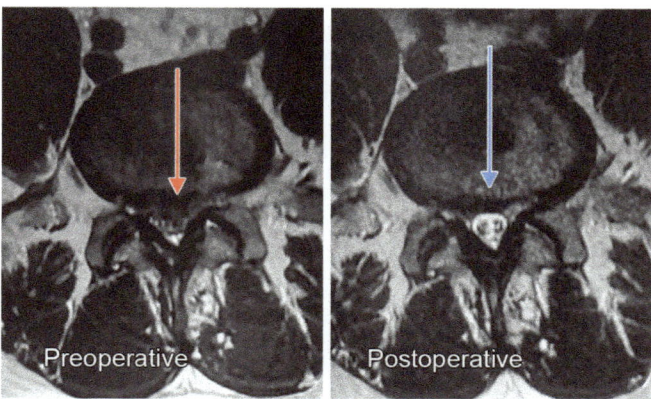

Fig. 26: *Image Courtesy:* Dr Manish Raj

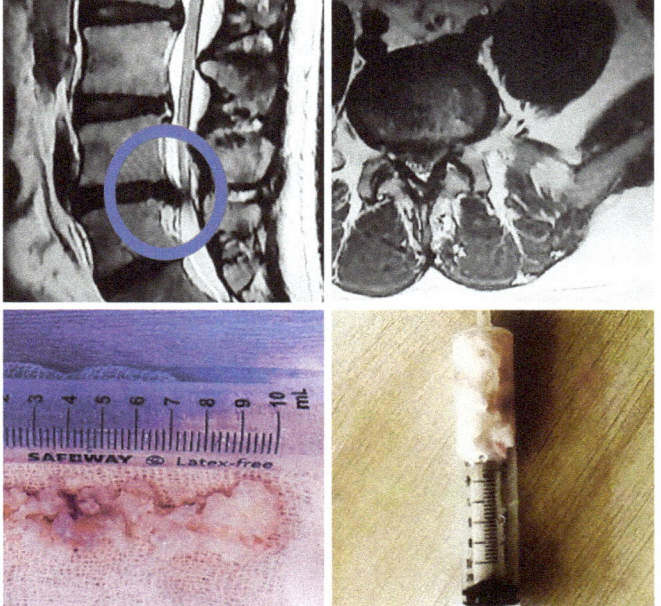

Fig. 27: *Image Courtesy:* Dr Manish Raj

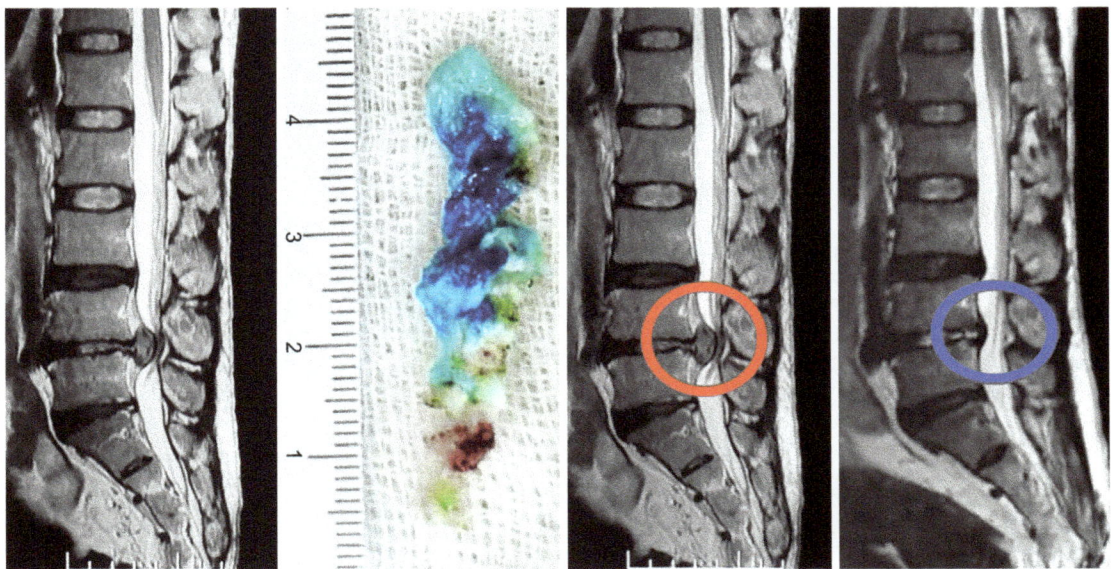

Fig. 28: *Image Courtesy:* Dr Manish Raj

CONCLUSION

- Various degrees and stages of lumbar disc prolapse can be treated effectively using endoscopic discectomy.
- Various approaches—transforaminal, interlaminar unilateral biportal techniques—are available.
- Technological advances made these procedures very effective, and most cases can be handled without opening the back of the patients.
- Learning curve is long and steep.
- In-depth knowledge of 3D anatomy of spine is required.
- Awake patient is the main advantage as it prevents major complications related to nerve injury.
- Once the adequate discectomy and foraminotomy is performed, free nerves are visible at the end of the procedure.
- Complications need to be explained preoperatively to the patients and the operator should be keeping vigilant before discharging the patient.

CHAPTER 57: Kyphoplasty

Samir Ranjit Jani

BASIC INFORMATION

- Acute compression fractures occur commonly in traumatic injuries (falls, motor vehicle accidents) as well as in susceptible patients (osteoporosis, malignancy/multiple myeloma)
- Standard conservative treatment is initially rest, nonsteroidal inflammatory drugs (NSAIDs), and bracing. Bracing often leads to exacerbation of other spine issues and is poorly tolerated by patients.
- If there is no improvement in 6–8 weeks, it is reasonable to consider kyphoplasty.
- Kyphoplasty involves creating a cavity in which polymethyl methacrylate (PMMA) is injected to cement fracture. This can be done using balloons or a curved stylet. Vertebroplasty is when the PMMA is injected without the creation of the cavity.
- The patient will require IV sedation at a minimum. Many operators perform this procedure under general anesthesia as well depending on the patient's needs.

PROCEDURES

Step 1: Procedure can be done under general anesthesia or IV sedation. Place patient in prone position **(Fig. 1)**. Prep and drape in usual sterile fashion. Take initial fluoroscopic image in both AP and lateral views. Often the lateral view is helpful to correctly identify the desired level **(Fig. 2)**. Take a 22G

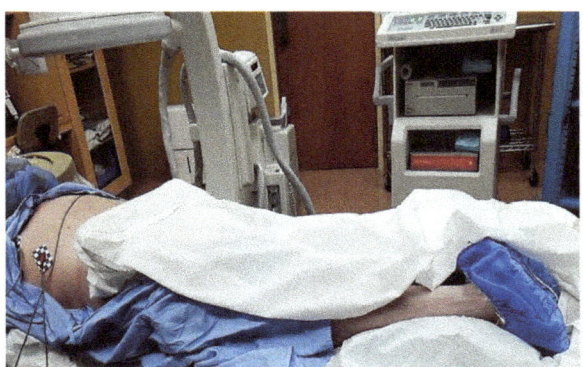

Fig. 1: Patient in prone position.

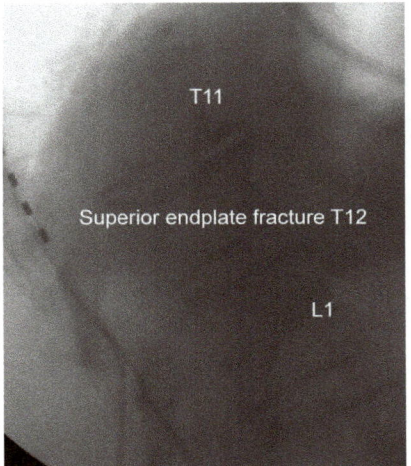

Fig. 2: Initial fluoroscopic image prior to procedure showing endplate fracture.

spinal needle and administer local anesthesia (Lidocaine 1–2% 5 mL) deep onto the periosteum of the corresponding pedicle you wish to enter.

Step 2: Using a scalpel, make a skin nick adequate for trocar placement.

Step 3: Push trocar under the skin **(Figs. 3A and B)**.

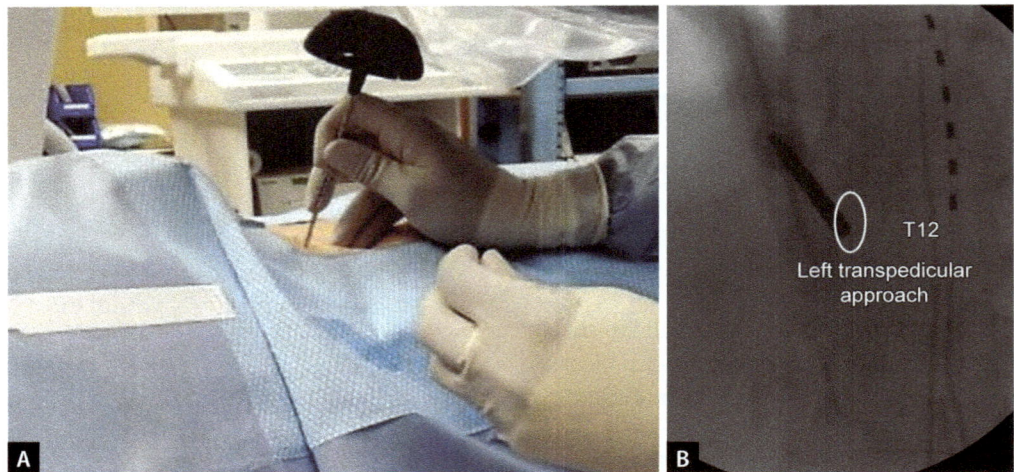

Figs. 3A and B: (A) Trocar under the skin; (B) Trocar at pedicle.

Step 4: Get trocar to purchase and take initial images to line up the trocar and pedicle **(Fig. 3B)**. It is useful to turn lateral to assess cephalad/caudal angulation as well (aim toward superior endplate if superior fracture or inferior endplate if inferior fracture). Ensure the trocar stays lateral to the pedicle's medial border. Epidural space is medial to this landmark **(Fig. 4)**. Continue to advance trocar with firm hammering with mallet alternating between anteroposterior (AP) and lateral views **(Fig 5)**. Once the trocar is confirmed to enter the vertebral body, the trocar/curved stylet can be driven toward the midline of the vertebral body. It is now safe to go medial past the pedicle's medial border in AP view.

Once the trocar is confirmed to enter the vertebral body, the trocar/curved stylet can be driven toward the middle of the vertebral body. It is now safe to go medial past the pedicle's medial border in AP view.

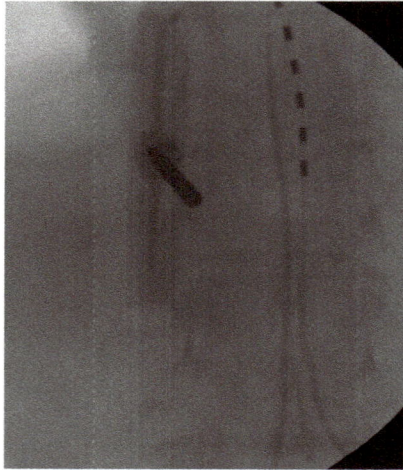

Fig. 4: Trocar stays lateral to the medial border of epidural space—anteroposterior view.

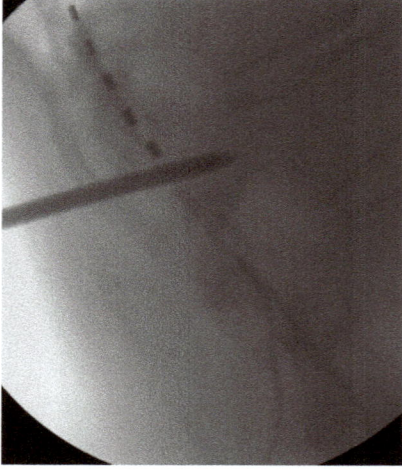

Fig. 5: Trocar in lateral view traversing epidural space safely.

Step 5: Use a mallet to direct trocar to point one-third to one-half of the way into the vertebral body in lateral view **(Fig. 6)**. Next, insert a curved stylet and direct this to the center of the vertebral body. Continue to alternate between AP and lateral views. Insert a cavity-creating device (either balloon or curved stylet) and ensure the cavity expands to fill the whole vertebral body in all planes (inferior/superior, anterior/posterior, medial/lateral). If using a bipedicle approach, repeat the procedure for the contralateral side.

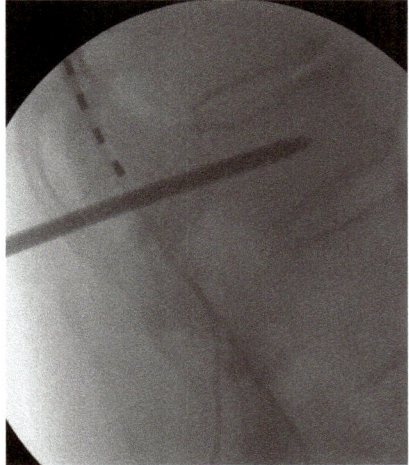

Fig. 6: Trocar in vertebral body.

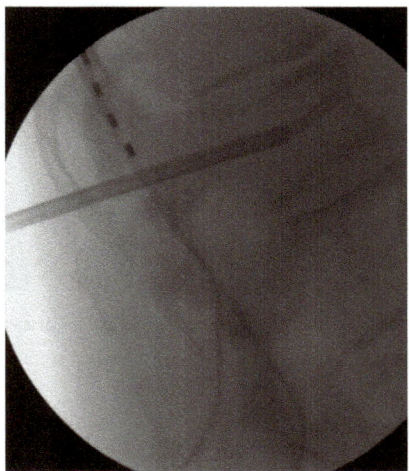

Fig. 7: Trocar with curved stylet in lateral view at the midline of the vertebral body.

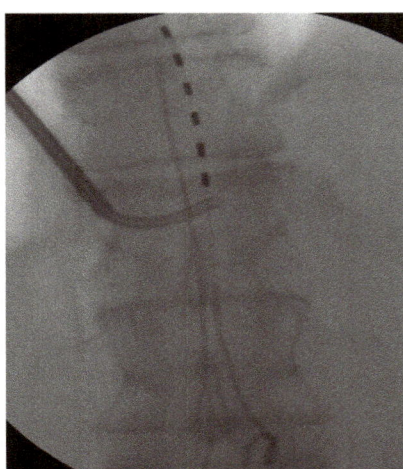

Fig. 8: Trocar with curved stylet in anteroposterior view advancing to anterior border.

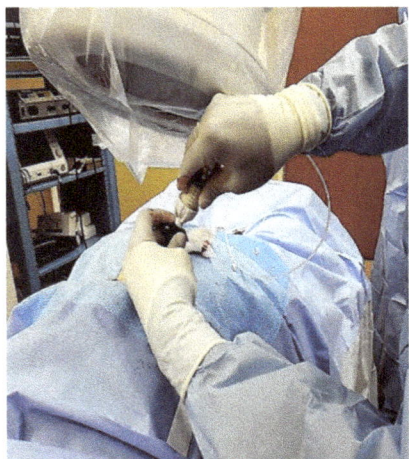

Fig. 9: Injecting methyl methacrylate.

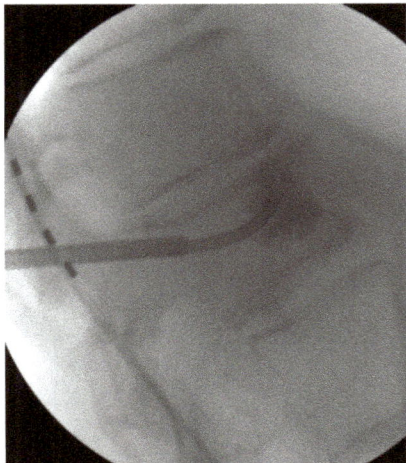

Fig. 10: Injecting methyl methacrylate—lateral view.

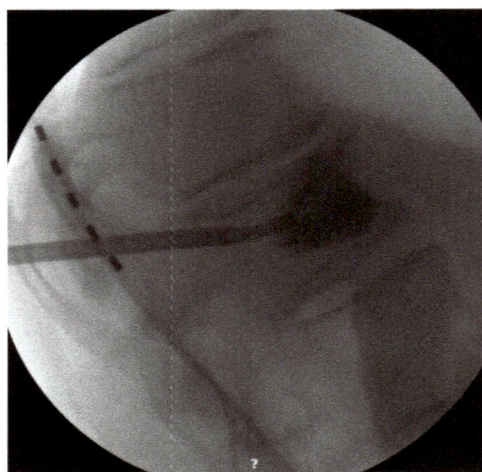

Fig. 11: Continued adequate fill ensuring no trocar cement tracking toward epidural space.

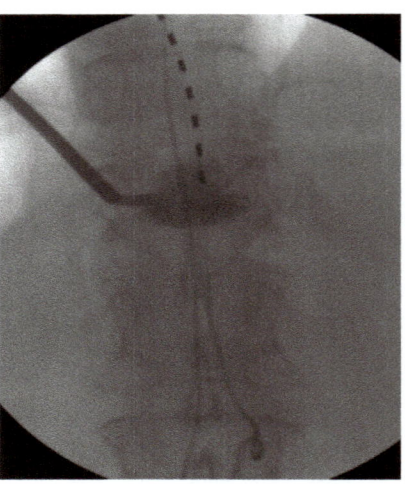

Fig. 12: Final AP view showing PMMA extending from pedicle to pedicle.

Step 6: Once an adequate cavity is created, attach premixed MMA. Note starting volume to ensure proper documentation of the amount of MMA injected.

Always inject PMMA in the lateral view. This is to ensure no posterior spread toward the epidural space/thecal sac. If seen, immediately stop any additional cement administration.

Periodically check AP view to ensure adequate medial to lateral fill of vertebral body; ideally PMMA is seen pedicle to pedicle **(Fig. 12)**. Start to remove instruments in lateral view. Confirm no trailing of PMMA toward thecal sac even while removing instruments.

Step 7: Remove trocar and take final picture. Apply small Band-Aid/dressing.

Tip: PMMA comes in both fast and slow hardening versions. If used too soon, PMMA is liquidity and increases the risk of inadvertent trailing. If used too late, it can harden making it impossible to inject. Consistency should be like toothpaste. Place approximately 2–4 mL per level. Only inject in lateral view; however, do alternative between AP and lateral views to ensure adequate fill in all dimensions. When completed, remove instruments in lateral view ensuring no PMMA trailing into the epidural space.

Index

Page numbers followed by *f* refer to figure, and *fc* refer to flowchart

A
Abdomen, lower 6*f*, 148*f*
Acetabular fractures 262
Acetabular landmark 176
Acetabular region 175
Acetabulum 200*f*, 201*f*
Acromioclavicular joint 36*f*
Acromion process 247
Adhesive pad 194*f*
Adjacent endplate edema 42*f*
Advance catheter 296
Advanced pain management 289
Alcohol 63
    injection of 179
Allergic reactions 60
Anaphylactoid reaction 60
Anemia 54
Anesthesia 177, 302
    general 69*f*
    local 59, 61, 139, 106*f*, 158*f*, 177, 200, 218*f*, 232, 252, 261, 265, 273*f*
Ankle 34*f*, 35*f*
Annular fibers 309*f*
Annulectomy 310, 310*f*
Anterior abdominal wall 258
Anterior superior iliac spine 268, 269, 277
Anterior syndesmotic ligaments 35*f*
Antibiotic wash 297
Anticoagulants 52, 132
Aorta 226
    side of 226
Appendectomy 103
Arachnoiditis 63
Artery
    carotid 219
    celiac 226*f*
    subclavian 244, 249, 251, 252
    suprascapular 246, 247*f*
Articular pillar 20*f*, 21*f*, 89*f*, 91, 94, 98
    anterior border of 97
    center of 89*f*, 93*f*
    left 17*f*, 18*f*, 83*f*
    right 17*f*, 18*f*, 83*f*
    waist of 89*f*
Ataxia 98
Atomic Energy Regulatory Board 46
Australia antigen 54
Axial scan technique 253
Axilla 309
Axon abnormalities 63

B
Backpain 283
Balloon compression 69*f*
Bending needle tip, advantage of 227
Bifid root 244
Bladder tumor 235
Bleeding
    disorders 88
    problems 111
    time 54
Block needle 4*f*, 5*f*
Blood
    aspirations for 279
    negative aspiration of 261
    thinners 111
Bone 144*f*
    contact 143*f*
    fractures, cancellous 56
    loss, slow 56
    scan 56*f*
        normal 56*f*
Bony Bankart lesion 42*f*
Bony structures 3
Botulinum toxin 175, 176
Bow-tie appearance 33*f*
Brachial plexus 244*f*, 249, 250*f*-252*f*, 296
    block 249
        procedure 249
    bundles 249, 252
    supraclavicular scanning of 249*f*
    upper trunk of 245*f*
Bronchospasm 60
Bucket-handle tear 43*f*
Bupivacaine 61, 175, 225, 229, 249
Burger's disease 232
Burns, bipolar 158
Buttock muscles 284*f*

C
C spine, parts of 89*f*
Calcaneal spur 210, 211*f*
    basic information 210
    causes 210
    injection 210
    physiotherapy 210
    procedure 210
    repetitive trauma 210
    treatment 210
Calcaneocuboid joint injection 37*f*
Calcaneofibular ligament 35*f*
Calcium, aspiration of 37*f*
Calf muscles 285*f*
Cancer
    pain
        relief of 253
        syndromes 72
    penile 235
Cannula 97*f*, 144*f*, 145*f*, 173, 173*f*
    over joint 172*f*
    superior view of 143*f*
    ventral tangs of 173
Carbohydrate 60
Carbolic acid 63
Cardiac device 132
Cardiovascular collapse 60
C-arm 139, 141, 157, 177
    caudal tilt of 134*f*
    craniocaudal tilt 74*f*
Carpometacarpal joint injection 37*f*
Caudal epidural
    block 146
        contraindications 146
        equipement and supplies 146
        indications 146
        medications 146
        procedure 146
    injection 127*f*
    space 130*f*, 147, 147*f*
Caudal tilt 7*f*, 19*f*, 22*f*
Caudal vertebra 300
Cavity creating device 319
Cefuroxime 299
Celiac plexus 226
    block 53*f*, 228, 229, 229*f* 286
        concentration 229
        contraindications 229
        drugs 229
        indications 229
        procedure 229
Cellulitis 294
Central canal stenosis, severe 41*f*
Cephalic direction 17*f*, 83*f*, 141*f*, 143
Cephalic tilt 6*f*, 13*f*, 22*f*, 148*f*
Cerebrospinal fluid 29*f*, 30, 263
    free flow of 296*f*
Cervical cordotomy 72, 72*f*
    percutaneous 72
    preparation for 72*f*
Cervical facet
    arthropathy 88
    joint
        pain 87*fc*, 97*f*
        radiofrequency 91
Cervical medial branch
    block 82, 87*fc*, 91
    radiofrequency ablation 88
Cervical nerve root 244, 244*f*, 245*f*
Cervical procedures 16*f*, 91
Cervical radiculopathy 291
Cervical radiofrequency denervation 91
Cervical segments 72
Cervical somatic referral pattern 82*f*

Index

Cervical spine 16, 16f-21f, 27f, 28f, 73f, 77, 82f, 83f, 85f, 244
    anteroposterior of 21f
    magnetic resonance imaging of 29f
    radiograph anteroposterior projection 27f
    sequence 40f
Cervical spondylosis 88, 91
Cervical vertebra 244f
Cervix, tumors of 235
Chemical neurolytic agents 59
Chemotoxic reactions 60
Chest 50, 101
Chronic neuropathic pelvic pain
    diagnosis of 177
    treatment of 177
Chronic pain 54, 59, 283
    management 253
Classical transversus abdominis 260, 260f
    plane
        block 260
        sonoanatomy of 260f
Clavicle, acromion of 246f, 247, 247f
Clonidine 61, 62f, 268
Clotting time 54
Coagulopathy 103, 232
Coccydynia 179
Coccygeal nerve block 179
    advanced options 179
    complications 179
    equipment 179
    indications 179
    medications 179
    procedure details 179
    treatment options 179
Coccygectomy 179
Coccygodynia 179
Coccyx
    anatomy of 180f
    anterior margin of 180, 180f
Colon, metastatic tumors of 235
Complete blood count 54
Complex regional pain syndrome 58, 58f, 215, 253, 291
Compression test 170
Computed tomography 55
Continuous fluoroscopy 12f, 151f, 155f
Cordotomy 72, 74f
    head rest 73f
    probe 72f, 75f
Coronal proton-density fat 42f
Cortical bone 56
Cortisol 60
COVID-19
    disease, cause of 54
    pandemic 52, 54
    related investigations 54
    safety 52
    test 50
Cranial fossa, middle 26f, 70f
Cruciate ligament, anterior 33f, 34, 43f
C-spine model 16f
CT-guided celiac plexus block 225
    complications 225
    contraindications 225
    drugs and concentration 225
    indications 225
    procedure 225

CT-guided splanchinc plexus block 223
    contraindications 223
    drugs and concentration 223
    indications 223
    procedure 223
Curve tip needle 114, 155f, 177f, 180f

D

Daily living, activities of 170, 177
Deltoid ligament 35f
Depression, cardiac 60
Dexamethasone 61, 61f, 111, 116, 146, 149f, 152f, 268, 299
Diabetes mellitus 60, 200, 232
    non-insulin dependent 60
Digital infrared thermal imaging 58
Disc
    access 15f
    forceps, insertion of 308f
    guidewire in 306f, 307f
    height, sever loss of 129f
    herniation, recurrent 299
    posterior one-third of 306f
    removal forceps 309f
    space, middle of 8f
Discogram 56, 304f
    normal 57f
Distraction test 170
Dorsal heel spur 210
Dorsal scapular
    artery 251
    nerve 244
Dorsolumbar spine, anteroposterior view of 55f
Double needle technique 14f, 150f, 155
Double posterior cruciate ligament 43f
Drugs, steroid group of 59
Dual-diagnostic fluoroscopic-guided local anesthesia 156
Dual-energy X-ray absorptiometry 55
Dural puncture, high-risk of 129
Dye spread 53f, 104f, 106f, 110f, 147f, 222f, 224f, 230f, 233f, 234f, 239f
    anteroposterior view 181f
    bilateral 226f
    lateral view 181f, 237f
Dysesthesias 62

E

Edema
    local 199
    subchondral 43f
Eighth cervical nerve root 249
Elbow
    joint 198
    strap 199
Electrodiagnostic studies 57
Electromyography 57
Electronic media 58
Endoscope, insertion of 307f
Endoscopic radiofrequency ablation 179
Epicondylitis, lateral 197
Epidural catheter 130
    fixation of 106f
Epidural fat 310f
    stippling 80f
    visualization of 308f

Epidural injection 39f
Epidural needle 130f
Epidural space 59, 116f, 119f, 128f, 309, 318f
Erector spinae muscle 263-265
Ethyl alcohol 62
Extensor digitorum 285
External defibrillator 132
External oblique 260
Eye 10f
    protection 49, 49f

F

Faber test 170
Facet joint 17f, 18f, 83f
    cyst 41f
    injection 8f, 10f
    pain 97f
Failed back syndrome 111
Fascia
    iliaca 268, 277
    lata 268, 277
    prevertebral 249
Fat
    metabolism 60
    saturated sequence 32f
Femoral artery 276-278
Femoral nerve 262, 277, 278
Femoral vein 276-278
Femur
    head of 200f, 203f
    mid-shaft of 201f
    shaft of 201f
Fentanyl 61
Fifth cervical nerve root 250, 251
Fifth cervical vertebra
    anterior tubercle of transverse process of 250
    posterior tubercle of transverse process of 250
    transverse process of 250
Flexor carpi
    radialis 198
    ulnaris 198
Flexor digitorum superficialis 198
Fluoroscope 89f
    anteroposterior position 88f
    bipolar 68f
Fluoroscopic assisted procedures 165f
Fluoroscopic-guided
    hip joint injection 38f
    subtalar joint injection 38f
Fluoroscopic screening 91
Fluoroscopy 3, 5f-10f, 16, 18f, 22, 25, 91 110, 200, 203
    basic principles 4f
    cephalad tilt of 185f
    guided 220, 229
    lumbar level 6f
Fogarty catheter 68f, 70f
Foramen 309
    medial quadrant of 187f
    ovale 25f, 26f, 68f-70f
    sleeve in 309f
    superior quadrant of 187f
Foraminal stenosis 40f
Foraminoplasty 300
Foraminotomy 305f

Fossa, supraclavicular 252*f*
Fourth cervical nerve root 250
Fracture, endplate 317*f*
Frostbite 232

G

Gaenslen test 170
Gait, abnormal 210
Gallbladder 223
   carcinoma of 105
Gasserian ganglion 67, 68
Gastrografin 59
Gauge spinal needle 136*f*
Glucocorticoids 60
Gluteal cleft 275*f*
Gluteus maximus 272, 284
Gluteus medius 203, 272
   tendon, attachment of 205*f*
Gluteus minimus 203, 272
   tendon, attachment of 205*f*
Glycerine 63
   phenol in 62*f*
Glycerol 62, 63
   gangliolysis 67
Golfer's elbow 197, 198, 199*f*
   pathophysiology 198
   physical therapy 199
   procedure details 199
   symptoms 198
   treatment 198
Greater sciatic
   foramen 270
   notch 271*f*, 272, 273*f*, 275*f*
Greater trochanter 200*f*, 204*f*, 271, 272, 274
Greater trochanteric
   bursa injection 203
   pain syndrome 203
Guidewire, insertion of 305*f*
Gun barrel technique 8*f*, 15*f*, 121*f*, 128*f*

H

Half-in-half-out technique 308
Hamstring muscles 285*f*
Head and neck 65
Headache 60
Heating spinal hardware, risk of 132
Heel spurs, symptoms of 210
Hematoma 112, 299
Hemipelvis, right 159*f*, 164*f*
Hemogram 175
Hernia repairs 258
Herniated disc 309
Herpes zoster 232
High osmolar contrast media 59
High-energy electromagnetic radiation 44
High-resolution computer tomography 55
Hip 175
   arthroscopy 262
   fractures, acute pain for 276
   joint 276
      injection 200
      ipsilateral 165*f*
      replacement 262
Horner's syndrome 217*f*
   ipsilateral 253
Human immunodeficiency virus 52, 54
Humeral head 38*f*

Hyaluronidase 61, 62*f*
Hydrocortisone 61
Hyperechoic articular process 256*f*
Hyperhidrosis 232
Hypertonic saline 62
Hypervolemia 60
Hypotension 253

I

Iatrogenic complication 235
Ileum 176
Iliac bone 272*f*
Iliac crest 15*f*, 160*f*, 187*f*, 260, 261*f*, 262*f*, 263, 264, 266, 301
Iliac spine
   anterior inferior 276-278
   posterior superior 162*f*, 262, 262*f*, 263, 264, 266, 271, 272, 274
Iliacus muscle 268, 277, 278
Iliopubic eminence 276, 278, 279
Ilio-pubic ramus 277
Ilium 173*f*
Impar block, ganglion of 238
Inadvertent intravascular injection 270
Infection 54, 103, 299
   local 103, 175, 232
Inferior articular process 7, 8*f*, 11, 113, 114
Infraneural technique 13*f*, 122*f*, 123*f*, 128*f*, 149*f*
Injection
   site of 198*f*
   types of 79
Inside-out technique 308
Intercostal drop technique 106*f*
Intercostal muscle 285
Intercostal nerve block 103
   complications 103
   contraindications 103
   equipment and drugs 103
   indications 103
   procedure details 103
Interlaminar cervical epidural block 79
   contraindications 79
   indications 79
   medications used 79
   risks 79
Interlaminar lumbar epidural block 109
Interlaminar lumbar epidural steroid
      injection 109
   contraindications 109
   equipment and supplies 109
   indications 109
   medications 109
   procedure 109
Internal carotid artery 244, 250
Internal jugular vein 219, 250
Internet explosion, era of 52
Interventional minimally invasive techniques 298
Interventional pain management 1, 58, 104
   informed consent for 50
   medications used for 59
   protocol for 52
   treatment 54, 59
Intervertebral disc 15*f*
Intervertebral foramen 9*f*, 12, 24*f*, 117*f*, 119*f*, 126*f*, 163*f*

Intervertebral foraminal ligamentum 300
Intra-articular pathologies 200
Intrapleural block 105
   contraindications 105
   drugs and concentration 105
   equipment 105
   indications 105
   procedure details 105
   sizes of needle 105
   types 105
Intrathecal catheter 296*f*
Intrathecal drug delivery system 294, 294*f*
   contraindications 294
   indications 294
   procedure 294
Intrathecal implants, implantation of 55
Intrathecal injection 112
Iodinated contrast media 59, 59*fc*
Iohexol 60*f*, 175, 179
Ionic contrast media 60*f*
Ischial spine 177, 177*f*, 178*f*
Ischium, posterior border of 272, 273*f*
Isteropac 59

J

Joint 171
   anterior 14*f*, 153*f*, 174
   atlanto-occipital 28*f*
   costotransverse 29*f*, 255*f*
   costovertebral 29*f*
   finder and pin 173
   line 95, 158
      perimeter of 154*f*
   medial border of 157
   posterior 14*f*, 153*f*, 154*f*, 171*f*, 174

K

Kambin's triangle 299, 300
Ketamine 61
Kidney 223
Knee 33*f*
   replacement 262
   sequence 43*f*
Kyphoplasty 317
   procedures 317

L

Laminectomy, left 42*f*
Landmark technique 193
Lateral femoral condyle 43*f*
Lateral femoral cutaneous nerve 262, 268, 269, 269*f*, 277
   block 268, 268*f*
Latissimus dorsi 285
Leads
   apron 47*f*
   fixation of 292*f*
   tunneling of 292*f*
Leap-frog technique 157*f*, 158*f*
Left sacroiliac joint 154*f*
   block 154*f*
Lidocaine 134, 157*f*, 175, 226
Ligaments 156
   posterior syndesmotic 35*f*
Lignocaine 61, 62*f*, 179, 229, 235
Limbs 291

Linea semilunaris 259
Liver 223
Local steroid injections 210
Longus coli 219
Low osmolality contrast media 59
Lower limb surgery, surgical anesthesia for 270
Lower lumbar vertebra 8*f*
Lower thoracic caudal tilt 6*f*
Lower trunk 251
Low-volume extension tubing 126*f*
Lumbar disc herniation 109, 111, 146
Lumbar endoscope 307*f*
Lumbar fluoroscopy 8*f*
Lumbar intervertebral disc 299
Lumbar lordosis 112*f*
Lumbar medial branch
    block and radiofrequency ablation 132
    radiofrequency
        denervation 138
        neurotomy 132
Lumbar plexus 262-265
    block 262
        complications 262
        contraindications 262
        indications 262
        ipsilateral 262
Lumbar radiculopathy 109, 111, 146, 291
Lumbar radiofrequency denervation, steps for 138
Lumbar spinal stenosis 109, 146
Lumbar spine 30*f*, 31*f*, 41*f*
    axial T2 sequence 31*f*
    coronal reformat 31*f*
    creates 8*f*
    lateral view of 55*f*
    plain radiography of 55
    sagittal T2 sequence 31*f*
    scoliosis of 129*f*
    sequence 41*f*, 42*f*
Lumbar spondylosis 123*f*
Lumbar sympathetic plexus block 232, 234
    contraindications 232
    indications 232
    procedure 232
Lumbar transforaminal epidural steroid injections 121
Lumbosacral spine 107, 109*f*, 175
    anteroposterior view of 121*f*
Lung 24*f*
    carcinoma of 105
Lymph edema 57
Lymphadenopathy, aortic 223

M

Magnetic resonance imaging 40, 55
Malignancy 317
Mandibular nerve 287
Maxillary sinus 25*f*
    inferior border of 69*f*
Medial branch
    block 8*f*, 95*f*
    radiofrequency 8*f*
        neurotomy 132
Medial longissimus 284
Medial meniscus 43*f*
Medial paravertebral muscles 284

Medical fraternity 58
Medicine, practice of 50
Meningitis 63
Methyl methacrylate 319*f*
Methylparaben 61
Methylprednisolone 61, 61*f*, 175, 200
Microdiscectomy 42*f*
Midazolam 61
Middle trunk 244, 245, 249-251
Mid-thoracic paravertebral region 254*f*, 256*f*, 257*f*
    paramedian transverse scan of 256*f*
Mid-thoracic spine 255*f*
Morphine 61
Motor stimulation 196*f*
Multilevel disc-osteophyte bars 40*f*
Multimodal analgesia, part of 258
Multimodal polypharmacy 59
Multiple myeloma 317
Muscle 264
    abdominal 286*f*
    anterior scalene 243, 244, 249-252
    masticatory 287, 287*f*
    paraspinal 255
    supraspinatus 246, 247
Myelogram 74*f*
Myelography 56
Myelomatosis 60
Myofascial trigger points 283

N

Nausea 60
Neck 200*f*, 201*f*
Needle entry 221, 230
    point 176*f*, 199*f*, 207*f*, 295*f*
Needle insertion 260*f*, 303*f*
    point of 262*f*, 264, 266
Needle placement 176, 151*f*, 207, 221
Needle tip 15*f*, 304*f*
    manipulation of 303*f*
    near celiac plexus 226*f*
    towards target 227*f*
Nerve entrapment, abdominal 103, 105
Nerve root 116*f*, 118*f*, 125*f*, 130*f*, 151*f*, 221
    damage 63
    injection 38*f*, 39*f*
    injury 112, 299
    left 41*f*
Neural foramen 137*f*
Neuralgia
    post-herpetic 103, 105, 291
    trigeminal 62, 67
Neurolysis 63
Neurolytic agent 62, 234
Neurolytic celiac plexus block, complications of 229
Neuromodulation 183, 185
Neuropathic pain 129, 291
    symptoms 177
Neuropathy 57
Neurostimulation 294
Neurotoxicity, severe 61
Nonopioid medications 294
Nonsteroidal inflammatory drugs 317
Normal electromyography tracings 57*f*
Nuclear medicine scanning 56
Nucleus, abnormal 308

O

Oblique muscles 286
Obturator nerve 262
Occipital nerve block 98
Omnipaque 68*f*, 179
Opiates 61
Oral morphine 285
Organs, radiation effects of 44*f*
Orofacial pain syndromes 215
Osteochondral injury 43*f*
Osteopenia 56
Osteophytes 126*f*
Osteoporosis 317
Osteoporotic bone 56
Oxygen saturation 52

P

Pacing electrodes 132
Pain 177
    block 50
    chronic 54, 59, 283
    group of 50
    management 50, 58
    maximum relief in 54
    neuropathic 129, 291
    physician
        magnetic resonance imaging for 40
        mandatory for 50, 52
    post-laminectomy 111
    post-thoracotomy 105
    practice 58
    radicular 114, 117, 121*f*, 124*f*, 285*f*
    relief 58, 239
    sharp 176
    shooting 311
    urogenital 232
Pancreas 223
Paracentral disc protrusion, left 148*f*
Paralysis 112, 299
Paramedian sagittal trident view approach 266
Paramedian transverse
    oblique approach 262, 263*f*
    scan 255*f*, 256, 257*f*
Paraplegia 112, 299
    temporary 235
Parasacral parallel shift 270, 271
Parasacral sciatic nerve block 270
Parasympathetic nervous systems 238
Partial lower extremity paralysis 235
Patella, medial aspect of 43*f*
Pelvic hematoma formation 270
Pelvic pain
    chronic 235
        neuropathic 177
Pelvis 6*f*, 148*f*
Peng block 278
Percutaneous balloon compression 67
Pericapsular nerve group block 276, 276*f*, 277*f*, 278*f*
Periodontal disease 57
Peripheral blocks 191
Peripheral vascular disease 232
Peroneal nerve 209
Personnel monitoring devices 46
Phantom limb 232

Phenol 63
Pheochromocytoma 60
Physical therapy 198
Pillow under pelvis 146f, 179f
Piriformis muscle 176, 176f, 273f, 275f
    anatomy of 175, 175f
Piriformis tendon 175
Plantar fasciitis 210
Platelet-rich plasma 197
Pleura 249, 285, 286f
Pleural puncture 253
Pneumothorax 103, 253
Polymethyl methacrylate 317
Popliteal nerve 208f
    block 206
        basic information 206
        complications 207
        contraindications 206
        drugs 206
        equipment 206
        indications 206
        preprocedure preparation 206
        procedure 207, 208
Post-annulus dissection 311f
Postcontrast injection static image 126f
Posterior transversus abdominis plane
    block 261
        probe position 261f
        sonoanatomy of 261f
Post-laminectomy syndrome 291
Post-mastectomy pain syndrome 285, 286f
Post-traumatic syndromes 215
Pregnancy 60, 111, 232
Prilocaine lignocaine mixture, application of 283
Probe, placement of 274f
Prostate malignancy 235
Protein 60
Proton density fat-saturated sequence 32f, 33f, 35f
Provocative diskogram 57, 57f
Pseudo-joint provoked concordant pain 15f
Pseudomeningocele 129f
Psoas
    major 263-267
        muscle 263
    muscle 262, 264
    tendon 277, 278
Pubic ramus, superior 276
Pudendal nerve 178f
    block 177
    pulsed radiofrequency 178
Pudendal neuralgia 177
    causes of 177
Pulsed radiofrequency procedure 177
Pump in situ 297f
Puncture skin 161f

Q

Quadratus lumborum 263, 264
    muscle 264, 265
Quadriceps muscle contraction 265

R

Racz catheter 130, 130f, 131f
Racz procedure 130

Radiation
    biological effects of 44fc
    detection 46
    effects of 45f
    exposure 45fc
    gloves 48, 48f
    protection 44, 46, 47f
        cardinal rules of 46f
        equipment 47
        principles of 46
    types of 44
Radiofrequency 95f
    cannula 95, 195f, 196f
    denervation 91, 97f
    electrodes 90f
    lesion 138, 138f
    lesioning tips 72
    needle 135f, 218f
    neurotomy 132, 193
    procedures 283
    rhizotomy 67
Radiopaque 59
    contrast 59
Radiotherapy, low-dose 210
Raynaud's disease 215, 232
Rectal
    abdominis 259
    malignancy 235
    sheath, anterior 259
Reflex sympathetic dystrophy 58
Refractory shoulder joint pain 193
Renal toxicity 60
Retrodiscal technique 13f, 122f, 123f, 128f, 149f
Rhomboids 285
Rib
    border of 104
    fractures, analgesia for 253
    inferior portion of 104
    lower border of 104f
Right sacroiliac joint 12f, 14f, 153f, 155f, 159f
    part of 153f
    posteroanterior view of 109f
Right transforaminal lumbar epidural block 116f
Ropivacaine 61, 62f, 175, 249

S

Sacral ala 157
Sacral foramen 160f
Sacral nerve stimulation 185
Sacral plate, posterior 161f
Sacral plexus 273f, 274
    block 270
        anatomy 270
        complications 270
        contraindications 270
        formation of 270f
Sacral promontory 236
Sacral roots, treatment of 179
Sacral segments 72
Sacrococcygeal ligament 146
Sacroiliac fusion, right 171f
Sacroiliac joint 14f, 42f, 59, 145, 153, 189f, 175
    block 153, 155
    fusion 170
        contraindications 170
        indications 170
        types of 170

    injection 14f
        bilateral 39f
    lower end of 13f
    medial border of 158f
    neuroanatomy of 156
    pain 153
    radiofrequency denervation 156
Sacrum 13f, 159f, 173f
    anatomy of 164f, 180f
    C-arm position of 157f
    lateral wall of 171f
Sartorius
    margin of 268
    muscle 268
Scalene muscle, middle 244, 245, 249-252
Scan technique 263, 264, 266
Scapula
    anteroposterior view of 195f
    edge of spine of 193f
    spine of 195f, 246f, 247
Sciatic nerve 175f, 208, 274, 274f
Sedation 232
Sensory stimulation 158, 178
Sepsis 294
Serratus anterior 285
Seventh cervical
    nerve root 250
    vertebra, posterior tubercle of transverse process of 250
Severe acute respiratory syndrome coronavirus 2 54, 55
Sexual dysfunction 234
Shamrock's approach 264, 265f
    sonoanatomy of 264f
Shin muscles 285f
Shoulder 32f, 309
    hydrodistension 38f
    sequence 42f
Sickle cell anemia 60
Simple myofascial pain syndrome 285
Sims' position 271f
Sixth cervical nerve root 250
    bifid root of 251
Sixth cervical vertebra
    anterior tubercle of transverse process of 250
    posterior tubercle of transverse process of 250
Skeleton, anatomy on 193f
Ski boot 20f, 21f
Skin
    burn 161f, 164f
    celiac plexus 226f
    entry point 98, 139, 142f, 144f, 303f
    incision 171f, 303f
    local anesthesia 259, 269
    markings 300
    puncture point 165f
Sleeve, passing of 306f
Sonoanatomy 246f, 247f, 249f, 266f, 273f, 275f, 276f
    muscles 284f
Spinal cord
    anterolateral quadrant of 74f
    infarcts 63
    stimulation 291, 295
        contraindications 291
        indications 291

Spinal hardware 132
Spinal needle 116, 216*f*
Spinal quadrant, anterior 72
Spinal stenosis, moderate-to-severe 129*f*
Spinalis multifidus 284
Spinolaminar line 80*f*
Spinothalamic tract 72, 75*f*
Splanchnic plexus block 220
    contraindications 220
    indications 220
    procedure 220
Spleen 223
Spondylolisthesis 41*f*
Sponge around needle 222*f*, 227*f*, 231*f*, 237*f*
Square off vertebral endplate 6*f*
Square vertebral endplates 113*f*
Staphylococcus aureus 303
Stellate ganglion 285
    anatomy of 215*f*
    block 215, 217
        contraindications 215
        indications 215
    radiofrequency ablation of 217, 217*f*
    ultrasound-guided block of 219
Stellate radiofrequency ablation 218*f*
Sternocleidomastoid muscle 244, 250, 251
Sternotomy 103
Steroids 60, 79, 127*f*, 200
    injection of 119*f*, 130
    types of 61, 61*f*
Stimuplex needle 176*f*
Stomach 223
Stump pain 232
Subacromial subdeltoid bursa 36*f*
Subcostal transversus abdominis plane block 258, 258*f*, 259*f*
Subcutaneous tissue 161*f*, 164*f*
Subpedicular block 148*f*
Subpedicular technique 11*f*, 114*f*, 119*f*, 122*f*-124*f*, 128, 128*f*, 151*f*
Superior articular
    facet 300
    process 5, 7, 8*f*, 11, 20*f*, 85*f*, 94, 113, 114, 133*f*, 135*f*, 139*f*, 144, 161*f*, 162*f*
Superior gemellus 284
Superior gluteal artery 272
Superior hypogastric plexus block 235
Superior transverse scapular ligament 246
Supraglenoid notch 247
Suprascapular fossa 246, 247, 247*f*
    sonoanatomy of 246*f*, 247*f*
Suprascapular nerve 146, 246, 245*f*, 246, 247, 247*f*, 249, 251
    block 243, 243*f*
        posterior approach landmark identification 246*f*
        injection site of 247*f*
    radiofrequency neurotomy of 193
Suprascapular notch 195*f*, 246*f*
Supraspinatous tear 42*f*
Surgeries, abdominal 258
Sympathetic block 59, 213
Sympatholysis, evidence of 232
Synovial recess, anterior 201*f*

T

Taha's technique 270, 274
Talofibular ligaments
    anterior 35*f*
    posterior 35*f*
Tendon
    attachment 197
    calcification 37*f*
    fibers 42*f*
Tennis elbow 197
    signs 197
    symptoms 197
    tender point for 197*f*
    treatment 197
Tensor fascia lata 268, 269, 269*f*
Thermistor probe 218*f*
Thermogram 58, 58*f*
Thermography 57
Thigh thrust test 170
Third occipital nerve 98, 98*f*
    block 21*f*, 86*f*
        lower targets for 21*f*
        middle targets for 21*f*
Thoracic fluoroscopy 22*f*-24*f*
Thoracic paravertebral block 253
    complications 253
    indications 253
Thoracic spine 24*f*, 29*f*, 30*f*
    area 22
    CT sagittal reformat 29*f*
    radiograph anteroposterior projection 29*f*
Thoracic spinous process 255
Thoracotomy 103
Thorax 101
Thrombosis 60
Thyroid shield 48, 48*f*
Thyrotoxicosis 60
Tibial nerve 209
Tight transforaminal lumbar epidural block 116*f*
Toxicity 63
Trabecular bone 56
Transducer, parasacral parallel shift of 272*f*
Transforaminal endoscopic discectomy 298
    anatomy 299
    complications 299
    contraindications 299
    drugs 299
    indications 298
Transforaminal epidural injection 5*f*, 11*f*, 12*f*, 24*f*, 127*f*, 285
Transforaminal lumbar
    endoscopic decompression 298
    epidural
        block 111, 112, 119*f*
        steroid injection 126*f*
Transient sciatic neuralgia 270
Transverse process 256*f*, 264, 265
Transversus abdominis 259-261
    aponeurosis 261*f*
    muscles 259
    plane block 258
        contraindications 258
        indications 258
        types of 258
Trapezius muscle 246, 247
Trench foot 232
Triamcinolone 61, 61*f*, 111, 200, 299
    acetonide 175
Trident sign 266
Trigeminal ganglion interventions 25
Trigeminal nerve
    block 67
    characteristics of 67
    sensory innervation of 67*f*
Trigeminal percutaneous balloon compression, equipment for 68*f*
Trocar 318*f*, 319*f*
Trochlear inclination, lateral 57*f*
Trunk, neuropathic pain of 291
Tubercle, anterior 244*f*
Tumor, testicular 235
Tunnel catheter 297
Tunnel vision 52*f*, 201*f*, 237*f*
Tuohy needle 80*f*, 81*f*, 110*f*

U

Ultrasound 204
Ultrasound-guided
    block 219, 241
    dry needling 281, 283
    technique popliteal block 208
    tibiotalar joint injection 37*f*
    transversus abdominis plane block 258
Upper abdominal surgeries 103, 105
Upper lumbar thoracic caudal tilt 6*f*
Upper trunk 244, 245, 250, 251
    anterior division 249
    formation of 251*f*
    posterior division 249
Urinary retention 270
Urografin 59
Uterus, tumors of 235

V

Vascular insufficiency 232
Vascular puncture 253
Vasculitis 215
Vasodilation 60
Vasomotor 60
Vasovagal reaction 60
Vertebral artery 250, 251
Vertebral body 41*f*, 126*f*, 263-265
    center of 93*f*
    middle of 19*f*
    midline of 319*f*
    osteophytes 5*f*
Vertebral disc osteophytes 5*f*
Vertebral end plates 9*f*, 15*f*
Vertebroplasty 8*f*
Visceral injury 270
Vital signs, monitoring of 180, 196, 234
Vomiting 60

W

Weakness 57

X

X-ray 44, 175
    technique 194
Xylocaine 303

Other Best-selling Books

UNDERSTANDING ANESTHETIC EQUIPMENT & PROCEDURES: A PRACTICAL APPROACH

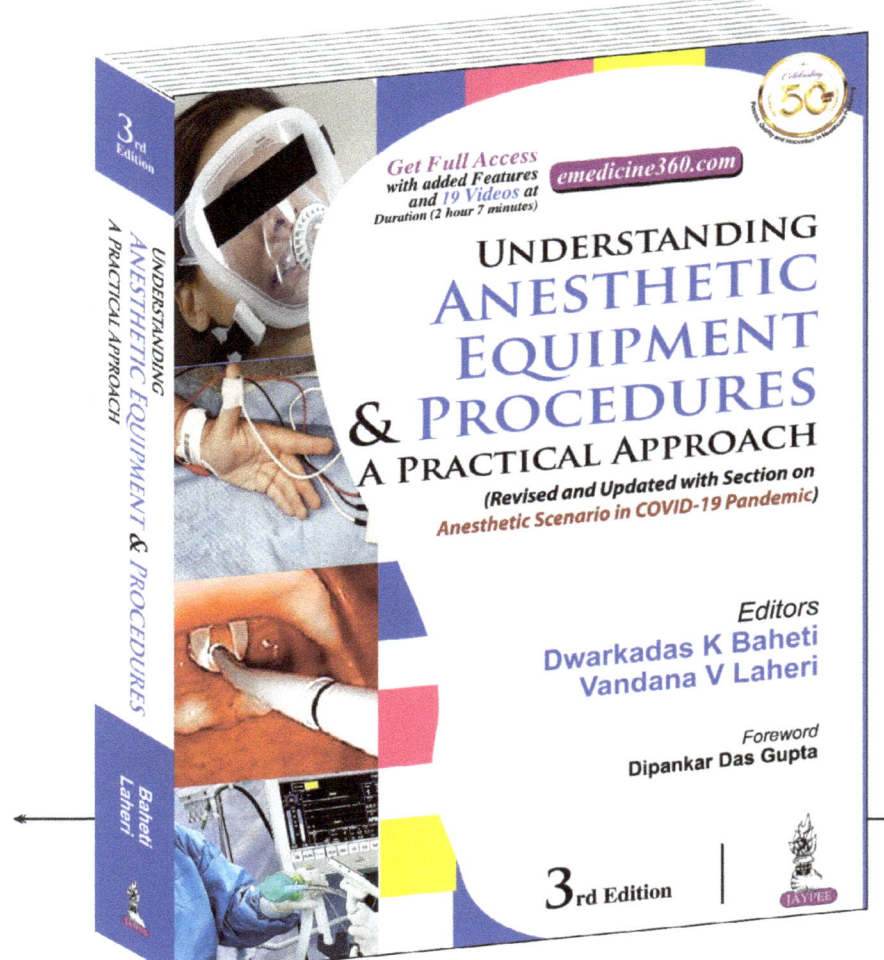

DK Baheti, *et al.*

Full Color | Soft Cover | 3/e, 2021
8.5" x 11" | 638 Pages | 9789354650062

JAYPEE
The Health Sciences Publisher

Please visit our website
www.jaypeebrothers.com or Scan the QR Code

EU GSPR Authorised Reprsentative
Logos Europe, 9 rue Nicolas Poussin
1700, La Rochelle, France
Phone: +33 (0) 6 67 93 73 78
E-mail: contact@logoseurope.eu